MOSBY'S
Canadian
Textbook
FOR THE
Support Worker

SHEILA A. SORRENTINO, RN, PHD
Curriculum and Health Care Consultant
Normal, Illinois

ROSEMARY GOODACRE, RN
Instructor and Co-ordinator, Personal Support Worker Program
Fleming College

First Canadian Edition

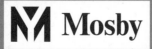

ISBN: 0-920513-48-4

Acquisitions Editor: Ann Millar
Editorial Manager: Zak Knowles
Publishing Services Manager: Gayle May
Production Manager: Joseph Selby
Production Editor: Marcel Chiera
Designer: Kathy Gosche
Printing and Binding: MaplePress

Elsevier Canada
1 Goldthorne Avenue, Toronto, ON, Canada M8Z 5S7
Phone: 1-866-896-3331
Fax: 1-866-359-9534

Printed in the United States of America

1 2 3 4 5   08 07 06 05 04

DEDICATION
To my parents and my brothers and sisters

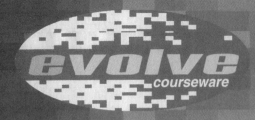

The Latest *Evolution* in Learning.

Evolve provides online access to free learning resources and activities designed specifically for the textbook you are using in your class. The resources will provide you with information that enhances the material covered in this book and much more.

Visit the Web address listed below to start your learning evolution today!

 LOGIN: *http://evolve.elsevier.com/Canada/Sorrentino/SupportWorker*

Evolve Online Courseware for Sorrentino: *Mosby's Canadian Textbook for the Support Worker* offers the following features:

- **Content Updates**
  New and updated information related to this textbook.

- **Additional Resources**
  Additional materials to enhance textbook content.

- **Links to Related Websites**
  Links to other sites related to content in this textbook.

- **Links to Related Products**
  See what else Elsevier Science has to offer in a specific field of interest.

Think outside the book . . . evolve

INTRODUCTION

This instructor's manual was developed to complement *Mosby's Canadian Textbook for the Support Worker*, First Canadian Edition. It is intended to assist you in your teaching responsibilities. The following content is included for your convenience.

1. Chapter objectives
2. Chapter key terms
3. Instructor preparation boxes for each chapter
4. Chapter outlines
   a. Boxes are referenced to the textbook page number
   b. Procedures are referenced with this icon: ▶
5. Lists of suggested classroom activities for each chapter
6. Homework assignments for each chapter
7. Student assignments for each chapter
8. Chapter quizzes
9. Final exams (two versions)
10. Answers to student assignments
11. Answers to chapter quizzes
12. Answers to the final exams
13. Answers to the study questions in *Mosby's Canadian Workbook for the Support Worker*, First Canadian Edition—Revised.

Students should be encouraged to actively participate in all learning activities. Assuming the role of the patient/resident when practicing and return demonstrating the procedures is a valuable learning experience. This role playing helps students to develop empathy for the persons they will care for.

Support workers are very important members of the health care team. It is necessary to provide them with the knowledge, skills, and confidence necessary to provide safe care to the whole person in a variety of health care settings.

INSTRUCTOR TIPS

Instructor preparation for class

1. Carefully review the chapter objectives. Your presentation should cover each of the objectives. You should also review the key terms and their definitions.

2. Read the chapter in the textbook. Review the questions at the end of the chapter. You should be able to answer these questions.

3. If you will be using the accompanying student workbook, review the workbook activities for the appropriate chapter.

4. Read the instructor's preparation box at the beginning of each chapter in the *Instructor's Manual.*

5. Review the outline in the *Instructor's Manual.*

6. Carefully review the classroom activities outlined in the *Instructor's Manual.*
   a. Gather all necessary equipment and supplies for each activity before class.
      (1) Make a checklist of the items you will need. Remember small items such as chalk, coloured markers, and notebook paper.
      (2) Arrange the items in the order you will use them.
   b. Prepare all copies, handouts, index cards, flip charts, and overhead transparencies before class.
      (1) Make sure you have enough handouts for each student.
   c. Gather and view any videos and/or slides you will be using in class.
   d. Make sure the equipment you will be using is available and in good working order before class.
   e. Make sure all arrangements for guest speakers and field trips are completed.
      (1) Always send a thank-you note to guest speakers and agencies that have provided field trip opportunities.

7. Arrive in the classroom at least 15 minutes before class is scheduled to begin.
   a. Organize your materials, arrange the classroom, and set up necessary equipment.
   b. Greet students as they arrive. You can also answer any questions that individual students may have.

Classroom tips

1. Always start and end on time.

2. Provide breaks at specified times. Stay on schedule.

3. Address each student by his or her preferred name. Let students know how you wish to be addressed.

4. Bring extra pens, pencils, and paper in case anyone has forgotten any of these items.

5. Provide students with written reminders of assignment expectations that include the day, date, and time each assignment is due.

6. Collect student assignments at the beginning of class.
   a. Review assignments with students. Clarify any wrong answers and answer questions.

7. Return any quizzes or tests from the previous class.
   a. Provide the correct answers. Clarify any wrong answers. Set up appointments with individual students as necessary.

8. Let students know when you will be available to them outside of classroom time. Provide them with a number where you can be reached.
   a. If you tell students that you will be available at a specific time, it is important to be available.

9. Provide students with the following information in writing when a field trip is planned: day, date, time, name and location of the agency.

Student evaluation tips

1. Student evaluations and grades are based on:
   a. Attendance
   b. Participation in classroom activities
   c. Completeness and accuracy of student assignments
   d. Demonstration of skills in performing procedures
   e. Quiz results
   f. Test results

2. It is important to present and clarify expectations on the first day of class. You must be consistent in applying expectations. If a student is having difficulty, address the problem in a timely, professional, and caring manner. Each student must be given the opportunity to succeed. Standards, however, must be maintained.

TEACHING TECHNIQUES

Promoting student self-esteem

How we as human beings feel about ourselves affects every aspect of the experience of living. How we function in school, at work, at leisure, and within relationships is directly related to our private vision of ourselves.

Creating a consistent habit in your classroom of validating students is one of the most important parts of your curriculum. Students learn better if they feel important, listened to, and capable of learning.

Actions you can take in the classroom to give your students a positive experience include the following:

1. *Be available to your students.* Let your students know that you are available to help with any problems they might have in your class. Give them your individual attention, making them feel that they are important to you.

2. *Be a good listener.* Do not interrupt students with your interpretation of what they are saying. Make sure you have heard the person correctly by paraphrasing what was said if you are uncertain. Make eye contact. Do not appear distracted and ready to go on to another activity. Try not to be critical or judgmental about what was said. Be gentle with your criticism if it is necessary.

3. *Remember names and details about students.* Let students know that you care about them as individuals as well as students.

4. *Share some of yourself with students.* You are a role model to your students. Look for things you share in common to talk about.

5. *Be sincere with compliments.* Identify unique and special qualities about each student and each class you teach. Let students know that you appreciate them and enjoy teaching them.

6. *Be careful with your negative feelings.* This can be a challenge. Some students may not be easy to teach. Try to be fair in your dealings with all students.

7. *Use a variety of teaching modalities in the classroom.* Utilizing a variety of teaching modalities in the classroom is necessary to accommodate the different learning styles of students. Variety can also counter classroom stagnation and boredom. The goal of all methods introduced into the classroom is to involve each student. The classroom activities in this manual utilize lecture, large and small group activities, the use of flip charts and the chalkboard, overhead transparencies, videos, slides, demonstrations, simulators and anatomical models, handouts, guest speakers, field trips, and a variety of health care equipment and supplies. Learning should be interesting and fun.

Guidelines for Answering Multiple Choice Questions

The following is a useful guide for students to help them understand and answer correctly multiple choice questions.

1. Always read the question or statement carefully. Do not scan or glance at a question. Scanning or glancing can cause you to miss important key words. Read each word of the question.

2. Before reading the answers, decide what the answer is in your own words. Then read each answer carefully. Select the one best answer. Choose your answer after you have read all four choices.

3. DO NOT READ THINGS INTO A QUESTION. Take the question as it is asked. Do not add your own thoughts or ideas to the question. Do not assume or suppose "what if." Just respond to the information provided.

4. Trust your common sense. If you are unsure of an answer, select your first choice. DO NOT CHANGE your answer unless you are ABSOLUTELY sure of the correct answer. Your first reaction is probably the best. Studies have proven that the first reaction is usually correct. Do not change the answer unless you are positive that your first choice was wrong.

5. Look for the key words in each question. Sometimes key words will be highlighted, underlined, or in italics. Common key words include the following: always, never, first, except, best, not, correct, incorrect, true, or false.

6. Be careful of answers with the following key words or phrases: always, never, every, only, all, none, at all times, or at no time. These words and phrases do not allow for exceptions. In nursing, many times there will be exceptions to an answer, but sometimes answers containing those words listed above are indeed correct. Here are a few examples. Which of the following are correct and

which are incorrect:
   a. Always use a turning sheet.
   b. Never shake linens.
   c. Never place linens on the floor.
   d. The cotton drawsheet must always cover the plastic drawsheet.
   e. The signal light must always be attached to the bed.
   f. Soap is used for all baths.

7. Omit those answers that are obviously wrong. Then choose the best of the remaining answers.

8. Pace yourself during the examination. Do not spend time on difficult questions. First answer all of the questions that you know. Then go back and answer the difficult ones. Sometimes you will remember the answer later. Or another test question may give you a clue to the one you skipped. Spending too much time on a question can cost you valuable time later.

9. Go back to the questions you skipped. Answer all questions by eliminating and narrowing your choices. Be sure to mark an answer even if you are not sure. The question will definitely be counted wrong if you do not choose an answer.

10. Review the test a second time for completeness and accuracy before turning it in.

11. Make sure you have answered each question. Also verify that you have only given one answer for each question.

12. Remember that the test has not been designed to trick or confuse you. The written competency evaluation tests what you know, not what you do not know. You know more than you will be asked.

13. Multiple choice tests do not require total recall. The answer has been provided. You only have to select the one best answer from the four choices.

14. Avoid last minute "cramming" when you study. Not only will it increase your stress level, but it will cause you to confuse facts and information.

CONTENTS

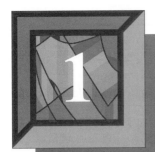

The Role of the Support Worker

Instructor's Preparation

I. Read Chapter 1 in the textbook. Carefully review chapter objectives, key terms, and review questions.

II. Read the outline in Chapter 1 of the instructor's guide. Carefully review the classroom activities, the student assignment, and the quiz.

III. If you are using the accompanying student workbook, review the activities for Chapter 1.

IV. Gather all necessary supplies and equipment for classroom activities and student assignments.
   A. Prepare the correct number of handouts
   B. Prepare appropriate flip charts
   C. Prepare overhead transparencies
   D. Prepare situation cards
   E. Gather coloured markers
   F. Gather any other items that will be needed for classroom activities
   G. Assemble items in the order they will be used

V. Make sure that the necessary equipment is available and in good working order.

Objectives

- Define the key terms listed in this chapter
- Explain the goal of support work
- Describe the five main responsibilities of support work
- Explain the goal of the health care team
- List the common members of a health care team
- Explain the difference between regulated and unregulated health care providers
- Explain why scope of practice is important to support work
- Explain what it means to have a professional approach to support work
- Identify the five priorities of compassionate care
- Identify four considerations when solving problems

Key Terms

activities of daily living (ADL)
assistive personnel
client
compassion
confidentiality
dignity
discretion
licensed practical nurse (LPN)
patient
professionalism
registered nurse (RN)
registered practical nurse (RPN)
rehabilitation
resident
scope of practice
support worker

Outline

The Role of the Support Worker

I. INTRODUCTION
  A. You will provide services to people in facilities and in the community
  B. Supervised by a nurse or other professional you work as part of the health care team
  C. Legislation, employer policies and the person's condition influence how you function and how much supervision you need
  D. Ultimate goal is to improve the person's quality of life
  E. While tending to physical needs you also relieve loneliness, provide comfort, encourage independence and promote self-respect (see Figure 1-1, p. 3)
II. SUPPORT WORK ACROSS CANADA
  A. Nature of support work differs across the country because of differences in training programs, work settings, job responsibilities and terms used to describe support workers
  B. Some sections of this book may not apply to your province or territory
  C. Support worker refers to the worker who provides personal care and support services
  D. Refer to page 4 in the textbook for a variety of titles
  E. Settings for support work
    1. Facility-based settings
      a. Long-term care facilities provide services to people who cannot care for themselves at home but do not need hospital care (see Figure 1-2, p. 4)
      b. Hospitals provide services to people requiring acute care
    2. Community-based settings
      a. Workplaces within the community where health care and support services are provided
      b. Most common setting is the person's home (see Figure 1-3, p. 4)
  F. Support worker responsibilities
    1. Tasks performed by support workers vary across Canada; generally grouped into following categories
      a. Personal Care—includes assisting with (ADL)
        (1) You help with eating, bathing, grooming, dressing, toileting, changing positions for people with limited mobility

        (2) Provide for the person's safety and physical comfort
        (3) You are not responsible for deciding what should or should not be done for a person; however, you must observe and report any changes in the person's behaviour or health as this is important information for the health care team
      b. Support for nurses and other health care professionals
        (1) You assist nurses or other health care team members by following the established care plan for each client
        (2) There will be many procedures that you will do and report
      c. Family support
        (1) In facilities, you may assist in admissions, introductions of family and client to others, help them settle
        (2) In private homes you will be assisting families care for loved ones
        (3) Family situations vary and your role will vary depending on needs
      d. Social support
        (1) You may help people participate in social activities, which provide the person with enjoyment and a chance to meet with friends.
        (2) You may also organize social activities or be hired to be a person's companion
      e. Housekeeping/home management
        (1) In facilities, you may do housekeeping tasks such as bed-making
        (2) In private homes, home management (housekeeping) duties vary depending on the needs of the client and may include light cleaning and meal preparation
        (3) Refer to the article "A day in the life of a Support Worker," p. 5 in the textbook
  G. People receiving health care and support services are known by different terms, depending on the workplace setting
    1. Patient, when in hospital

2. Resident, when in long-term care facility
3. Client, when in the community
4. Always remember that he or she is first and foremost a person and every person is unique
5. They have a variety of needs, life experiences, situations, wants, and opinions, and come from a variety of cultures (see Chapter 11)
6. Part of your job is to respect diversity (see various Respecting Diversity boxes throughout the textbook)
7. People you support include:
   a. Older adults
      (1) Aging is a normal process and many older adults enjoy good health, however the body normally changes with age, and risks of serious illness and disability increase with age
      (2) Most remain at home as long as possible; others are unable to care for themselves and move into residential facilities
   b. People with disabilities
      (1) May be disabled due to illness, injury, or conditions present at birth
      (2) May affect physical or mental functioning, or both
      (3) Many adults with disabilities work and live independently
      (4) You may assist with ADL
   c. People with medical problems
      (1) May include illness, diseases, or injuries
      (2) May be short-term, long-term, or progressive and life threatening
   d. People having surgery
      (1) May involve preoperative support or postoperative care such as preventing complications, relieving pain
      (2) Some recover in hospitals and others at home.
   e. People with mental health problems
      (1) Vary from mild (need help making decisions or coping with stress) to severe (need assistance with ADL)
   f. People needing rehabilitation
      (1) A process of restoring a person to the highest level of functioning possible through use of therapy, exercise, or other methods
      (2) May need to regain functions following surgery, illness, or accident
      (3) Some hospitals have special units but many people receive support at home
   g. Children
      (1) When hospital care is needed, children are admitted to the pediatric unit
      (2) Some areas of Canada hire support workers to be with the children (see Figure 1-4, p. 9)
      (3) Most support work occurs in community settings
      (4) May receive care for physical or intellectual disabilities, or because a parent is ill, disabled, or has a new baby
   h. Mothers and newborns
      (1) Complications and difficulties can occur during pregnancy, or 6 to 8 weeks following delivery
   i. People receiving special care
      (1) Some hospitals hire support workers to provide care in special care units such as coronary care units, kidney dialysis units, burn units, etc.
      (2) May transport people from one unit to another, assist with special procedures, provide personal care
      (3) In some parts of Canada, support workers do not provide care to patients in unstable or critical condition

III. THE HEALTH CARE TEAM
   A. Includes workers with a variety of skills and knowledge who work together to meet the client's needs and to provide quality care
   B. Many professionals are involved in the care of one person
   C. The support worker, the client, and the family are important members of the team
   D. The client is always the focus (see Figure 1-5, p. 9)
      1. Regulated workers
         a. A regulated profession is self-governing and has a professional organization (college) that sets education and

license requirements

b. Establishes scope of practice, codes of ethics, and standards of conduct and legislation that details roles and responsibilities

c. The college also disciplines members guilty of misconduct

2. Unregulated workers

a. Unregulated professions have no college or legislation, no official education or training programs, and no code of ethics

b. Support workers are unregulated

c. You are accountable to your supervisor, your employer, and your clients

d. Table 1-1, p. 11 in the textbook, describes the titles and position of common health care members

3. Scope of practice

a. To protect the client from harm you must know what you can and what you cannot do, and the legal limits of your role

b. Never perform a function or task that you have not been trained to do or is beyond legal limits of your role

c. Can cause harm to a client and serious legal problems for yourself and your employer

d. Sources of information about your scope of practice:

(1) Your training program includes information for support workers in your province or territory

(2) Your employer's policies— written policies you need to read carefully, to know what you can and cannot do

(3) Your supervisor—always ask for directions if unsure

4. Supervision of support workers

a. In most settings, nurses or other professionals supervise support workers

b. The Registered Nurse (RN) is licensed and regulated by the province or territory to maintain overall responsibility for planning and provision of care

c. RN may have university or college diplomas

d. RN assesses, develops nursing plans, implements and evaluates care, and carries out physician's orders

e. RN directs work of the registered

practical nurse (RPN), support workers, and other assistive personnel

f. RPN, or licensed practical nurse (LPN), is licensed and regulated to carry out basic nursing care

g. RPN or LPN may have college certificate or diploma

h. RPN or LPN usually functions under supervision of RN, needs little supervision caring for stable clients, and assists RN with care of seriously ill clients

i. In some provinces or territories, RPNs or LPNs supervise support workers

j. Depending on the situation, support workers may be supervised by another health professional such as a social worker, agency supervisor, recreational therapist, or the client themselves

k. Be aware of provincial or territorial legislation that limits tasks and procedures that you can perform (see Chapter 10)

IV. BEING A PROFESSIONAL

A. Professionalism

1. Demonstrate respect for others, commitment, competence, and appropriate behaviour

2. Be cheerful and friendly, work when scheduled, perform tasks competently, and help others

3. Demonstrate a positive attitude

a. Believe your work is very important, valuable, show enthusiasm, consideration, courtesy, honesty, and cooperativeness

b. Think before you speak, do not gossip

c. Box 1-1, p. 12 in the textbook, lists negative statements to avoid

4. Demonstrate a sense of responsibility

a. Admit your mistakes and don't blame others

b. Accept constructive criticism and learn from others

c. Always report to work on time when scheduled

d. Finish assigned tasks or tell supervisor immediately if unable to finish

e. Call your supervisor if unable to work or will be late

5. Have a professional appearance

a. Your appearance shows respect and includes paying attention to your clothes, grooming, and hygiene (see Box 1-2 and Figure 1-6, p. 12)

6. Show discretion about client information
   a. Discretion means good judgment and being careful about what you say, how you say it, when you say it, and where you say it
   b. Confidentiality means respecting and guarding personal and private information about another person
   c. Information should only be shared among team members involved in the client's care
   d. Information about your employer, your co-workers, and other clients is private
7. Show discretion about personal matters
   a. No matter how well you know a client, do not discuss personal matters with them (see Chapter 6), nor discuss problems with others (see Box 1-3, p. 13)
8. Use acceptable speech and language
   a. Do not use foul, vulgar, abusive, slang language; instead speak gently and clearly and never argue or fight with a client, family, or co-workers

V. THE PRIORITIES OF SUPPORT WORK: COMPASSIONATE CARE
   A. Compassion means caring about another person's misfortune and suffering
   B. Providing compassionate care means treating people with respect, kindness, and understanding as they are coping with illness, disability, and perhaps personal problems
   C. No matter what kind of care or support you provide, most clients have the following needs.
      1. To preserve their dignity
      2. To live independently
      3. To express their preferences
      4. To preserve their privacy (see Figure 1-7, p. 13)
      5. To be safe from harm
   D. People who are disabled, or suffer a serious illness, depend on others to meet their needs
   E. Not all people have the same needs, however, most have at least some to the needs discussed
   F. See Providing Compassionate Care boxes throughout the textbook for priorities of support work

G. The acronym DIPPS will remind you of these five priorities: Dignity, Independence, Preference, Privacy, and Safety

VI. DECISION MAKING AND PROBLEM SOLVING
   A. You make decisions every day, and most decisions involve solving problems
   B. When solving problems, consider the following:
      1. The priorities of support work—solutions should not compromise DIPPS
      2. The client's viewpoint—involve clients in solving problems that concern them
      3. Your scope of practice—learn and observe the rules of your workplace
      4. Your supervisor's viewpoint—can you handle this problem or should your supervisor
   C. Crucial to your role but difficult when just starting (see Support Workers Solving Problems boxes throughout the textbook)

Classroom Activities

1. If possible, gather job descriptions for support workers from various settings. Distribute these to students. Give students 15 minutes to read the job descriptions. Then ask the following questions:
   a. Is there anything in the job description that you do not understand
   b. Is there anything in the job description that you would be unable to do for any reason? Explain.
   c. What do you like about the job description?
   d. What do you not like about the job description?

2. List on the board the different groups of people support workers may care for. Ask the students to identify why each group may need care.

3. List the six aspects below, about being a professional, on index cards. Divide the class into six groups and assign each group a task to demonstrate.
   a. A positive attitude
   b. A sense of responsibility
   c. A professional appearance
   d. Discretion about client information
   e. Discretion about personal matters
   f. Acceptable speech and language.

4. Write DIPPS on the board and ask the class to discuss how they could promote each of these aspects.

5. Draw a small circle on the board and ask the students to identify the main focus of the health care team. Write "client" in the first circle, then ask who should be in next circle. Draw a larger circle around the small circle and write family in second circle. Ask the class to identify any professional or non-professional who may be an important member of the team. Remember even a family pet could be very important to the client and should be included in the plan.

Homework Assignments

Ask students to answer the questions at the end of Chapter 1 in the textbook. Tell students the date and time that this assignment must be completed and turned in.

If the accompanying workbook is being used, assign the Chapter 1 workbook exercises. Tell students the date and time that this assignment must be completed and turned in.

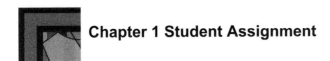

Name _____

Date _____

The Role of the Support Worker

Match the terms with the correct definitions.

a. Dietician
b. Occupational therapist (OT)
c. Activities director
d. Physical therapist (PT)
e. Support worker
f. Registered practical nurse (RPN)
g. Physician (doctor)
h. Occupational therapy assistant
i. Registered nurse (RN)
j. Medical records technician
k. Speech-language pathologist
l. Podiatrist
m. Pharmacist
n. Medical laboratory technician (MLT)
o. Medical technologist (MT)
p. Social worker
q. Radiographer/radiological technologist
r. Cleric
s. Audiologist
t. Respiratory therapist

1. _____ Assesses, plans, and implements recreational needs

2. _____ Assists RNs and LPNs in giving care; must be supervised by a nurse

3. _____ Tests hearing; prescribes hearing aids; works with hearing impaired persons

4. _____ Assists persons with their spiritual needs

5. _____ Assesses and plans for nutritional needs

6. _____ Provides direct patient care under the direction of an RN

7. _____ Collects samples and performs laboratory tests on blood, urine, and other body fluids, secretions, and excretions

8. _____ Maintains medical records

9. _____ Performs complicated laboratory tests on blood, urine, and other body fluids, secretions, and excretions

10. _____ Assists persons to learn or retain skills needed to perform activities of daily living

11. _____ Performs tasks and services supervised by an OT

12. _____ Fills medication orders written by a doctor; monitors and evaluates drug interactions

13. _____ Assists persons with musculoskeletal problems; focuses on restoring function and preventing disability from illness or injury

14. _____ Diagnoses and treats diseases and injuries

15. _____ Prevents, diagnoses, and treats foot disorders

16. _____ Takes x-rays and processes film for viewing

17. _____ Assesses, makes nursing diagnoses, plans, implements, and evaluates nursing care; supervises RPNs and support workers

18. _____ Assists in treatment of lung and heart disorders; gives respiratory treatments and therapies

19. _____ Helps patients and families with social, emotional, and environmental issues affecting illness and recovery

20. _____ Evaluates speech and language and treats persons with speech, voice, hearing, communication, and swallowing disorders

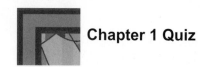

Chapter 1 Quiz

Name _____

Date _____

The Role of the Support Worker

True or False

Mark **T** *for true or* **F** *for false.*

1. _____ Rehabilitation helps persons return to their highest level of physical and psychological functioning.

2. _____ The goal of health promotion is to reduce the risk of illness.

3. _____ Long-term care centers only provide care to the frail elderly.

4. _____ The nursing team is managed by the doctor.

Multiple Choice

Circle the BEST answer.

5. Resident is a term used to describe a person who is receiving care at:
   a. Home
   b. A long-term facility
   c. An outpatient clinic
   d. A hospital

6. The main focus of health care team is to :
   a. find a cure for the client's illness or condition
   b. see as many clients as possible
   c. complete assigned tasks as quickly as possible
   d. provide quality care for the client

7. Support workers are:
   a. unregulated health care workers
   b. licensed health care workers
   c. members of a professional college
   d. member of a regulatory body

8. Scope of practice means:
   a. the tasks that are assigned by your supervisor
   b. the task that a client asks you to perform
   c. the effort you put into performing a task
   d. the legal limits of your role

9. Compassion means:
   a. caring about another's misfortune and suffering
   b. keeping one's feeling to oneself
   c. taking pity on those who are less fortunate
   d. approaching your work with enthusiasm

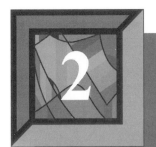

2

The Canadian Health Care System

Instructor's Preparation

   I. Read Chapter 2 in the textbook. Carefully review chapter objectives, key terms, and review questions.

  II. Read the outline in Chapter 2 of the instructor's guide. Carefully review the classroom activities, the student assignment, and the quiz.

 III. If you are using the accompanying student workbook, review the activities for Chapter 2.

 IV. Gather all necessary supplies and equipment for classroom activities and student assignments.
     A. Prepare the correct number of handouts
     B. Prepare appropriate flip charts
     C. Prepare overhead transparencies
     D. Prepare situation cards
     E. Gather colored markers
     F. Gather any other items that will be needed for classroom activities
     G. Assemble items in the order they will be used

  V. Make sure that the necessary equipment is available and in good working order.

 VI. Contact guest speakers to confirm the day, date, time, and location that they are expected.
     A. Ask the speakers if they require any special equipment or supplies. Make sure these are available.

Objectives

• Define the key terms listed in this chapter
• Describe medicare and how it has evolved
• Identify the federal, provincial and territorial roles in the health care system
• Explain the five principles of medicare described in the *Canada Health Act*
• Identify how the focus of the Canadian health care system is shifting
• Explain why health promotion and disease prevention are important functions of the Canadian health care system
• Recognize the emerging importance of home care and your role in providing some of the services

Key Terms

Canada Health Act (1984)
disease prevention
health promotion
home care
medicare

Outline

The Canadian Health Care System

  I. INTRODUCTION
    A. Canada's national health insurance system (Medicare) ensures that all Canadians have access to quality health care
    B. Uses provincial/territorial and federal taxes to pay for care
    C. Faced with increasing costs, Canadians are

re-examining health care spending and priorities

D. Support workers play an important role in the system

II. THE EVOLUTION OF CANADA'S HEALTH CARE SYSTEM

A. In the first part of last century, individuals paid their own hospital and doctor's bills

B. No set fees; if they couldn't afford to pay, they needed to find a charity organization (i.e. Red Cross)

C. During the Great Depression in the 1930s, families couldn't afford care; many ill and disabled people depended on family members or neighbours for care (see Box 2-1, p. 17)

D. In 1947 Saskatchewan had the first hospital insurance plan

E. By 1961, ten provinces and two territories agreed to provide in-patient hospital care; costs were split between federal and provincial governments

F. By 1972, insurance extended to cover medical services outside the hospital

III. THE MODERN HEALTH CARE SYSTEM

A. The federal role

1. Deliver health care to Aboriginal people, people living on reserves, military personnel, veterans, inmates of federal jails, and members of the RCMP

2. Develop and carry out government policy and programs that promote health and prevent disease

3. Transfer tax money to provinces and territories to share costs of medical care

4. Ensure that the same quality and type of care is provided to all—the *Canada Health Act* (1984) clarifies the types of health care services that are insured

5. Box 2-2, p. 17 in the textbook, outlines five principles that must be met in order for provinces and territories to qualify for federal money

A. The provincial/territorial role

1. Develop and administrate health care insurance

2. Finance and plan health care services following the five basic principles in the *Canada Health Act*

3. Pay for hospital and physician costs and some costs of rehabilitation

4. Varies across country

5. People can purchase extra insurance to cover costs not included in their area

IV. HEALTH CARE REFORM

A. Many challenges to the country's ability to provide quality health care

B. Many rural or remote areas face severe shortages of physicians, nurses, and other health care workers

C. Long wait lists for surgeries and diagnostic testing

D. High price for drugs and technology currently being developed

E. In the 1990s, changes to the system were designed to reduce costs—health promotion and disease prevention, and home care

1. Health promotion and disease prevention

a. Health promotion refers to strategies that improve or maintain health and independence

b. Disease prevention refers to strategies that prevent the occurrence of disease or injury

c. Key factors determining a person's health:
(1) Income and social status
(2) Social support networks (see Chapter 4)
(3) Education
(4) Employment and working conditions
(5) Environment
(6) Personal health practices and coping skills

d. Government policy promotes health and prevents illness by improving these areas

e. Examples of policies include immunization programs, prenatal and parenting classes, information campaigns and measures to improve living conditions for those in need

2. Home care

a. Partly to save money and partly as a result of technological advance, patients are sent home sooner following hospital procedures

b. Fewer patients stay in hospital overnight or for extended time

c. To support patients governments increased spending for home care, which is now the most common community-based service

d. Home care provides services to a wide range of clients and offers a wide range of services

e. Services include nursing care, PT, OT,

speech therapy, nutrition counselling, social work, respiratory therapy, and other professional services
f. Support services include personal care, assistance with ADL, and home management
g. Support workers provide most support services for home care and are employed by either a private or not-for-profit agency
h. Volunteer agencies also provide services (see Figure 2-3, p. 19)
i. Publicly funded home care programs are available across Canada, but the range of services varies (see Table 2-1 and Box 2-3, p. 20)
j. All offer the following:
 (1) Client assessment
 (2) Case coordination and management (see Chapter 7)
 (3) Nursing services
 (4) Support services
k. Eligibility and hours of services provided also vary depending on the province or territory

Classroom Activities

1. The federal, provincial, and territorial health acts are available on the Internet. Download these acts and discuss their implications on support workers.

2. Invite an older person to talk to the class about health care as they remember years ago.

3. Write on the board "Home Care." Ask students to list the possible tasks they might perform to allow a client to remain in their home.

Homework Assignments

Ask students to answer the questions at the end of Chapter 2 in the textbook. Tell students the date and time that this assignment must be completed and turned in.

If the accompanying workbook is being used, assign the Chapter 2 workbook exercises. Tell students the date and time that this assignment must be completed and turned in.

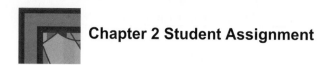 **Chapter 2 Student Assignment**

Name _____

Date _____

The Canadian Health Care System

1. List the support services offered through home care.

    a. _____

    b. _____

    c. _____

2. Health Promotion refers to:

_____

3. Disease Prevention refers to:

_____

4. List the key factors that determine a person's health.

    a. _____

    b. _____

    c. _____

    d. _____

    e. _____

    f. _____

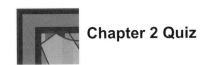 **Chapter 2 Quiz**

Name _____

Date _____

The Canadian Health Care System

| **True or False** | **Multiple Choice** |

Mark **T** *for true or* **F** *for false.*

1. _____ Canadians believe that quality health care should be available to all.

2. _____ Provincial government transfers tax dollars to other provinces and territories to share the cost of health care services.

3. _____ The provincial government finances and plans health care services following the five principles of the *Canada Health Act.*

4. _____ The Provincial Government decides on location of hospitals and LTC facilities.

Circle the BEST answer.

5. The *Charter of Rights and Freedoms* guarantees our right to:
   a. Mobility
   b. Vote
   c. Life, liberty and security
   d. All of the above

6. There are many advantages of home care. Which is *not?*
   a. Lower costs
   b. Greater comfort
   c. Slower rate of recovery
   d. Lower risk of infection

7. Immunization programs are an example of:
   a. Home care services
   b. Disease prevention
   c. Facility-based treatment
   d. Medicare

8. The most pressing cause of health care reform has been:
   a. Rising costs of providing technology, drugs, and services
   b. The depression
   c. Lack of available technology
   d. Lack of accessibility

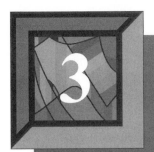

Workplace Settings

Instructor's Preparation

I. Read Chapter 3 in the textbook. Carefully review chapter objectives, key terms, and review questions.

II. Read the outline in Chapter 3 of the instructor's guide. Carefully review the classroom activities, the student assignment, and the quiz.

III. If you are using the accompanying student workbook, review the activities for Chapter 3.

IV. Gather all necessary supplies and equipment for classroom activities and student assignments.

    A. Prepare the correct number of handouts

    B. Gather any other items that will be needed for classroom activities

    C. Assemble items in the order they will be used

V. Make sure that the necessary equipment is available and in good working order.

Objectives

- Define the key terms listed in this chapter
- Differentiate between community-based care and facility-based care
- List work settings where support workers are employed
- Differentiate between residential facilities and other medical facilities
- Describe the various types of residential facilities
- Identify the issues and challenges support workers encounter in the workplace

Key Terms

acute care
acute illness
adult daycare
assisted-living facility
chronic illness
community-based services
community day program
convalescent care
group home
hospice

inpatient
long-term care
long-term care facility
mental health services
outpatient
palliative care
rehabilitation services
residential facility
respite care
retirement residence
supportive housing facility
subacute care

Outline

Workplace Settings

I. INTRODUCTION
  A. Support workers are employed in different settings with different goals and services
  B. Wherever you work, you provide people with vital services that enable them to be as safe, comfortable, dignified, and independent as possible
II. WORKING IN COMMUNITY-BASED SETTINGS
  A. Current trends aim to decrease hospital costs and increase resources in community-based services
  B. Home care agencies and day programs are most likely to hire support workers
    1. Home care
      a. A vital part of Canada's health care system (see Chapter 2)
      b. Support workers play a central role in care
      c. Provide a range of care (see Figure 3-1, p. 24)
      d. Hired full-time, part-time, or casual basis
      e. Must follow agency policies and procedures
      f. Box 3-1, p. 24 in the textbook, describes some of the issues and challenges associated with working in home care
    2. Community day programs (also called adult day care)
      a. Programs for people with physical and/or mental health problems or older adults who need assistance
      b. Day programs, which can be held in a variety of settings, meet the client's needs and provide a break for family caregivers

      c. Each program is unique in the services provided, including recreational activities in many cases (see Figure 3-2, p. 25)
      d. Support workers provide personal care and assistance with recreational and social activities to those attending
      e. Follow employer policies and procedures
      f. Box 3-2, p. 25 in the textbook, lists common issues and challenges when working in community day programs
    3. Working directly for clients
      a. Support workers may be hired by the client or the client's family, and these people select and supervise their own support workers
      b. Box 3-3, p. 25 in the textbook, describes issues and challenges associated with working directly for clients
III. WORKING IN A FACILITY
  A. Hospitals and other medical facilities
    1. Patients in hospitals usually have serious illnesses or injuries and require skilled professional care and complex equipment
    2. The role of the support worker varies from territory to territory, province to province, and city to city, depending on the hospital's needs
    3. Hospitals and other medical facilities provide a variety of services
    4. Services include:
      a. Acute care—provided for short time, intended to diagnose and treat an immediate health issue; provided mainly in a hospital
      b. Subacute care (convalescent care)
        (1) Health care or rehabilitation for people recovering from surgery, injuries, or serious injury
        (2) Condition is stable but still needs care, requiring complex equipment and procedures
        (3) Many hospitals and long-term care facilities provide subacute care
      c. Long-term care
        (1) Provided over the course of months or years to people who cannot care for themselves
        (2) Many people in care suffer from chronic illness (on-going illness, slow or gradual onset and continues to grow worse)

(3) Goal is to help person cope with challenges of living with a long-term illness or disability

d. Respite care

(1) Temporary care of a person with a serious illness or disability

(2) Gives caregivers a break and is provided in home by support workers, in hospitals, or in other facilities

e. Rehabilitation services

(1) Therapies and educational programs designed to restore or improve the person's independence and functional abilities

f. Palliative care

(1) Services for people living with progressive, life-threatening illnesses or conditions that aim to relieve or reduce uncomfortable symptoms but not produce a cure

(2) Goal is to meet the needs of clients and families

(3) May be offered in hospitals, facilities, or hospices (facilities that provide palliative care)

(4) May also be offered in the home (see Chapter 46)

g. Mental health services

(1) Services for persons with mental disorders

(2) May be within a facility, a hospital or health centre, or as community-based care and support

(3) Offer assessment and treatment programs as inpatient or outpatient

B. Residential facilities

1. Provide living accommodations, care, and support services

a. Vary in size and levels of care

b. People using residential facilities are called residents

c. Temporary or permanent home

d. provide care in comfortable home-like setting (see Figure 3-3, p. 27)

e. Those requiring care include:

(1) Frail, older adults

(2) People of all ages who have physical or mental disabilities, or both

(3) People with mental illness

(4) People with alcohol or drug problems

2. Assisted-living facilities

a. Also called supportive housing facilities

b. Facilities where people live in their own apartments and are provided support services

c. Usually apartment buildings providing support to older adults who require minimal care

d. May cook their own meals and receive:

(1) 24-hour monitoring and emergency services

(2) Social/recreational programs

(3) One or two daily meals

(4) Housekeeping and laundry services

3. Group homes

a. Provide supervision, care and/or support to a small number of people with physical and/or mental disabilities

b. Share a house in a residential neighborhood (see Figure 3-4, p. 27)

c. Receive 24-hr. supervision, meals, etc.

d. Residents can include adolescents, elderly, abused women, or people suffering from alcohol abuse

e. Number and type of staff depends on type of home

f. Approved and licensed by provincial or territorial government

g. Partially funded by government

h. Level of assistance and supervision depends on type and size of home

4. Retirement residences

a. Provide accommodation and supervision for older adults

b. Have own bedrooms and bathrooms and share common living and dining areas (Figure 3-5, p. 28)

c. Do not require nursing care and receive minimal assistance

d. Goal is to allow older people to live as independently as possible while providing security, support-services, and varying degree of care as needed

(1) Regulations vary; privately owned in some provinces

(2) Not regulated or financed by government

(3) Residents are not ill or disabled and most can meet their own care needs

(4) Support workers may be hired by

the facility or resident
      (5) The type of care required depends on the client and facility
  4. Long-term care facilities
     a. Also called nursing homes, homes for the aged, long-term care homes, and special care homes.
     b. Provide higher levels of care
     c. 24-hour professional nursing care and support services for people who cannot care for themselves at home but do not need hospital care
     d. Most are frail, older adults with many health problems
     e. Some are young and middle-aged with severe chronic health conditions or disabilities
     f. Goals are to maintain health and independence to greatest extent possible
     g. May stay in a ward, or a private or semi-private room, and may have their own bathroom or share; tubs and showers are in common rooms
     h. Licensed, regulated, and funded by province or territory; medicare pays some of the costs and residents pay a monthly fee and for extra service charges
     i. Some are privately owned; some are-operated by government or charitable organizations as not-for-profit
     j. Work environment is highly structured and RNs plan and coordinate resident care
     k. Support workers report to a nurse and provide ADL care (see Figure 3-6, p. 28)
IV. Issues and challenges associated with facility-based care
   1. Working in a facility also presents issues and challenges to the support worker (see Box 3-4, p. 29)

Classroom Activities

1. Ask the students to discuss their experiences with any type of community-based setting or facility.

2. List on the board the services hospitals and other medical facilities offer (acute care, long-term care, etc.) and ask the students to describe the type of care each service provides.

3. Divide students into groups of 4 and ask them to come up with a list of challenges and issues they might find when working in a facility, working directly for clients, or working with a community day program. Ask for one person in each group to report their responses. Allow 20 minutes for discussion. After each group reports, ask for suggestion on how to resolve the issues and challenges. Allow 15 minutes for discussion. Compare the students' responses with the issues and challenges in covered in Chapter 3.

4. On the board, write "assisted-living facilities," "retirement residences," and "long-term care facilities." Ask the students to describe the care required by clients in each of these settings

Homework Assignments

Ask students to answer the questions at the end of Chapter 3 in the textbook. Tell students the date and time that this assignment must be completed and turned in.

If the accompanying workbook is being used, assign the Chapter 3 workbook exercises. Tell students the date and time that this assignment must be completed and turned in.

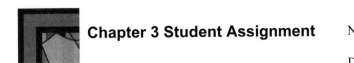

Name _____

Date _____

Workplace Settings

Fill in the Blanks.

1. List 5 types of settings you may be employed in:

   a. _____

   b. _____

   c. _____

   d. _____

   e. _____

2. Identify the differences between acute and chronic illness

   Acute:

   a. _____

   b. _____

   c. _____

   d. _____

   e. _____

   Chronic:

   a. _____

   b. _____

   c. _____

   d. _____

   e. _____

3. List two issues and challenges associated with working with:

   Community day programs:

   a. _____

   b. _____

   Directly for clients:

   a. _____

   b. _____

   In a facility:

   a. _____

   b. _____

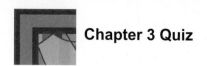

Name _____

Date _____

Workplace Settings

| True or False | Multiple Choice |

True or False

*Mark **T** for true or **F** for false.*

1. _____ Subacute care is another name for convalescent care.

2. _____ A chronic illness can be cured.

3. _____ An acute illness occurs over a long period of time.

4. _____ A hospice provides palliative care to people who are dying.

5. _____ In group homes people with similar physical or mental disabilities live together in a house.

6. _____ If the support worker is employed in a facility, shift work is required.

Multiple Choice

Circle the BEST answer.

7. What type of service provides a temporary break to family caregivers?
   a. Acute-care facility
   b. Palliative care
   c. Respite care
   d. Out-patient services

8. Residents in LTC facilities generally require:
   a. 24-hour nursing care and support services.
   b. Supervision and limited support services.
   c. Adult care.
   d. Housekeeping.

9. What is the role of the Community Access Centre?
   a. Free hotline.
   b. Co-ordinate services in home.
   c. Move you into a LTC facility.
   d. Co-ordinate appropriate services needed.

10. Rehabilitation takes place:
    a. Only in LTC.
    b. Only in hospitals.
    c. Only in specialized facilities.
    d. In a variety or facility of community settings.

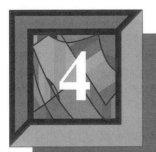

4

Health, Wellness, Illness, and Disability

Instructor's Preparation

I. Read Chapter 4 in the textbook. Carefully review chapter objectives, key terms, and review questions.

II. Read the outline in Chapter 4 of the instructor's guide. Carefully review the classroom activities, the student assignment, and the quiz.

III. If you are using the accompanying student workbook, review the activities for Chapter 4.

IV. Gather all necessary supplies and equipment for classroom activities and student assignments.
   A. Prepare the correct number of handouts
   B. Prepare overhead transparencies
   C. Prepare situation cards
   D. Gather any other items that will be needed for classroom activities
   E. Assemble items in the order they will be used

V. Make sure that the necessary equipment is available and in good working order.

Objectives

- Define the key terms listed in this chapter
- Learn how definitions of health have changed
- Understand the concept of holism and explain how it affects your role
- Explain the current concepts of health and wellness
- Understand how health can be achieved in all dimensions of life
- Explain common reactions to illness and disability
- Describe change and loss associated with illness and disability
- Explain the effects of stigma and discrimination on people who are ill and disabled

Key Terms

disability
discrimination
emotional health
health
holism
illness
intellectual health
physical health
prognosis
social health

social support system
spiritual health
stigma
wellness

Outline

Health, Wellness, Illness, and Disability

I. HEALTH AND WELLNESS
  A. Definitions of health have changed over the years
  B. At end of the 1800s, it meant not being sick
  C. Communicable diseases were leading causes of death
  D. During the first half of the 20th century, with the discovery of antibiotics and vaccines, people started to live longer, and were sick less often
  E. During the latter part of 20th century, people started to realize that lifestyle and the environment affect health
  F. New emphasis on holistic (whole) health
  G. Health is now considered a state of well-being in all dimensions of one's life (see Figure 4-1, p. 33)
  H. Wellness is achieving the best health possible in all five dimensions
  I. Many people try to achieve wellness but few do; many are healthy physically but not emotionally
  J. Health is a continuum (see Figure 4-2, p. 33) and a person's place shifts during their lives
    1. Physical health
      a. Influenced by genetics and lifestyle, and achieved when the body is strong, fit, and free of disease
      b. The following factors contribute to physical health:
        (1) Following a nutritious diet (see Chapter 25)
        (2) Exercising regularly
        (3) Living in a smoke-free environment
        (4) Drinking alcohol moderately or not at all
        (5) Having a good night's sleep
        (6) Following safety practices, e.g. seat belts
        (7) Seeking medical attention when needed
    2. Emotional health
      a. Results when people:
        (1) Feel good about themselves
        (2) Have strong self-esteem, self-control and self-awareness
        (3) Accept help and give help to others
      b. Emotions will vary throughout one's life depending on misfortune and suffering
      c. You will deal with emotionally healthy and unhealthy individuals; avoid judging and learn to read their emotions so that you respond in a caring manner
    3. Social health
      a. Achieved through stable and satisfying relationships
      b. Socially healthy people approach others with respect, warmth, openness and trust
      c. Few people enjoy social health throughout life
      d. Feelings of isolation and loneliness are common among older adults, those who have suffered losses of people close to them, and new immigrants
      e. Most people need and have a social support system (an informal group of people who help each other)
      f. A social support system can help ill and frail people stay in their homes longer (see Figure 4-3, p. 34)
      g. Support workers may be key members of the support system
    4. Spiritual health
      a. Achieved through the belief in a purpose greater than the self
      b. May or may not involve participation in a formal religion or even believing in a higher being
      c. Gives a belief of right and wrong; behaviour reflects this belief
      d. Elements are compassion, honesty, humility, forgiveness, and charity
      e. For some, closely linked with religion
      f. Support workers must respect client's beliefs, items representing their religion, and if responsible for getting them to religious services it is done on time (see Respecting Diversity box, p. 35)
    5. Intellectual health
      a. Achieved through an active, creative mind
      b. Intellectually healthy people are inter-

ested in what is happening around them

c. They analyze, reason, and solve problems, and are open-minded and eager to learn.

d. Many residential facilities have recreational programs, which encourage residents to remain active through many different programs such as games, outings, etc. (see Figure 4-4, p. 35)

e. Support workers can encourage clients to remain active by talking to them about community and world events (see Support Workers Solving Problems box, p. 36)

II. ILLNESS AND DISABILITY

A. Illness is the loss of physical or mental health

B. A disability is the loss of physical or mental function

C. Some are acute (broken arm, influenza) or chronic (paraplegia), some can be progressive, and some can be managed to prevent further medical problems

1. Table 4-1, p. 36 in the textbook, lists medical conditions that many clients have

D. See Chapters 31, 33-36, and 38 for complete descriptions of common illness and disabilities

E. Always remember the client is a whole person

III. THE EXPERIENCE OF ILLNESS AND DISABILITY

A. Usually affects all aspects of a person's life

1. No two people experience illness and disability in the same way

2. Some have never known life any other way, some adjust well, and others have a very difficult time

3. Box 4-1, p. 38 in the textbook, lists common reactions

4. Factors affecting a person's experience include:

a. Nature of illness or condition

b. Age

c. Level of physical fitness

d. Amount and degree of pain and discomfort

e. Prognosis

f. Emotional, social, intellectual and spiritual health

g. Personality and ability to cope with difficulties

h. Culture (see Chapter 11)

i. Presence of emotional, social and financial support

B. Change and loss associated with illness and disability

1. Change in routine—almost always changes

2. Change in work life (see Box 4-2, p. 38)

3. Change in family life

4. Change in sexual function

5. Loss of independence

6. Loss of dignity

7. Change in self-image

a. Support workers need to understand how the condition affects every aspect of the client's life

b. Do not make assumptions or judge behaviour, but do provide warmth, acceptance, and respect (see Providing Compassionate Care box, p. 39)

C. Attitudes of others toward illness and disability

1. Some people are uncomfortable or fearful and may stare or avoid eye contact with ill or disabled people.

2. Some ill and disabled people experience stigma (marks a person as different or flawed) or discrimination (treats people unfairly based on their group membership)

3. Those with AIDS, mental illness, and substance abuse disorders are more vulnerable to discrimination. Can result in isolation, loneliness, and depression

Classroom Activities

1. Make transparencies of the continuum of health (see Figure 4-2, p. 33). Display on an overhead projector. Ask the class to identify where on the continuum people suffering from the following may be:

a. Someone who has just lost their partner

b. Someone who has had a heart attack

c. Someone who is depressed

d. A client confined to bed

e. Someone new to a country and unable to speak the language

Homework Assignments

2. Ask the class to list the changes people may face with a serious illness or recent disability. Write their answers on the board then divide the class into groups of four and ask them to make a list of examples for each identified change.

3. Write DIPPS on the board and ask the class how they can provide compassionate care for people with serious illness and disability using this acronym.

4. Divide the class into groups of 4 and ask each group to list factors that could influence a person's experience of illness or disability. Have a spokesperson report their results, and write the list on the board.

Ask students to answer the questions at the end of Chapter 4 in the textbook. Tell students the date and time that this assignment must be completed and turned in.

If the accompanying workbook is being used, assign the Chapter 4 workbook exercises. Tell students the date and time that this assignment must be completed and turned in.

Chapter 4 Student Assignment

Name _____

Date _____

Health, Wellness, Illness, and Disability

Match the following terms with the correct definitions.

a. Physical health

b. Emotional health

c. Social health

d. Spiritual health

e. Intellectual health

1. _____ Achieved through stable and satisfying relationships.

2. _____ Achieved through belief in a purpose greater than the self

3. _____ Achieved when the body is strong, fit, and free of disease

4. _____ Achieved through an active, creative mind

5. _____ results when people feel good about themselves

6. List the factors, which could affect a person's experience of illness and disability:

a. _____

b. _____

c. _____

d. _____

e. _____

f. _____

g. _____

h. _____

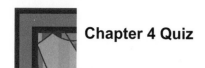

Name _____

Date _____

Health, Wellness, Illness, and Disability

True or False	Multiple Choice

*Mark **T** for true or **F** for false.*

1. _____ Health and wellness mean the same thing.

2. _____ Most people are not affected by a serious illness.

3. _____ People facing a loss are usually sad.

4. _____ Daily routines are almost always affected by illness or disability.

5 _____ Chronic means permanent.

6. _____ Older people are not interested in recreational programs.

7. _____ Religion is important to many people.

Circle the BEST answer.

8. The term discrimination means:
   a. Denial
   b. A characteristic that marks a person as different or flawed
   c. Behaviour that treats people unfairly based on their group membership
   d. A refusal to admit the truth

9. To help clients who are ill or disabled you should:
   a. not make assumptions.
   b. not judge the person's behaviour.
   c. communicate with warmth and care.
   d. All of the above.

10. A holistic approach to health care means:
    a. Focussing on the person's spiritual health
    b. Focussing on the person's physical health
    c. Focussing on the person's mental health
    d. Focussing on the whole person

11. The definition of health is now:
    a. A state of well being in all dimensions of one's life.
    b. Absence of disease or illness.
    c. Perfect balance of body, mind, and spirit.
    d. None of the above.

5 Working with Others: Teamwork, Supervision, and Delegation

Instructor's Preparation

I. Read Chapter 5 in the textbook. Carefully review chapter objectives, key terms, and review questions.

II. Read the outline in Chapter 5 of the instructor's guide. Carefully review the classroom activities, the student assignment, and the quiz.

III. If you are using the accompanying student workbook, review the activities for Chapter 5.

IV. Gather all necessary supplies and equipment for classroom activities and student assignments.

   A. Prepare the correct number of handouts

   B. Prepare appropriate flip charts

   C. Prepare overhead transparencies

   D. Prepare situation/index cards

   E. Gather correct video

   F. Gather coloured markers

   G. Gather any other items that will be needed for classroom activities

   H. Assemble items in the order they will be used

V. Make sure that the necessary equipment is available and in good working order.

Objectives

- Define the key terms listed in this chapter
- List the benefits and challenges to working on a health care team
- Explain your role on the health care team
- Describe how teams function in different health care settings
- Explain how delegating applies to you
- Describe the delegation process and your role in it

Key Terms

accountable
assigning
authority
case manager
delegation
family conference
multidisciplinary team
task
transfer of function

Outline

Working with Others:
Teamwork, Supervision, and Delegation

I. THE HEALTH CARE TEAM
  A. In most health care settings you work as a team—a group of people who work together toward a common goal (see Chapter 1)
    1. Teams must have holistic approach and promote all five dimensions of person's life
    2. Team members depend on each other to perform their roles and communicate effectively with each other
    3. Members of the health care team vary according to settings and clients needs
    4. Can vary from two to fifteen people on a team
    5. Support workers are part of a multidisciplinary team.
  B. Benefits of working on a team
    1. Opportunities for collaboration
      a. Support workers often find new ways of comforting clients, which needs to be shared with other workers
    2. Opportunities for communication
      a. Box 5-1, p. 43 in the textbook, demonstrates a meeting
    3. A wide array of abilities, skills, and perspectives
      a. Support workers are valuable in meetings, as they are often the only member who may see the client daily
    4. Better decision making and problem solving
    5. A positive, trusting atmosphere
      a. Team members learn to trust and respect each other
  C. Challenges of working on a team
    1. Recognizing role boundaries
      a. Never attempt any task you are not allowed to perform
      b. Be aware of your scope of practice and your employer's policies and procedures
    2. Being flexible, perhaps by exchanging shifts or assisting with certain tasks
    3. Handling conflict
      a. Team members should feel comfortable addressing problems to the team leader
      b. May also mean apologizing to a team member whose feelings are hurt or admitting mistakes
    4. Expressing your needs and views
      a. Support workers are important members of a team and should not be intimidated by physicians and nurses in meetings
      b. You are the one spending the most time with the client
  D. Teamwork in facilities
    1. Teams vary as much as settings themselves
    2. However, they have one thing in common: they all work in the same place, which makes communication easy
    3. Long-term care facilities
      a. Most use multidisciplinary team approach and are led by an RN
      b. Support workers are important members, as they know the residents well.
      c. The resident and family are part of the team
      d. Other members on a team depend on the resident's needs (see Figure 5-1, p. 44)
    4. Hospitals
      a. Functions and members vary from hospital to hospital and department to department
      b. Members of the team are determined by the patient's needs
    5. Hospices and palliative care units
      a. Most use multidisciplinary approach
      b. Members are usually nurses, support workers, physicians, social workers, the client and family, and any other person the client wishes
      c. Facilities are also considered community-based services
      d. Support workers are sometimes asked to join a family conference held with the team and family members to discuss the client's care, and are often called when difficulties arise
    6. Assisted-living facilities
      a. Usually located in a single building, which makes communication easier
      b. Staff is small and is often multidisciplinary
      c. Members depend on the client's needs and are led by a supervisor.
  E. Teamwork in community settings
    1. Home care
      a. Team usually includes the client, family, case manager (who assesses,

monitors, and evaluates a client's needs and coordinates care), physician, nurses, support workers and their supervisor

    b. Do not meet regularly, and communicate by telephone or written reports

  2. Community day programs

    a. Rehabilitation program team may include a supervisor (often nurse or other health care professional), other professionals, and support workers

    b. A recreational program team may include a supervisor (usually a recreational or occupational therapist) and support workers

    c. Regular opportunities to discuss the client's progress

    d. May meet before program starts, after it is over, or weekly

II. WORKING UNDER SUPERVISION

  A. You are responsible to the client, co-workers and your supervisor

    1. Supervisor is usually an RN

    2. Some provinces allow RPNs to supervise support workers in long-term care facilities

    3. In community settings, support workers may occasionally be supervised by an RPN, a social worker, or another health care professional

  B. Supervision in a facility

    1. Team leader is usually an RN who has overall responsibility for the client's care, the work of other RNs, RPNs, support workers, and assistive personnel

    2. If RN is not on duty, support workers report to the charge nurse

  C. Supervision in a community setting

    1. Support workers are responsible to a supervisor who works for the same agency

    2. Agency may be hired by a health district, access centre, or community services organization

    3. A case manager communicates with the supervisor who then gives the support worker instruction about the client's care

    4. Agency may be hired by the client or client's family who will give the supervisor instructions regarding care needed

    5. Supervisor will relay instructions to the support worker

    6. In some cases, clients hire their own support workers, and the client is the supervisor

  D. Respecting your supervisor and employer

    1. Support workers must respect supervisors and employers

    2. Avoid talking about clients or co-workers

    3. Speak to supervisor if you are having difficulties and use some of the strategies discussed in Chapters 8 and 12

    4. Do not talk to clients about work problems

    5. A negative attitude could destroy trust the client has in the agency

III. DELEGATION

  A. Nurse practice acts give RNs and RPNs certain responsibilities and the authority to perform nursing tasks

    1. A responsibility is a duty or obligation to perform some act or function

    2. A task is a function, procedure, activity, or work that does not require an RN's professional knowledge or judgement

    3. Your supervisor assigns most of your daily tasks

     a. Assigning means giving responsibility for providing care or support

     b. Assigned tasks do not require a nurse's education and professional judgement

     c. Some tasks could harm a client if done by unqualified workers

    4. To delegate means to authorize another person to perform a task

  B. Who can delegate?

    1. RNs delegate to RPNs and support workers

    2. Some provinces and territories allow RPNs to delegate to support workers

     a. The delegating nurse remains accountable for the delegated task

      (1) Accountable means being responsible for one's actions and the actions of others who perform delegated tasks

     b. Support workers are not allowed to delegate tasks

  C. Delegation in a facility

    1. When RNs delegate a task in a facility they are required to:

     a. Teach the support worker the task

     b. Assess their performance

     c. Monitor the support worker over time to ensure they remain able to perform the task correctly and safely

    2. Support workers cannot assign or delegate, which means a co-worker can help

with a task assigned but cannot do the task himself or herself

D. Delegation in the community
  1. If your supervisor is an RN, they will follow the same delegation process used in facilities
  2. If not an RN, the agency will send out an RN to instruct the support worker, and to assesse and monitor performance
  3. Some agencies provide educational programs for support workers where certain tasks are taught
     a. Students graduate only once they are successful at completing the task
     b. The agency is responsible to monitor the task
  4. If asked to perform tasks by a professional who is not an RN, use judgement but refuse the task if you have concerns about your ability to perform the task or if it is beyond your scope of practice
  5. Know your employer's policies and never perform a task that is beyond your scope of practice

E. Delegation process
  1. Tasks must be within the legal limits of what support workers can do
  2. Before delegation, the nurse must know:
     a. What your province or territory allows
     b. The tasks included in your job description
     c. What you were taught in your training program
     d. What skills you learned and how they were evaluated
     e. About your work experience
  3. It is wise for the nurse to get to know you and for you to get to know the nurse
  4. Agency policies, guidelines, and your job description state what tasks nurses can delegate
  5. Provincial or territorial legislation determines tasks that can be delegated as well as when and how tasks can be delegated
  6. Across the country there are similarities but each province or territory has its own rules (see Box 5-2, p. 46)
  7. The RN makes delegation decisions after considering the factors listed in Box 5-3, p. 48 in the textbook
  8. The nurse decides whether to delegate or not
  9. Do not be offended if not allowed to per-

form a task that is part of your job description
  10. The nurse makes the decision that is best for the person
  11. The person's circumstances are central factors in making delegation decisions
  12. The five rights of delegation:
     a. The right task
     b. The right circumstances
     c. The right person
     d. The right directions and communication
     e. The right supervision

F. Your role in delegation
  1. Delegated tasks are performed for or on a person
  2. There are two choices: agree or refuse to do the task
     a. Use the "five rights" of delegation to make your choice
  3. Accepting a task
     a. When you agree to perform a task, you are responsible for your actions
     b. The task must be completed safely
     c. Report to the nurse what you did and your observations
  4. Refusing a task
     a. You have the right to say no
     b. Refuse to perform a task when:
        (1) The task is beyond the legal limits of your role
        (2) The task in not in your job description
        (3) You are not prepared to perform the task safely
        (4) The task could harm the person
        (5) The person's condition has changed
        (6) You do not know how to use supplies or equipment
        (7) Directions are unethical, illegal, or against agency policies
        (8) Directions are unclear or incomplete
        (9) A nurse is not available for supervision
     c. Use common sense
     d. Do not ignore an order or request
     e. You must communicate your concerns to the nurse
     f. You must have sound reasons for your refusal

Classroom Activities	**Homework Assignments**

Classroom Activities

1. Ask the class to identify the different types of facilities they may be working in. Write the list on the board. Ask them to describe the possible team members for each facility.

2. Invite someone from your local access centre to explain to the class their role and how they co-ordinate care.

3. Obtain from your provincial nursing regulating college, a list of the tasks, which an RN can delegate to support workers. Discuss this list with the class and explain why each task would be on the list. For example, catheterization is introducing an instrument into a body orifice.

4. Divide the class into groups of 4. Write the five rights of delegation on the board. Ask each group to describe what each right means. Have one person from each group report their discussions.

Homework Assignments

Ask students to answer the questions at the end of Chapter 5 in the textbook. Tell students the date and time that this assignment must be completed and turned in.

If the accompanying workbook is being used, assign the Chapter 5 workbook exercises. Tell students the date and time that this assignment must be completed and turned in.

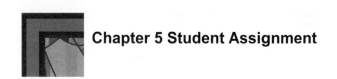

Name _____

Date _____

Working with Others: Teamwork, Supervision, and Delegation

Fill in the definitions for the following terms.

1. A task is:

_____.

2. Delegation means:

_____.

3. A family conference is:

_____.

4. An assignment is:

_____.

5. A multidisciplinary team is:

_____.

When should you refuse a delegated task? (Write in the nine different situations when you should refuse to do a task.)

6. _____

7. _____

8. _____

9. _____

10. _____

11. _____

12. _____

13. _____

14. _____

Chapter 5 Quiz

Name _____

Date _____

Working with Others: Teamwork, Supervision, and Delegation

True or False	Multiple Choice

Mark **T** *for true or* **F** *for false.*

1. _____ Support workers can supervise other support workers.

2. _____ A case manager provides hands on nursing.

3. _____ You may be supervised by an RPN if allowed in your province or territory.

4. _____ Accountable means being responsible for the outcome.

Circle the BEST answer.

5. A procedure can be delegated to you by:
   a. the client.
   b. a physician.
   c. a social worker.
   d. an RN.

6. Scope of practice means:
   a. The tasks that are assigned by your supervisor.
   b. The task that a client asks you to perform.
   c. The effort you put into performing a task or procedure.
   d. The legal limits of your role.

7. Delegation means:
   a. To give responsibility for providing care.
   b. To authorize another worker to perform a task.
   c. To transfer responsibility to another worker.
   d. To give another worker the power or right to enforce an act, function or role.

Fill in the Blanks

8. Identify 3 of the 5 Rights of Delegation:

   a. _____.

   b. _____.

   c. _____.

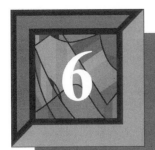

6

Working with Clients and Their Families

Instructor's Preparation

I. Read Chapter 6 in the textbook. Carefully review chapter objectives, key terms, and review questions.

II. Read the outline in Chapter 6 of the instructor's guide. Carefully review the classroom activities, the student assignment, and the quiz.

III. If you are using the accompanying student workbook, review the activities for Chapter 6.

IV. Gather all necessary supplies and equipment for classroom activities and student assignments.

  A. Prepare the correct number of handouts

  B. Prepare appropriate flip charts

  C. Prepare overhead transparencies

  D. Prepare situation/index cards

  E. Gather correct video

  F. Gather coloured markers

  g. Gather any other items that will be needed for classroom activities

  H. Assemble items in the order they will be used

V. Make sure that the necessary equipment is available and in good working order.

Objectives

- Define the key terms listed in this chapter
- Recognize that each client is an individual and a whole person
- Describe Erikson's developmental stages
- Explain how Maslow's hierarchy of needs applies to support work
- Explain the difference between a professional helping relationship and a friendship
- Explain independence, dependence and interdependence
- Describe common family patterns
- Explain how the health care team assists the family

Key Terms

compassion
competence
dependence
empathy
family
independence
interdependence
need
primary caregiver
psychosocial health
relationship
respect
self-actualization
self-awareness
self- esteem

Outline

Working with Clients and Their Families

I. INTRODUCTION
- A. The patient or resident is the most important person.
  1. The person is important and special
  2. The person is treated as someone who thinks, acts, feels, and makes decisions
  3. Each person has fears, needs, and rights
  4. The client is usually part of a family, and it is important to understand your role

II. CARING FOR THE PERSON
- A. To provide good care, you must be aware of the whole person
- B. Holism means whole (see Chapter 4)
  1. The person has physical, social, psychological, and spiritual parts
  2. Each part relates to and depends on the others

III. PSYCHOSOCIAL HEALTH
- A. Well being in the social, emotional, intellectual and spiritual dimensions of one's life
- B. Factors that influence psychosocial health include:
  1. Personality
  2. Family background
  3. Environment
  4. Life circumstances

IV. ERIKSON'S DEVELOPMENTAL STAGES
- A. Psychologist who strongly influenced ideas about the development of psychosocial health
- B. Theory that people move through a series of stages throughout their lives (see Table 6-1, p. 52)
- C. Each stage is necessary and must be completed before moving on to the next task

V. MASLOW'S HIERARCHY OF NEEDS
- A. A need is something necessary or desirable for maintaining life and mental well-being
- B. Lower level needs must be met before higher level need
- C. Physical needs such as oxygen, food, water, elimination, rest, and shelter are required for life
  1. These are the most important needs for survival
  2. They must be met before higher level needs
- D. Safety needs include safety and security, protection from harm, danger, and fear
  1. Many people are afraid of health care

2. People feel safe and secure if they understand procedures
3. People should know:
  a. Why a procedure is done
  b. Who will do it
  c. How it will be performed
  d. What sensations and feelings to expect
- E. Love and belonging needs relate to love, closeness, affection, belonging, and meaningful relationships
  1. These needs can be met by family, friends, and health care workers
- F. Self-esteem needs relate to thinking well of yourself and being thought well of by others
  1. People often lack self-esteem when ill or injured
- G. Self-actualization needs involve learning, understanding, creating, and experiencing one's potential
  1. The highest need
  2. Rarely, if ever, is it totally met

VI. YOUR RELATIONSHIP WITH THE CLIENT
- A. A relationship is the connection between two or more people
- B. A professional helping relationship
  1. You must maintain a professional helping role with your clients, which is different from a friendship (a personal social relationship that benefits both involved)
  2. Box 6-1, p. 54 in the textbook, compares a professional helping relationship with a friendship
  3. When working with clients always demonstrate the following (see Box 6-1, p. 54)
    a. Respect
    b. Compassion (see Support Workers Solving Problems box, p. 54)
    c. Empathy
    d. Competence
    e. Self-awareness (see Support Workers Solving Problems box, p. 55)
- C. Independence, dependence, and interdependence
  1. Independence: state of not depending on others for control or authority
  2. Dependence: state of relying on others or support
  3. Interdependence: state of depending on each other
  4. Goal of most clients' care is to achieve or maintain as much independence as possible (see Figure 6-2, p. 56)

5. You must respect the client's choices to do some things independently and to accept help with other things even if you do not understand their decisions

D. Independence and self-esteem
   1. Self-esteem can suffer when independence is limited or lost
   2. People's roles and identifies can change when they are no longer in control of their lives (see Chapter 4)
   3. You must be sensitive to how people feel
   4. They need to find ways to rebuild their self-esteem, and need support and encouragement with honest, constructive feedback in a gentle, supportive manner

E. Independence and Balance of Power
   1. A strong, independent person may control the vulnerable, dependent person and in some situations, this leads to abuse (see Chapter 19)
   2. Be aware of the balance of power and avoid controlling behaviour; instead of imposing your will on clients, involve them in solving problems

VII. THE CLIENT'S FAMILY
A. Close personal relationships are central to the lives of most people and involve some forms of dependency
   1. A family is a biological, legal, or social network of people who provide support for one another
   2. May include people related by blood or marriage, or unrelated people
   3. You and your client may have different ideas about what is a family and you must respect their definition and not impose your values

B. Your role in assisting the family: many different situations
   1. You may provide care to infants, mothers, children, or adults of all ages
   2. You may provide respite for a primary caregiver (see Focus on Home Care box, p. 57)
      a. By providing basic care, you enable family members to invest time in the relationship
   3. Changes arise in a family when illness or disabilities occur (see Chapter 4)
      a. Can be difficult changes with new patterns of dependency
   4. The ill person may feel angry becoming a

dependent; the caregiver may feel angry because of added responsibilities
   5. Professionals on the care team can help families cope with the changes and stress

C. Families in conflict
   1. Some families are already dealing with conflict when illness or disability occurs; this stress adds to the conflict
   2. There may be bickering, arguments, etc. or the conflict may be hidden
   3. Sometimes the health care team can help families resolve these conflicts, but you must realize that this is not your role
   4. Be aware or family relationships, conflicts, etc. (see Figure 6-3, p. 57)
   5. Observe and report on family interactions (see Box 6-2, p. 58)
   6. Be alert for signs of abuse (see Chapter 19)

Classroom Activities

1. Make a transparency of Erikson's Theory of Psychological Development listing stages, ages, and psychosocial task. Ask the students to describe what each stage might represent. Then compare with description of task in Table 6-1, p. 52 in the textbook.

2. Draw a large triangle on the board and divide into 5 parts. Write in Maslow's hierarchy of needs. Ask the class to identify what needs are met in each level.

3. Divide the class into groups of 3-4 and have each group develop a list of qualities a support worker needs to have with the client to ensure a professional relationship happens. Allow 15 minutes for discussion, then ask one person from each group to report to the class.

4. Write the definition of self-esteem on the board. Ask the class how the following scenarios could affect them in all areas of their life:
   a. Loss of an arm
   b. Diagnosis of cancer
   c. A stroke which leaves you unable to communicate
   d. Bedrest for 6 months

5. Write the word "family" on the board. Ask the class to identify all of the different combinations

of families they are aware of. Compare to the list on page 56 and discuss different ideas of family and respect for the client's values.

Homework Assignments

Ask students to answer the questions at the end of Chapter 6 in the textbook. Tell students the date and time that this assignment must be completed and turned in.

If the accompanying workbook is being used, assign the Chapter 6 workbook exercises. Tell students the date and time that this assignment must be completed and turned in.

Name _____

Date _____

Working with Clients and Their Families

Fill in the definitions for the following terms.

1. Respect is:

   _____.

2. A relationship is:

   _____.

3. A primary caregiver is:

   _____.

4. Empathy is:

   _____.

5. Compassion is:

   _____.

Give examples of the needs identified in Maslow's hierarchy of needs:

6. Physical needs:

   a. _____.

   b. _____.

   c. _____.

7. Safety needs:

   a. _____.

   b. _____.

   c. _____.

8. Love and belonging:

   a. _____.

   b. _____.

   c. _____.

How can you help your clients meet the following needs?

9. Self-esteem needs:

   a. _____.

   b. _____.

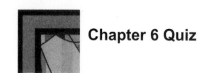

Name _____

Date _____

Working with Clients and Their Families

True or False

Mark T for true or F for false.

1. _____ It is acceptable to have a friendship and professional relationship with your client.

2. _____ A peer group is a group of friends or acquaintance.

3. _____ Empathy involves judging others.

4. _____ Children develop self-esteem when they learn to control their bodies.

5. _____ Families are composed of many different networks of people.

6. _____ A caregiver can feel angry at their new role.

7. _____ A professional helping relationship is established to benefit the client.

8. _____ Independence means depending on other.

9. _____ Conflicts among families can be hidden

10. _____ Reporting is always done in writing.

Multiple Choice

Circle the BEST answer.

11. Compassion means:
    a. Caring about another's misfortune and suffering.
    b. Keeping one's feelings to oneself.
    c. Taking pity on those who are less fortunate.
    d. Approaching your work with enthusiasm.

12. Common courtesy is a sign of:
    a. pity.
    b. respect.
    c. compassion.
    d. self-awareness.

13. Maslow's most basic need includes:
    a. oxygen, food, water, and shelter.
    b. oxygen, elimination, food, rest, and belonging.
    c. shelter, self worth, oxygen, water, rest, and food.
    d. oxygen, food , water, elimination, rest, and shelter.

14. Psychological aspects include:
    a. personality behaviour.
    b. sexuality.
    c. growth and development.
    d. life span.
    e. all of the above.

15. Which is not part of Erikson's theory of psychosocial development?:
    a. People move through a series of stages throughout their lives.
    b. People must successfully complete a task in each stage before moving on to the next.
    c. Babies must learn to trust that their needs will be met.
    d. Moving to unfamiliar surroundings creates love and belonging needs.

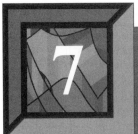

7

Client Care: Planning, Processes, Reporting, and Recording

Instructor's Preparation

I. Read Chapter 7 in the textbook. Carefully review chapter objectives, key terms, and review questions.

II. Read the outline in Chapter 7 of the instructor's guide. Carefully review the classroom activities, the student assignment, and the quiz.

III. If you are using the accompanying student workbook, review the activities for Chapter 7.

IV. Gather all necessary supplies and equipment for classroom activities and student assignments.
   A. Prepare the correct number of handouts
   B. Prepare overhead transparencies
   C. Prepare situation cards
   D. Gather any other items that will be needed for classroom activities
   E. Assemble items in the order they will be used

V. Make sure that the necessary equipment is available and in good working order.

Objectives

- Define the key terms listed in this chapter
- Explain the steps in the care planning process in facilities
- Explain the steps in the care planning process in the community
- Explain the function of the care plan
- Describe you role in the care planning process
- Explain why observation is an important part of the support worker's role
- Explain the difference between objective data and subjective data
- Explain what makes an observation effective
- Explain how reporting differs in a facility and a community setting
- List four functions of charts
- Identify the types of documents found in a client's chart
- List the basic rules for recording
- Use the 24-hour clock
- Explain why confidentiality is important to the care planning process
- Explain how computers have affected the care planning process

Outline

Client Care: Planning, Processes, Reporting, and Recording

I. THE CARE PLANNING PROCESS IN FACILITIES
  A. The method used by nurses to plan and deliver nursing care
  B. Five steps: assessment, nursing diagnosis, planning, implementation, and evaluation
  C. Each step is important; the purpose is to meet the person's nursing needs
  D. The nursing process is ongoing
    1. It constantly changes as new information is gathered and the person's needs change
    2. Assessment involves collecting information about the person
      a. Information is gathered from:
        (1) Nursing history
        (2) Family history
        (3) Information from the physician
        (4) Past medical records
        (5) Test results
        (6) Physical assessment
        (7) Mental status assessment
        (8) Observations made by support workers
    3. Nursing diagnosis is a statement describing a health problem that is treated by nursing measures
      a. The RN uses information from the assessment to make a nursing diagnosis

      b. Nursing diagnoses and medical diagnoses are different
        (1) Medial diagnosis is the identification of a disease or condition by a doctor
      c. A person may have more than one nursing diagnosis
        (1) Nursing diagnoses involve the person's physical, emotional, social, and spiritual needs
        (2) Use North American Nursing Diagnosis list (see Box 7-1, p. 62)
    4. Planning involves setting priorities and goals and developing measures or actions to help the client meet these goals
      a. The person, family, and nursing team help the RN plan
      b. Priorities relate to what is most important for the person
        (1) Once the client and nurse decided on the client's needs they decide on priorities
        (2) Family members and the health care team often take part
        (3) Nurses use Maslow's theory of needs to set priorities (see Chapter 6)
        (4) Needs for life and survival must be met first
      c. A goal is that which is desired in or by a person as a result of nursing care
        (1) Goals are practical, achievable, measurable results (see Figure 7-1, p. 63)
        (2) Aimed at the person's highest level of well-being and functioning
        (3) Promote health and prevent health problems
        (4) Promote the person's rehabilitation
      d. Nursing interventions are chosen
        (1) An action or measure taken by the nursing team to help the person reach a goal
      e. Establishing the care plan
        (1) Is a written document about the care a person should receive
        (2) Has the person's nursing diagnoses, goals, and interventions
        (3) The care plan has several important functions:
          (a) Lists care and services the person receives

(b) Ensures care is consistent

(c) Enables health care team to communicate details about person's care

(4) Care plan is not a finished document; change it as the client's needs, condition, and progress change

(5) Has the measures or actions for each goal

(6) The RN usually has responsibility for care plan changes

(7) The plan must be carried out

5. Implementation means to perform or carry out

a. Care is given in this step

b. Nursing measures range from simple to complex

c. Nurse in charge assigns or delegates tasks

d. Tasks must be within legal limits of your role and job description

e. Nurse uses an assignment sheet to tell you what tasks need to be done for each person

f. Main functions of implementation process

(1) Provide care

(2) Observing the person during care

(3) Reporting and recording the care completed

(4) Reporting and recording observation made during care

g. Providers must report and record their actions and observations after care is completed, according to employer policy

h. Report and record after giving care, not before

i. Know about changes in the nursing care plan so you can give correct care

6. Evaluation means to measure and assess

a. This step involves measuring if the goals in the planning step were met

b. Goals may be met totally, in part, or not at all

c. Changes in nursing diagnoses, goals, and the care plan may result from evaluation

d. The nursing process never ends

e. Your observations are used for the evaluation step

f. Team meetings are often part of the evaluation

II. THE CARE PLANNING PROCESS IN COMMUNITY SETTINGS

A. Assessment

1. The case manager meets with the client and family to identify client's problems and needs

2. Family important as serious illness and disability affect family life (see Chapter 4)

3. Case manager considers family's needs, health, training etc., and what services and equipment will be needed to care for the client at home

4. Case manager also considers if the home is a safe environment and if other specialists need to assess the home for safety

B. Planning

1. Can be lengthy and complicated

2. Once case manager has met with client and family, identified priorities, set goals and determined available resources, a master care plan and health care team are put together (see Figure 7-2, p. 64)

3. Case manager determines how much publicly funded home care the client and family are eligible for and if the family is able to pay for additional help if needed

4. If the client needs help from a support worker, the case manager will contact your agency and your supervisor will assign you to provide the care needed

5. Agencies and other professionals involved with the client may each develop their own care plan but the case manager is in charge of the master plan

6. Some clients choose to coordinate and manage their own care

C. Implementation

1. Agency staff provides care and service on dates and times arranged by the case manager

2. If unforeseen needs arise, the client or family will contact the case manager who will then contact your agency

D. Evaluation

1. Case manager meets with the client and family periodically to assess progress

2. Case manager meets with and receives reports from other providers who will be monitoring and evaluating their own care plans

III. YOUR ROLE IN THE CARE PLANNING PROCESS

A. Developing observation skills

1. Support workers are often with the clients more than any other care providers
2. May be the first to observe changes, and are expected to make accurate and careful observation for use in the care plan
3. Use all of senses when observing the client—sight, hearing, touch, and smell; two types of observations:
   a. Objective data (signs)
      (1) Information you observe (i.e., you feel a pulse or see urine)
   b. Subjective data (symptoms)
      (1) Information reported by the client (i.e., nausea, pain)
4. When reporting subjective data use the person's exact words
5. Box 7-2, p. 66 in the textbook, is a guide to follow when making observations
6. Focus your observations on the person's physical, mental, emotional, and social conditions, plus any new conditions that you observe

B. Describing your observations
1. Your observations are critical to care planning as nurses and case mangers use your observations for assessment and evaluation.
2. Be precise and accurate
3. Do not interpret or make assumptions
4. Box 7-3, p. 67 in the textbook, contains examples of ineffective and effective descriptions of observations

IV. VERBAL REPORTING
A. Introduction
1. Verbal report is the spoken account of care provided and observation you have made
2. Employers use different methods for verbal reporting so know your employer's policies
3. Box 7-4, p. 68 in the textbook, describes circumstances when you must contact your supervisor
4. Remember the rules of confidentiality when verbally reporting

B. Verbal reporting in a facility
1. Your reports to the charge nurse must be prompt, thorough, and accurate, and must identify the client by name (room and bed number)
2. Report only what you have done or observed, and start with the most important information

3. Always immediately report any change in client's condition
4. Charge nurses usually give a report at end of the shift to the staff starting shift so ensure they have accurate information

C. Verbal reporting in a community setting
1. Agencies have their own policies for verbal reports, which may include calling the agency daily
2. Always call if something out of the ordinary occurs
3. Follow agency policy and guidelines (see Box 7-4 and Box 7-5, p. 68)

V. CHARTS (ALSO KNOWN AS A RECORD)
A. Introduction
1. Written account of client's condition, illness, and responses to care
2. It is a permanent, legal record that provides:
   a. Communication for health care teams (see Figure 7-3, p. 68)
   b. Currency as the care plans change, as client's needs change
   c. Accountability, since charts are signed and dated by members of the health care team
   d. Continuity of care, as it provides information of past health problems and may detect patterns and changes in client's health

B. Documents used in charts
1. Will vary depending on the employer; common documents are:
   a. Data forms—details about physical, emotional, social, and intellectual health, plus interests, medications, etc.
   b. Assessment forms
   c. Home assessment forms—document any changes needed to be made to the client's home (see Box 32-3, p. 562)
   d. Care plans—contain goals and intervention
   e. Progress notes—vary depending on employer and if health care team members all use same forms or have their own
   f. ADL check lists and flow sheets (also called tick sheets)—describe daily care (see Figure 7-5, p. 71)
   g. Task sheets—used by agencies in community settings to record provided care and services (see Figure 7-6, p. 72)

h. Graphic sheets—record measurements and observations made every shift, or three or four times a day (see Figure 7-7, p.73)

i. Other flow sheets—record frequent measurements or observations

j. Summary reports—may be monthly, or over a longer period of time

k. Incident reports (occurrence report—Chapter 16) written accounts of accident, error, or unexpected event

l. Kardex—card file that summarizes information in the chart and is a quick reference

C. Recording (charting)

1. Documenting care and observations

   a. Employers have their own policies including when to record, how often, what can be recorded, who should record, colour of ink, etc.

   b. Make sure everything you record is dated, accurate, and relevant

   c. Use guidelines in Box 7-6, p. 74 in the textbook, and follow employer's policies

2. Recording time

   a. The 24-hour clock is used to document care

   b. Involves using a four digit number (see Figure 7-8, p. 74)

   c. First two digits are for hours and last two digits are for minutes

   d. Box 7-7, p. 74 in the textbook, shows morning hours (similar to conventional clock) and afternoon hours (add 12 to first two digits)

   e. Makes communication more accurate

   f. Terminology and abbreviations (see Chapter 48)

D. Recording in a facility

1. In acute-care setting, you will most likely document care on graphic sheets, flow sheets, and/or progress notes

2. In long-term care settings, you will likely document care on checklists or flow sheets; summary reports on care provided may also be required

E. Recording in the community

1. Every agency and case manager keep separate client charts

2. Some charts are kept in the home in a binder

3. Policies regarding support workers

charting vary from agency to agency

4. Most agencies have client care task sheets that are taken to each assignment (see Figure 7-6, p. 72)

   a. New task sheet for each client

   b. Check off as each task is completed.

5. Most have space to record observations, verbal reports you make to your supervisor, and phone instructions you receive from your supervisor

6. The frequency task sheets are submitted to your supervisor depends on agency policy

F. Confidentiality

1. The chart is confidential and you are ethically and legally bound to keep client information confidential

2. All employers have strict guidelines about confidentiality

3. Only health care team members involved in the client's care have access to confidential information

4. Be very careful transporting a document and do not become distracted from your task

G. Computers in health care

1. Systems collect, send, record, and store information

2. Medical records and care plans are on computer in many agencies

   a. Recordings are more accurate, legible, and reliable (see Figure 7-9, p. 75)

3. Computers are also used to monitor certain measurements such as blood pressure, temperatures, heart rates, and heart function

4. Doctors can use computers when diagnosing

5. Computers save time

6. Computer information is easy to access

7. Follow ethical and legal considerations related to privacy, confidentiality, and defamation

Classroom Activities

1. Obtain documentation forms used by support workers in the agencies to which students will be assigned. Share and discuss the correct use of these forms with students.

   a. Ask students to spend 15 minutes completing the forms. Collect the completed forms. Correct and return to the students at the beginning of the next class. Be available to answer questions and to clarify any incorrect entries.

2. Make transparencies of a mock patient or resident record that contains documentation errors. Display on an overhead projector. Ask students to identify the errors.

3. Write the following steps of the nursing process on the chalkboard. Then ask students to identify what each step involves. Write the correct answers under each step. Allow time for discussion.
   a. Assessment
   b. Nursing diagnoses
   c. Planning
   d. Implementation
   e. Evaluation

4. Place the following items on a paper towel:
   a. A tablespoon of ketchup
   b. A small glass of apple juice
   c. A tablespoon of peanut butter
   d. A tablespoon of mayonnaise

5. Ask each student to make observations about each item and to record their observations. Then have each student report the observations to the class.

Discuss the importance of being clear and concise when you are making, reporting, and recording observations.

6. Display a diagram of the 24-hour clock on an overhead transparency. Discuss how to convert time using the 24-hour clock.
   a. Randomly call on students to convert the following times using the 24-hour clock:
   (1) 2:05 am
   (2) 3:15 am
   (3) 1:06 pm
   (4) 12:10 pm
   (5) 6:35 am
   (6) 10:36 pm

Homework Assignments

Ask students to answer the questions at the end of Chapter 7 in the textbook. Tell students the date and time that this assignment must be completed and turned in.

If the accompanying workbook is being used, assign the Chapter 7 workook exercises. Tell students the date and time that this assignment must be completed and turned in.

Chapter 7 Student Assignment

Name _____

Date _____

Client Care: Planning, Processes, Reporting, and Recording

Match the following terms with the correct definitions.

a. Nursing diagnosis
b. Reporting
c. Symptoms
d. Signs
e. Nursing intervention
f. Nursing process
g. Recording

1. _____ A statement describing a health problem that can be treated by nursing measures

2. _____ The method used by nurses to plan and deliver nursing care

3. _____ Writing or charting patient or resident care and observations

4. _____ Objective data—information that can be seen, heard, felt, or smelled by another person

5. _____ Subjective data—that which is reported by a person

6. _____ An action or measure taken by the nursing team to help the person reach a goal

7. _____ A verbal account of person care and observations

Identify which of the following symptoms is objective data and which is subjective data.
(O=objective data; S=subjective data)

8. _____ backache

9. _____ itching

10. _____ pale skin

11. _____ blurred vision

12. _____ drainage from the eyes

13. _____ productive cough

14. _____ belching

15. _____ pain when breathing

16. _____ bad taste in the mouth

17. _____ dry, cracked lips

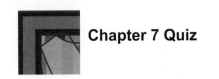
Name _____

Date _____

Client Care: Planning, Processes, Reporting, and Recording

True or False

*Mark **T** for true or **F** for false.*

1. _____ The medical diagnosis and the nursing diagnosis are always the same.

2. _____ The medical record is a permanent legal document.

3. _____ Everyone who works at an agency has the right to read the patient's or resident's records.

4. _____ Assessment involves setting priorities and goals.

5. _____ You may share your computer password with other members of the health team.

Multiple Choice

Circle the BEST answer.

6. The written guide giving directions about the nursing care a patient should receive is the:
   a. Kardex.
   b. Medical record.
   c. Nursing care plan.
   d. Chart.

7. Flow sheets are:
   a. Completed when the person is admitted to the agency.
   b. Card files used to summarize information.
   c. Used only by RNs.
   d. Used to record frequent measurements or observations.

8. During which step of the nursing process is care given?
   a. Planning
   b. Evaluation
   c. Implementation
   d. Assessment

9. Which is incorrect when recording on a patient's or resident's chart?
   a. Communicate clearly and concisely.
   b. Use a pencil in case you make a mistake.
   c. Record in a logical manner.
   d. Record only what you observed and did yourself.

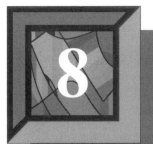

8

Managing Stress, Time, and Problems

Instructor's Preparation

I. Read Chapter 8 in the textbook. Carefully review chapter objectives, key terms, and review questions.

II. Read the outline in Chapter 8 of the instructor's guide. Carefully review the classroom activities, the student assignment, and the quiz.

III. If you are using the accompanying student workbook, review the activities for Chapter 8.

IV. Gather all necessary supplies and equipment for classroom activities and student assignments.
   A. Prepare the correct number of handouts
   B. Prepare appropriate flip charts
   C. Prepare overhead transparencies
   D. Prepare situation/index cards
   E. Gather correct video
   F. Gather coloured markers
   G. Gather any other items that will be needed for classroom activities
   H. Assemble items in the order they will be used

V. Make sure that the necessary equipment is available and in good working order.

VI. Contact guest speakers to confirm the day, date, time, and location that they are expected.
   A. Ask the speakers if they require any special equipment or supplies. Make sure these are available.

Objectives

- Define the key terms listed in this chapter
- Understand how stress can affect all dimensions of life
- List signs of stress
- Discuss defence mechanisms
- Describe common stressors
- Describe how to manage stress
- Define SMART goals
- Describe methods that will improve your decision-making and problem-solving abilities
- Explain how to deal with conflict

Key Terms

anxiety
burnout
conflict
defence mechanism
stress
stressor

Outline

Managing Stress, Time, and Problems

I. STRESS
   A. Introduction
      1. Normal part of life
      2. Stress is the emotional, behavioural, or physical response to an event or situation
      3. The event or situation that causes stress is called a stressor
      4. New situations or illness can cause stress
      5. Some stress can be good (for example,

stress caused by a busy schedule can make you work more effectively)

6. Long-term stress can lead to burnout (state of physical, emotional, and mental exhaustion)

7. Affects the whole person and can have positive or negative effect on all dimensions(see Table 8-1, p. 78)

B. Responses to stress

1. A person's responses to stressors are influenced by several factors including:
   a. health
   b. temperament or personality
   c. past experiences with the same or similar stressors
   d. the number of other stressors the person is experiencing
   e. the nature, severity, and duration of the stressors

2. Physical responses are usually similar (see Box 8-1, p. 79)

3. Emotional and behavioural responses vary from person to person (see Box 8-2, p. 79)

4. Important to recognize stress in yourself and your client

5. Tell your supervisor if you observe signs of stress in your client; remember, your role is to observe and report, not assess or diagnose

6. Professionals can help the client cope with stress

C. Defence mechanism

1. An unconscious reaction that blocks unpleasant or threatening feelings

2. Most people occasionally use as it can help relieve stress

3. Learning to recognize and understand defence mechanisms clients use will enable you to provide compassionate care
   a. Conversion—changing an emotion into a physical complaint
   b. Denial—refusing to accept an unpleasant or threatening reality
   c. Displacement—directing emotions toward a person or thing that seems safe, instead of the source of emotions
   d. Projection—assigning one's feelings to someone or something else
   e. Rationalization—making excuses for one's behaviour or situation while ignoring the real reason

f. Reaction formation—acting in a way that is opposite to what one feels

g. Regression—reverting or moving back to earlier behaviours

h. Repression—keeping unpleasant or painful thoughts or experiences from the conscious mind

D. Sources of stress

1. Change—positive or negative

2. Pressure—feeling pushed beyond one's limits or abilities (see Figure 8-1, p. 80)

3. Lack of Control—people feel stress when they cannot control what happens to them or around them

4. Conflict—a clash between opposing interests and ideas

5. Daily irritations—depending on the person's reaction, any frustrating incident can cause stress

6. See Focus on Older Adult and Focus on Children boxes, p. 81

E. Managing stress in your life

1. Burnout is common among health care workers as support work can be physically and emotionally demanding

2. Managing stress is essential; don't ignore signs of stress, built up stress can result in burnout, illness, or taking your stress out on clients

3. Good communication with your supervisor will help relieve stress, if you talk about the stressors

4. Strategies that will help you manage stress in your life:
   a. develop self-awareness
   b. take care of your needs
   c. think positively
   d. assert yourself
   e. ask others for help and support
   f. practise calming exercises (see Boxes 8-3 and 8-4, p. 82)

II. TIME MANAGEMENT

A. Introduction

1. Managing your time effectively can reduce stress in all aspects of your life

2. Identify your priorities

3. Providing competent, compassionate care at work is a priority

4. To determine your priorities outside of work, ask the questions listed on page 83 in the textbook, then assign a number to each

B. Setting smart goals
  1. Setting goals for youself will help you manage time and reduce stress
  2. Do not set more than ten goals
  3. Each goal should be SMART:
    a. Specific
    b. Measurable
    c. Achievable
    d. Realistic
    e. Timely
C. Planning your life and your work
  1. Well-organized people include their personal and professional goals in weekly and daily planning
  2. Reviewing your assignment the day before or before your shift starts helps you gain valuable time with clients
  3. If possible, plan how much time each task may take (see Box 8-5, p. 83)

III. DECISION MAKING
A. Support workers make many decisions every day as they organize their workday and personal life
B. Skills you need to make decisions
  1. Focus—requires concentration, involvement, and commitment (see Figure 8-2, p. 84)
  2. Flexibility—be flexible and responsive, and involve clients in decisions that involve them, when possible
  3. Decisiveness—stick to your decisions, unless they are not working
C. Decision making in different health care settings
  1. In facilities, you need to decide which person's needs to meet first
  2. In the community, you must plan your time so that you are not late for the next client

IV. PROBLEM SOLVING—A PROCESS
A. Identify the problem—you must first determine if you have a problem, and what the problem is
B. Analyze the problem
  1. Once you know you have a problem, you need to decide if it is one you can solve on your own or need to contact your supervisor
  2. You must follow your employer's policies about contacting your supervisor
  3. Analyzing a problem involves communication, both verbal and nonverbal (see

Support Workers Solving Problems box, p. 85)
C. Devise a plan
  1. Think of as many solutions as you can
  2. Decide which is the most practical and helpful
  3. Be creative, but make sure it is safe (see Support Workers Solving Problems box, p. 86)
D. Dealing with conflict
  1. Some problems can be resolved at once, others take longer
  2. Conflict in the workplace can occur when people bring their own values, attitudes, stress, etc. to work
  3. Conflict arises over issues or events and must be worked out otherwise the work environment becomes unpleasant and care is affected
  4. Report all conflicts with your clients to your supervisor, even if the conflict is resolved
  5. Conflicts with co-workers need only be reported if you cannot resolve them
  6. The guidelines listed in Box 8-6, p. 86 in the textbook, can help you deal with conflict

Classroom Activities

1. Write the word "stress" on the board. Ask the students to write on a sheet of paper ten things that have caused them stress in the last two months. Ask the students to share some of their stressors, if comfortable to do so.

2. On the board, write the list of defence mechanisms listed on p. 79 in the textbook and give an example of each. Ask the students if they can give more examples of each defence mechanism.

3. Ask the students to list ways they have heard of or tried to manage stress.

4. Ask the students to list their top five current stressors, and identify how they might reduce the stress from each stressor. Give the students 15 minutes for this exercise. Ask the students to try the se methods for one month and submit a summary of their success.

5. Write goals and then SMART on the board. Ask

the students to describe what each letter in smart stands for and give an example.

6. Give the class examples of workplace conflicts and ask them to problem solve each scenario.

Ask students to answer the questions at the end of Chapter 8 in the textbook. Tell students the date and time that this assignment must be completed and turned in.

If the accompanying workbook is being used, assign the Chapter 8 workbook exercises. Tell students the date and time that this assignment must be completed and turned in.

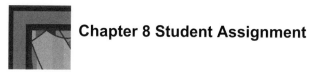

Name _____

Date _____

Managing Stress, Time, and Problems

Write your answers in the spaces provided.

1. When faced with a problem with a client, list five circumstances when you should call your supervisor for help with the problem.

   a. _____

   b. _____

   c. _____

   d. _____

   e. _____

2. What does SMART stand for when setting goals?

   a. _____

   b. _____

   c. _____

   d. _____

   e. _____

3. What questions can you ask yourself to determine if you have a problem?

   a. _____

   b. _____

   c. _____

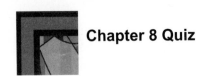

Name _____

Date _____

Managing Stress, Time, and Problems

True or False	Multiple Choice

Mark **T** *for true or* **F** *for false.*

1. _____ People respond to stress with physical and/or emotional responses.

2. _____ Stress is a normal part of life.

3. _____ Physical effects of stress might include N/V/D/.

4. _____ Time obligations must be carried out as part of your regular day to day routine.

5. _____ A child shows different signs of stress than an adult.

6. _____ You do not need to report conflicts with clients to your supervisor if you resolve them.

7. _____ Daily planning can help you meet your goals.

Circle the BEST answer.

8. Emotional and behavioural signs of stress include:
   a. rapid speech
   b. difficulty sleeping
   c. sore muscles
   d. fatigue
   e. any of the abov

9. The defence mechanism referred to as projection means:
   a. refusing to accept an unpleasant reality
   b. assigning one's feelings to someone else
   c. making excuses for one's behaviour
   d. changing emotion into a physical symptom

10. The first step in the problem solving process is to:
   a. call for help
   b. learn to say no
   c. identify the problem
   d. think of as many solutions as you can

11. Which is not involved in the problem solving process:
   a. setting goals
   b. identify the problem
   c. analyze the problem
   d. devise a plan
   e. dealing with conflict

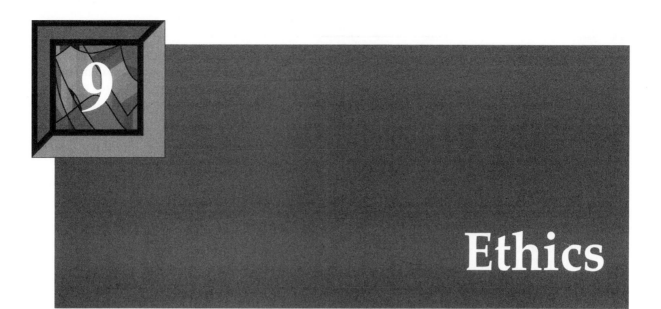

9

Ethics

Instructor's Preparation

I. Read Chapter 9 in the textbook. Carefully review chapter objectives, key terms, and review questions.
II. Read the outline in Chapter 9 of the instructor's guide. Carefully review the classroom activities, the student assignment, and the quiz.
III. If you are using the accompanying student workbook, review the activities for Chapter 9.
IV. Gather all necessary supplies and equipment for classroom activities and student assignments.
  A. Prepare the correct number of handouts
  B. Prepare appropriate flip charts
  C. Prepare overhead transparencies
  D. Prepare situation/index cards
  E. Gather correct video
  F. Gather coloured markers
  G. Gather any other items that will be needed for classroom activities
  H. Assemble items in the order they will be used
V. Make sure that the necessary equipment is available and in good working order.

Objectives

- Define the key terms listed in this chapter
- Explain the purpose of a code of ethics
- Identify the four basic principles of health care ethics
- Describe how each of the four principles applies to support work
- Apply the principles to solve ethical dilemmas

Key Terms

autonomy
beneficence
ethics
health care ethics
justice
nonmaleficence
self-determination

Outline

Ethics

I. INTRODUCTION
  A. Ethics refers to the moral principles or values that guide us when deciding what is right and what is wrong, what is good and what is bad
  B. Your ethics will have a great impact on your personal and professional relationships
  C. You will rely on your ethics to help you make difficult choices and decisions

II. CODE OF ETHICS
- A. Health care teams form professional helping relationships with clients and have developed ethical standards to guide interactions
- B. Regulated professions have codes of ethics provided by their governing college
- C. Support workers do not have a formal code of ethics, but many employers have informal codes of ethics that describe the values and personal qualities to guide your work
- D. See Box 9-1, p. 89 in the textbook, for a sample code of ethics for support workers

III. THE PRINCIPLES OF HEALTH CARE ETHICS
- A. Health care ethics is the philosophical study of what is morally right and wrong when providing health care services
  1. Four basic principles of health care ethics are:
     - a. Autonomy
     - b. Justice
     - c. Beneficence
     - d. Nonmaleficence
- B. Autonomy (also called self-determination)
  1. Means having free choice involving decisions that affect one's life
  2. As long as a person is mentally competent, they have their right to make decisions concerning lifestyle, medical care, and services affecting them; this right is protected by laws (see Chapter 10)
  3. You must always respect your client's choices and preferences even with routine tasks; it is unethical to ignore choices and preferences
  4. It becomes very complicated when your client's decision could cause themselves-risks; always consult your supervisor if you have concerns about a client's safety
  5. Respecting your client's autonomy also means that you do not judge their choices or lifestyle by your own values or standards
  6. Never express your disapproval of their choices or preferences, politics, religion, or lifestyle
- C. Justice
  1. Means that all people should be treated in a fair and equal manner
  2. In Canada it means that all Canadians, regardless of ability to pay, receive access to the same medical services
  3. Some people are easier to work with than others, so you may want to spend less

time with demanding people or people whose lifestyle you don't agree with, but this is unjust and unethical
  4. Treating people justly also means that you do not betray their trust
  5. Clients trust you to handle their possessions with care, respect their privacy, perform your services competently and skillfully, and keep all conversations and health information confidential (see Chapter 10)
- D. Beneficence
  1. Means doing or promoting good; these principles are central to your work
  2. Support work is about promoting wellness, helping people in the daily lives, and supporting them during difficult times
  3. The client's needs come before those of his or her family
  4. If you feel a family member's request goes against the needs of the client, contact your supervisor for guidance
  5. You must always stay within your boundaries of a professional helping relationship (see Chapter 6)
  6. Do not ask clients to do something that is in your interests rather than theirs
  7. You must always remain professional and not become involved in family disagreements, or take advantage of a strained family relationship
  8. To do the most good for your clients:
     - a. Always give your best effort
     - b. Finish your tasks on time
     - c. Be careful, alert, and exact when following instructions
     - d. Be compassionate and empathetic
     - e. Avoid using work time for your own interests (e.g. watching TV, drinking coffee)
- E. Nonmaleficence
  1. Means seeking to do no harm
  2. Harm can be intentional (abuse) or unintentional (accidental injury or negligence)
  3. Perform only those tasks that you have been trained to do, and recognize the limits of your role and knowledge
  4. Family and clients may innocently ask you to perform tasks that are not in your scope of practice, and could cause harm to the client if you are not trained to do the task
  5. Refer all questions about treatment plans,

diagnosis, and all medical information to your supervisor; discussing or giving medical information is outside your scope of practice

6. Keep your skills and knowledge current, support work is constantly changing; the more knowledge and practice you have, the safer your skills will be

7. You can protect your clients by applying the guidelines in Chapter 18 and Chapter 16

IV. DEALING WITH ETHICAL DILEMMAS

A. Codes of ethics provide guidelines for ethical behaviour, but cannot give answers or rules for every situation

B. When making an ethical decision, consider all the possible options to the dilemma, and carefully consider the following:

1. Does the option respect the client's wishes and preferences?

2. Does the option provide the client with a short-term or long-term benefit?

3. Could the option cause harm or increase the client's risk of harm?

4. Does the option treat the client justly and fairly?

C. Answers to these questions often contradict each other; for example, the client's preference may increase the risk of harm

1. You must involve your supervisor in the solution

D. See the Support Workers Solving Problems box, p. 92 in the textbook

E. Remember to consider the four principles of health care ethics when making your decisions

Classroom Activities

1. Collect from various agencies and facilities the codes of ethics they have established for their support workers. Divide the class into groups of four and ask them to compare the codes of ethics and report back to the total class any differences they have identified.

2. Write on the board the words "autonomy", "justice", "beneficence", and "nonmaleficence." Ask the students to define what these terms mean to them. Divide the class into small groups. Ask each group to develop two examples of how they can apply these principles in their work in a long-term care facility and two examples in their work in the community.

3. Write the words "Professional Relationship" on the board. Ask the students to list as many examples as possible how they can make sure they maintain this type of relationship with their clients.

Homework Assignments

Ask students to answer the questions at the end of Chapter 9 in the textbook. Tell students the date and time that this assignment must be completed and turned in.

If the accompanying workbook is being used, assign the Chapter 9 workbook exercises. Tell students the date and time that this assignment must be completed and turned in.

Chapter 9 Student Assignment

Name _____

Date _____

Ethics

Fill in the blanks.

1. The four basic principles of health care ethics are:

    a. _____

    b. _____

    c. _____

    d. _____

2. List five examples of behaviour that might be included in a code of ethics for support workers:

    a. _____

    _____

    b. _____

    _____

    c. _____

    _____

    d. _____

    _____

    e. _____

    _____

3. List four ways you can ensure you are meeting the principle of justice with your client:

    a. _____

    _____

    b. _____

    _____

    c. _____

    _____

    d. _____

    _____

Chapter 9 Quiz

Name _____

Date _____

Ethics

<hr>

| **True or False** | **Multiple Choice** |

*Mark **T** for true or **F** for false.*

1. _____ Ethics means doing or promoting good.

2. _____ Self-determination means the same thing as autonomy.

3. _____ Always take your client's side to show support if there is a family dispute.

Circle the BEST answer.

4. Respecting personal preference is an example of:
   a. Autonomy
   b. Justice
   c. Beneficence
   d. Nonmaleficence

5. Which member of the health team is not responsible to ensure that the client has been informed before any procedure is done?
   a. Support worker
   b. Nurse
   c. Physician
   d. Social worker

6. Handling your client's possessions with care and respect is which principle of ethics?
   a. Autonomy
   b. Justice
   c. Beneficence
   d. Nonmaleficence

7. Keeping your skills and knowledge current supports which principle of ethics?
   a. Autonomy
   b. Justice
   c. Beneficence
   d. Nonmaleficence

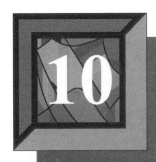

10

Legislation: The Client's Rights and Your Rights

Instructor's Preparation

I. Read Chapter 10 in the textbook. Carefully review chapter objectives, key terms, and review questions.

II. Read the outline in Chapter 10 of the instructor's guide. Carefully review the classroom activities, the student assignment, and the quiz.

III. If you are using the accompanying student workbook, review the activities for Chapter 10.

IV. Gather all necessary supplies and equipment for classroom activities and student assignments.
   A. Prepare the correct number of handouts
   B. Prepare appropriate flip charts
   C. Prepare overhead transparencies
   D. Prepare situation/index cards
   E. Gather correct video
   F. Gather coloured markers
   G. Gather any other items that will be needed for classroom activities
   H. Assemble items in the order they will be used

V. Make sure that the necessary equipment is available and in good working order.

Objectives

- Define the key terms listed in this chapter
- Explain the basic rights protected by the *Canadian Charter of Rights and Freedoms* and the provincial and territorial human rights codes.
- Describe client rights
- Identify ways you can respect your client's rights
- Describe the difference between criminal and civil laws
- Describe how negligence, defamation, assault, battery, false imprisonment, and invasion of privacy apply to your job
- List the types of legislation that address support workers' rights and duties

Key Terms

act
assault
autonomy
battery
civil law
consent
crime
criminal law
defamation
false imprisonment
harassment
informed consent
invasion of privacy

legislation
liable
libel
negligence
regulation
right
self-determination
slander
substitute decision maker
tort

Outline

Legislation:
The Client's Rights and Your Rights

I. INTRODUCTION
  A. Ethics concerns what you should or should not do
  B. Legislation tells you what you can and cannot do and is a body of laws that govern the behaviour of a country's residents
  C. Courts protect the client and the support worker's rights

II. UNDERSTANDING RIGHTS
  A. A right is something to which a person is justly entitled
  B. Moral rights are based on a sense of fairness or ethics and are based on moral principles
  C. Legal rights are based on rules and principles outlined in the law and enforced by society

III. BASIC HUMAN RIGHTS IN CANADA
  A. All provinces and territories have legislation that addresses the rights of people using health care services
    1. They vary across the country and are constantly being revised
    2. Box 10-1, p. 96 in the textbook, shows examples of legislation
  B. Legislation consists of acts (specific laws) and regulations (detailed rules that implement the requirements of the act)
  C. Most health care acts consist of general requirements for maintaining health, safety, and well-being
    1. Box 10-2, p. 97 in the textbook shows an example of regulations in British Columbia
  D. If a province or territory does not have regulations they lay out detailed standards.
  E. All residential facilities must abide by the rules or risk losing their license

IV. BILLS OF RIGHTS
  A. Introduction
    1. Provinces such as Manitoba and Ontario have created a bill of rights for clients
    2. Box 10-3, p. 98 in the textbook, lists Ontario's *Resident's Bill of Rights* for long-term care
    3. Box 10-4, p. 99 in the textbook, lists the *Bill of Rights* for community care clients
    4. Some facilities and agencies write their own bills of rights
    5. You must know your provincial or territorial laws, and your employer's policy regarding client's rights
    6. In general, all clients have the following rights:
      a. The right to be treated with dignity and respect
      b. The right to privacy and confidentiality
      c. The right to give or withhold informed consent
      d. The right to autonomy
  B. The right to be treated with dignity and respect
    1. This is an ethical principle and legal obligation
    2. Most health care legislation refers to the client's right to be treated with dignity
    3. A long-term facility is the resident's home and should provide the same freedoms as the resident's own home
      a. Many have policies, acts, or regulations that recognize the resident's rights:
        (1) To live in a safe and clean environment
        (2) To be properly sheltered, fed, clothed, groomed, and cared for according to their needs
        (3) To keep and display personal possessions
        (4) To have family present 24 hours per day if the person is dying
        (5) To be free from emotional, physical, sexual, and financial abuse
        (6) To discuss problems with, or suggest changes, to any aspect of the services provided to them
    4. Respecting the person's dignity and independence is a basic and important part of support work
    5. Treating a person with dignity provides emotional support and greatly contributes to quality of life
    6. Box 10-5, p. 100 in the textbook, list

ways to show respect for the client's dignity

C. The right to privacy and confidentiality
   1. People have the right to receive care in private, and in a way that does not expose their body unnecessarily
   2. Only those involved in the person's care should see, handle, or examine a person's body
   3. Information about the client's care, treatment, and condition is confidential; all provinces and territories have privacy and confidential legislation
   4. Box 10-6, p. 101 in the textbook, lists measures that show respect for privacy and confidentiality

D. Informed consent recognizes the person's right to decide what will and will not be done to his or her body, and who can touch his or her body
   1. Consent is informed when a person clearly understands:
     a. The reason for treatment
     b. What will be done
     c. How it will be done
     d. Who will do it
     e. The expected outcomes
     f. Other treatment options
     g. The effects of not having the treatment
   2. A parent or legal guardian gives consent for persons under the age of 18
   3. A responsible party gives consent for:
     a. A mentally incompetent person
     b. Persons who are unconscious, sedated, or confused
     c. Persons with certain mental health disorders
   4. A form is signed giving general consent to treatment when the person enters the agency
   5. Special consent forms are required for surgery and other complex and invasive procedures
   6. The doctor is responsible for informing the person about all aspects of treatment
   7. You are never responsible for obtaining written consent

E. The right to autonomy
   1. People using health care have the right to make decisions and choices concerning their care and lifestyle, as well as their admission, discharge, or transfer to or from a facility (see Focus on Long-Term Care box, p. 102)
   2. All clients have the right to participate in assessing and planning their own care and treatment
   3. They need to have complete and accurate information about their condition, care, and treatment; if the client has questions about their condition, inform your supervisor, do not discuss diagnosis or health conditions with clients
   4. Personal choice is important for quality of life, dignity, and self-respect; you must allow the client to make choices whenever safely possible

V. UNDERSTANDING LEGAL ISSUES
A. Laws tell you what you can and cannot do
   1. Law is a rule of conduct made by a government body
   2. Criminal laws are concerned with offenses against the public and against society
     a. Violation is called a crime
   3. Civil laws deal with relationships between people

B. Torts are part of civil law
   1. Unintentional torts
     a. Negligence means the person did not mean or intend to cause harm
       (1) The negligent person failed to act in a reasonable and careful manner
     b. Malpractice is negligence by professionals
     c. Box 10-7, p. 103 in the textbook, lists common negligent acts of support workers
     d. Remember:
       (1) You are legally responsible for your own actions
       (2) Sometimes refusing to follow a nurse's directions is your right and duty
   2. Intentional torts are acts meant to be harmful
     a. Defamation is injuring the name and reputation of a person by making false statements to a third person
     b. Libel is making false statements in print, writing, pictures, or drawings
     c. Slander is making false statements orally
     d. Assault is intentionally attempting or threatening to touch a person's body

without consent
  e. Battery is touching a person's body
     without the person's consent
     (1) The person must consent to any
         procedure, treatment, or other act
         that involves touching the body
     (2) The person has the right to with-
         draw consent at any time
     (3) Consent must be informed to be
         valid
     (4) Consent can be verbal or a ges-
         ture
  f. False imprisonment is unlawful re-
     straint or restriction of a person's
     freedom of movement
     (1) Threat of restraint or actual phys-
         ical restraint is false imprison-
         ment
  g. Invasion of privacy is exposing a
     person's name, photograph, or private
     affairs without the person's permission
  h. Fraud is saying or doing something to
     trick, fool, or deceive another person
     (1) Giving inaccurate or incomplete
         information
VI. YOUR LEGAL RIGHTS
  A. Federal, provincial, and territorial legislation
     ensures that Canadian workers receive fair
     wages and work in a fair and safe environ-
     ment
  B. There are laws that protect workers' rights
     and clarify their requirements and duties
  C. These laws have different names across the
     country
  D. These laws address:
     1. Human rights legislation—protects
        worker's basic human rights of equality
        and nondiscrimination, and freedom from
        harassment
     2. Occupational health and safety legisla-
        tion—outlines the rights and responsibili-
        ties of workers, employers, and supervi-
        sors in creating and maintaining a safe
        work environment
     3. Employment standards and legislation—
        state minimum acceptable employment
        standards within the workplace
     4. Labour relations legislation—addresses
        how employers and employees can re-
        solve workplace issues, and ensures that
        employees have the right to form or join
        a union
     5. Workers' compensation legislation—ad-
        dresses how workers are financially com-

pensated for accidental injuries on the job
     6. Long-term care facilities legislation—ad-
        dresses basic rights of residents and de-
        scribes requirements for operating the fa-
        cility
     7. Community services legislation—sets out
        the rules and procedures for accessing
        and providing community services

Classroom Activities

1. Distribute copies of your provincial or territorial
   human rights code. Ask the class to identify the
   areas this code protects for support workers and
   clients.

2. Distribute copies of the *Canadian Charter of
   Rights and Freedoms.* Divide the class into small
   groups and ask them to summarize the basic rights
   and freedoms protected by this act (allow 15 minutes). Have the groups report their list to the class.

3. Write on the board "The Right to be Treated with
   Dignity and Respect." Ask the class to list ways
   they can provide this right to residents in long-
   term care settings, and then prepare a second list
   for clients in the community.

4. Divide the class into small groups and ask each
   group to list five ways of providing autonomy for
   residents in long-term facilities and five ways of
   providing autonomy for clients in the community.
   Allow 20 minutes for this activity and then ask
   each group to report their lists to the class. Write
   all answers on the board.

5. Write "Assault and Battery" on the board and ask
   the class to define and give examples of each.

6. Discuss with the class the causes of negligence
   and its possible effects on their clients, themselves, and their agencies.

Homework Assignments

Ask students to answer the questions at the end of
Chapter 10 in the textbook. Tell students the date and
time that this assignment must be completed and
turned in.

If the accompanying workbook is being used, assign
the Chapter 10 workbook exercises. Tell students the
date and time that this assignment must be completed
and turned in.

Chapter 10 Student Assignment

Name _____

Date _____

Legislation: The Client's Rights and Your Rights

Write your answers in the spaces provided.

1. Generally each long-term care facility has a Resident's Bill of Rights. List four general rights.

   a. _____

   b. _____

   c. _____

   d. _____

2. What are two Bills of Rights for Persons in the Community?

   a. _____

   b. _____

3. List the ways you can protect the person's right to privacy.

   a. _____

   b. _____

   c. _____

   d. _____

Match each term with the correct definition.

a. negligence
b. malpractice
c. fraud
d. invasion of privacy
e. assault
f. battery
g. slander
h. false imprisonment

4. _____ a threat or unsuccessful attempt to commit bodily harm to another person

5. _____ an unintentional wrong causing harm to patient or damage to their property

6. _____ restraining someone without proper consent

7. _____ negligence on the part of a professional

8. _____ to trick, fool, or deceive another and cause harm

9. _____ talking about a patient by name in a public area

10. _____ unauthorized touching of a person's body without consent

11. _____ speaking falsely of someone else

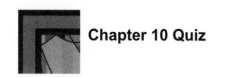

Name _____

Date _____

Legislation: The Client's Rights and Your Rights

| **True or False** | **Multiple Choice** |

Mark **T** *for true or* **F** *for false.*

1. _____ Employment standards and legislation protects you from harassment.

2. _____ Self-determination and autonomy mean the same thing.

3. _____ Tort is another name for a specific law.

4. _____ Rights are based on moral principles.

5. _____ Civil laws deal with relationships between people.

6. _____ Slander means making false statements in print.

7. _____ If your client gives you permission to do a procedure you are not trained to do, you will be protected from legal action since you have their consent.

Circle the BEST answer.

8. A signed consent is not needed:
   a. before surgery.
   b. on admission to a facility.
   c. when medical treatment is done.
   d. when a support worker gives a routine bath.

9. Battery is:
   a. Intentionally attempting to touch a person's body
   b. Intentionally threatening to touch a person's body
   c. Touching the person's body without consent
   d. Unlawful restraint

10. If you are injured at work, which legislation will determine how you will be financially compensated?
    a. Occupational health and safety
    b. Human rights legislation
    c. Workers' compensation legislation
    d. Labour relations legislation

11. If you do not wipe up a spill and a client falls, you are guilty of:
    a. Assault
    a. Battery
    a. Slander
    d. Negligence

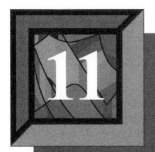

Caring about Culture

Instructor's Preparation

I. Read Chapter 11 in the textbook. Carefully review chapter objectives, key terms, and review questions.

II. Read the outline in Chapter 11 of the instructor's guide. Carefully review the classroom activities, the student assignment, and the quiz.

III. If you are using the accompanying student workbook, review the activities for Chapter 11.

IV. Gather all necessary supplies and equipment for classroom activities and student assignments.

    A. Prepare the correct number of handouts

    B. Prepare appropriate flip charts

    C. Prepare overhead transparencies

    D. Prepare situation/index cards

    E. Gather correct video

    F. Gather coloured markers

    G. Gather any other items that will be needed for classroom activities

    H. Assemble items in the order they will be used

V. Make sure that the necessary equipment is available and in good working order.

Objectives

- Define the key terms listed in this chapter
- Understand the differences between race, ethnicity, and culture
- Recognize the factors that influence a person's culture
- Appreciate that culture influences a person's attitudes and behaviours in many areas
- Describe how culture may affect communication, family organization, religious convictions, and perceptions about illness and health care
- Reflect on how your own cultural biases may affect your relationships with your clients
- Discuss how you can provide culturally sensitive care

Key Terms

culture
discrimination
ethnicity
personal space
prejudice
race
stereotype

Caring about Culture

I. RACE, ETHNICITY AND CULTURE
- A. Race refers to groups of people who share similar features such as skin colour, facial characteristics, and bone structure
- B. Ethnicity refers to groups of people who share a common history, language, geography, national origin, religion, and identity
  - 1. Canada has many racial and ethnic groups (see Table 11-1, p. 108)
- C. Culture refers to the characteristics of a group of people—the language, values, beliefs, habits, ways of life, rules of behaviour, and traditions that are passed from one generation to the next
- D. Everyone has a culture; some people can belong to many cultures at the same time
  - 1. Figure 11-1, p. 107 in the textbook, shows factors that shape a person's culture

II. EFFECT OF CULTURE
- A. Culture will affect how a person deals with daily situations and problems
  - 1. Canada has so many different cultures you cannot feasibly understand all of them, but you need to know that culture can affect the person's beliefs and behaviours in:
    - a. Communication
    - b. Family and social organization
    - c. Religion and worship
    - d. Health care practices and reactions to illness
- B. Culture and communication
  - 1. Your community may have many clients who speak different languages or dialects
  - 2. You may be working with an interpreter or may have to rely on nonverbal cues (see Respecting Diversity box, p. 109)
  - 3. Touch—can be an important part of nonverbal communication
    - a. Can convey comfort, caring, love, affection, concern, reassurance, etc.
    - b. Often, people are comforted by touch
    - c. Many cultures have rules or expectations about who can touch, when to touch, and where on the body they can be touched (see Figure 11-2, p. 109)
    - d. Some cultures embrace touch while

others are embarrassed, offended, or uncomfortable
    - e. Support workers should try to obtain information about their client's culture in order to provide the appropriate greetings and touch
  - 4. Personal space
    - a. The area immediately around one's body
    - b. The exact distance requirements will vary depending upon the individual, the situation, and the culture
    - c. Be aware of your client's reactions to you; if they step back, or move their body away from you, you may be invading their personal space
  - 5. Eye Contact—has different meanings within different cultures
    - a. In Western culture, it is a sign of good self-concept, attention, and honesty; lack of eye contact can communicate dishonesty, shyness, embarrassment, or guilt
    - b. In Asian and Aboriginal cultures, eye contact is considered disrespectful and an invasion of privacy
  - 6. Facial Expressions
    - a. Many facial expressions are universal, but you must understand the cultural background of your client
    - b. In some cultures they may smile to hide negative emotions
    - c. Other cultures use many facial expressions and gestures to communicate
  - 7. Silence
    - a. The use of silence varies greatly by cultural groups
    - b. It is very important that support workers are aware of the cultural background of their clients
    - c. Silence can mean agreement, privacy, or time for the listener to understand in different cultures
    - d. You must be aware of what your silence or your client's silence may indicate
- C. Culture and the family
  - 1. Culture affects family structure and roles and responsibilities of various members during times of illness
  - 2. In Western culture, the nuclear family usually consists of parents and children

(see Figure 11-3, p. 110)

3. Children are encouraged to be self-sufficient, and most young adults leave the family home
4. Care of relatives outside the nuclear family is usually entrusted to others
5. In Asian, Aboriginal, and South Asian cultures, extended families are common (see Figure 11-4, p. 110)
6. Families usually care for elders and sick family members
7. Sometimes first-generation children rebel against the culture of their parents, which can cause great stress for the parents (see Box 11-1, p. 111)

D. Culture and religion
1. Religion relates to spiritual beliefs, needs, and practices
2. May promote beliefs and practices related to daily living habits, behaviour, relationships with others, diet, healing, days of worship, birth and birth control, medicine and death
3. Many people rely on religion for support and comfort during illness; a visit from their spiritual leader or adviser may be helpful
4. Be sure to let your supervisor know if your client requests a visit and provide privacy during the visit
5. Always respect the client's beliefs, practices, and religious symbols
6. Never try to convert your clients to your own belief system

E. Culture and perceptions of health care and illness
1. In Western culture, the general belief is that disease is caused by biological or environmental factors, that illness and disease can often be prevented, and that people can be cared for or cured using scientifically proven methods
2. Some cultures believe that supernatural forces cause illness
3. People may use charms, rituals, alternative medicines, or traditional or folk medicine, which may include ancient remedies passed down many generations
4. Some folk remedies either help the person or have no effect on the person's health
5. If the practice does not harm the client,

the nurse or case manager may include it in the care plan
6. Some practices may interfere with the client's medical treatment, for example, some herbal medicines may interact with prescription drugs
7. The health care team must be aware of all health care practices to ensure they are not harmful to the client (see Support Workers Solving Problems box, p. 112)
8. Tell your supervisor if:
   a. Your client tells you that he or she is using alternative or folk remedies
   b. You observe a client using alternative or folk remedies

III. PROVIDING CULTURALLY SENSITIVE CARE
A. People respond to their cultural influences in their own unique way
B. Never use stereotypes to judge your client
C. Stereotypes are overly simple or exaggerated impression of a person or group based on a person's ethnicity, religion, or other factor
D. Stereotypes are often associated with prejudice—an attitude that judges a person based on his or her membership in a group
E. Making assumptions is always wrong, and often hurtful
F. Prejudice frequently leads to discrimination—a behaviour that treats people unfairly based on their group membership
G. Your attitudes and behaviours are shaped by your culture
H. Some people react negatively or fearfully to cultural differences
I. You don't have to agree with the client's beliefs and practices, but you must be tolerant and not make judgements about them
J. In order to accept people of different cultures, it is important to learn from them; respect and show interest in their traditions, foods, dress, and customs

Classroom Activities

1. Write the words "Race", "Ethinicity", and "Culture" on the board. Ask the class to define each word and list as many examples as possible for each term.

2. Draw a circle on the board and write the word "Culture" inside the circle. Ask the class to name

as many factors as possible that can influence culture. List the factors outside the circle (see Figure 11-1, p. 107).

3. Divide the class into small groups of 3 or 4. Ask the students to list as many religions as they can, and describe all traditions, beliefs, practices that they know about for each religion. Have a member from each group report back to the class.

4. Ask each student in the class to list their ethnic background (British, Latin, Asian, etc.) and write the list on the board.

5. From the University of Toronto Web site (http://cwr.utoronto.ca/cultural/english), download cultural profiles, which are available for many countries. These profiles include information on communicating, family life, eating, world of work, health care, learning, spirituality, and religion. Download one profile for each student. Ask the students to read each profile (allow 20 minutes) and summarize for the class the information, which may be helpful in caring for a person from that culture.

Homework Assignments

Ask students to answer the questions at the end of Chapter 11 in the textbook. Tell students the date and time that this assignment must be completed and turned in.

If the accompanying workbook is being used, assign the Chapter 11 workbook exercises. Tell students the date and time that this assignment must be completed and turned in.

Chapter 11 Student Assignment   Name _____

                                     Date _____

Caring about Culture

Write your answers in the spaces provided.

1. List and describe 2 different types of families.

   a. _____

      _____

      _____

   b. _____

      _____

      _____

2. The most important thing to remember with culturally diverse clients is:

   _____

   _____

   _____

3. List 3 significant characteristics of different cultures.

   a. _____

   b. _____

   c. _____

Complete the sentences.

4. Race refers to:

   _____

5. Culture refers to:

   _____

6. Personal space is:

   _____

7. A stereotype is:

   _____

8. Prejudice is:

   _____

9. An extended family may include:

   _____

10. Discrimination is:

   _____

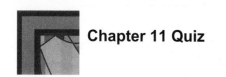

Chapter 11 Quiz

Name _____

Date _____

Caring about Culture

True or False

*Mark **T** for true or **F** for false.*

1. _____ All cultures are comfortable with physical touch.

2. _____ Some children rebel against the culture of the parents.

3. _____ You should never try to convert your clients to your own beliefs.

4. _____ All folk remedies are harmless.

5. _____ Casual touching from strangers is uncomfortable in Chinese culture.

6. _____ Eye contact is considered disrespectful in Aboriginal culture.

7. _____ Culture refers to the characteristics of a group of people.

Multiple Choice

Circle the BEST answer.

8. Which of the following statements about culture and religion is false?
   a. A person's cultural background probably influences health and illness practices.
   b. Dietary practices may be influenced by culture and religion.
   c. A person's cultural and religious practices are not allowed in the health care facility.
   d. A person may follow all of the beliefs and practices of his/her religion or culture.

9. Culture
   a. Includes language, beliefs, traditions, and dress
   b. Is influences by family and media technology
   c. Is totally learned
   d. a, b, and c
   e. None of the above

10. Ethnicity is
    a. Based on race, religion, national origin
    b. Influenced by identification with ancestral homeland
    c. a and b above

11. To identify someone by "race" includes what physical characteristics:
    a. Skin colour
    b. Eye colour
    c. Facial features
    d. a and b only
    e. a, b, and c

12. Which is false?
    a. Prejudice is an attitude that judges people based on their group membership.
    b. In some situations, prejudice is acceptable.
    c. Prejudice frequently leads to discrimination.
    d. Stereotypes are often associated with prejudice.

72

Interpersonal Communication

Instructor's Preparation

   I. Read Chapter 12 in the textbook. Carefully review chapter objectives, key terms, and review questions.

   II. Read the outline in Chapter 12 of the instructor's guide. Carefully review the classroom activities, the student assignment, and the quiz.

   III. If you are using the accompanying student workbook, review the activities for Chapter 12.

   IV. Gather all necessary supplies and equipment for classroom activities and student assignments.
     A. Prepare the correct number of handouts
     B. Prepare appropriate flip charts
     C. Prepare overhead transparencies
     D. Prepare situation/index cards
     E. Gather correct video
     F. Gather coloured markers
     G. Gather any other items that will be needed for classroom activities
     H. Assemble items in the order they will be used

   V. Make sure that the necessary equipment is available and in good working order.

Objectives

- Define the key terms listed in this chapter
- Describe the communication process
- Describe verbal and nonverbal communication
- Explain the methods of and barriers to effective communication
- Explain how to communicate with an angry client
- Explain why assertive communication is important
- Demonstrate how to explain procedures and tasks to clients

Key Terms

active listening
assertiveness
body language
closed questions
empathetic listening
focusing
interpersonal communication
nonverbal communication
open-ended questions
paraphrasing
verbal communication

Outline

Interpersonal Communication

  I. INTRODUCTION
    A. Good interpersonal communication is needed to provide safe and effective care

B. Health care teams need to share information about what was done for the client, what needs to be done, and response to care and treatments

C. Through communication you get to know your client and you express your thoughts and ideas

II. THE COMMUNICATION PROCESS

A. Interpersonal communication is the exchange of information between two people

B. It involves the sender, message, receiver and, response to the message (feedback); during the exchange, each person acts as both sender and receiver

C. If the receiver does not understand the message or misinterprets the message, mistakes or misunderstanding can occur

D. There are factors that can influence good communication:
   1. Perceptions
   2. Experiences
   3. Physical and mental health
   4. Emotions
   5. Values
   6. Beliefs
   7. Culture

E. The relationship between the sender and receiver also affects communication

F. Easier if people involved respect each other (see Figure 12-1, p. 116)

G. To effectively communicate with your clients:
   1. Understand and respect them
   2. Be sensitive to their situation and needs
   3. Accept their culture and religion
   4. Appreciate their stress, problems, and frustrations
   5. Understand their meaning rather than just their words

III. VERBAL COMMUNICATION

A. Messages are sent through the spoken word

B. Sometimes symbols substitute for the spoken word such a sign language

C. To effectively communicate with words you need to:
   1. Choose you words carefully
   2. Use simple, everyday language
   3. Speak clearly, slowly, and distinctly
   4. Control the volume and tone of your voice
   5. Be brief and concise
   6. Present information in a logical manner
   7. Ask one question at a time
   8. Determine understanding

   9. Do not pretend to understand

IV. NONVERBAL COMMUNICATION (DOES NOT INVOLVE WORDS)

A. Gestures, facial expressions, posture, body movements, touch, and smell are examples
   1. Nonverbal messages more accurately reflect the person's feelings

B. Body language
   1. Body language includes posture, gait, facial expressions, eye contact, hand movements, gestures, body movements, and appearance
   2. People send messages with their body language
      a. Posture, protecting a body part
   3. You also send messages by the way you act and move
      a. Your body language should show interest and enthusiasm
      b. Your body language should show caring and respect

C. Touch
   1. Conveys comfort, caring, love, affection, interest, trust, concern, and reassurance
   2. The meaning of touch depends on a person's age, gender, life experience, and culture
      a. See the article Caring About Culture, p. 109 in the textbook
      b. All cultural groups have rules or practices about touch
   3. Some people do not like being touched
   4. Touch should be gentle, not hurried or rough
   5. Touch should not be sexual in nature

D. Silence
   1. The use of silence also conveys messages
   2. Can convey acceptance, rejection, fear, or a need to think
   3. During sad times you may not need to say anything
   4. Useful when making difficult decisions and when a person is upset
   5. Silence can show respect and empathy (see Box 12-1, p. 117)

V. COMMUNICATION METHODS

A. Listening means being attentive to the person's verbal and nonverbal communication
   1. Use the senses of sight, hearing, touch, and smell
   2. Concentrate on what the person is saying and observe nonverbal clues
   3. Nonverbal communication supports what

the person says or shows other feelings
4. Listening requires that you care and have interest
5. Guidelines for listening include:
   a. Face the person
   b. Have good eye contact
   c. See Caring About Culture, p. 109 in the textbook, for eye contact practices of other cultures
   d. Lean toward the person
   e. Respond to the person
   f. Avoid communication barriers (see pp. 120-121 in the textbook)
B. Paraphrasing is restating the person's message in your own words
   1. Paraphrasing serves three purposes:
      a. It shows you are listening
      b. It lets the person see if you understand the message sent
      c. It promotes further communication
C. Empathetic listening means being attentive to a person's feelings.
   1. Empathy means being open to and trying to understand the experiences and feelings of others
   2. Can help reduce feelings of loneliness
   3. Can create trust between you and the client
D. Asking closed questions
   1. Focus on specific information
   2. Some closed questions have "yes" or "no" answers
   3. Others require brief responses
E. Open-ended questions lead or invite the person to share thoughts, feelings, or ideas
   1. The person chooses what to talk about
   2. Responses are longer and give more information than direct questions
F. Clarifying lets you make sure that you understand the message
   1. Ask the person to repeat the message
G. Focusing is dealing with a certain topic
   1. Useful when a person rambles or wanders in thought

VI. COMMUNICATION BARRIERS
A. Some barriers such as vision and hearing problems cannot be avoided; you must learn to work around these (see Figure 12-3, p. 120, and Chapters 35 and 36)
B. Cultural differences can also interfere
C. Clients may attach different meanings to verbal and nonverbal communications (see Chapter 11)

D. Factors in the environment can also affect communication, such as loud noises
E. Improve communication by avoiding:
   1. Interrupting
   2. Answering your own questions
   3. Giving advice
   4. Minimizing problems
   5. Using patronizing language (see Box 12-2, p. 121)
   6. Failing to listen

VII. COMMUNICATION WITH ANGRY PEOPLE
A. Anger is a common emotion seen in clients, residents, and families
B. Causes of anger include fear, pain, and death and dying
C. Loss of function and losing control of one's health and life can also cause anger
D. Anger is a symptom of some diseases
E. Persons who abuse alcohol and drugs are likely to show anger
F. Some people are generally angry
G. Anger is communicated verbally and nonverbally and violence can occur
H. Good communication is important to prevent and deal with anger
I. Follow the guidelines for dealing with angry person listed in Box 12-3, p. 122 in the textbook

VIII. COMMUNICATING ASSERTIVELY
A. A style of communication in which thoughts and feelings are expressed positively and directly without offence to others
B. You stand up for your rights while respecting the rights of others
C. Being assertive is different from being aggressive
D. When assertive you are confident, calm, and composed; when aggressive you are upset, cold, or angry
E. Be confident and assertive when communicating with all members of the health team including physicians
F. Box 12-4, p. 123 in the textbook, describes three responses to a situation

IX. EXPLAINING PROCEDURES AND TASKS
A. Clients feel safer and more secure if they understand what is going to happen before you start a procedure, since some procedures may be unfamiliar or frightening to them
B. They should be told why the procedure is needed, who will do it, how it will be done, and what sensations they might feel
C. You may help clients practice tasks they have

been shown by health care professionals, or you may be expected to teach clients simple tasks

D. You must give clear, precise explanations and instructions that your client can understand

E. Use the following four-step teaching method:
1. Tell the client the steps in the task
2. Show the client how to do each step
3. Have the client try each step
4. Review the client's success with each step

F. Follow the guidelines listed in Box 12-5, p. 124 in the textbook

G. Break tasks into steps and teach one step at a time

H. Remember, people learn at different rates and in different ways

Classroom Activities

1. Write on the board "A large city" and "A small city." Instruct the students to write down on a piece of paper what they would consider the population for a large city and a small city. Ask the students to share their answers. Discuss how their definition and how a client's definition can vary depending on their background, previous travel experience, etc. This exercise will show the students the importance of choosing words carefully.

2. On separate index cards write: angry, happy, in pain, smelling a bad odour, sad, frustrated, unable to understand what if being said. Place the cards in a basket. Ask each student to draw a card and through body language demonstrate the emotion on the card. Students should put the card back in the basket for other students to draw. Allow 20 minutes.

3. Ask students to discuss how verbal and nonverbal communication is used in their daily lives.

4. Discuss how verbal and nonverbal communications are being used in the classroom.

5. Ask the students to give examples of open-ended and closed questions. Discuss the advantages and disadvantages of each type of question.

Homework Assignments

Ask students to answer the questions at the end of Chapter 12 in the textbook. Tell students the date and time that this assignment must be completed and turned in.

If the accompanying workbook is being used, assign the Chapter 12 workbook exercises. Tell students the date and time that this assignment must be completed and turned in.

Chapter 12 Student Assignment   Name _____

Date _____

Interpersonal Communication

Write your answers in the spaces provided.

1. Identify which communication technique is being used in the following examples:

   a. " Mr. Lopez do you want to get up now?"

   _____

   b. "Tell me about your pain?"

   _____

   c. Using your senses: concentrate on what the person is saying, using good eye contact.

   _____

   d. Not saying anything—just being with the person to show you care.

   _____

2. Match the word to the meaning.
   ___ Paraphrasing
   ___ Direct Questions
   ___ Open Ended Questions
   ___ Clarifying
   ___ Focusing

   a. Focus on specific information
   b. Useful when a person rambles or wanders in conversation
   c. Restating message in your own words
   d. Allow a person to share thoughts and feelings
   e. Allows you to make sure you understand

3. The function of communication is:

   _____

4. The purpose of communication is:

   _____

5. List the qualities of voice that affect communication:
   a. _____

   b. _____

   c. _____

   d. _____

6. The communication process consists of:

   a. _____

   b. _____

   c. _____

   d. _____

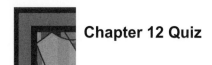
Name _____

Date _____

Interpersonal Communication

True or False	Multiple Choice

*Mark **T** for true or **F** for false.*

1. _____ Verbal messages more accurately reflect a person's feelings than non-verbal messages.

2. _____ Everyone likes to be touched.

3. _____ Open-ended questions lead the person to share thoughts, feelings, or ideas.

4. _____ Giving your opinion promotes effective communication.

5. _____ Listen and use silence when dealing with an angry person.

6. _____ Assertive communication involves expressing your feelings and thoughts comfortably and confidently.

7. _____ Aggressive communication involves being confrontational to get what you want.

*Circle the **BEST** answer.*

8. Restating the person's message in your own words is called:
   a. Paraphrasing
   b. Non-verbal communication
   c. Focusing
   d. A direct question

9. Which of the following does not promote effective communication?
   a. Speak clearly, slowly, and distinctly
   b. Control the loudness and tone of your voice
   c. Ask several questions at once
   d. Repeat information as needed

10. Communication that uses the spoken word is:
    a. Non-verbal communication
    b. Focusing
    c. Body language
    d. Verbal communication

11. Which does not promote effective listening?
    a. Facing the person
    b. Sitting back in the chair with your arms crossed
    c. Good eye contact
    d. Asking questions

12. Direct questions are used to:
    a. Show the person that you care
    b. Make sure you understand what was said
    c. Focus on specific information
    d. Allow the person time to think

78

13

Body Structure and Function

Instructor's Preparation

I. Read Chapter 13 in the textbook. Carefully review chapter objectives, key terms, and review questions.

II. Read the outline in Chapter 13 of the instructor's guide. Carefully review the classroom activities, the student assignment, and the quiz.

III. If you are using the accompanying student workbook, review the activities for Chapter 13.

IV. Gather all necessary supplies and equipment for classroom activities and student assignments.

    A. Prepare the correct number of handouts

    B. Prepare appropriate flip charts

    C. Prepare overhead transparencies

    D. Prepare situation/index cards

    E. Gather the following transparencies: TA1 through TA25

    F. Gather coloured markers

    G. Gather anatomical models

    H. Gather any other items that will be needed for classroom activities

    I. Assemble items in the order they will be used

V. Make sure that the necessary equipment is available and in good working order.

Objectives

- Define the key terms listed in this chapter
- Identify the basic structures of the cell, and explain how cells divide
- Describe four types of tissue
- Identify the structures of each body system
- Describe the functions of each body system

Key Terms

artery
capillary
cell
digestion
hemoglobin
hormone
immunity
menstruation
metabolism
organ
peristalsis
respiration
system
tissue
vein

Outline

Body Structure and Function

I. INTRODUCTION
   A. You help clients meet their basic needs
   B. A basic knowledge of the body's normal structure and functions will help you provide safer, more efficient care

II. CELLS, TISSUES, AND ORGANS
   A. A cell is the basic unit of body structure
      1. Cells need food, water, and oxygen to live and perform their functions.
      2. Basic structure (see Figure 13-1, p. 128)
         a. The cell membrane is the outer covering that encloses the cell and helps it hold its shape
         b. The nucleus is the control center of the cell; it directs the cell's activities
         c. Cytoplasm surrounds the nucleus
         d. Protoplasm refers to all the structures, substances, and water within the cell
         e. Chromosomes are threadlike structures within the nucleus that contain genes
         f. Genes are contained within chromosomes; they control the physical and chemical traits inherited by children from their parents
         g. Cells reproduce by dividing in half—a process called mitosis (see Figure 13-2, p. 128)
      3. Cells are the body's building blocks
   B. Tissue is groups of cells with similar functions
      1. The body has four basic types of tissue:
         a. Epithelial tissue—covers internal and external body surfaces
         b. Connective tissue—anchors, connects, and supports other body tissues
         c. Muscle tissue—allows the body to move by stretching and contracting
         d. Nerve tissue—receives and carries impulses to the brain and back to the body parts
   C. Organs are formed by groups of tissues
      1. An organ performs one or more functions
      2. Examples are the heart, brain, liver, lungs, and kidneys
   D. Systems are formed by organs that work together to perform special functions (see Figure 13-3, p. 130)

III. THE INTEGUMENTARY SYSTEM
   A. The skin and its appendages—hair, nails, and sweat and oil glands
   B. largest system in the body
   C. The body's natural covering (integument means covering)
   D. Two layers (see Figure 13-4, p. 129)
      1. Epidermis is the outer layer; it contains living cells and dead cells
         a. Living cells contain pigment that gives the skin its color
      2. Dermis is the inner layer of skin made up of connective tissue
         a. Blood vessels, nerves, sweat and oil glands, and hair roots are found in the dermis
   E. The skin has many important functions:
      1. Provides a protective covering for the body
      2. Prevents bacteria and other substances from entering the body
      3. Prevents excess loss of water from the body
      4. Protects the body from injury because cold, pain, touch, and pressure are sensed
      5. Appendages
         a. Entire body except palms of the hands and soles of the feet are covered in hair
         b. Hair in the nose and ears and eyelashes protects these organs from dust, insects and foreign bodies
         c. Nails protect the tips of fingers and toes
         d. Sweat glands help the body regulate temperature
         e. Sweat consists of water, salt and small amount of wastes, secreted through pores in skin; the body is cooled as sweat evaporates
         f. Oil glands lie near hair shafts. Secrete oil into space near shaft and the oil travels to surface to keep hair and skin soft and shiny.

IV. THE MUSCULOSKELETAL SYSTEM
   A. Provides the framework for the body and allows the body to move
   B. Protects and gives the body shape
      1. Besides bones and muscels, the system has ligaments, tendons, and cartilage
   C. Bones
      1. The body has 206 bones (see Figure 13-5, p. 130)
      2. Four types of bones:
         a. Long bones bear the weight of the

body
  b. Short bones allow skill and ease in movement
  c. Flat bones protect the organs
  d. Irregular bones are the vertebrae in the spinal column
  3. Bones are hard, rigid structures covered by a membrane called periosteum
  4. Blood cells are manufactured in bone marrow
D. Joints
  1. A joint is the point at which two or more bones meet
  2. Allow movement (see Chapter 22)
  3. Cartilage cushions the joints
  4. Synovial membrane lines the joints
  5. Three types of joints:
    a. Ball and socket joint allows movement in all directions
    b. Hinge joint allows movement in one direction
    c. Pivot joint allows turning from side to side
E. Muscles
  1. The body has more than 500 muscles (see Figure 13-7 and Figure 13-8, pp. 132-33)
  2. Voluntary muscles can be consciously controlled
    a. Skeletal muscles are voluntary; they are striated
  3. Involuntary muscles work automatically and cannot be consciously controlled
    a. Also called smooth muscles
    b. Cardiac muscle appears striated
  4. Perform three important body functions:
    a. Movement of body parts
    b. Maintenance of posture
    c. Production of body heat
  5. Tendons connect muscles to bones
V. THE NERVOUS SYSTEM
A. Controls, directs, and coordinates body functions. There are two main divisions: the central nervous system and the peripheral nervous system
  1. Some nerve fibers have a protective covering call a myelin sheath
B. The central nervous system
  1. Consists of the brain and the spinal cord (see Figure 13-9, p. 134)
    a. The brain is covered by the skull and has three main parts (see Figure 13-11, p. 135)
      (1) The cerebrum

      (a) The largest part
      (b) The center of thought and intelligence
      (c) Right hemisphere controls the left side of the body
      (d) Left hemisphere controls the right side of the body
      (e) Cerebral cortex is the outside of the cerebrum; it controls the highest functions of the brain
      (2) The cerebellum regulates and coordinates body movements
      (3) The brain stem connects the cerebrum to the spinal cord
        (a) Made up of the midbrain, pons, and medulla
    b. The spinal cord
      (1) Lies within the spinal column
      (2) Contains pathways that conduct messages to and from the brain
    c. The brain and spinal cord are covered by three layers of connective tissue called meninges
      (1) Dura mater is the outer layer; next to the skull
      (2) Arachnoid is the middle layer
      (3) Pia mater is the inner layer
    d. Arachnoid space is the space between the middle and the inner layers; it is filled with cerebrospinal fluid
      (1) Cerebrospinal fluid protects the central nervous system
C. The peripheral nervous system (see Figure 13-10, p. 135)
  1. Has 12 pairs of cranial nerves and 31 pairs of spinal nerves
  2. Autonomic nervous system controls involuntary muscles and certain body functions that occur automatically; it is divided into the sympathetic and parasympathetic nervous systems
    a. Sympathetic nervous system tends to speed up functions
    b. Parasympathetic nervous system slows down functions
D. The sense organs (senses are sight, hearing, taste, smell, and touch)
  1. Receptors for taste on the tongue are called taste buds
  2. Receptors for smell are in the nose
  3. Touch receptors are found in the dermis
  4. The eye (see Figure 13-12, p. 136)

a. Has three layers:
- (1) The sclera is the white of the eye; the outer layer
- (2) The choroid is the second layer; contains blood vessels, the ciliary muscle, and the iris
  - (a) Iris gives the eye color
  - (b) Pupil is the opening in the middle of the iris
- (3) The retina is the inner layer; contains receptors for vision and nerve fibers of the optic nerve

b. Light enters the eye through the cornea and passes to the lens behind the pupil; light is then reflected to the retina and carried to the brain by the optic nerve

c. The aqueous chamber separates the cornea from the lens
- (1) Filled with a fluid called aqueous humor

d. The vitreous body is behind the lens; supports the retina and maintains the eye's shape

5. The ear (see Figure 13-13, p. 137)
a. Functions in hearing and balance
- (1) The external ear is the outer part; called the pinna or auricle
  - (a) Sound waves are guided through the external ear to the auditory canal
  - (b) The auditory canal extends about 1 inch to the eardrum
  - (c) The eardrum (tympanic membrane) separates the external ear from the middle ear
- (2) The middle ear
  - (a) Contains the eustachian tube and three small bones called ossicles
  - (b) The eustachian tube connects the middle ear and the throat
  - (c) The ossicles amplify sound and transmit sound to the inner ear
    - (i) The malleus looks like a hammer
    - (ii) The incus resembles an anvil
    - (iii) The stapes is shaped like a stirrup

- (3) The inner ear
  - (a) Consists of semi-circular canals and the cochlea
  - (b) The cochlea contains fluid; the fluid carries sound waves to the auditory nerve; the auditory nerve carries the message to the brain
  - (c) The three semi-circular canals are involved with balance

VI. THE CIRCULATORY SYSTEM
A. Made up of the blood, the heart, and the blood vessels
B. The blood consists of blood cells and a liquid called plasma
1. Plasma
- a. Carries blood cells to other body cells
- b. Carries substances needed by cells for proper functioning

2. Red blood cells are called erythrocytes
- a. Give the blood its red color
- b. Pick up hemoglobin in the lungs
- c. Hemoglobin carries oxygen to the cells
- d. Hemoglobin picks up carbon dioxide (as waste) from the cells
- e. Red blood cells are destroyed by the liver and spleen as they wear out
- f. Bone marrow produces new red blood cells

3. White blood cells are called leukocytes
- a. Protect the body against infection
- b. The number of white blood cells increases when there is an infection in the body
- c. White blood cells are produced by the bone marrow

4. Platelets are called thrombocytes
- a. Necessary for the clotting of blood
- b. Produced by the bone marrow
- c. Live about 4 days

C. The heart (see Figure 13-15, p. 138)
1. A muscle that pumps blood through the blood vessels to tissues and cells
2. Lies in the middle-to-lower part of the left chest cavity (see Figure 13-14, p. 138)
3. Is hollow and has three layers
- a. Pericardium is the outer layer; a thin sac covering the heart
- b. Myocardium is the second layer; the

thick, muscular portion of the heart
  c. Endocardium is the inner layer; the membrane lining the inner surface of the heart
 4. The heart has four chambers
  a. Right atrium receives blood from body tissues
  b. Left atrium receives blood from the lungs
  c. Right ventricle pumps blood to the lungs for oxygen
  d. Left ventricle pumps blood to all parts of the body
 5. Valves are located between the atria and ventricles
  a. Valves allow blood to flow in one direction
  b. Tricuspid valve is between the right atrium and right ventricle
  c. Mitral valve (bicuspid) is between the left atrium and left ventricle
 6. There are two phases of heart action:
  a. Diastole is the resting phase; the heart chambers fill with blood
  b. Systole is the working phase; blood is pumped through the blood vessels when the heart contracts
 D. The blood vessels
 1. Blood flows to body tissues and cells through blood vessels
 2. Three groups of blood vessels: (arteries, capillaries, and veins)
  a. Arteries carry oxygen-rich blood away from the heart
   (1) The aorta is the largest artery
   (2) An arteriole is the smallest branch of an artery; arterioles connect with blood vessels called capillaries
   (3) Food, oxygen, and other substances pass from capillaries into cells
   (4) Waste products are picked up from cells by capillaries and carried back to the heart by veins
  b. Veins
   (1) Return blood to the heart
   (2) Are connected to capillaries by venules
   (3) Two main veins empty into the right atrium
    (a) Inferior vena cava carries

blood from the legs and trunk
    (b) Superior vena cava carries blood from the head and arms
   (4) Venous blood contains little oxygen and a lot of carbon dioxide
  c. Blood flows through the circulatory system (see Figure 13-16, p. 139)
VII. THE RESPIRATORY SYSTEM
 A. Oxygen is needed for survival
 B. The respiratory system brings oxygen into the lungs and eliminates carbon dioxide (see Figure 13-17, p. 140)
 1. The process is called respiration
  a. Inhalation (inspiration) is breathing in
  b. Exhalation (expiration) is breathing out
 2. The process of respiration:
  a. Air enters the body through the nose
  b. Air then passes into the pharynx (throat)
  c. Air passes from the pharynx into the larynx (voice box)
  d. A piece of cartilage called the epiglottis acts like a lid over the larynx; prevents food from entering the airway
  e. Air passes from the larynx into the trachea (windpipe)
  f. The trachea divides into the right and left bronchus; each bronchus enters a lung
  g. Upon entering the lungs, the bronchi divides into bronchioles
  h. Eventually bronchioles subdivide into tiny air sacs call alveoli
  i. Alveoli are supplied by capillaries
  j. Oxygen and carbon dioxide are exchanged between alveoli and capillaries
 C. The right lung has three lobes; the left lung has two lobes
 D. The lungs are separated from the abdominal cavity by a muscle called the diaphragm
 E. Each lung is covered by a two-layered sac called the pleura
 1. The pleura secretes a fluid that prevents the layers from rubbing together
 F. A bony framework consisting of the ribs, sternum, and vertebrae protects the lungs
VIII. THE DIGESTIVE SYSTEM (ALSO CALLED THE GASTROINTESTINAL SYSTEM)
 A. It breaks down food so it can be absorbed for

use by the cells
  1. This process is called digestion
B. It also eliminates solid wastes from the body
C. The digestive system consists of the alimentary canal (GI tract) and the accessory organs of digestion (see Figure 13-18, p. 141)
D. The alimentary canal
  1. A long tube extending from the mouth to the anus
  2. Digestion begins in the mouth (oral cavity)
  3. Teeth cut, chop, and grind food
  4. The tongue aids in chewing and swallowing
  5. Taste buds on the tongue sense sweet, sour, bitter, and salty tastes
  6. Salivary glands secrete saliva, which moistens food for easier chewing and begins digestion in the mouth
  7. The pharynx is a muscular tube that contracts during swallowing and pushes food into the esophagus
  8. Involuntary muscle contractions (peristalsis) move food down the esophagus into the stomach
    a. The esophagus is a muscular tube about 25 centimetres (10 inches) long
  9. The stomach is a muscular, pouch-like sac. Stomach muscles stir and churn food to break it into smaller particles
  10. Food is mixed and churned with gastric juices to form chyme
  11. Peristalsis pushes chyme from the stomach into the small intestine
  12. The small intestine is about 6 metres (20 feet) long; the first part is called the duodenum
  13. More digestive juices are added to the chyme in the duodenum
  14. Digestive juices chemically break down food so it can be absorbed
  15. Peristalsis moves the chyme through the jejunum and ilium; villi, which line the small intestine, absorb digested food into capillaries
  16. Undigested chyme passes from the small intestine to the large intestine (large bowel or colon)
  17. The colon absorbs most of the water from the chyme
  18. The remaining semi-solid material (feces) passes into the rectum and out of the body through the anus as solid waste
IX. THE URINARY SYSTEM
  A. Functions:

  1. To remove waste products from the blood
  2. To maintain water balance within the body
B. Structures (see Figure 13-19, p. 142)
  1. The kidneys are two bean-shaped organs in the upper abdomen
    a. Each kidney has over a million tiny nephrons
      (1) The nephron is the basic working unit of the kidney
    b. Nephrons separate nutrients and minerals in the blood (water, sodium, amino acids, glucose) from the toxins and waste products
    c. Most water and other necessary substances are reabsorbed by blood and recirculated
    d. The rest of the fluid and waste products form urine
    e. Urine flows through the tubule into a collecting tubule that drains into the renal pelvis within the kidney
    f. A tube called the ureter is attached to the renal pelvis
    g. The ureters carry urine to the bladder
    i. Urine is stored in the bladder until the desire to urinate is felt (usually occurs when there is about 250 ml of urine in the bladder)
    j. Urine passes from the bladder through the urethra
    k. Urine then passes from the body through the meatus (opening at the end of the urethra)
X. THE REPRODUCTIVE SYSTEM
  A. The difference between the male and female reproductive systems allows for the process of reproduction
  B. The male reproductive system
    1. Structures (see Figure 13-20, p. 143)
      a. Testes (testicles) are the male sex glands; also called gonads
        (1) Male sex cells (sperm) are produced in the testes
        (2) The male hormone (testosterone) is also produced in the testes
        (3) The testes are suspended between the thighs in a sac called the scrotum
      b. Sperm travel from the testes to the epididimis (a coiled tube)
      c. From the epididimis, sperm travel through a tube called the vas deferens; each vas deferens joins a seminal vesicle

d. The two seminal vesicles store sperm and produce semen (the fluid that carries the sperm from the male reproductive tract)

e. The ducts of the seminal vesicles unite to form the ejaculatory ducts

f. The ejaculatory duct passes through the prostate gland

g. The prostate gland secretes fluid into the semen

h. As the ejaculatory ducts leave the prostate, they join the urethra (the urethra is the outlet for urine and semen)

i. The urethra is contained within the penis

j. The penis is outside the body and has erectile tissue

k. When a man is sexually excited, blood fills the erectile tissue, the penis becomes enlarged, hard, and erect

l. The erect penis can enter the vagina; semen is released into the vagina

C. The female reproductive system

1. Structures (see Figure 13-21, p. 144)

a. The female gonads are two almond-shaped organs called ovaries

(1) One on each side of the uterus in the abdominal cavity

(2) Ovaries contain the female sex cells (ova or eggs)

(3) One ovum is released monthly during the reproductive years

(a) This is called ovulation

(4) The ovaries also secrete the female hormones estrogen and progesterone

(5) The released ovum travels through a fallopian tube

(a) One is located on each side of the uterus and is attached at one end to the uterus

b. The ovum travels through the fallopian tube to the uterus (a hollow, muscular pear-shaped organ)

c. The sex cells from the male and female unite into one cell; that cell implants into the lining of the uterus (endometrium) where it grows into a baby

d. The uterus serves as a place for the unborn baby to grow and receive nourishment

e. The cervix (neck) of the uterus projects into the vagina

f. The vagina opens to the outside of the body and receives the penis during sexual intercourse; it also serves as part of the birth canal

g. Glands in the vaginal wall keep it moist

h. In young girls, the vaginal opening is partially closed by a membrane called the hymen

2. External genitalia (vulva)

a. The mons pubis is a fatty pad over a bone called the symphysis pubis (covered with hair in the adult female)

b. The labia majora and labia minora are folds of tissue on each side of the vaginal opening

c. The clitoris is a small organ composed of erectile tissue (becomes hard when sexually stimulated)

d. Mammary glands (breasts) secrete milk after childbirth

(1) Made up of glandular tissue and fat

3. Menstruation

a. The endometrium is rich in blood to nourish an unborn baby (fetus)

b. If pregnancy does not occur, the endometrium breaks up and is discharged through the vagina and outside the body (menstruation)

c. The cycle occurs about every 28 days

d. Menstrual flow usually lasts 3 to 7 days

e. Ovulation occurs on or about day 14 of the cycle

f. The female hormones estrogen and progesterone cause the endometrium to thicken for possible pregnancy

g. If pregnancy does not occur, the hormones decrease and the endometrium breaks up and is discharged through the vagina

D. Fertilization

1. For reproduction to occur, a male sex cell (sperm) must unite with a female sex cell (ovum)

2. The uniting of the sperm and ovum is called fertilization

XI. THE ENDOCRINE SYSTEM

A. Made up of glands called the endocrine glands (see Figure 13-24, p. 146)

B. Endocrine glands secrete chemical substances

called hormones into the bloodstream
C. Hormones regulate the activities of other organs and glands in the body
D. The pituitary gland (master gland)
  1. Located at the base of the brain behind the eyes
  2. Divided into two lobes
    a. The anterior pituitary lobe
      (1) Secretes growth hormone needed for growth of muscles, bones, and other organs
      (2) Thyroid stimulating hormone (TSH) is needed for proper functioning of the thyroid gland
      (3) Adrenocorticotropic hormone (ACTH) stimulates the adrenal glands
      (4) Also secretes hormones that regulate growth, development, and function of male and female reproductive systems
    b. Posterior pituitary lobe
      (1) Secretes an antidiuretic hormone that prevents kidneys from excreting excessive amounts of water
      (2) Oxytocin causes uterine muscles to contract during childbirth
E. The thyroid gland
  1. Located in the neck in front of the larynx
  2. Secretes thyroid hormone (TH)—regulates metabolism (burning of food for heat and energy by the cells)
F. The parathyroid glands
  1. Four glands—two located on each side of the thyroid gland
  2. Secrete parathyroid hormone, which regulates the body's use of calcium
    a. Insufficient calcium causes tetany (a state of severe muscle contraction and spasm)
G. The adrenal glands
  1. One is located on the top of each kidney
  2. Has two parts
    a. The adrenal medulla secretes epinephrine and norepinephrine (stimulates the body for quick energy in emergencies)
    b. The adrenal cortex secretes:
      (1) Glucocorticoids, which regulate metabolism of carbohydrates; also control the body's response to stress and inflammation
      (2) Mineralocorticoids, which regulate the amount of salt and water absorbed and lost by the kidneys
      (3) Small amounts of male and female sex hormones
H. The pancreas
  1. Secretes insulin
    a. Regulates the amount of sugar in the blood available for use by cells
    b. If sugar cannot enter the cells, excess amounts build up in the blood; this condition is called diabetes mellitus
I. The gonads
  1. Glands of human reproduction
    a. Male glands (testes) secrete testosterone
    b. Female glands (ovaries) secrete estrogen and progesterone

XII. THE IMMUNE SYSTEM
A. Protects the body from disease and infection
B. Defends against threats inside and outside the body
C. Functions to provide the body with immunity
  1. Specific immunity is the body's reaction to a specific threat
  2. Non-specific immunity is the body's reaction to anything it does not recognize as normal
D. Special cells and substances function to produce immunity
  1. Antibodies are normal body substances that recognize and attack abnormal or unwanted substances
  2. Antigens are abnormal or unwanted substances
  3. Phagocytes are white blood cells that digest and destroy unwanted substances
  4. Lymphocytes are white blood cells that produce antibodies
  5. B lymphocytes (B cells) cause the production of antibodies that circulate in plasma
  6. T lymphocytes (T cells) function to destroy invading cells
E. When the body senses an antigen, the immune system is activated

Classroom Activities

1. Explain to students why a basic understanding of the body parts and how they work is important in meeting patient/resident needs. Give the following example:
  a. Knowing about the types of muscles and joints, and how each works is necessary to move and

position a person comfortably and safely.
  b. Call on students. Ask them to give other –examples. Write their responses on the chalkboard.

2. Display an overhead transparency showing the organization of the body, from cells to tissues to organs to systems to the whole person
  a. Call on students to provide the definition of:
    (1) A cell
    (2) Tissues
    (3) Organs
    (4) Systems

  Write the correct responses on the chalkboard.

3. Display an overhead transparency showing an unlabeled cell
  a. Call on students to identify the parts of the cell.

4. Display an overhead transparency showing the four types of tissue.
  a. On a flip chart write the name of each type of tissue. Write each type in a different color. Leave space after each type to write in the function.
    (1) Call on students to describe the function of each type of tissue. Write the correct answers on the flip chart.

5. Display an overhead transparency showing the layers of the skin. Use this as a basis to discuss the functions of the skin.

6. Divide students into groups of three or four. Give each group 5 minutes to list the important functions of the skin.
  a. Call one student from each group to give one function. Write the correct answers on the chalkboard.

7. Introduce the musculoskeletal system. Explain the purpose of this system.
  a. Display overhead transparencies showing the anterior and posterior view of the muscles and bones of the body. This gives the students an overview of what the entire system looks like.
  b. If possible, use an anatomical skeleton to assist you in teaching this system. Allowing students to touch and manipulate the skeleton provides an excellent opportunity to learn how the body is put together and how joints move. It also provides a more realistic view of how the bones look and feel.

  c. Write each of the four types of bones on the chalkboard. Call on students to describe the function of each type of bone. Write the correct answers on the chalkboard.
  d. Divide students into groups of three or four. Give each group 10 minutes to:
    (1) List and define the three types of joints.
    (2) List each body joint and identify each type of joint.

Call on one student from each group to identify one type of joint and list all the joints in the body of that type. Write the correct answers on the chalkboard.

8. Discuss the difference between voluntary and involuntary muscles. Call on students to gives examples of each.

9. Write on the chalkboard: "The muscles perform three important body functions." Call on students to provide the three functions. Write the correct answers on the chalkboard.

10. Introduce the nervous system. Define the purpose of the nervous system. Ask students to identify the two main divisions of the nervous system. Write the correct answers on a flip chart. Use a separate sheet and a different color for each. Then ask students what the central nervous system consists of and what the peripheral nervous system consists of. Write the correct answers on the appropriate flip chart.
  a. Display an unlabeled overhead transparency showing the brain and spinal cord.
    (1) Call on students to identify each part and describe its function.
  b. Display an overhead transparency showing the peripheral nervous system. This allows students to visualize how complex this system is.
    (1) Ask students to define the following terms: Write the correct answers on the chalkboard.
      (a) Autonomic nervous system
      (b) Sympathetic nervous system
      (c) Parasympathetic nervous system

11. Call on a student to write the five senses on the chalkboard.
  a. Display an overhead transparency of the eye. Use this as a basis to discuss the eye and its functions.
    (1) If available, use an anatomical model of the eye to help teach this section. Allow

students to handle the model. This will help students identify and remember the structures of the eye.

b. Display an overhead transparency of the ear. Use this as a basis to discuss the ear and its function.

  (1) If available, use an anatomical model of the ear to help teach this section. Allow students to handle the model. This will help students identify and remember the structures of the ear.

12. Introduce the circulatory system. Write on the chalkboard: "The circulatory is made up of…." Ask students to complete the sentence. Write the correct answer on the chalkboard.

a. Write the following components of the blood on a separate sheet of a flip chart:

  (1) Plasma

  (2) Red blood cells (Erythrocytes)

  (3) White blood cells (Leukocytes)

  (4) Platelets (Thrombocytes)

Call on students to describe the function of each. Write the correct answers on the appropriate sheet of the flip chart.

b. Display an overhead transparency showing the structures of the heart. Use this as a basis to discuss the functions of the heart.

c. Divide students into groups of three. Write the following items on the chalkboard:

  (1) Define the function of the heart.

  (2) List and define the three layers of the heart.

  (3) List and describe the function of the four chambers of the heart.

  (4) Name and describe the location of the heart valves.

  (5) Name and describe the two phases of heart action.

Provide each group with several sheets of notebook paper. Ask each group to discuss the information asked for above. Allow them 15 minutes to complete the exercise and write the answers on the notebook paper provided. Starting with the first item on the list, call on one student from each group to read an answer. Clarify any wrong answers. Write the correct answers under the appropriate item on the chalkboard.

a. Display an overhead transparency showing the arterial and venous systems. Use this as a basis to discuss the blood flow through each system.

Call on students to answer the following questions:

  (1) What is the function of arteries?

  (2) What is the name of the largest artery?

  (3) What is the smallest branch of an artery called?

  (4) What is the function of capillaries?

  (5) What is the function of veins?

  (6) What connects veins to capillaries?

  (7) Name the two main veins and describe their functions.

13. Introduce the respiratory system.

a. Call on students to describe the function of the respiratory system.

b. Display an overhead transparency showing the respiratory system. Use this as a basis to discuss the processes involved in respiration.

c. Divide students into pairs. Allow each pair 10 minutes to outline the process of respiration. Call on one pair to place their outline on the chalkboard. Ask all the students to check the outline for correctness and completeness. Students may change the outline when appropriate until it is correct.

d. Call on students to answer the following questions:

  (1) How many lobes does each lung have?

  (2) What is the name of the muscle that separates the lungs from the abdominal cavity?

  (3) What is the name of the two-layered sac that covers each lung?

14. Introduce the digestive system.

a. Call on students to answer the following questions:

  (1) What is the function of the digestive system?

  (2) What organs make up the digestive system?

b. Display an overhead transparency showing the digestive system. Use this a basis to discuss the process of digestion.

c. Write the following terms on a flip chart: Mouth, teeth, tongue, taste buds, salivary glands, pharynx, peristalsis, esophagus, stomach, small intestine, duodenum, villi, large intestine, rectum, anus. Use a variety of colored markers. Leave space after each term. Call on students to come forward and write in the function of each term in the digestive process. A different student should be chosen for each term. Clarify any wrong answers.

15. Introduce the reproductive system
    a. Display an overhead transparency showing the male reproductive system. Use this as a basis to discuss the structures and function of the male reproductive system.
    b. Ask students the following question:
       (1) What is the name and the function of the male sex glands?
    c. Display an overhead transparency showing the female reproductive system. Use this as a basis to discuss the structures and function of the female reproductive system.
    d. Ask students the following question:
       (1) What is the name and function of the female gonads.
    e. Display an overhead transparency showing the male and female reproductive cells.
       (1) Explain the process of intercourse, fertilization, and pregnancy.
       (2) Explain the menstrual cycle and how it relates to fertilization and pregnancy. Allow time for questions.

16. Introduce the endocrine system.
    a. Write on the chalkboard or flip chart:
       (1) "The endocrine system is made up of endocrine glands." Then ask students:
          (a) What do endocrine glands secrete?
          (b) What function do hormones have?
    b. Display an unlabeled overhead transparency showing the location of the endocrine glands. Call on students to identify the location of each of the endocrine glands. Write in the correct answers.

    c. Write the name of each endocrine gland on an index card. Divide students into groups of three. Distribute one card to each group. Ask each group to compile information about the gland on their card. Allow 15 minutes. Call on one student from each group to report to the class. Allow time for questions and discussion.

17. Introduce the immune system
    a. Ask students why this system is so important.
    b. Write the names of the following cells and substances that produce immunity. Ask students to describe the function of each.
       (1) Antibodies
       (2) Antigens
       (3) Phagocytes
       (4) Lymphocytes
       (5) B lymphocytes
       (6) T lymphocytes

Homework Assignments

Ask students to answer the questions at the end of Chapter 13 in the textbook. Tell students the date and time that this assignment must be completed and turned in.

If the accompanying student workbook is being used, assign the Chapter 13 workbook exercises. Tell students the date and time that this assignment must be completed and turned in.

Name _____

Date _____

Body Structure and Function

1. Label the parts of a cell

   a. _____

   b. _____

   c. _____

2. List and define the four basic types of tissue:

   a. _____

   _____

   _____

   b. _____

   _____

   _____

   c. _____

   _____

   _____

   d. _____

   _____

   _____

3. Fill in the blanks:

   a. Groups of tissues form _____.

   An organ performs _____.

4. Describe the function of each system:

   a. The integumentary system—_____

   _____

   b. The musculoskeletal system—_____

   _____

   c. The nervous system—_____

   _____

   d. The circulatory system—_____

   _____

   e. The respiratory system—_____

   _____

   f. The digestive system—_____

   _____

   g. The urinary system—_____

   _____

   h. The reproductive system—_____

   _____

   i. The endocrine system—_____

   _____

   j. The immune system—_____

   _____

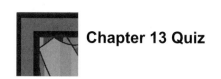

Chapter 13 Quiz

Name _____

Date _____

Body Structure and Function

<table>
<tr><td>

True or False

*Mark **T** for true or **F** for false.*

1. _____ The digestive system is the largest system of the body.

2. _____ The ball-and-socket joint allows movement in all directions.

3. _____ The action of the stomach is controlled by involuntary muscles.

4. _____ The peripheral nervous system is made up of the brain and spinal cord.

5. _____ The liquid part of the blood is called plasma.

6. _____ During systole, the heart chambers fill with blood.

7. _____ The smallest branch of an artery is a capillary.

8. _____ In the lungs, oxygen and carbon dioxide are exchanged between the alveoli and capillaries.

9. _____ The urinary system removes solid waste from the body.

10. _____ Male sex cells are called sperm.

11. _____ Ovaries secrete the female hormones estrogen and progesterone.

12. _____ The uniting of the sperm and ovum into one cell is called menstruation.

13. _____ The pancreas is called the master gland.

14. _____ Leukocytes are necessary for the clotting of blood.

</td><td>

Multiple Choice

Circle the BEST answer.

15. The basic unit of body structure is:
    a. An organ.
    b. A cell.
    c. Tissue.
    d. Mitosis.

16. The type of bone that bears the weight of the body is:
    a. Long bone.
    b. Flat bone.
    c. Irregular bone.
    d. Short bone.

17. Muscles perform all of the following functions except:
    a. Movement of body parts.
    b. Protect the body against infection.
    c. Maintenance of posture.
    d. Production of body heat.

18. The largest part of the brain and the center of thought and intelligence is:
    a. The cerebellum.
    b. The midbrain.
    c. The brain stem.
    d. The cerebrum.

19. The substance in red blood cells that carries oxygen and gives blood its color is:
    a. Protoplasm.
    b. Plasma.
    c. Hemoglobin.
    d. Leukocytes.

20. Which heart chamber pumps blood to the lungs?
    a. The right atrium
    b. The left ventricle
    c. The left atrium
    d. The right ventricle

</td></tr>
</table>

Name _____

Date _____

Body Structure and Function

21. Where does digestion begin?
    a. In the stomach
    b. in the esophagus
    c. In the mouth
    d. In the duodenum

22. Food mixed with gastric juice to form a semi-liquid substance is called:
    a. Chyme.
    b. Peristalsis.
    c. Bile
    d. Feces.

23. Urine passes from the bladder through the:
    a. Ureter.
    b. Urethra.
    c. Kidney.
    d. Glomerulus.

24. The lining of the uterus is called:
    a. The cervix.
    b. Ovulation.
    c. The endometrium.
    d. The hymen.

25. The system that protects the body from disease and infection is called the:
    a. Endocrine system.
    b. Immune system.
    c. Respiratory system.
    d. Integumentary system.

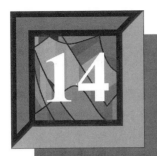

14

Growth and Development

Instructor's Preparation

I. Read Chapter 14 in the textbook. Carefully review chapter objectives, key terms, and review questions.

II. Read the outline in Chapter 14 of the instructor's guide. Carefully review the classroom activities, the student assignment, and the quiz.

III. If you are using the accompanying student workbook, review the activities for Chapter 14.

IV. Gather all necessary supplies and equipment for classroom activities and student assignments.

   A. Prepare appropriate flip charts

   B. Prepare situation/index cards

   C. Gather coloured markers

   D. Gather any other items that will be needed for classroom activities

   E. Assemble items in the order they will be used

V. Make sure that the necessary equipment is available and in good working order.

Objectives

- Define the key terms listed in this chapter
- Understand the principles of growth and development
- Identify the stages of growth and development and the normal age ranges for each stage
- Identify the developmental tasks of each age-group
- Describe the normal growth and development for each age-group

Key Terms

adolescence
development
developmental task
ejaculation
growth
menarche
menopause
primary caregiver
puberty
reflex

Outline

Growth and Development

I. INTRODUCTION
- A. A basic understanding of growth and development helps you give better care
- B. Primary caregiver is used in this chapter (the person mainly responsible for providing or assisting with a child's basic needs)

II. PRINCIPLES
- A. Growth is the physical changes that are measured and occur in a steady and orderly manner
- B. Development refers to changes in psychological and social functioning
- C. A person behaves and thinks in certain ways at different stages of development
- D. Growth and development:
    1. Overlap
    2. Depend on each other
    3. Occur at the same time
- E. Basic principles:
    1. Growth and development occur from fertilization until death
    2. The process proceeds from the simple to the complex
    3. Growth and development occur in certain directions:
        a. From head to foot
        b. From the center of the body outward
    4. Growth and development occur in a sequence, order, and pattern
        a. Certain developmental tasks must be completed during each stage
    5. The rate of growth and development is uneven, not at a set pace
    6. Each stage has its own characteristics and developmental tasks

III. INFANCY (BIRTH TO 1 YEAR)
- A. Developmental tasks:
    1. Learning to walk
    2. Learning to eat solid foods
    3. Beginning to talk and communicate with others
    4. Beginning to have emotional relationships with the primary caregiver and siblings
    5. Developing sleep and feeding patterns
- B. Neonatal period is the first 28 days after birth
    1. The average newborn is 19 to 21 inches long and weighs 7 to 8 pounds
    2. The newborn's head is large compared to the rest of the body
    3. The central nervous system is not well developed
    4. Newborns have certain reflexes (involuntary movements)
        a. The Moro reflex (startle reflex) occurs when a baby is frightened by a loud noise; the arms are thrown apart, the legs extend, and the head is thrown back
        b. The rooting reflex is stimulated when the infant's cheek is touched near the mouth; the head turns toward the touch (helps guide the baby's mouth to a nipple)
        c. The sucking reflex is produced by touching the cheeks or side of the lips
        d. The grasping reflex occurs when the infant's palm is stimulated (the fingers close around the object)
- C. Infants sleep most of the time during the first few weeks of life
- D. Body movements are uncoordinated and without purpose
- E. At 1 month, infants can hold their head up
- F. At 2 months, infants can smile and follow objects with their eyes
- G. Three-month-old infants can raise their heads and shoulders when lying on their stomachs
- H. Infants 4months of age should be able to roll over, sit up if supported, and shed tears when crying
    1. Moro and rooting reflexes have disappeared
- I. At 5 months, infants grasp objects and play with their toes; teeth start to come through the gums
- J. At 6 months, there are usually two lower teeth
- K. At 7 months, the upper teeth start to erupt; babies respond to their name
- L. At 8 months, babies may be able to stand when holding on to something
- M. Nine-month-old infants crawl
- N. At 10 months, infants can walk around when holding on to objects; they understand "bye-bye," "mama," and "daddy"
- O. Many infants start to walk at 1 year; they can hold a cup and shake their head "no"

IV. TODDLERHOOD (1 TO 3 YEARS)
- A. Developmental tasks:
    1. Tolerating separation from the primary caregiver
    2. Gaining control of bowel and bladder

functions

3. Using words to communicate with others
4. Becoming less dependent on the primary caregiver

B. The toddler years are known as "the terrible twos"

C. The ability to move about and walk increases

D. Toddlers are very curious about their surroundings

E. The toddler learns to climb

F. Increased hand coordination gives toddlers new skills
   1. Right or left handedness is seen during the second year

G. Toilet training is a major developmental task
   1. Children must be psychologically and physically ready
   2. Bowel control is easier than bladder control

H. Speech and language skills increase
   1. By 3 years of age, children speak in short sentences

I. Play ability increases
   1. The toddler is possessive; the word "mine" is often used

J. Temper tantrums and saying "no" are common

K. Toddlers start to explore their environments

L. If the primary caregiver is consistently present when needed, a child learns to feel secure

V. PRESCHOOL (3 TO 6 YEARS)

A. Children grow taller but gain little weight

B. Developmental tasks:
   1. Increasing ability to communicate and understand
   2. Performing self-care activities
   3. Learning the difference between the sexes; developing sexual modesty
   4. Learning right from wrong and good from bad
   5. Learning to play with others
   6. Developing family relationships

C. The 3-year-old child
   1. Becomes more coordinated
      a. Walks on tiptoes; balances on one foot
   2. Personal care skills increase
   3. Can draw circles and crosses
   4. Knows about 1000 words
      a. Talks and asks questions constantly
      b. Likes talking dolls and musical toys
   5. Play is important
   6. They know their own sex
   7. The concept of time develops

a. "Yesterday" and "tomorrow" are confusing

8. Is less fearful of strangers
9. Things are done to please primary caregivers

D. The 4-year-old child
   1. Can hop, skip, and throw and catch a ball
   2. Can bathe with help and usually attend to their own toilet needs
   3. Vocabulary increases to about 1500 words
      a. Can sing simple songs, repeat four numbers, count to three, name a few colors
   4. May tend to attack others
      a. Tease, tattle, and tell fibs
   5. Can play cooperatively
   6. Enjoys playing "dress up"
   7. Plays in groups of two or three
   8. Curiosity about the opposite sex continues
      a. Enjoys playing "doctor and nurse"
   9. Strongly prefers the caregiver of the other sex
   10. Rivalries occur; 4-year old children try to run away from home

E. The 5-year-old child
   1. Continues to develop coordination
   2. Can use a pencil and copy diamond and triangle shapes
   3. Has a vocabulary of about 14,000 words
   4. Is more responsible and truthful and quarrels less
   5. Has greater awareness of rules
   6. Is proud of his or her accomplishments
   7. Enjoys simple number and word games
   8. Imitates adults during play
   9. Also enjoys activities with the primary caregiver of the same sex
   10. Tolerates brothers and sisters well

VI. MIDDLE CHILDHOOD (6 TO 8 YEARS)

A. Preschoolers often have nursery school and kindergarten experiences

B. Enter the world of peer groups, games, and learning

C. Developmental tasks:
   1. Developing social and physical skills needed for playing games
   2. Learning to get along with peers
   3. Learning behaviors and attitudes appropriate to one's own sex
   4. Learning basic reading, writing, and arithmetic skills

5. Developing a conscience and morals
6. Developing a good feeling and attitude about oneself

D. The 6-year-old child
1. Grows about 2 inches and gains 3 to 6 pounds
2. Loses baby teeth
3. Seems to be constantly on the go
4. Enters first grade
   a. The world of school, activities, and other children
5. Often described as bossy, opinionated, charming, argumentative, and "know-it-all"
6. Plays well with children of both sexes
   a. May have a best friend
   b. Tattling is common
7. Has a vocabulary of about 16,500 words
8. Knows the alphabet, begins to read and spell
9. Starts collections of odds and ends

E. The 7-year-old child
1. Grows 2 inches in height; weighs 49 to 56 pounds
2. Hand coordination increases
3. Learns to write
4. Is more serious and less stubborn
5. More aware of self, his or her body, and the reactions of others
6. Likes going to school, learning, and reading
7. Reading skills increase and learns to tell time
8. Plays in groups
   a. Boys prefer to play with boys and girls prefer to play with girls
   b. May join scouting groups

F. The 8-year-old child
1. Growth in height and weight continues
2. More permanent teeth appear
3. Peer groups, activities, and opinions are important
4. Gets along with adults
5. Boys and girls play separately
6. Gives advice but does not take criticism well
7. Is curious about science, history, and other places
8. Is friendly and affectionate

VII. LATE CHILDHOOD (9 TO 12 YEARS)
A. Pre-adolescence
B. Developmental tasks are similar to those of middle childhood; is expected to be more re-

fined and mature in achieving the following tasks:
1. Becoming independent of adults; learning to depend on oneself
2. Developing and keeping friendships with peers
3. Understanding physical, psychological, and social roles of one's sex
4. Developing moral and ethical behavior
5. Developing greater muscle strength, co-ordination, and balance
6. Learning how to study

C. Boys grow about 1 inch per year; girls grow about 2 inches per year
1. Girls are usually taller than boys

D. Skill in team sports becomes important
E. Body change occurs as the onset of puberty nears
1. Genital organs begin to grow

F. Factual sexual education is needed
1. Information is shared among friends
2. Parents and children may be uncomfortable discussing sex with each other

G. Peer groups are the center of activities
1. The group begins to affect the child's attitude and behavior

H. Arguments between boys and girls are common

I. Is more aware of the mistakes and weaknesses of adults
1. Rebellion against adults is common
2. Disagreements between parents and children increase

J. By age 12, the child understands about 50 000 words in reading

VIII. ADOLESCENCE (12 TO 18 YEARS)
A. A time of rapid growth and psychological and social maturity
B. Begins with puberty
1. The reproductive organs begin to function
2. The secondary sex characteristics appear
3. Girls experience puberty between ages 10 and 14
4. Boys reach puberty between ages 12 and 16

C. Developmental tasks:
1. Accepting changes in the body and appearance
2. Developing appropriate relationships with males and females of the same age
3. Accepting the male or female role appropriate for one's age

4. Becoming independent from parents and adults
5. Developing morals, attitudes, and values needed for functioning in society
D. Menarche is the beginning of menstruation
  1. Marks the onset of puberty in girls
  2. Secondary sex characteristics appear
    a. Increase in breast size
    b. Appearance of pubic and axillary hair
    c. Slight deepening of voice
    d. Widening and rounding of the hips
E. Ejaculation (the release of semen)
  1. Signals the onset of puberty in boys
  2. Nocturnal emissions (wet dreams) occur
  3. Other secondary sex characteristics appear
    a. Appearance of facial hair
    b. Pubic and axillary hair
    c. Hair on arms, chest, and legs
    d. Deepening of the voice
    e. Increase in neck and shoulder size
F. A growth spurt occurs
G. Is described as the awkward stage
H. Changes in appearance are often hard to accept
I. Emotional reactions vary from high to low
J. Need to become independent from adults, especially parents
  1. Must learn to function, make decisions, and act in a responsible manner
  2. May get a job
K. Judgement and reasoning are not always sound
  1. Guidance, discipline, and emotional and financial support from parents is still needed
  2. Disagreements with parents are common
L. Both sexes are interested in parties, dances, and other social activities
M. Dating begins
  1. Parents worry that dating will lead to sexual activity, pregnancy, and sexually transmitted diseases
N. Begins to think about careers and what to do after high school
O. Needs to develop morals, values, and attitudes for living in society
P. Parents, peers, culture, religion, television, school, and movies are factors that influence adolescents
Q. Drug abuse, unwanted pregnancy, alcoholism, and criminal acts are common problems of troubled adolescents

IX. YOUNG ADULTHOOD (18 TO 40 YEARS)
A. There is little physical growth
B. Developmental tasks:
  1. Choosing education and an occupation
  2. Selecting a marriage partner
  3. Learning to live with a partner
  4. Becoming a parent and raising children
  5. Developing a satisfactory sex life
C. Education and occupation are closely related
D. Employment is necessary for economic independence and supporting a family
E. Most adults marry at least once
  1. Others choose to remain single
  2. May live alone, with friends of the same sex, or with persons of the opposite sex
  3. Gay and lesbian persons may commit to a partner
F. Many factors affect choosing a marriage partner
  1. Age, religion, interests, education, race, personality, and love
  2. Partners must learn to live together
  3. Open and honest communication help create a successful partnership
G. Adults need to develop a satisfactory sex life
  1. Sexual frequency, desire, practices, and preferences vary
H. Most couples decide to have children
  1. They need to agree on child rearing practices and discipline methods
  2. They need to adjust to the child and the child's needs

X. MIDDLE ADULTHOOD (40 TO 65 YEARS)
A. This stage is more stable and comfortable
B. There are fewer worries about children and money
C. Developmental tasks:
  1. Adjusting to physical changes
  2. Having grown children
  3. Developing leisure-time activities
  4. Relating to aging parents
D. Several physical changes occur
  1. Energy and endurance begin to slow down
  2. Weight control becomes a problem
  3. Facial wrinkles and gray hair appear
  4. The need for eyeglasses is common
  5. Hearing loss may begin
  6. Menopause means menstruation stops; women can no longer have children
  7. Many illnesses and diseases can develop
E. Children leave home

F. May have more spare time for hobbies and other interests

G. May need to provide care for parents who are aging and developing poor health

H. Often have to deal with the death of parents

XI. LATE ADULTHOOD (65 YEARS AND OLDER)

A. Developmental tasks:

1. Adjusting to a decrease in physical strength and loss of health
2. Adjusting to retirement and reduced income
3. Coping with the death of a partner
4. Developing new friends and relationships
5. Preparing for one's own death

Classroom Activities

1. Write the basic principles of growth and development on separate pages of a flip chart. Use this as a basis for discussion.

   a. Call on students to explain the difference between growth and development.

2. Write each stage of growth and development on an index card. Place each index card in a basket or box. Divide students into groups of three. Have each group pick an index card from the basket or box. Ask each group to discuss and list the physical changes and developmental tasks related to

the stage written on their index card. Then have each group report to the class. Allow time for discussion.

3. Ask students to share how they are dealing with the developmental tasks that relate to their particular age group.

   a. If they have children, what developmental tasks are they involved in?

   b. What developmental tasks are older parents or relatives involved in?

4. Call on students to discuss how a basic knowledge of the principles of growth and development will help them provide better care to patients and residents?

   a. Ask students how a knowledge of developmental tasks will effect the care they give.

Homework Assignments

Ask students to answer the questions at the end of Chapter 14 in the textbook. Tell students the date and time that this assignment must be completed and turned in.

If the accompanying student workbook is being used, assign Chapter 14 workbook exercises. Tell students the date and time that this assignment must be completed and turned in.

Chapter 14 Student Assignment   Name _____

Date _____

Growth and Development

List the basic principles of growth and development.

1. _____

2. _____

3. _____

4. _____

5. _____

6. _____

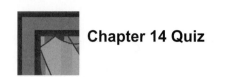

Name _____

Date _____

Growth and Development

True or False

*Mark **T** for true or **F** for false.*

1. _____ Development relates to physical changes that are measured and occur in a steady and orderly manner.

2. _____ The rate of growth and development is even and at a set pace.

3. _____ The newborn's head is large in comparison to the rest of the body.

4. _____ Adolescence is a time of rapid growth and psychological and social maturity.

5. _____ Puberty is the time when menstruation stops

Multiple Choice

Circle the BEST answer.

6. Newborns have certain reflexes. Which reflex is necessary for feeding? (It guides the baby's mouth to the nipple.)
   a. Sucking reflex
   b. Rooting reflex
   c. Startle reflex
   d. Grasping reflex

7. Toilet training is a major developmental task for:
   a. Infants.
   b. Toddlers.
   c. Preschool children.
   d. Six-year-old children.

8. At what stage should children receive factual sex education?
   a. Toddlerhood
   b. Preschool age
   c. Middle childhood
   d. Late childhood

9. Which is not a developmental task of adolescence?
   a. Accepting change in appearance
   b. Becoming independent from parents and adults
   c. Developing leisure time activities
   d. Developing morals, values, and attitudes needed to function in society

10. Adjusting to retirement and reduced income is a developmental task of:
    a. Adolescence.
    b. Young adulthood.
    c. Late adulthood.
    d. Middle adulthood.

15

Caring for Older Adults

Instructor's Preparation

I. Read Chapter 15 in the textbook. Carefully review chapter objectives, key terms, and review questions.

II. Read the outline in Chapter 15 of the instructor's guide. Carefully review the classroom activities, the student assignment, and the quiz.

III. If you are using the accompanying student workbook, review the activities for Chapter 15.

IV. Gather all necessary supplies and equipment for classroom activities and student assignments.
    A. Prepare the correct number of handouts
    B. Prepare appropriate flip charts.
    C. Prepare overhead transparencies
    D. Gather coloured markers

E. Gather any other items that will be needed for classroom activities
F. Assemble items in the order they will be used

V. Make sure that the necessary equipment is available and in good working order.

VI. Contact guest speakers to confirm the day, date, time, and location that they are expected.
    A. Ask the speakers if they require any special equipment or supplies. Make sure these are available.

VII. Confirm all plans for the field trip.
    A. Contact the agency to confirm location, day, date, and time.
    B. Prepare an index card for each student with the location day, date, and time of the field trip. Include special instructions (i.e., dress code).

Objectives	Key Terms
• Define the key terms listed in this chapter	ageism
• Describe the effects of retirement	discrimination
• Identify the social changes common in older adulthood	dysphagia
	dyspnea
• Describe how a partner's death affects the survivor	geriatrics
• Describe the changes that occur in the body's systems during aging and the care required	gerontology
	middle-old
• Explain how aging affects sexuality in older adults	old-old
• Describe how the health care team promotes the client's sexuality	stereotype
	young-old
• Explain the effect of ageism on older adults	

Outline

Caring for Older Adults

I. INTRODUCTION
  A. The number of older persons is increasing
    1. People live longer and are healthier and more active than ever before
  B. Late adulthood is broken down into three age ranges:
    1. Young-old—persons 60 to 74
    2. Middle-old—persons 75 to 84
    3. Old-old—people over age 85
  C. Gerontology is the study of the aging process
  D. Geriatrics is the care of the aged
  E. Normal changes occur in body structure and function
    1. Usually changes are gradual
  F. Psychological and social changes also occur
  G. Developmental tasks of late adulthood:
    1. Adjusting to decreased physical strength and loss of health
    2. Adjusting to retirement and reduced income
    3. Coping with the death of a partner
    4. Developing new friends and relationships
    5. Preparing for one's own death
II. EMOTIONAL AND SOCIAL CHANGES
  A. Gray hair, wrinkles, and slower movements are physical reminders of growing old
  B. Retirement and death of a partner, family, and friends are social reminders
  C. Retirement
    1. Most people look forward to retirement
    2. Is a reward for a lifetime of hard work
    3. Some must retire because of chronic disease or disability
      a. Can make retirement difficult
    4. Some people need work for psychological and social fulfillment
      a. Retirement can be hard for them
    5. Some retired people have part-time jobs or do volunteer work
    6. Retirement usually means reduced income
      a. Expenses are not less
      b. Reduced income may force life-style changes
    7. Some people plan for retirement through savings, investments, retirement plans, and insurance
  D. Social relationships
    1. Change throughout life (see Respecting Diversity box, p. 162)
      a. Children grow up, leave home, and have families
      b. Older friends and family members move away, die, or become disabled
      c. Most older people have regular contact with family and friends
    2. Separation from children and lack of companionship is a common cause of loneliness in older persons
    3. Many older persons adjust to these changes with:
      a. Hobbies
      b. Church and community activities
      c. New friends (see Figure 15-2, p. 162)
    4. Being a grandparent brings great love and enjoyment
    5. Children often care for their older parents
      a. Parents and children change roles
  E. Death of a partner
    1. Women live longer then men
      a. Many women will become widows
    2. When the death of a partner occurs, the loss is crushing
      a. The person loses a lover, friend, companion, and confidant
      b. The survivors grief may be great
      c. Serious physical and mental health problems can result
      d. The surviving partner may attempt suicide
III. PHYSICAL CHANGES
  A. Certain physical changes are a normal part of aging (see Table 15-1, p. ~~151~~) 164
  B. The rate and degree of change varies with each person
  C. Influencing factors include:
    1. Diet
    2. General health
    3. Exercise
    4. Stress
    5. Environment
    6. Heredity
  D. Some have physical changes caused by disease, illness, or injury
  E. The integumentary system
    1. Skin loses elasticity and fatty tissue layer
      a. Skin sags; folds, lines, and wrinkles appear
    2. Dry skin develops
    3. The skin is fragile and easily injured (see Chapter 41)
    4. The skin has fewer nerve endings

5. Loss of fatty tissue increases sensitivity to cold
6. Nails become thick and tough (see Chapter 28)
7. Feet usually have poor circulation
8. Dry skin is easily damaged and causes itching
    a. Baths are taken less frequently
    b. Only mild soaps are used
    c. Lotions, oils, and creams prevent drying and itching
9. Older persons may complain of cold feet
    a. Hot water bottles and heating pads are not used
        (1) The risk of burns is great
10. White or gray hair is common
11. Hair thins in both men and women
12. Growth of facial hair may occur in women
13. Hair is dryer

F. The musculoskeletal system
1. Muscles atrophy and decrease in strength
2. Bones lose strength, become brittle, and break easily
3. Joints become stiff and painful
4. These changes result in a gradual loss of height, loss of strength, and decreased mobility
5. Older persons need to be as active as possible
    a. A regular exercise program is helpful
6. Diet should be high in protein, calcium, and vitamins
7. The person is protected from injury and falls (see Chapter 16)
8. Turn and move the person gently and carefully
9. Range-of-motion exercises are helpful (see Chapter 22)

G. The nervous system
1. Changes occur in the senses
    a. Hearing and vision losses occur (see Chapter 36)
    b. The senses of taste and smell dull
    c. Touch and sensitivity to pain and pressure are reduced
    d. The ability to feel heat and cold is reduced
        (1) Safety measures are practiced when applying heat and cold (see Chapters 27 and 41)
        (2) Good skin care is provided
    e. Blood flow to the brain is reduced

        (1) There is a progressive loss of brain cells
        (2) Memory is often shorter
        (3) The ability to respond is slowed
        (4) Confusion, dizziness, and fatigue may occur
    f. Less sleep is needed
        (1) Sleep periods are shorter

H. The cardiovascular system
1. The heart muscle becomes less efficient
2. Arteries lose their elasticity and become narrow
    a. Poor circulation occurs in many body parts
    b. Rest periods are needed during the day
    c. Daily activities are planned to avoid overexertion
3. Moderate exercise helps to stimulate circulatory, respiratory, digestive, and musculoskeletal functions
4. Exercise helps prevent thrombi in leg veins
5. Active or passive range-of-motion exercises are needed if the person is confined to bed (see Chapter 22)

I. The respiratory system
1. Respiratory muscles weaken and lung tissue becomes less elastic and more rigid
2. Difficulty in breathing (dyspnea) may occur with activity
3. The person may not have enough strength to cough and clear the upper airway
    a. Respiratory infections and diseases may develop
4. Normal breathing is promoted
    a. Heavy bed linens should not cover the chest
    b. Turning, repositioning, and deep breathing help prevent respiratory complications from bedrest
    c. The person should be as active as possible

J. The digestive system
1. Salivary glands produce less saliva
    a. This can cause difficulty swallowing (dysphagia)
2. Secretion of digestive juices decreases
3. Loss of teeth and ill-fitting dentures affect chewing
4. Decreased peristalsis results in slower emptying of the stomach and colon
    a. Flatulence and constipation are

common
5. Dry, fried, and fatty foods are avoided
6. Good oral hygiene and denture care improve the ability to taste
7. High-fiber foods are hard to chew and can irritate the intestines
   a. Foods providing soft bulk are ordered for persons with chewing problems or constipation
      (1) Whole-grain cereals, and cooked fruits and vegetables
8. Aging requires diet changes
   a. Older people need fewer calories than young people do
   b. More fluids are needed
   c. The person needs foods to prevent constipation and bone changes
   d. High protein foods are needed
      (1) These foods are usually costly
K. The urinary system
   1. Kidney function decreases with age
   2. The kidneys shrink (atrophy)
   3. Removal of body wastes is less efficient
   4. Urine is more concentrated
   5. Bladder muscles weaken
   6. Bladder size decreases
   7. Urinary incontinence may occur (see Chapter 29)
   8. In men, the prostate gland enlarges
      a. Difficulty urinating or frequent urination are common problems
   9. Older persons are at risk for urinary tract infections
      a. Adequate fluids are necessary
         (1) Personal choice in beverages is important
         (2) Most fluids should be ingested before 1700 hrs. (5:00 P.M.)
   10. Bladder training programs may be necessary
   11. Indwelling catheters are sometimes needed
L. Reproductive organs change with aging
   1. In men:
      a. The hormone testosterone decreases
      b. It takes longer for erection to occur
      c. The phase between erection and orgasm is longer
      d. Orgasm is less forceful than in younger years
      e. After orgasm, erection is lost quickly
      f. The time between erections is longer
      g. Older men may need the penis stimu-

lated for sexual arousal
   h. Changes result in decreased frequency of sexual activity
   i. Mental and physical fatigue, overeating, and excessive drinking affect erections
   j. Some men fear performance problems and avoid sex
2. In women:
   a. Menopause occurs at about age 50 (menstruation stops/reproductive years end)
   b. The hormones estrogen and progesterone decrease
   c. The uterus, vagina, and external genitalia atrophy (shrink)
   d. Thin vaginal walls and vaginal dryness may cause uncomfortable or painful intercourse
   e. Sexual arousal takes longer
   f. The time between excitement and orgasm is longer
   g. Orgasm is less intense
   h. The pre-excitement state returns more quickly
3. Frequency of sexual activity decreases for many men and women
   a. Reasons relate to weakness, mental and physical fatigue, pain, and reduced mobility
   b. Some people cannot have sexual intercourse
      (1) This does not mean sexual needs or desires are lost
   c. Some persons lose their sexual partner to death or divorce
4. Focus on older persons
   a. Sexual relationships are important for older persons
      (1) They fall in love, hold hands, embrace, and have sex
      (2) They need sex, love, affection
   b. Love, affection, and intimacy are needed throughout life
   c. As other losses occur, feeling close to another person is more important
M. Meeting the person's sexual needs
   1. Sexuality is part of the total person
   2. Sexual activity does not always mean sexual intercourse
   3. The nursing team must allow and support the meeting of sexual needs
      a. The measures listed in Box 15-1, p.

166 in the textbook, promote sexuality
4. Focus on long-term care
   a. Married couples are allowed to share the same room
      (1) They can share the same bed if their conditions permit
   b. A single resident may develop a relationship with another single resident
      (1) They are allowed time together
5. Older persons have the right to be sexual

IV. CARING FOR OLDER CLIENTS
   A. Western Culture values youth and this is reflected in media messages, advertisements, greeting cards, and cartoons
   B. Media images like to depict older adults as stereotypes, which encourages discrimination and is based on ageism
   C. Remember that every person is unique, and develops and ages in his or her own way
   D. If you treat older adults without respect, their dignity is threatened and they may feel no longer useful, productive members of society
   E. Remember that many older people are coping with loss of loved ones, friends and health, dignity, self-esteem
   F. Support workers must be aware of all the changes that occur with aging (see Providing Compassionate Care box, p. 167).

Classroom Activities

1. Write the following terms on the chalkboard:
   a. Young-old
   b. Middle-old
   c. Old-old
      (1) Call on students to provide the age ranges for each term. Write in the correct answers.

2. Display an overhead transparency showing the developmental tasks of late adulthood. Use this as a basis to review and discuss the tasks with students.

3. Divide students into three groups. Provide each group with several sheets from a flip chart and colored markers. Assign each group to make a list of the changes that occur with aging in one of the following categories:
   a. Physical
   b. Psychological
   c. Social
      (1) Allow students 10 minutes to complete the list. Then call on one student from each

group to display the group's list and review it with the class. Allow time for discussion.

4. Ask students to share any personal experiences with change and loss.
   a. What factors influenced how they adjusted to the change and/or loss.

5. Write the words Sex and Sexuality on the chalkboard. Then call on students to describe the difference between the two words.
   a. Ask students to discuss the factors that affect their attitudes about sex and sexuality.

6. Divide students into two groups. Provide each group with a flip chart and colored markers.
   a. Ask one group to identify and list the age-related changes in the male reproductive system. They should also identify how these changes impact sex and sexuality for men.
   b. Ask one group to identify and list the age-related changes in the female reproductive system. They should also identify how the changes impact sex and sexuality in women
   Allow 15 minutes for this exercise. Then call on one student from each group to report to the class. Allow time after each presentation for questions and discussion.

7. Display measures to promote sexuality (see Box 15-1, p. 166) on an overhead transparency. Use this as a basis for discussion.

8. Invite an older person or persons to speak to the class about aging. Ask them to share both positive and negative experiences. Encourage students to ask questions.
   a. Provide time after the presentation for the older person(s) and the students to socialize. Provide a beverage and snack.

Homework Assignments

Ask students to answer the questions at the end of Chapter 15 in the textbook. Tell students the date and time that this assignment must be completed and turned in.

If the accompanying student workbook is being used, assign the Chapter 15 workbook exercises. Tell students the date and time that this assignment must be completed and turned in.

Name _____

Date _____

Caring for Older Adults

Write your answers in the spaces provided.

1. List three physical changes that are a normal part of aging for each of the following systems.
   Integumentary system:
   a. _____

   b. _____

   c. _____

   Nervous system:
   a. _____

   b. _____

   c. _____

   Respiratory system:
   a. _____

   b. _____

   c. _____

2. List three ways to respect and promote your client's sexuality.
   a. _____

   b. _____

   c. _____

3. Late adulthood is broken down into three age ranges. List the ranges.
   a. _____

   b. _____

   c. _____

4. How are sex and sexuality different?

   _____

   _____

   _____

Chapter 15 Quiz

Name _____

Date _____

Caring for Older Adults

True or False

Mark **T** *for true or* **F** *for false.*

1. _____ Gerontology is the study of the aging person.

2. _____ Growing old is only a physical process.

3. _____ All persons age at the same rate.

4. _____ As people age, muscles atrophy and strength decreases.

5. _____ The senses of smell and taste decrease with age.

6. _____ Older persons become more and more farsighted.

7. _____ Older persons do not enjoy sexual activity.

8. _____ Sexuality is not important for older persons.

9. _____ Attitudes and sex needs stay the same as a person ages.

10. _____ Injury and illness can affect sexual function.

11. _____ The nursing team has an important role in meeting the person's sexuality needs

Multiple Choice

Circle the BEST answer.

12. Aging requires certain dietary changes. Which is true?
    a. Older people need more calories than younger people.
    b. Less fluids are needed.
    c. High protein foods should be avoided.
    d. Older persons need foods that prevent constipation and musculoskeletal changes.

13. A resident refuses a bath. You must:
    a. Call the resident's family.
    b. Get help and give the bath.
    c. Report the refusal to the nurse.
    d. Change the resident's care plan.

14. The inability of the male to have an erection is:
    a. Transvestite.
    b. Impotence.
    c. Intercourse.
    d. Masturbation.

15. Female hormones decrease with menopause. Which is not an effect of reduced hormone levels?
    a. The uterus, vagina, and external genitalia atrophy.
    b. Intercourse may be uncomfortable.
    c. Arousal takes longer.
    d. Sexual desire is lost.

16. Sexual activity:
    a. Always involves intercourse.
    b. Is not allowed in nursing centers.
    c. Involves handholding, touching, and embracing.
    d. Is unhealthy for older persons.

17. You promote sexuality by:
    a. Helping a patient apply make up.
    b. Draping and screening the person appropriately.
    c. Allowing privacy for masturbation.
    d. All of the above.

18. The time when menstruation stops is called:
    a. Menopause.
    b. Impotence.
    c. Orgasm.
    d. Testosterone.

Safety

Instructor's Preparation

I. Read Chapter 16 in the textbook. Carefully review chapter objectives, key terms, and review questions.

II. Read the outline in Chapter 16 of the instructor's guide. Carefully review the classroom activities, the student assignment, and the quiz.

III. If you are using the accompanying student workbook, review the activities for Chapter 16.

IV. Gather all necessary supplies and equipment for classroom activities and student assignments.

   A. Prepare the correct number of handouts

   B. Gather the following transparency: TA26

   C. Gather coloured markers

   D. Gather restraints

   E. Gather any other items that will be needed for classroom activities

   F. Assemble items in the order they will be used

V. Make sure that the necessary equipment is available and in good working order.

VI. Contact guest speakers to confirm the day, date, time, and location that they are expected.

   A. Ask the speakers if they require any special equipment or supplies.

Objectives

- Define the key terms listed in this chapter
- Describe accident risk factors
- Describe the safety measures for preventing falls, burns, poisoning, and suffocation
- Explain how to prevent equipment accidents
- Identify fire prevention measures
- Explain what to do during a fire
- Describe how identifying the client, providing call bells, and using bed rails correctly promote client safety
- Explain how to protect yourself in the workplace

Key Terms

call bell
hazardous material
incident report
occurrence report
OH&S (occupational health and safety) legislation
suffocation
Workplace Hazardous Material Information System (WHMIS)
workplace violence

Outline

Safety

  I. INTRODUCTION

    A. Safety is a basic need

    B. In a safe setting, a person has little risk of illness or injury

    C. The person feels safe and secure physically

and mentally
  D. Your employer is also responsible for providing a safe working environment for you

II. ACCIDENT RISK FACTORS
  A. Awareness of surroundings
    1. Some persons are unconscious or in a coma
      a. Cannot react or respond to people, places, or things
    2. Confused and disoriented persons
      a. May not understand what is happening
      b. Can harm themselves and others
  B. Vision
    1. People with poor vision are at risk for falls
    2. Can trip on items
    3. Can take wrong medications, wrong doses, or poisons
  C. Hearing
    1. Hearing impaired persons have problems hearing explanations and instructions
    2. May not hear fire alarms, sirens, weather warnings, horns, and oncoming cars
      a. The person does not know to move to safety
  D. Smell, touch, and taste
    1. The person may have problems smelling smoke or gas
    2. They may have problems sensing heat or cold; can get burned
    3. Diminished taste and smell may cause someone to eat spoiled food or not smell a gas leak
  E. Impaired mobility
    1. Being unable to move out of danger is a serious risk
    2. Even minor changes (e.g. sore knee) could prevent a person from recovering from a stumble and they may fall
    3. Paralyzed persons may not sense pain, heat, or cold
    4. They may be unable to move to safety
  F. Medications
    1. Drugs have side effects
      a. Loss of balance, dizziness, lightheadedness, vision changes, confusion, etc.
  G. Age
    1. See Focus on Children
    2. See Focus on Older Adults
      a. Movements are slower and less steady
      b. Balance may be affected
      c. Decreased sensitivity to heat and cold
      d. Poor vision and hearing

      e. Decreased sense of smell

III. SAFETY MEASURES
  A. You must protect patients and residents, yourself, and co-workers from accidents and injuries
  B. Preventing falls—children
    1. Falls are the leading causes of injuries in children (see Box 16-1, p. 172)
  C. Preventing falls—older adults and others at risk
    1. Most falls occur in bedrooms and bathrooms
    2. Needing to urinate is a major cause of falls
    3. The risk of falling increases with age (see Box 16-2, p. 172)
      a. Most falls are in persons between the ages of 65 and 85
      b. A history of falls increases a person's risk
    4. Most falls occur in the evening
      a. Also during shift changes
    5. Accident risk factors are listed on p. 170 in the textbook
    6. Facilities have fall prevention programs.
    7. Box 16-3, p. 173 in the textbook, lists safety measures that prevent falls
    8. The nursing care plan lists measures for the person's specific risk factors
  D. Hand rails and grab bars (see Figure 16-4, p. 174)
    1. Provide support for persons who are weak or unsteady when walking
    2. Provide support for sitting down or getting up from the toilet
    3. Used when getting into and out of the tub
  E. Preventing burns
    1. Burns are a leading cause of death, especially among children and older persons
    2. Many burns to older adults occur in the kitchen; commonly caused by loose fitting sleeves dangling over the burner
    3. Next common cause is bathwater and heating pads
    4. Box 16-5, p. 176 in the textbook, lists safety measures to prevent burns
  F. Preventing poisoning
    1. Children are often victims of poisoning
    2. Aspirin, cigarette butts, vitamins, and household products are common poisons
    3. Poisoning in adults may be from carelessness, poor vision, confusion, or disorientation

4. Sometimes poisoning is a suicide attempt
5. Confused or disoriented adults may eat poisonous or contaminated food (see list on p. 174)
6. Box 16-4, p. 175 in the textbook, lists the safety measures that prevent poisoning

G. Preventing suffocation
1. Suffocation is when breathing stops from lack of oxygen
2. Common causes include choking on an object, drowning, inhaling gas or smoke, strangulation, electrical shock, and carbon monoxide poisoning
3. Children under 1 year of age and clients with serious mobility or mental impairements are at greatest risk
4. Box 16-6, p. 177 in the textbook, list-safety measures to help prevent suffocation

H. Preventing equipment accidents
1. All equipment is unsafe if broken, not used correctly, or not functioning properly
   a. Check glass and plastic items for cracks, chips, and sharp or rough edges
2. Do not use or give damaged items to patients or residents
3. Electrical equipment must work properly and be in good repair
   a. Frayed cords or overloaded outlets can cause electrical shocks (see Figure 16-7, p. 178)
   b. Three-pronged plugs are used on all electrical items (see Figure 16-9, p. 178)
      (1) Immediately report shocks
   c. Warning signs of faulty electrical items:
      (1) Shocks
      (2) Loss of power or power outage
      (3) Dimming or flickering of lights
      (4) Sparks
      (5) Sizzling or buzzing sounds
      (6) Burning odor
      (7) Loose plugs
4. Box 16-7, p. 178 in the textbook, lists safety measures to help prevent equipment accidents

IV. PREVENTING FIRES
A. The entire health team must prevent fires (see Box 16-8, p. 179)
1. They must act quickly and responsibly.

2. Oxygen systems are widely used in facilities and home care settings
3. Supplied through portable oxygen tanks, wall outlets, or oxygen concentrators (see Chapter 43)
4. Oxygen is highly flammable
5. Special safety measures are needed (see Box 16-9, p. 178)

B. Preventing fires
1. Box 16-8, p. 179 in the textbook, summarizes fire prevention measures
2. Focus on home care
   a. Smoke detectors are important
   b. Space heaters present fire hazards
      (1) Follow manufacturers instructions
      (2) Keep 3 feet away from curtains, drapes, and furniture
      (3) Do not place heaters where people walk
      (4) Protect yourself and others from burns
      (5) Keep heaters away from children and other persons
      (6) Keep heaters away from water
      (7) Make sure cords are in good repair
      (8) Do not leave heaters unattended
      (9) Store kerosene outside in the original container

C. What to do if a fire occurs
1. Know your agency's policies and procedures
2. Know the locations of fire alarms, fire extinguishers, and emergency exits
3. Facilities conduct fire drills to practice emergency fire procedures
4. Remember the word RACE when fire occurs
   a. R—rescue persons in immediate danger
   b. A—(alarm) sound the nearest alarm and notify the switchboard operator
   c. C—confine the fire by closing doors and windows; turn off oxygen or electrical equipment in the area of the fire
   d. E—(extinguish) use extinguishers on a small fire that has not spread
5. Clear equipment from all regular and emergency exits
6. See Focus on Home Care box, p. 179
7. Using a fire extinguisher
   a. Different extinguishers are used for

different kinds of fires
   b. Using a Fire Extinguisher ▶ p. 180
8. Evacuating
   a. Facilities have policies and proce-
      dures.
   b. Box 16-10, p. 181 in the textbook, de-
      scribes safety measures for both home
      and facility
   c. Persons closest to the danger are taken
      out first
   d. Those who can walk are given blan-
      kets and escorted to a safe place by a
      staff member
   e. Figure 16-11, p. 182 and Figure 16-12,
      p. 183 in the textbook, show how to
      rescue non-ambulatory persons
V. PROVIDING SAFE CARE DURING PROCE-
   DURES
   A. Identifying the client
      1. You must follow your employer's policies
         and procedures to identify clients as life
         and health are threatened if the wrong
         care is give.
      2. In the community you are providing care
         to only one person but make sure you
         have the right care plan with you
      3. In long term care facilities you will often
         get to know the residents over time, but
         until then, be sure to check the resident's
         name and room number before adminis-
         tering care; some facilities have photo
         IDs
      4. Know your employer's policies and pro-
         cedures
      5. In hospitals, patients have ID bracelets
         (see Figure 16-13, p. 184)
      6. Compare the name on the treatment card
         or assignment sheet with the name on the
         ID bracelet (see Figure 16-14, p. 184)
   B. Using the call bell
      1. A safety device that lets the client call for
         assistance
      2. Different facilities have different call sys-
         tems such as:
         a. Cord attached to the bed or chair with
            a button on its end (see Figure 16-15,
            p. 184)
         b. Pressing a button that switches on a
            light above door (see Figure 16-16A,
            p. 185) or connects to the intercom
            (see Figure 16-16B, p. 185)
         c. If the client has limited hand mobility,
            some devices can be activate by tap-

ping (see Figure 16-17, p. 185)
         d. If your clients cannot use a call system
            (due to confusion, or coma, etc.),
            check on them often and check care
            plan carefully for special communica-
            tion methods
         e. See Focus on Home Care box, p. 185
            in the textbook
         f. Whenever you leave the client's room
            (1) Keep the call bell within the
                client's reach or within reach of
                visitors and staff
            (2) Place the call bell on the client's
                strong side
            (3) Remind the client to use it when
                help is needed
            (4) Answer the call bell promptly
   C. Bed rails
      a. Bed rails are 1/2, 3/4, or full length
      b. Your supervisor and the care plan tell
         you when to raise bed rails
      c. They are necessary for persons who
         are unconscious or sedated.
      d. May be used for some confused or dis-
         oriented people.
         (1) If the person requires bed rails,
             the rails are always kept up, ex-
             cept when bedside care is being
             given
      e. Bed rails are hazards for persons trying
         to get out of bed without help (see
         Figure 16-20, p. 186)
      f. Gaps in bed rails can occur (Figure
         16-20, p. 186)
      g. If a client falls into a gap, an injury to
         the neck, head, chest, etc., may occur
      h. Sometimes, padding or gap protectors
         are used (see Figure 16-22, p. 187)
      i. Follow manufacturer and employer
         policy
      j. Form of environmental restraint (see
         Chapter 17).
      k. Must have the client's or substitute de-
         cision maker's consent
      l. Check the client frequently
VI. Promoting your personal safety
   A. Creating a safe workplace—each province
      has occupational health and safety (OH&S)
      legislation designed to protect employees
      from injuries and accidents in the workplace
      1. The name and details of the legislation
         vary across the country
      2. It assumes that all people in the work-

place are responsible for health and safety and have certain rights and duties

B. Responsibilities of the employer and the supervisor
1. They must take every reasonable precaution to protect your health and safety
2. See Focus on Home Care box, p. 187
3. Your employer is responsible for
   a. Having written policies that promote safety
   b. Training and educating you about these policies
   c. Creating a health and safety committee to identify hazards in the workplace and investigate accidents
   d. Respond to reports of hazards
   e. Warn you about hazards and correct when possible
   f. Report all accidents promptly to the government responsible for OH&S
   g. All necessary equipment is available and in working order

C. Employee's responsibilities
1. Follow all safety policies and procedures
2. Use recommended protective equipment and clothing
3. Report all safety hazards and concerns to your supervisor
4. Complete an incident report, which once completed is submitted to your employer (see Box 16-11, p. 188)
5. You have the right to refuse to do unsafe work but can not refuse to work if the danger is a normal part of the job or refusing to work could endanger the client

D. Reducing personal security risks
1. Workplace violence is any physical assault or threatening behaviour that occurs in a work setting
2. Home care workers are at risk due to the fact that they work alone
3. Clients, family members, or any person in the home could turn violent
4. Box 16-12, p. 191 in the textbook, lists personal safety measurers you should always follow

VII. HANDLING HAZARDOUS SUBSTANCES
A. OH&S requires that health care employees understand the risks of hazardous substances and how to handle them safely
B. A hazardous substance is any chemical that presents a physical hazard or a health hazard in the workplace

C. Exposure can occur under normal working conditions or during certain emergencies
D. Hazardous substances include:
1. Drugs used in cancer therapy
2. Gases used to give anesthesia
3. Gases used to sterilize equipment
4. Oxygen
5. Disinfectants and cleaning solutions
6. Mercury (found in some thermometers and blood pressure devices)
E. Labels
1. WHMIS labels provide information for safe handling (Figure 16-23 and Figure 16-24, p. 189)
2. Supplier (or manufacturer) applies label; or the employer, if they make the product
3. Warning labels include
   a. product information
   b. supplier information
   c. hazard symbols
   d. risk factors
   e. precautionary statements
   f. first aid measures
   g. references to the MSDS

Classroom Activities

1. Introduce the topic of safety.
   a. Write the word "SAFETY" on the chalkboard.
   b. Ask students to define safety and a safe environment. Write their answers on the board.

2. Display a list of the following accident risk factors on an overhead transparency. Use it as a basis for discussion.
   a. Awareness of surroundings
   b. Vision
   c. Hearing
   d. Smell and touch
   e. Paralysis
   f. Medications
   g. Age

3. Ask students to identify and discuss:
   a. Common causes of falls.
   b. Factors that increase the risk of falls.
      (i) Display Box 16-2, p. 172 in the textbook, on an overhead transparency as a basis for discussion.
   c. Safety measures to prevent falls.
      (i) Display Box 16-1, p. 172 in the textbook, on an overhead transparency as a basis for discussion.

4. Divide students into groups of three. Ask each group to discuss the use of bed rails. Tell them to write the answers to the following questions on a piece of notebook paper. Allow 10 minutes. Then call on students from each group to answer the questions. Clarify any wrong answers.
   a. Are bed rails considered a restraint? Explain.
   b. When are bed rails used?
   c. What safety precautions are taken when bed rails are used?

5. Using the information in Boxes 9-4, 9-5, and 9-6 in the textbook discuss safety measures to prevent burns, poisoning, and suffocation. Encourage students to ask questions.

6. Write the following on the chalkboard: "Warning signs of faulty electrical equipment."
   a. Call on students to list the signs. Write the correct answers on the chalkboard.

7. Invite a representative from OH&S to discuss:
   a. The requirements for handling hazardous substances
      (1) Encourage students to ask questions
      (2) Ask students to write down key points in a notebook

8. Invite a representative from the fire department to:
   a. Discuss fire safety in the home and in health care settings.
   b. Demonstrate the proper use of a fire extinguisher.
      (1) Ask students to write key points in a notebook.
      (2) Allow time for questions and discussion.

9. Invite a representative from the police department to discuss:
   a. Workplace violence.
   b. Personal safety practices.
      (1) Encourage students to ask questions.

10. Discuss the importance of reporting accidents and errors.

Homework Assignments

Ask students to answer the questions at the end of Chapter 16 in the textbook. Tell students the date and time that this assignment must be completed and turned in.

If the accompanying workbook is being used, assign the Chapter 16 workbook exercises. Tell students the date and time that this assignment must be completed and turned in.

Chapter 16 Student Assignment

Name _____

Date _____

Safety

Write your answers in the spaces provided.

1. List medication side effects that increase a person's risk for falls.

   a. _____

   b. _____

   c. _____

   d. _____

   e. _____

   f. _____

   g. _____

   h. _____

   i. _____

2. Common causes of burns are:

   a. _____

   b. _____

   c. _____

   d. _____

   e. _____

3. Common causes of suffocation include:

   a. _____

   b. _____

   c. _____

   d. _____

   e. _____

4. What safety precautions are practiced where oxygen is used and stored?

   a. _____

   b. _____

   c. _____

   d. _____

   e. _____

   f. _____

   g. _____

   h. _____

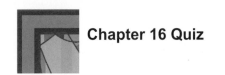

Chapter 16 Quiz

Name _____

Date _____

Safety

True or False	Multiple Choice

Mark **T** *for true or* **F** *for false.*

1. _____ The physical changes of aging decrease the older person's risk for injury.

2. _____ Most falls occur in bedrooms and bathrooms.

3. _____ The bed is in the lowest horizontal position except when giving bedside care.

4. _____ Bed rails are safe for patients trying to get out of bed without help.

5. _____ Aspirin and household products are common poisons.

6. _____ Pillows are used to position infants.

7. _____ Calling the person by name is a safe way to identify the person.

8. _____ Bed wheels are unlocked when giving bedside care.

9. _____ Two-pronged cords are used on all electrical equipment.

10. _____ Assaults are uncommon in health care settings.

11. _____ If you feel threatened in a person's home, you should leave and call your supervisor.

Circle the BEST answer.

12. You notice a frayed electrical cord on a patient's bed. You should:
   a. Call someone to fix it.
   b. Report it to the nurse immediately.
   c. Tell the patient.
   d. Report it at the end of your shift.

13. You must check the MSDS before:
   a. Using a hazardous substance.
   b. Cleaning up a leak or spill.
   c. Disposing of the substance.
   d. All of the above.

14. Which practice does not promote safety where oxygen is used?
   a. Turning electrical equipment off after it is unplugged.
   b. Removing smoking materials from the room.
   c. "No Smoking" signs.
   d. Removing wool blankets and synthetic fibers from the person's room.

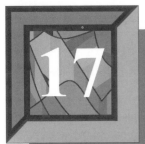

Restraint Alternatives and Safe Restraint Use

Instructor's Preparation

I. Read Chapter 17 in the textbook. Carefully review chapter objectives, key terms, and review questions.

II. Read the outline in Chapter 17 of the instructor's guide. Carefully review the classroom activities, the student assignment, and the quiz.

III. If you are using the accompanying student workbook, review the activities for Chapter 27.

IV. Gather all necessary supplies and equipment for classroom activities and student assignments.

    A. Prepare the correct number of handouts

    B. Gather appropriate flip charts

    C. Prepare overhead transparencies

    D. Prepare situation/index cards

    E. Gather correct video

    F. Gather coloured markers

    G. Gather any other items that will be needed for classroom activities

    H. Assemble items in the order they will be used

V. Make sure that the necessary equipment is available and in good working order.

Objectives

- Define the key terms listed in this chapter
- Describe the purpose of using restraints
- Describe complications from restraint use
- Identify restraint alternatives
- Demonstrate how to use restraints safely

Key Terms

chemical restraints
environmental restrains
physical restraints
restraint

Outline

Restraint Alternatives and Safe Restraint Use

I. INTRODUCTION

    A. Used to protect people from harming themselves or others

    B. Every effort is made to protect clients without using restraints

    C. They can cause emotional harm and physical injury and should only be used as a last resort

    D. Restraints require a physician's order and the RN will teach you how to apply the restraints properly and safely

        1. Support workers never decide if restraints

are to be used.
II. USE OF RESTRAINTS IN CANADA
   A. Use of restraints is a sensitive issue
      1. Current research shows that restraints may cause more harm than good
      2. People who are restrained show signs of severe emotional distress and their quality of life suffers
      3. Canadian hospitals and long-term care facilities have strict limits on the use of restraints and have written policies and procedures based on legal guidelines and standards
      4. Generally facilities have a "least restraint policy"
      5. Restraints are never used for discipline, punishment, or staff convenience
      6. Restraints are not used in community settings; physicians will recommend admission to a facility if the client is at risk for harming themselves or others
      7. Restraints are used only when necessary to treat a client's medical symptoms
      8. There are often causes and reasons for harmful behaviours
      9. The health care team must determine the cause of harmful behaviour and all alternatives to restraints (see Box 17-1, p. 196).
      10. If the alternatives to restraints do not protect the client, the physician may, as a last resort, order restraints
   B. Types of restraints
      1. Physical restraints—garments or devices used to restrict movement of the whole body or parts of the body
      2. Environmental restraints—barriers, furniture or devices that prevent free movement (see Figure 17-4, p. 197, and Bed Rails, Chapter 16)
      3. Chemical restraints—medications used to control behaviour or movement not otherwise required for the person's medical condition
III. COMPLICATIONS OF RESTRAINT USE
   A. Box 17-2, p. 197 in the textbook, lists complications from restraint use
   B. Injuries can occur when people try to free themselves, when the wrong restraint is used, or if the restraint not applied correctly
   C. Most serious risk is death from strangulation
   D. Many emotional effects to the client such as loss of dignity, self-esteem, embarrassment,

anger and depression
   E. See Providing Compassionate Care box, p. 198
IV. SAFETY GUIDELINES
   A. The least restrictive method is chosen, which allows the greatest amount of movement possible
   B. Follow the safety measures listed in Box 17-3, p. 199 in the textbook
   C. Always remember:
      1. Restraints are used to protect the client, not for staff convenience or discipline
      2. Restraints require a physician's order
      3. Use the least restrictive method
      4. Use restraints only after all other alternatives have been tried
      5. Unnecessary restraints is false imprisonment (see Chapter 10)
      6. Informed consent is needed
      7. Manufacturer's instructions must be followed
      8. Restraints are applied by knowledgeable workers
      9. The client's basic needs are met
      10. More than one staff member may be needed to safely apply the restraint
      11. Quality of life is protected
      12. The client is observed every 15 minutes, or more often, as required by the care plan
      13. The restraint is removed, the client is repositioned, and basic needs are met at least every 2 hours
      14. Information about restraints is recorded in the client's chart
   D. When caring for a restrained client, you need to report verbally (to your supervisor) or record on the chart the following information:
      1. Type of restraint used
      2. Reason for application
      3. Safety measures taken
      4. Time applied
      5. Time remove
      6. Care given when restrained
      7. Skin colour and condition
      8. Pulse felt in restrained part
      9. Complaints of pain, numbness, tingling (report these immediately)
V. APPLYING PHYSICAL RESTRAINTS
   A. Wrist restraints
      1. Limit movements of arms
   B. Mitt restraints
      1. Prevent finger use, but do not prevent

hand, wrist, or arm movements (see Figure 17-15, p. 203)
C. Vest and jacket restraints are applied to the chest
   1. Are always applied over a gown, pajamas, or clothes
   2. The person cannot get out of the bed or chair
   3. Jacket restraints have sleeves
   4. Vest restraints always cross in front
   5. Death can occur from strangulation
     a. You are advised to only assist the nurse in its application (see Figure 17-6, p. 200)
D. Belt restraints
   1. Used for the same reasons as vest restraints
   2. Always applied over clothes, a gown, or pajamas (see Figure 17-16, p. 204)
E. Elbow restraints
   1. The person cannot bend the elbows (see Figure 17-17, p. 205)

Classroom Activities

1. Introduce the subject of restraints. It is very important that students understand the guidelines for restraint use.
   a. Display the definition of a restraint on an overhead transparency. Use this as a basis for discussion.
   b. Call on students to answer the following questions:
     (1) When are restraints used?
     (2) What is meant by "staff convenience?"
     (3) When are drugs considered a chemical restraint?
   c. Divide students into two groups. Provide each group with several sheets of notebook paper. Ask one group to discuss and list the complications of restraints. Ask the other group to discuss and list restraint alternatives. Allow each group 15 minutes.
     (1) Call on one student from each group to report to the class. Encourage students to ask questions and provide additional input.

2. Have available the types of restraints described in this chapter.
   a. Ask students to handle each type. Encourage students to ask questions about the use and application of each type of restraint.
   b. Use the procedure checklists provided.
     (1) Demonstrate each procedure. Have each student practice and perform a return demonstration of each procedure.
     (2) During the return demonstrations on application of restraints, have each student take a turn being the patient or resident. Ask each student to be restrained for 15 to 20 minutes. Then discuss the following:
       (a) How did the restraint feel?
       (b) Did the student feel safe and secure?
       (c) Were self-esteem needs met? How?

Homework Assignments

Ask students to answer the questions at the end of Chapter 17 in the textbook. Tell students the date and time that this assignment must be completed and turned in.

If the accompanying workbook is being used, assign the Chapter 17 workbook exercises. Tell students the date and time that this assignment must be completed and turned in.

Name _____

Date _____

Restraint Alternatives and Safe Restraint Use

Write your answers in the spaces provided.

1. List 6 complications of restraint use.
   a. _____
   b. _____
   c. _____
   d. _____
   e. _____
   f. _____

2. Restraints are never used to:
   a. _____
   b. _____
   c. _____

3. List 10 safety measures when using restraints:
   a. _____
   b. _____
   c. _____
   d. _____
   e. _____
   f. _____
   g. _____
   h. _____
   i. _____
   j. _____

Match the description with the correct restraint.

a. active physical restraint
b. chemical restraint
c. vest restraint
d. passive physical restraint
e. geriatric chair
f. mitt restraint
g. wrist restraint

4. ____ A drug that is given to treat the individual's behaviour

5 ____ An attached tray to keep the individual from getting up

6. ____ Hands are covered to prevent the individual from removing a dressing

7. ____ If this is applied incorrectly, the individual can strangle or suffocate

8. ____ With this restraint, skin and circulation should be checked every 15 minutes

9. ____ This restraint attaches an individual's body to a non-movable object

10. ____ This restraint does not restrict freedom and allows access to certain body parts

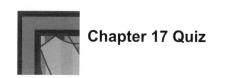

Chapter 17 Quiz

Name _____

Date _____

Restraint Alternatives and Safe Restraint Use

True or False

*Mark **T** for true or **F** for false.*

1. _____ Restraints are safe and are always used to prevent falls.

2. _____ Restraints are used only after trying all other alternatives.

3. _____ Restraints can increase a person's confusion and agitation.

4. _____ Vest restraints always cross in the front.

5. _____ Some medications are restraints.

6. _____ An RN can decide that a restraint is needed.

7. _____ Support workers can decide to put on a restraint if the resident is not co-operating in their care.

8. _____ Informed consent must be obtained from the client or substitute decision maker before a restraint can by used.

Multiple Choice

Circle the BEST answer.

9. A restraint attached to the person's body and a stationary object is a :
   a. chemical restraint
   b. passive physical restraint
   c. active physical restraint
   d. full bed rail

10. Which is not a safety measure for using a restraint?
    a. use the correct size of restraint
    b. use a sheet to restrain a person on the toilet
    c. crisscross vest restraints in front
    d. position the person in good body alignment before applying the restraint.

11. When applying a physical restraint, you
    a. must have physician's consent
    b. must have client or family consent
    c. tie in a slipknot
    d. use whatever restraint is available
    e. a and b
    f. a, b, and c
    g. a, b, and d

Preventing Infection

Instructor's Preparation

I. Read Chapter 18 in the textbook. Carefully review chapter objectives, key terms, and review questions.

II. Read the outline in Chapter 18 of the instructor's guide. Carefully review the classroom activities, the student assignment, and the quiz.

III. If you are using the accompanying student workbook, review the activities for Chapter 18.

IV. Review appropriate sections of video # 1, in Mosby's Nursing Assisting Video Series.

V. Gather all necessary supplies and equipment for classroom activities and student assignments.
- A. Prepare appropriate flip charts
- B. Prepare overhead transparencies
- C. Gather correct video
- D. Gather the following transparencies: TA27, TA28
- E. Gather coloured markers
- F. Gather all equipment and supplies needed to demonstrate and have each student return demonstrate the procedures in this chapter
- G. Gather any other items that will be needed for classroom activities
- H. Assemble items in the order they will be used

VI. Make sure that the necessary equipment is available and in good working order.

VII. Contact guest speakers to confirm the day, date, time, and location that they are expected.
- A. Ask the speakers if they require any special equipment or supplies; make sure these are available.

Objectives

- Define the key terms listed in this chapter
- Distinguish between pathogens and nonpathogens.
- Explain what microbes need to live and grow.
- Recognize the signs and symptoms of infection
- Describe the chain of infection
- List ways in which microbes are transmitted
- List risk factors for infection
- Describe common aseptic practices
- Explain why hand washing is so important
- Describe when to wash your hands and general guidelines for hand washing
- Describe cleaning, disinfection, and sterilization methods
- Understand the principles and practices of Standard Precautions and Transmission-Based Precautions
- Explain how to use personal protective equipment (PPE)
- Describe the principles and practices of surgical asepsis
- Perform the procedures described in this chapter

Key Terms

asepsis
aseptic techniques
biohazardous waste
clean technique
communicable disease
contagious disease
contamination
disinfection
infection
infection control
isolation precautions
medical asepsis
microbe
microorganism
multi-resistant organism (MRO)
nonpathogen
nosocomial infection
pathogen
personal protective equipment (PPE)
reservoir
Routine Practices
sharp
Standard Precautions
sterile
sterile field
sterile technique
sterilization
surgical asepsis
vaccine
transmission-based precautions

Outline

Preventing Infection

I. INTRODUCTION
   A. Infection is a major safety and health hazard
   B. Some infections cause only minor symptoms while other are serious.
   C. May delay recovery, create long-term problems or cause death.
   D. Older adults, people who are ill and people with disabilities are at great risk.
   E. Easily spread.
   F. All health care members must protect clients and themselves from infection.
   G. Must follow your employer's infection control policies.
II. MICROORGANISMS (microbes)
   A. A microbe is a small living plant or animal seen only with a microscope
      1. Microbes are everywhere
   B. Pathogens are microbes that are harmful and cause infection
   C. Nonpathogens are microbes that do not usually cause infection
   D. Types of microbes
      1. Bacteria are microscopic plant life that multiply rapidly
         a. Often called germs
      2. Fungi are plants that live on other plants or animals
      3. Protozoa are microscopic one-celled animals
      4. Rickettsiae are microscopic forms of life found in insects
         a. Transmitted to humans by insect bites
      5. Viruses are extremely small microscopic organisms that grow in living cells
   E. Requirements of microbes
      1. A reservoir or host is the environment where a microbe lives and grows
         a. Microbes get water and nourishment from the reservoir
         b. Most microbes need oxygen to live
         c. A warm, dark environment is needed
         d. Most microbes are destroyed by heat and light
   F. Normal flora
      1. Microbes that usually live and grow in a certain area
      2. When a nonpathogen is transmitted from its natural site to another site or host, it becomes a pathogen
   G. Multi-resistant organisms
      1. Bacteria reproduce very quickly and in

large numbers, they can change to protect themselves from antibiotics (known as MROs), and certain strains of bacteria are now very difficult to treat

    a. Becoming increasingly common

    b. Serious threat to patients and residents in health care facilities, and can be fatal

    c. Easily spread

    d. The two most common are MRSA (methicillin-resistant *Staphylococcus aureus*) and VRE (vancomycin-resistant *Enterococci*)

    e. You will be trained to follow special precautions when in contact with clients with these infections

III. THE SPREAD OF PATHOGENS

    A. A disease state resulting from the invasion and growth of microbes in the body

    B. A local infection is in one part of the body

    C. A systemic infection involves the whole body

    D. Box 18-1, p. 212 in the textbook, lists signs and symptoms of infection (see Focus on Older Adults box, p. 212)

       1. Pathogens do not always cause infections

    E. The chain of infection (see Figure 18-1, p. 213)

       1. Infection is a process involving:

          a. A pathogen—a microbe capable of causing disease

          b. A reservoir—a place for the pathogen to grow and multiply

          c. A portal of exit—a path the pathogen uses to leave the reservoir (e.g., respiratory, GI, urinary, and reproductive tracts; breaks in the skin; and blood)

          d. Methods of transmission—how the pathogen travels from the portal of exit to the next reservoir or host (see Figure 18-1, p. 214)

          e. A portal of entry—where the pathogen enters the new host's body

          f. A susceptible host—a person at risk for infection is needed for the microbe to grow and multiply

       2. Ability to resist infection depends on age, nutritional status, stress, fatigue, general health, medications, and presence of disease or injury (see Box 18-2, p. 215)

    F. Nosocomial infection

       1. An infection acquired during a stay at a hospital, health-care facility, or community setting

       2. Caused by normal flora or by pathogens transmitted from another source

       3. Microbes can enter the body through equipment used in treatments, therapies, and diagnostic tests

       4. Staff can transfer microbes

       5. Most common infections within health care settings include respiratory tract infections, urinary tract infections, gastrointestinal tract infection and skin infections.

       6. Sick, frail, and older clients have a hard time fighting infections

       7. The following help prevent the spread:

          a. Medical asepsis

          b. Isolation precautions

          c. Surgical asepsis

       8. The health team must prevent the spread of nosocomial infection by practicing:

          a. Medical and surgical asepsis

          b. Isolation precautions

IV. MEDICAL ASEPSIS

    A. Asepsis is being free of disease-producing microbes

    B. Medical asepsis (clean technique)

       1. Prevent the spread of microbes from one person or place to another

       2. The number of pathogens is reduced

    C. Surgical asepsis (sterile technique)

       1. Practices that keep equipment and supplies free of all microbes

       2. Sterile means the absence of all microbes

       3. Sterilization is the process that destroys all microbes

       4. Both pathogens and nonpathogens are destroyed

    D. Contamination is the process of being exposed to pathogens

    E. Hand washing

       1. Handwashing with soap and water is the easiest and most important way to prevent the spread of infection (see Box 18-4, p. 216)

       2. Wash your hands before and after giving care (see Box 18-3, p. 215)

       3. Focus on Home Care box, p. 217 in the textbook, discusses hand washing

       4. Handwashing ▶ p.218

    F. Care of supplies and equipment

       1. Single use, disposable items are discarded after use

       3. Some items (bedpans, urinals, water pitchers, etc.) are reused by the same client and must be decontaminated

5. Cleaning
   a. Removes debris and organic material
   b. Follow these guidelines:
      (1) Wear personal protective equipment
      (2) Rinse the item in cold water first
      (3) Wash the item with soap and hot water
      (4) Scrub thoroughly; use a brush if necessary
      (5) Rinse the item in warm water
      (6) Dry the item
      (7) Disinfect or sterilize the item
      (8) Disinfect equipment and the sink used in cleaning
      (9) Discard personal protective equipment
6. Disinfection
   a. The process of destroying pathogens—except spores
   b. Spores are killed by extremely high temperatures
   c. Germicides are disinfectants applied to skin, tissues, and nonliving objects
   d. Chemical disinfectants are used to clean nondisposable items
      (1) They can burn and irritate the skin
      (2) Wear utility gloves or rubber household gloves to prevent skin irritation
      (3) Check the MSDS before handling a disinfectant (see Chapter 16)
   e. Focus on home care
      (1) Detergents and hot water are common disinfectants
      (2) Many commercial products are available
      (3) Vinegar can also be used
7. Sterilization
   a. Destroys all nonpathogens and pathogens including spores
   b. Very high temperatures are used
      (1) Boiling water, radiation, liquid or gas chemicals, dry heat, and steam under pressure are methods
   c. Focus on home care
      (1) Boiling water is a simple way to sterilize items in the home
G. Other aseptic measures
   1. Box 18-5, p. 220 in the textbook, lists aseptic measures useful in home, work, and everyday activities

V. ISOLATION PRECAUTIONS
   A. Sometimes barriers are needed to prevent the escape of pathogens
   B. The Centers for Disease Control and Prevention (CDC) has guidelines for isolation precautions
      1. These precautions have been accepted by Health Canada and are currently in use in most Canadian health care facilities and community care agencies
      2. They recognize that all body fluids, including blood, secretions, and excretions, can transmit pathogens
      3. Two tiers are practiced—Standard Precautions and Transmission-Based Precautions
      4. Standard Precautions and Transmission-Based Precautions prevent the spread of communicable or contagious diseases
   C. Isolation precautions are based on clean and dirty
      1. Clean areas or objects are not contaminated
      2. Dirty areas or objects are contaminated
      3. If a clean area or object has contact with something dirty, it is contaminated
      4. Clean and dirty also depend on how the pathogen is spread
   D. Standard Precautions
      1. Box 18-7, p. 222 in the textbook, explains precautions
      2. Used in the care of all persons
      3. They prevent the spread of infection from:
         a. Blood
         b. All body fluids, secretions, and excretions (except sweat)
         c. Nonintact skin
         d. Mucous membranes
   E. Transmission-Based Precautions
      1. Highly contagious infections
      2. Additional isolation precautions are required to protect staff, visitors and other clients
      3. These precautions are followed in addition to Standard Precautions
      4. Three types—Airborne Precautions, Droplet Precautions, and Contact Precautions (see Box 18-8, p. 223) the one used depends on how the pathogen is spread

5. You must understand how certain infections are spread (see Table 18-1, p. 214)
6. The rules in Box 18-9, p. 224 in the textbook, are a guide for giving safe care
7. Your employer may have these or other guidelines
8. Know your policies

F. Protective measures
1. Box 18-9, p. 224 in the textbook, lists guidelines for giving safe care when isolation precautions are used
2. Standard Precautions and Transmission-Based Precautions involve wearing personal protective equipment (gloves, mask, gown, and/or eye protection)
3. Your supervisor and employer policy will guide you about when to use PPE
4. Box 18-10, p. 224 in the textbook, lists the proper order for putting on and taking off a full set of PPE
5. Wearing gloves
   a. Wear gloves whenever contact with blood, body fluids, secretions or excretions, mucous membranes, and nonintact skin is likely
   b. Gloves are not required for most routine care activities
   c. Some people are allergic to latex gloves, which can cause skin rashes, asthma, shock, difficulty breathing, and other ractions
   d. If you or your client are allergic, wear latex-free gloves
   e. Be sure you do not tear gloves when putting them on
   f. Remember the following about wearing gloves:
      (1) Gloves are easier to put on when your hands are dry
      (2) You need a new pair for every person
      (3) Remove and discard torn, cut, or punctured gloves immediately
      (4) Wear gloves only once
      (5) Put on clean gloves before touching mucous membranes or nonintact skin
      (6) Put on new gloves when gloves become contaminated
      (7) Make sure gloves cover your wrists; if you wear a gown, gloves must cover the cuffs

      (8) Remove gloves so the inside part is on the outside
      (9) Wash your hands after removing gloves
   d. Removing Gloves ▶ p. 225
6. Wearing masks and respiratory protection
   a. Masks prevent the spread of microbes from the respiratory tract
      (1) Used for airborne and droplet precautions
      (2) Disposable masks are used
      (3) A wet or moist mask is contaminated
      (4) Apply a new mask when contamination occurs
      (5) A mask should fit snugly over the nose and mouth
      (6) Wash your hands before putting on a mask
      (7) Only touch the ties during removal
      (8) Respiratory protection refers to special face masks that filter the air
      (9) The N95 respirator is an example (see Figure 18-12, p. 227)
      (10) Such protection is used for clients under airborne isolation
      (11) Follow employer policy
   b. Wearing a Mask ▶ p. 227
7. Wearing eye protection and face shields
   a. Protect the mucous membranes of your eyes, nose, and mouth from the person's pathogens (see Figure 18-9, p. 223)
   b. You may need protection when giving care, cleaning instruments, or disposing of contaminated fluids
   c. Discard disposable eye wear after use
   d. Reusable eye wear is cleaned before reuse
8. Bagging items
   a. Contaminated items are bagged to remove them from the person's room
   b. Leakproof plastic bags are used
      (1) They are labeled with the biohazardous symbol
   c. Biohazardous waste is items contaminated with blood, body fluids, secretions, or excretions (see Figure 18-15, p. 231)

d. Follow employer policy for bagging and transporting linen
   (1) Do not overfill bags
   (2) Tie the bag securely
e. Trash also is placed in a container labeled with the biohazardous symbol
   (1) Follow agency policy for bagging and transporting trash, equipment, and supplies
f. One bag is usually adequate
g. Double bagging
   (1) Two staff members are needed
   (2) The person in the room places contaminated items into a bag; the bag is sealed securely
   (3) The person outside the room holds open another bag with a wide cuff to protect hands from contamination
   (4) The contaminated bag is placed in the clean bag at the doorway
   (5) Double Bagging (see Figure 18-16, p. 231)

9. Wearing protective apparel (gowns, plastic aprons, shoe covers, boots, and leg coverings)
a. Gowns
   (1) Must completely cover clothing
   (2) Sleeves are long with tight cuffs
   (3) Open at the back
   (4) The inside and neck are clean
   (5) The outside and waist strings are contaminated
   (6) They are used only once
   (7) A wet gown is contaminated
b. Donning and Removing a Gown ▶ p. 229

10. Transporting persons
a. Special treatments or tests may require transporting the person to another area
b. A safe transport means that other persons, staff, and visitors are protected from infection
c. Guidelines for safe transport are listed on p. 232 in the textbook

G. Basic needs and Transmission-Based Precautions
1. Love, belonging, and self-esteem needs are often unmet
2. Visitors and staff often avoid the person
a. Wearing protective apparel takes extra effort

b. Fears about getting the disease are common
3. Self-esteem easily suffers
4. Sometimes visitors and staff may unknowingly make the person feel ashamed and guilty about having a contagious disease
5. How to help:
a. Remember that the pathogen is undesirable, not the person
b. Treat the person with respect, kindness, and dignity
c. Provide reading materials
d. Provide hobby materials if possible
e. Place a clock in the room
f. Encourage use of the telephone
g. Provide a current TV guide
h. Organize your work so you have time to visit
i. Say hello from the doorway often
6. Remember to disinfect or discard items that become contaminated
7. Focus on children
a. Infants and children do not understand isolation
b. Simple explanations are given to the child
c. Let the child see your face before putting on a mask or goggles
d. Say hello and tell the child your name
8. Focus on older persons
a. Personal protective equipment may increase confusion in persons with confusion and dementia
   (1) Let the person see your face when possible
   (2) Tell the person who you are and what you are going to do
   (3) Report signs and symptoms of confusion to the nurse
9. Focus on home care
a. Standard Precautions are always practiced
b. Sometimes Transmission-Based Pprecautions are needed

VI. SURGICAL ASEPSIS (STERILE TECHNIQUE)
A. Sterile technique is the practices that keep equipment and supplies free of all microbes
B. Is required anytime the skin or sterile tissues are penetrated (catharization, IV, suctioning)
C. Support workers are not normally authorized

to do these procedures, but they may be delegated to you

D. Principles of surgical asepsis
   1. Sterile gloves are needed
   2. You wear personal protective equipment as needed
   3. For sterile procedures, all items in contact with the person are kept sterile
   4. If any item is contaminated, the person is at risk for infection
   5. Maintain a sterile field (a work area free of pathogens and nonpathogens)
   6. Box 18-11, p. 233 in the textbook, lists the principles and practices of surgical asepsis
      a. Follow them to maintain a sterile field

E. Donning and removing sterile gloves
   1. Sterile gloves are put on after setting up the sterile field
      a. After putting on sterile gloves, you can handle sterile items within the sterile field
      b. Touch nothing outside the sterile field
   2. Always keep sterile gloved hands above your waist and within your vision
   3. If gloves become contaminated, remove them and put on a new pair
   4. Replace gloves that are torn, cut, or punctured
   5. Donning and Removing Sterile Gloves ▶ p. 234

Classroom Activities

1. Write on the chalkboard: "Infection is a major safety and health hazard."
   a. Discuss the role the support worker plays in infection control.
   b. Call on students to define the following terms:
      (1) Microbe
      (2) Pathogen
      (3) Nonpathogen
      (4) Normal flora
      (5) Infection
      (6) Nosocomial infection
      Explain to students the importance of learning these definitions.

2. Display an overhead transparency showing the chain of infection. Use this as a basis for discussion.

a. Call on students to describe common aseptic practices used in daily activities to prevent infection and the spread of microbes.

3. Show the following sections of video #1 in Mosby's Nursing Assisting Video Series:
   a. Infection precautions
   b. Handwashing
   c. Rules of Universal Precautions
   d. Isolation procedures
   e. Double bag technique
      (1) Ask students to write down key points in a notebook for future reference.
      (2) Allow time for questions and discussion following each portion of the video.

4. Write the following terms on the chalkboard:
   a. Medical asepsis
   b. Surgical asepsis
   c. Isolation Precautions
   d. The Bloodborne Pathogen Standard
   e. Contamination

Call on students to define and discuss each term. Write the correct answers on the chalkboard.

Clarify any wrong answers. Stress the importance of understanding the meaning of these terms.

5. Call on students to define the differences among cleaning, disinfecting, and sterilizing.

6. Ask students to identify and discuss the difference between Standard Precautions and Transmission-based Precautions.
   a. Write on a flip chart: "Standard Precautions prevent the spread of infection from:
      (1) _____
      (2) _____
      (3) _____
      (4) _____

Call on students to provide the answers. Write in the correct answers. Clarify any wrong answers.

7. Divide students into groups of three. Ask students to discuss how it might feel to be in isolation. Ask

them to identify ways to meet the person's needs for love, belonging, and self-esteem. Allow 15 minutes for discussion

a. Call on one student from each group to report to the class. Allow time for questions and discussion.

b. Ask them to include any special needs of children and older persons.

Homework Assignments

Ask students to answer the questions at the end of Chapter 18 in the textbook. Tell students the date and time that this assignment must be completed and turned in.

If the accompanying student workbook is being used, assign the Chapter 18 workbook exercises. Tell students the date and time that this assignment must be completed and turned in.

Preventing Infection

Write your answers in the blanks provided.

1. List the signs and symptoms of infection.

   a. _____

   b. _____

   c. _____

   d. _____

   e. _____

   f. _____

   g. _____

   h. _____

   i. _____

   j. _____

   k. _____

   l. _____

2. Define these terms:

   a. Exposure incident— _____

   _____

   b. Parenteral— _____

   _____

   c. Source individual— _____

   _____

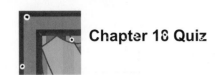

Name _____

Date _____

Preventing Infection

True or False

Mark **T** *for true or* **F** *for false.*

1. _____ To properly wash your hands, hold your hands and forearms higher than your elbows throughout the procedure.

2. _____ Clean technique keeps equipment and supplies free of all microbes.

3. _____ A systemic infection involves the whole body.

4. _____ Transmission-based Precautions are used in the care of all persons.

5. _____ The easiest and most important way to prevent the spread of infection is surgical asepsis.

6. _____ A wet gown is contaminated.

7. _____ Gloves are easier to put on when hands are wet.

8. _____ Wash your hands before putting on a mask.

9. _____ Wear gloves to pick up broken glass with your hands.

Multiple Choice

Circle the BEST answer.

10. A microbe that is harmful and causes infection is:
    a. A reservoir.
    b. A pathogen.
    c. A nonpathogen.
    d. Normal flora.

11. An infection acquired during a stay in a health care agency is a:
    a. Communicable disease.
    b. Nosocomial infection.
    c. Nonpathogen.
    d. Hepatitis infection.

12. The process of becoming unclean is:
    a. Asepsis.
    b. Disinfection.
    c. Contamination.
    d. Immunity.

13. The process of cleaning:
    a. Removes debris and organic materials.
    b. Destroys pathogens.
    c. Destroys spores.
    d. Uses very high temperature.

14. An item contaminated with blood, body fluids, secretions, and excretions that may be harmful to others is called:
    a. Biohazardous waste.
    b. A microorganism.
    c. Droplet precaution.
    d. Personal protective equipment.

15. Masks prevent the spread of microbes from:
    a. The gastrointestinal tract.
    b. The skin.
    c. The respiratory tract.
    d. All of the above.

16. Mrs. Adams is in isolation. Which is incorrect?
    a. Say hello from the doorway often.
    b. Treat her with respect, kindness, and dignity.
    c. Provide hobby materials if possible.
    d. Spend as little time in her room as possible.

19

Abuse

Instructor's Preparation

I. Read Chapter 19 in the textbook. Carefully review chapter objectives, key terms, and review questions.

II. Read the outline in Chapter 19 of the instructor's guide. Carefully review the classroom activities, the student assignment, and the quiz.

III. If you are using the accompanying student workbook, review the activities for Chapter 19.

IV. Gather all necessary supplies and equipment for classroom activities and student assignments.

   A. Prepare the correct number of handouts

   B. Prepare a ppropriate flip charts

   C. Prepare overhead transparencies

   D. Prepare situation/index cards

   E. Gather correct video

   F. Gather coloured markers

   G. Gather any other items that will be needed for classroom activities

   H. Assemble items in the order they will be used

V. Make sure that the necessary equipment is available and in good working order.

Objectives

- Define the key terms listed in this chapter
- Describe the types of abuse
- Describe the cycle of abuse
- Describe spousal abuse, child abuse, and abuse of older adults
- Describe how clients and health care workers can be abused
- Explain what to do if you have an abusive client
- Identify signs of abuse
- Explain your legal responsibilities when reporting abuse
- Describe what to do if a client tells you that he or she is being abused

Key Terms

abuse
ageism
emotional abuse
financial abuse
neglect
physical abuse
psychological abuse
sexual abuse
sexual harassment

Outline

Abuse

I. INTRODUCTION
   A. Abuse is physical or mental harm caused by someone in a position trust – such as a family member, partner, or caregiver
   B. Abuser has control over the victim so children, spouses, older adults, and people with disabilities are at risk for abuse
   C. Occurs in all social levels, in all races, and in all cultures
   D. You must know how to recognize and report suspected abuse

II. TYPES OF ABUSE
   A. Physical abuse – force or violence that causes pain, injury, and sometimes death
   B. Sexual abuse – unwanted sexual activity including sexual harassment (any conduct, comment, gesture, threat, or suggestion that is sexual in nature)
   C. Emotional abuse (psychological abuse) – words or actions that inflict mental harm
   D. Financial abuse – the misuse of a person's money or property, usually for the abuser's financial gain
   E. Neglect – failing to meet the basic needs of a dependent person

III. CYCLE OF ABUSE
   A. Abuse occurs over and over again (see Figure 19-1, p. 239)
   B. Often follows a pattern
      1. The tension-building phase
      2. The abusive phase
      3. The honeymoon phase
   C. There may be weeks, months, or years between events but usually the time between episodes gradually shortens and the abuse becomes more frequent and intense

IV. Abusive Relationships
   A. Abuse can occur in many different kinds of relationships, which are very complex, and there is usually no single cause for the abuse
   B. Spousal abuse
      1. Occurs in relationships, both women and men can be abuse by their partners
      2. One partner has power and control over the other
      3. Types of abuse include physical, sexual, verbal, economic, or social
         a. Physical abuse is unwanted punching, slapping, biting, hair pulling, or kicking
            (1) Death is a constant threat
         b. Sexual abuse is unwanted sexual contact
         c. Verbal abuse involves unkind and hurtful remarks
         d. Economic abuse involves controlling money
         e. Social abuse is controlling friendships and relationships
      4. The victim often hides the abuse and protects the abusive partner
      5. Some stay because they believe they deserve the abuse, or have nowhere to go
  C. Child abuse
      1. Occurs at every social level
      2. The abuser is usually a household member or someone known to the family
      3. Risk factors include:
         a. Stress
         b. Family crisis
         c. Drug or alcohol abuse
         d. Abuser history of being abused as a child
         e. Discipline beliefs that include physical punishment
         f. Lack of emotional attachment to the child
         g. A child with birth defects or chronic illness
         h. A child with personality or behaviors that are unacceptable to the abuser
         i. Unrealistic expectations for the child's behavior
         j. Families that move frequently
      4. Types of child abuse
         a. Abuse differs from neglect
             (1) Physical neglect involves depriving a child of food , clothing, shelter, and medical care
             (2) Emotional neglect involves not meeting a child's need for affection and attention
         b. Physical abuse is intentionally injuring a child
             (1) Death can occur
         c. Sexual abuse is using, persuading, or forcing a child to engage in sexual conduct
             (1) Rape is forced sexual inter-course
             (2) Molestation is sexual advances, such as kissing, touching, and fondling
             (3) Incest is sexual activity between family members

(4) Child pornography is photographing or videotaping a child involved in sexual acts

(5) Child prostitution is forcing a child to engage in sexual activity for money

D. Abuse of older adults

1. Are at risk for all types of abuse

2. Financial and emotional abuse are the most common types

3. Abusers are usually family members; the older adult does not report the abuse out of fear of the abuser, or fear of being moved to a facility, or may not know how to report abuse, or may be unable to report because of physical or mental disability

4. Family caregivers are more likely to be abusive when they resent their role

5. Ageism is another cause of abuse (see Chapter 15)

E. Abuse of clients

1. Can happen in facilities or home care settings by any member of the health care team, or by a visitor

2. Clients are at risk for all types of abuse, including violating a client's rights such as providing care against the person's wishes

3. Abuse often happens when support workers are under stress, either personal or work related

4. Some clients are abusive and difficult to work with; support workers must be able to recognize when they are feeling stressed and report this to the supervisor, and avoid becoming abusive to the client in response

5. If necessary request an assignment change (see Chapter 8)

F. Abuse of health care workers

1. Support workers are at risk for physical or verbal abuse from clients, their family members, or other members of the health care team

2. Especially at risk from clients with a mental illness or condition that affects behaviour, clients who have problems with drugs or alcohol, or those being placed in restraints

3. Never ignore or accept abuse

4. Your employer will have policies describing what to do if you have an abusive client

5. Box 19-1, p. 241 in the textbook, lists general safety measures

G. The sexually aggressive client

1. Some persons want their sexual needs met by the health team

a. This often embarrasses or angers the staff member

2. Often there are reasons for the person's behavior

a. Illness, injury, surgery, or aging often threaten a male's sense of manhood

b. Confusion or disorientation are causes

c. Touch may be a way to get attention

3. Masturbation is viewed as sexually aggressive behavior

a. It may be for sexual pleasure

b. Urinary or reproductive system disorders can cause genital soreness or itching

c. Poor hygiene and being wet or soiled also cause itching

4. Sexual advances may be intentional (the purpose is sexual)

a. Be professional

(1) Ask the person not to touch you; state the places you were touched

(2) Tell the person that you will not do what he or she wants

(3) Tell the person that those behaviors make you uncomfortable and ask the person not to act that way

(4) Allow privacy if the person is becoming sexually aroused

(5) Discuss the situation with the nurse

H. Sexual harassment

1. Is a form of sexual abuse if the behaviour offends you or makes you uncomfortable

2. Includes sexual comments, gestures, threats, or suggestions

3. Could be from a client's family member or a co-worker

4. Tell the person firmly and assertively that their behaviour is unacceptable and unwelcome

5. If the harassment persists tell your supervisor—in Canada employers are legally required to prevent sexual harassment at work

V. RECOGNIZING SIGNS OF ABUSE

A. Introduction

1. Box 19-2, p. 243 in the textbook, lists signs of various kinds of abuse

2. Support workers are not qualified to

judge whether or not your client is
abused.
3. Noticing one or two signs of possible
abuse does not necessarily mean abuse
has occurred -- it is only a possibility
4. Know your employer's procedures on reporting observation or suspicions
5. Immediately report to your supervisor
any concerns
B. Your legal responsibilities
1. You are legally responsible to report if
you witness or suspect child abuse
2. All provinces and territories require wit-
nessed or suspected child abuse to be reported directly to child protection author-
ities.
3. Consult with your supervisor before
making a report, but remember, in some
provinces failure to report child abuse
can result in fines or imprisonment; if
you have reasonable grounds, no legal action can be taken against you should your
suspicions prove to be wrong
4. Across Canada there are different laws requiring how, and to whom, abuse is reported
5. Know your employer's policies and your
provincial or territorial laws for reporting
abuse
6. In community settings (other than Nova
Scotia and Newfoundland), there are no
legal responsibilities to report abuse of an
adult living in the community; however,
you must report your suspicions to your
supervisor immediately
C. How to report abuse
1. Your employer will have specific rules for
how to report your observations
2. It is very important to record all your observations and to make your reports in
writing
3. Keep all your notes in case you are asked
to remember details at a later date
4. Record
a. Alleged victim's name, address, phone
number, age, and sex
b. Alleged abuser's name, address, phone
number, and relationship to victim
c. Description of abuse and neglect, suspicions, and evidence obtained to date
d. Record the date, time, and place; only
state the facts that you know
5. Protect the client's privacy and only tell
the people who need to know

D. When clients speak of abuse
1. Follow your employer's guidelines and
policies
2. Follow these general guidelines:
a. Listen attentively
b. Reassure the client that you believe
them
c. Assure the person that you will do
what you can to help
d. Provide emotional support for the
client whatever they may decide to do

Classroom Activities

1. Divide the class into small groups. Write on the
board "physical abuse, sexual abuse, financial
abuse, emotional abuse, and neglect." Ask each
group to identify 5 examples of each type. Allow
15 minutes for this activity. Have a spokesperson
report back to the class.

2. Reproduce Figure 19-1, p. 239 in the textbook, on
a transparency and explain to the class to cycle of
abuse.

3. Contact a representative from your local Child
Protection Agency to speak to the class about the
signs and symptoms of child abuse.

4. Many areas have an Elder Abuse Committee. Ask
a representative to speak to the class about the
types of abuse of the elderly occurring in your
area.

5. Ask the students to identify some of the possible
causes for sexually aggressive behaviour. Write
the list on the board. Then ask the class to suggest
ways they can handle a situation with a sexually
aggressive client.

Homework Assignments

Ask students to answer the questions at the end of
Chapter 19 in the textbook. Tell students the date and
time that this assignment must be completed and
turned in.

If the accompanying workbook is being used, assign
the Chapter 19 workbook exercises. Tell students the
date and time that this assignment must be completed
and turned in.

Chapter 19 Student Assignment

Name _____

Date _____

Abuse

Fill in the blanks below with the correct terms related to the types of elderly abuse.

1. _____ involves hitting, slapping, kicking, pinching, and beating.
2. _____ is the use of oral or written words or statements that speak badly of, sneer at, criticize, or condemn the person; this includes unkind gestures.
3. _____ is confining the person to a specific area.
4. _____ is when the elderly person's money is used by another person.
5. _____ includes humiliation, harassment, and threats of being punished or deprived of needs such as food, clothing, care, a home, or a place to sleep.
6. _____ is when the person is harassed about sex or is attacked sexually.

Fill in the blanks below with the correct terms related to the types of child abuse.

7. _____ means not meeting the child's need for affection and attention.
8. _____ is intentionally injuring the child.
9. _____ is using, persuading, or forcing a child to engage in sexual conduct.
10. _____ is forced sexual intercourse.

11. _____ involves sexual advances toward a child; this includes kissing, touching, or fondling sexual areas.
12. _____ is sexual activity between family members.
13. _____ involves photographing or video taping a child involved in sexual acts.
14. _____ is forcing a child to engage in sexual activity for money.
15. List five examples of abusive situations that might occur in a facility or a home:

    a. _____

    b. _____

    c. _____

    d. _____

    e. _____

16. Why do abused older adults choose not to complain about the abuse?

    a. _____

    b. _____

    c. _____

    d. _____

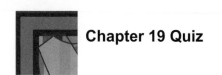

Chapter 19 Quiz

Name _____

Date _____

Abuse

True or False

Mark **T** *for true or* **F** *for false.*

1. _____ Ageism is a cause of abuse.

2. _____ Sexual harassment is not considered sexual abuse.

3. _____ Financial and emotional abuse are the most common types of elder abuse.

4. _____ More women than men are abused by their partner.

5. _____ The time between episodes of abuse becomes longer as time passes.

6. _____ Unless you are certain that abuse has occurred it is better not to say anything to your supervisor.

7. _____ If you witness abuse within a facility you must report this to your supervisor.

8. _____ Pressure sores are a sign of neglect.

Multiple Choice

Circle the best answer.

9. The cycle of abuse includes all *except*:
   a. tension-building
   b. neglect
   c. abusive phase
   d. honeymoon

10. You suspect an adult client is being abused. What should you do?
    a. Tell the family
    b. Tell your supervisor
    c. Call the police
    d. Ask the person if he or she was abused

11. Sexually aggressive behaviours can be caused by all but:
    a. dementia
    b. fever
    c. endocrine disorder
    d. acquired brain injury

12. Which is *not* a sign of emotional abuse?
    a. a change in behaviour
    b. person seems fearful
    c. private conversations are not allowed
    d. avoidance of touch

138

20

The Client's Environment: Promoting Well-Being, Comfort, and Rest

Instructor's Preparation

I. Read Chapter 20 in the textbook. Carefully review chapter objectives, key terms, and review questions.

II. Read the outline in Chapter 20 of the instructor's guide. Carefully review the classroom activities, the student assignment, and the quiz.

III. If you are using the accompanying student workbook, review the activities for Chapter 20.

IV. Gather all necessary supplies and equipment for classroom activities and student assignments.
   A. Prepare the correct number of handouts
   B. Prepare appropriate flip charts
   C. Prepare overhead transparencies
   D. Prepare situation/index cards
   E. Gather correct video
   F. Gather coloured markers
   G. Gather any other items that will be needed for classroom activities
   H. Assemble items in the order they will be used

V. Make sure that the necessary equipment is available and in good working order.

Objectives

- Define the key terms listed in this chapter
- Explain how to promote well-being during the admission, transfer, and discharge procedures
- Explain why comfort is important
- Describe four types of pain
- List the signs and symptoms of pain
- List the care plan measures that relieve pain
- Explain why rest and sleep are important
- Describe the factors that affect sleep
- Describe common sleep disorders
- List care plan measures that promote sleep
- Demonstrate the procedures described in this chapter

Key Terms

acute pain
admission
chronic pain
discharge
insomnia
phantom pain
radiating pain
transfer

The Client's Environment: Promoting Well-Being, Comfort, and Rest

I. INTRODUCTION
  A. Admission to a health care facility or agency often causes anxiety and fear
    1. The person and family may worry about the need for treatment or surgery and its outcome
    2. People admitted to facilities have fears about not returning home
    3. Many people are unfamiliar with health care agencies and facilities
  B. Transfers cause similar concerns
  C. Discharge is usually a happy time
    1. However, the person may need to adapt to other changes
  D. You must be courteous, kind, and respectful
II. WELL-BEING DURING TRANSITIONS
  A. Transitions are difficult for most people
  B. Elderly people or those who are unwell may feel anxious, unsettled, and alone
  C. Moving can cause or increase signs of confusion
  D. Support workers can help their clients during this process
III. ADMITTING A PERSON TO A FACILITY
  A. Admission is the official entry of a person into a health care facility
  B. Long-term care facilities
    1. The admission is made as simple and easy as possible
    2. Often admission procedures are completed 2 or 3 days before the person enters the facility
    3. Residents may arrive by ambulance, wheelchair, van, or private car
    4. This is a critical and emotional time for the resident and family
     a. The facility is now the person's home
    5. At some time, a photograph is taken and the person is given an ID bracelet
    6. Persons with dementia and their families may need special help
     a. Confusion may increase in a new setting
     b. The person may become fearful and agitated and want to leave
     c. The health care team works together to help the resident and family feel safe

and welcome.
    7. Admitting the person
     a. A nurse usually greets and admits the person
     b. It may be your responsibility to greet the person if the person has no serious discomfort or distress
      (1) Greet the person by name
      (2) Introduce yourself by name and title
     c. Admission procedures include:
      (1) Completing an admission checklist
      (2) Weighing and measuring the person
      (3) Obtaining a urine specimen if ordered
      (4) Orienting the person to the room, nursing unit, and hospital
     d. The resident needs to feel comfortable, safe, and secure
      (1) Avoid rushing
      (2) Treat the resident and family as guests
      (3) Tell them good things about the center
      (4) Introduce the person to other residents
       (a) Other residents are a source of comfort and support
      (5) Help the resident make the room as homelike as possible
       (a) Help the person unpack
      (6) When the resident is comfortable, the admission procedures are completed
       (a) A nurse or social worker explains the resident's rights to the resident and family
        (i) They are also given a booklet explaining these rights
      (7) Admitting the Person ▶ p. 249
  C. Except in emergencies, the admission process in a hospital starts in the admitting office
    1. Identifying information is obtained
    2. The person is given an identification number and an ID bracelet
    3. Admitting papers and a general consent for treatment are signed at this time
    4. The nursing unit is notified of the admission and is told the person's room and

bed number
IV. TRANSFERS
   A. Moving a person from one room or nursing unit to another
      1. Moves are usually related to changes in condition
      2. Sometimes the person requests a room change
   B. Reasons for transfer are explained by the doctor, nurse, or social worker
      1. The family and business office are notified
   C. You may assist with transfers or carry out the entire procedure
   D. The person is transported by wheelchair, stretcher, or bed
      1. Transferring the Person to Another Nursing Unit ▶ p. 250
V. DISCHARGES
   A. Discharge is the official departure of the person from an a hospital or other health care facility
      1. Usually planned in advance
   B. Persons are discharged to another hospital, a facility, or home
   C. The health team members plan the person's discharge
      1. They teach the person and family about diet, exercise, drugs, and how to perform care procedures or give treatments
      2. They arrange for home care and special therapy and equipment
      3. Doctor's appointments are made
   D. You will help the person pack belongings and dress
   E. The doctor must write a discharge order
      1. The nurse tells you when the person can leave and how to transport him or her
      2. If the person leaves by ambulance, ambulance attendants bring the stretcher to the room
   F. A resident may want to leave the facility without the doctor's permission
      1. Notify the nurse immediately
      2. The nurse handles the situation
   G. Discharging the Person ▶ p. 252
VI. COMFORT
   A. Temperature and ventilation
      1. Heating, air conditioning, and ventilation systems maintain a comfortable temperature and provide fresh air
      2. A temperature range of 20° C to 23° C is comfortable for most healthy people
      3. Stale room air and lingering odors can affect comfort and rest
      4. To protect persons from drafts:
         a. Make sure they wear enough clothing
         b. Cover them with blankets
         c. Provide lap robes to cover their legs
         d. Move them from drafty areas
      5. Older persons are more sensitive to cold
   B. Odors
      1. Good nursing care, good ventilation, and good housekeeping practices help eliminate odors
      2. To reduce odors:
         a. Empty and clean bedpans, urinals, commodes, and kidney basins promptly
         b. Change soiled linens and clothing promptly
         c. Dispose of soiled linens and clothing
         d. Clean persons who are wet or soiled
         e. Dispose of incontinent products promptly
         f. Dispose of ostomy products promptly
         g. Keep soiled laundry containers closed
         h. Provide good personal hygiene for the person
         i. Use room deodorizers when necessary and if allowed
      3. If you smoke, follow the employer's policy
         a. Wash your hands after handling smoking materials and before giving care
         b. Give attention to your uniform, hair, and breath
   C. Noise
      1. Ill people are sensitive to noises and sounds around them
      2. Common health care sounds may disturb them
         a. Clanging of equipment
         b. Clatter of dishes and trays
         c. Loud talking and laughing in hallways and at the nurse's station
         d. Television, radios, telephones, and buzzing intercoms
         e. Wheels on carts and other equipment
      3. Patients and residents may find sounds dangerous, frightening, or irritating
      4. What is noise to one person may not be noise to another

D. Lighting
  1. Good lighting is needed for safety and comfort
  2. People usually relax and rest better in dim light
  3. A bright room is more cheerful and stimulating
  4. Lighting is adjusted to meet the person's changing needs
  5. Bright lighting is helpful when giving care
  6. Always keep light controls within the person's reach
E. Room furniture and equipment
  1. Rooms are furnished and equipped for the person's basic needs
    a. Comfort
    b. Sleep
    c. Elimination
    d. Nutrition
    e. Personal hygiene
    f. Activity
    g. Communication
  1. The right to privacy is considered
  2. The bed
    a. Hospital beds are adjusted electrically or manually
    b. Many home care clients have regular beds
    c. The overbed table
      (1) Positioned over the bed by sliding the base under the bed
      (2) Height is adjusted for the person in bed or in a chair
      (3) Used for meals, writing, reading, and other activities
      (4) Many have moveable tops with storage areas underneath
      (5) The nursing team uses the overbed table as a work area
        (a) Only clean and sterile items are placed on the table
        (b) The table is cleaned after being used
        (c) Never place bedpans, urinals, or soiled linen on the overbed table
F. The bed side furniture (see Figure 20-3, p. 254)
  1. Is next to the bed
  2. Is a storage area for personal items and personal care equipment

  3. The top of the stand is used for tissues, the telephone, and other personal items
    a. For example: radio, clock, pictures, telephone
  4. Some stands have a rod at the side or back for towels and wash cloths
G. Chairs (see Figure 20-4, p. 254)
  1. The person's unit usually has one or two chairs
  2. Nursing facilities residents may bring their own chairs from home
H. Privacy curtains
  1. Rooms have privacy curtains
    a. They are pulled completely around the bed while care is given (see Figure 20-5, p. 254)
    b. They do not block sound or prevent conversations from being heard
  2. Portable screens can be used to provide privacy in the home setting (see Figure 20-6, p. 254)
I. The bathroom
  1. Many agencies have a bathroom in each room; some have a bathroom between two rooms
  2. A toilet, sink, call system, and mirror are standard equipment
  3. Handrails are installed by the toilet for the person's safety
  4. In some facilities, the toilet seats are higher than standard height
    a. Makes transfer easier
    b. Helpful for persons with joint problems
  5. Towel racks, toilet paper, soap, paper towel dispensers, waste basket, and call system are in the bathroom
J. Closet and drawer space
  1. Provided for the person's clothing
  2. Government regulations state that residents must have free access to the closet and its contents
K. Medical equipment
  1. Many agencies furnish rooms with other equipment
    a. For example: television, radio, clock
    b. Many rooms have telephones
    c. Some have wall mounted blood pressure equipment, oxygen tanks, portable suction equipment, IV poles, outlets for oxygen and suction (see Figure 20-7, p. 255)

VII. PAIN
A. Discomfort and Pain
    1. Means to ache, hurt, or be sore
    2. Comfort and discomfort are subjective
        a. You cannot see, hear, touch, or smell the person's comfort or discomfort
        b. You must rely on what the person tells you
    3. Report complaints to the nurse (used for the nursing process)
    4. Pain is personal
        a. If differs for each person
        b. If the person complains of pain or discomfort, the person has pain or discomfort
    5. Pain is a warning from the body
        a. It means there is damage to body tissue
        b. It often causes the person to seek health care
B. Types of pain
    1. Acute pain is felt suddenly, lasts a short time, decreases with healing
    2. Chronic pain lasts longer than 6 months, remains after healing, and is constant or occurs "on and off"
    3. Radiating pain is felt at the site of tissue damage and in nearby areas
    4. Phantom pain is felt in a body part that is no longer there
C. Factors affecting pain
    1. Past experience
        a. Knowing what to expect can help or hinder how the person handles pain
        b. If a person has not had pain before, the person may be very afraid and anxious
    2. Anxiety relates to feelings of fear, dread, worry, and concern
        a. The person feels uneasy and tense
        b. Pain and anxiety are related
        c. Anxiety increases how much pain the person feels
        d. Lessening anxiety helps reduce pain
        e. Knowing the cause of pain and what to expect helps reduce anxiety
    3. Rest and sleep
        a. Rest and sleep restore energy
        b. Rest and sleep reduce body demands and allow the body to repair itself
        c. Lack of rest and sleep affects how the person deals with pain
        d. Pain seems worse when the person is tired or restless
        e. A person usually pays more attention to pain when unable to sleep
    4. Attention
        a. The more a person thinks about pain, the worse it can seem
        b. Pain often seems worse at night
            (1) Environment is quiet and less activity occurs
    5. Personal and family duties
        a. Dealing with pain often relates to personal and family obligations
        b. Pain may be ignored or denied if it interferes with caring for family or earning a living
    6. The value or meaning of pain
        a. Some people view pain as a sign of weakness
        b. Sometimes pain results in pleasure (childbirth)
        c. Pain is used to avoid certain persons or things
        d. Pain can be used to get attention
    7. Support from others
        a. Pain is often easier to deal with when family and friends offer support and comfort
        b. Touch is comforting to some
        c. Some people must deal with pain alone
            (1) Being alone can increase anxiety
            (2) Facing pain alone is hard for everyone
    8. Culture
        a. Affects how a person responds to pain
        b. See Respecting Diversity box, p. 256 in the textbook
    9. Focus on children
        a. Children may not understand pain
        b. They have fewer ways of dealing with pain
            (1) They rely on adults for help
        c. Young children have difficulty alerting adults to pain
            (1) Adults must be alert for behaviors and situations that signal pain
  10. Focus on older persons
        a. Older person may have decreased pain sensations
            (1) This places them at greater risk for undetected disease or injury

b. Chronic pain may mask new pain
c. They often deny or ignore pain because of what it may mean
d. Thinking and reasoning are affected in some older persons
   (1) Changes in behavior may indicate pain
   (2) Nursing staff must be alert for signs of pain
   (3) Report changes in the person's usual behavior to the nurse
D. Signs and symptoms
1. Promptly report to the RN any information you collect about pain (use the person's exact words)
2. The nurse needs the following information:
   a. Location—where is the pain? (ask the person to point to the area of the pain)
   b. Onset and duration—when did it start and how long has it lasted?
   c. Intensity—does the person complain of mild, moderate, or severe pain
   d. Description—ask the person to describe the pain
   e. Box 20-2, p. 257 in the textbook, lists some words used to describe pain
   f. Factors causing pain—what was the person doing before the pain started and when the pain started?
   g. Vital signs—increases often occur with pain
   h. Other signs and symptoms—Box 22-2, p. 537 in the textbook, lists signs and symptoms that often occur with pain
E. Measures to Relieve Pain
1. The RN uses the nursing process to promote comfort and relieve pain
2. Box 20-3, p. 257 in the textbook, lists the nursing measures that are often part of care plans
3. Other measures are often needed to control pain (the nurse may ask you to assist or instruct you on how to perform them properly)
   a. Distraction means to change the person's center of attention
      (1) Attention is moved away from the pain
   b. Relaxation means to be free from mental or physical stress
      (1) Reduces pain and anxiety
      (2) A comfortable position and a quiet room are necessary
   c. Guided imagery is creating and focusing on an image; the person is asked to create a pleasant scene
      (1) Use a calm voice and soft music
4. Doctors often order drugs to control or relieve pain
   a. Such medication can cause orthostatic hypotension, drowsiness, dizziness, and coordination problems
      (1) Protect the person from injury
      (2) The nurse and the care plan alert you to safety measures

VIII. REST AND SLEEP
A. Being at Rest
1. Being calm, at ease, and relaxed
   a. The person is free from anxiety and stress
   b. It may involve physical inactivity or doing something calming
2. Basic needs must be met for a person to rest
   a. You can promote rest by meeting physical needs
3. Safety and security needs must be met
4. Many people have rituals and routines before resting
   a. Follow routines and rituals whenever possible
5. Love and belonging are important for rest
   a. The person knows that others care
6. Meeting esteem needs is important
   b. Relates to feeling good about oneself
7. Some persons need long rest periods, others are refreshed after resting 15 to 20 minutes
8. Ill or injured persons need to rest more often
   a. Allow rest periods as they are needed
   b. Do not rush the person
9. Plan and organize care so the person can rest without interruptions
10. If bedrest is ordered, complications are prevented (see Chapter 22)
11. A state of unconsciousness, reduced voluntary muscle activity, and lowered metabolism
   a. The unconsciousness is temporary
12. Sleep is a basic need
   a. The body saves energy during sleep

b. Body functions slow

c. The vital signs fall

d. Tissue healing and repair occur

e. Sleep lowers stress, tension, and anxiety

f. The person regains energy and mental alertness

13. Sleep requirements

   a. The amount of sleep needed varies for each age-group

     (1) The amount needed decreases with age (see Table 20-1, p. 259)

14. Factors affecting sleep

   a. Illness

     (1) Increases the need for sleep

     (2) Signs and symptoms of illness can interfere with sleep

     (3) Treatments and therapies can interfere with sleep

     (4) The emotional effects of illness can affect sleep

   b. Nutrition

     (1) Weight loss or gain can affect sleep

     (2) Some foods affect sleep

   c. Exercise

     (1) Usually helps the person sleep well

     (2) Exercising right before bedtime interferes with sleep

       (a) There should be at least 2 hours between exercise and bedtime

   d. Environment

     (1) People adjust to their usual sleeping environment (bed, pillow, noise, lighting, sleeping partner)

     (2) Changes in environment can affect the amount and quality of sleep

   e. Drugs and other substances

     (1) Some drugs promote sleep (sleeping pills); these drugs also decrease the length of REM sleep

       (a) Behavior problems and sleep deprivation can occur

       (b) Persons under the influence of alcohol may awaken during sleep; difficulty returning to sleep is common

       (c) Caffeine prevents sleep

     (2) The side effects of some drugs effect sleep

   f. Life-style changes

     (1) Life-style relates to a person's daily routine and way of living

       (a) Work, school, play, and social events

   g. Emotional problems

     (1) Fear, worry, depression, and anxiety

     (2) Losses are stressful and affect sleep

B. Sleep disorders

1. Involve repeated sleep problems

2. The amount and quality of sleep are affected

3. Box 20-4, p. 259 in the textbook, lists the signs and symptoms that occur

4. Insomnia

   a. A chronic condition in which the person cannot sleep or stay asleep

   b. Three forms:

     (1) Unable to fall asleep

     (2) Unable to stay asleep

     (3) Early awakening and unable to fall back asleep

   c. Emotional problems are common causes

   d. The fear of dying during sleep is another cause

   e. The fear of not being able to sleep is a cause

   f. The RN plans measures to promote sleep

     (1) Emotional or physical problems are also treated

5. Sleep deprivation

   a. The amount and quality of sleep are decreased

   b. Sleep is interrupted

   c. Illness and hospital care are common causes

6. Sleepwalking

   a. The person leaves the bed and walks about

   b. The person is not aware of sleepwalking

   c. Children sleepwalk more than adults

   d. Stress, fatigue, and some drugs can cause sleepwalking

   e. The person needs protection from injury

f. Guide sleepwalkers back to bed
g. Sleepwalkers startle easily; awaken them gently

IX. Promoting sleep
1. The RN assesses the person's sleep patterns
2. Your observations are important
   a. Report any of the signs and symptoms listed in Box 20-5, p. 260 in the textbook
3. Check the care plan to ensure you give the correct care

Classroom Activities

1. Write the following terms on the chalkboard:
   a. Admission
   b. Discharge
   c. Transfer
   Call on students to define each term. Write the correct definition for each term on the chalkboard.

2. Call on students to discuss the admission process.
   a. What anxieties and fears do persons being admitted to a health care agency experience?
   b. Ask students to share any personal experience related to being admitted to a health care agency.

3. Divide students into groups of three. Provide each group with several sheets of notebook paper.
   a. Ask students to discuss and identify the special needs of persons being admitted to a long-term care center. Allow 15 minutes.
      (1) Call on one student from each group to report to the class
      (2) Allow time after the reports for discussion

4. Write the following on a flip chart:
   a. Admitting the person involves:
      (1) Greeting the person by name
      (2) Introducing yourself
      (3) Completing an admission checklist
      (4) Weighing and measuring the person
      (5) Obtaining a urine specimen if ordered
      (6) Orienting the person
   b. Use this list as a basis to discuss the admission process.
   c. Call on students to describe what happens during each step of the process.

5. Obtain sample admission checklists from a local hospital and a local long-term care center. Distribute one of each to each student. Review each form with students. Answer any questions.
   a. Tell students to keep these forms. They will complete them when they return demonstrate the admission procedure.

6. Review the transfer and discharge process with students. Discuss the role of the nursing assistant in each process.

7. Use the procedure checklists provided. Demonstrate each procedure in this chapter.
   a. Ask each student in return to demonstrate each procedure in this chapter. Each student should take a turn in the role of patient or resident.
   b. Stress the importance of accuracy when obtaining, reporting, and recording height and weight. Accuracy is also important when completing the admission checklist.

8. Arrange a field trip to a local hospital and a local long-term care facility. The goal is to provide students the opportunity to see a patient and resident room (an empty hospital room and an occupied resident room).
   a. Remember, you must ask permission to enter an occupied room.
   b. Ask students to take a notebook along. Ask them to observe and note the following about each unit:
      (1) Temperature and ventilation
      (2) Odors
      (3) Noise
      (4) Lighting
      (5) Room furniture and equipment
         (a) The bed
         (b) The overbed table
         (c) The bedside stand
         (d) Chairs
         (e) Privacy curtains
      (6) Personal care items
      (7) The call system
      (8) The bathroom
      (9) Closet and drawer space
      (10) Other equipment
   c. Ask students to note the differences in the unit in the hospital and the long-term care facility.

9. Ask students to make a list of the things they would have to give up if they were to live in a nursing center.
   a. What items are most important to them and why?

10. Discuss the importance of personal space.
    a. Ask students to discuss ways they can help persons feel at home. What can they do to respect the person's space and belongings?
    b. Divide students into groups of three. Provide each group with several sheets of notebook paper.
       (1) Allow each group 15 minutes to discuss how they can protect the right to privacy and choice when providing care in the hospital, nursing center, and the home. One member of each group should take notes.
       (2) Call on one student from each group to report to the class.

11. Call on students to define comfort and discomfort or pain.

12. Write the following terms on a flip chart. Use a different color marker for each term. Allow space after each term to write in the definition.
    b. Acute pain
    b. Chronic pain
    c. Radiating pain
    d. Phantom pain
    Call on students to define each term. Write the correct answer after each term.

13. Divide students into groups of three. Provide each group with several sheets of notebook paper. Ask each group to list and describe the factors affecting pain.
    a. Allow 15 minutes for students to complete this exercise.
    b. Call on one student from one group to report to the class. Students from other groups can provide input as appropriate.
    c. Allow time for questions.
    d. Discuss various nursing measures to promote comfort and relieve pain.
    e. Ask students to share personal experiences with pain and the measures they use to relieve pain.

14. Call on students to identify special needs of children and older persons who experience pain.

15. Write the following on the chalkboard: "What information does the nurse need about pain?"
    a. Call on students to list the information. Write the correct answers on the chalkboard.

16. Invite a professional with expertise in relaxation techniques and guided imagery to visit the class. Have the person perform relaxation techniques and guided imagery with the students.
    a. Discuss the experience with the students.
    b. How did the techniques help them relax?

17. Ask students to identify and discuss the measures used to promote rest and sleep in health care settings.
    a. Ask students to share the measures they use in their personal lives to promote sleep.

18. Ask students to share any rituals and/or routines they may have at bedtime.
    a. How do these rituals and routines help them sleep?
    a. What happens if these rituals and routines are disturbed?

Homework Assignments

Ask students to answer the questions at the end of Chapter 20 in the textbook. Tell students the date and time that this assignment must be completed and turned in.

If the accompanying workbook is being used, assign the Chapter 20 workbook exercises. Tell students the date and time that this assignment must be completed and turned in.

Name _____

Date _____

The Client's Environment

Write your answers in the spaces provided.

1. Define the following terms:

   a. Admission:

   _____
   _____

   b. Discharge:

   _____
   _____

   c. Transfer:

   _____
   _____

2. What do admissions procedures involve?

   a. _____
   _____

   b. _____
   _____

   c. _____
   _____

   d. _____
   _____

3. List measures used to control odors when providing care.
   a. _____
   b. _____
   c. _____
   d. _____
   e. _____
   f. _____
   g. _____
   h. _____
   i. _____

4. Rooms are furnished for the person's basic needs. There is furniture and equipment for:
   a. _____
   b. _____
   c. _____
   d. _____
   e. _____
   f. _____
   g. _____

5. List words used to describe pain.
   a. _____
   b. _____
   c. _____
   d. _____
   e. _____
   f. _____
   g. _____
   h. _____
   i. _____
   j. _____
   k. _____
   l. _____
   m. _____
   n. _____
   o. _____

6. What behaviors are signs of pain?
   a. _____
   b. _____
   c. _____
   d. _____
   e. _____
   f. _____
   g. _____
   h. _____
   i. _____
   j. _____
   k. _____
   l. _____
   m. _____
   n. _____

Name _____

Date _____

The Client's Environment

True or False

Mark **T** *for true or* **F** *for false.*

1. _____ Admission to a health care agency often causes anxiety and fear.

2. _____ The admission process begins when the person arrives on the nursing unit.

3. _____ The person is fully dressed when his or her weight is measured.

4. _____ Persons may request a room change.

5. _____ The person will feel safer and more secure if you explain what you are doing and why.

6. _____ Reasons for a transfer are explained to the person by assistive personnel.

7. _____ Residents of long-term care facilities are encouraged to keep some personal items and arrange them as they choose.

8. _____ If you smoke, you must wash your hands after handling smoking materials.

9. _____ Light controls should be within the person's reach.

10. _____ Bed wheels are kept locked at all times, except when moving the bed.

11. _____ The urinal is placed on the overbed table.

12. _____ The signal light is always kept within the person's reach.

13. _____ Mr. Jones hoards food in the drawer of his bedside stand. You must wait until he leaves the room and remove the food.

14. _____ Illness and injury decrease the need for rest and sleep.

15. _____ Acute pain is felt suddenly and generally lasts less than 6 months.

16. _____ Pain is personal. It differs for each person.

17. _____ Amount of sleep needed increases with age.

18. _____ Changes in a person's usual environment can affect amount and quality of sleep.

19. _____ Clients in long-term care facilities have the right to choose what measures are helpful to promote comfort, rest, and sleep.

20. _____ Exercising right before bedtime promotes sleep.

Multiple Choice

Circle the BEST answer.

21. You are admitting a person who is ambulatory. Which is correct?
    a. Make a surgical bed.
    b. Open the bed and lower it to its lowest position.
    c. Raise the bed to the highest position.
    d. Keep the bed closed and in the highest position.

22. A person with dementia is being admitted to a nursing center. Which is correct?
    a. Family members are asked to leave to help the person adjust.
    b. Complete the admission process as quickly as possible.
    c. The person's confusion may increase in new surroundings.
    d. All of the above.

23. You are admitting Mrs. Dillan. While you are taking her vital signs, she complains of severe abdominal pain. You should:
    a. Call the doctor.
    b. Finish the admissions process. Then report Mrs.

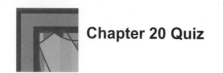

Chapter 20 Quiz

Name _____

Date _____

The Client's Environment

Dillan's complaint of pain to the nurse.
c. Call the nurse immediately.
d. Tell Mrs. Dillan not to worry because her doctor will see her soon.

24. Mrs. Lynn wishes to leave the hospital without the doctor's permission. You should:
a. Help her dress and pack.
b. Notify the nurse immediately.
c. Ask her why she wants to leave, and try to persuade her to stay.
d. Call her family.

25. The person's unit:
a. Is arranged for staff convenience.
b. Should always have dim lighting.
c. Should be as personal and homelike as possible.
d. Is kept clean by the person.

26. You help control noise by:
a. Answering telephones and signal lights promptly.
b. Talking and laughing at the nurse's station.
c. Using equipment that needs repair or oil.
d. All of the above.

27. To use the patient or resident bed safely, do all of the following except:
a. Keep the wheels locked except when moving the bed.
b. Lower the bed to the lowest horizontal position to give care.
c. When using an electric bed, teach the person how to use the controls.
d. When using a manual bed, make sure cranks are left down when not in use.

28. To provide full visual privacy, you must:
a. Provide care with the room door open.
b. Pull the curtain around the bed only if the person has a roommate.
c. Pull the curtain around the bed only if the person asks you to.
d. Always pull the curtain completely around the person's bed when care is given.

29. Leaving one's home is difficult. Therefore, it is important to:
a. Make the person's unit as homelike as possible.
b. Allow the person to bring some personal items.
c. Help the person in choosing the best place for personal items.
d. All of the above.

30. A chronic condition in which a person cannot sleep or stay asleep is:
a. Discomfort.
b. Enuresis.
c. Insomnia.
d. NREM sleep.

31. You promote comfort by:
a. Keeping the bed linens tight and wrinkle free
b. Giving a back massage.
c. Positioning the person in good body alignment.
d. All of the above.

32. Pain that is felt in a part of the body that is no longer there is:
a. Acute pain.
b. Phantom pain.
c. Radiating pain.
d. Chronic pain.

33. During sleep:
a. There are no voluntary arm or leg movements.
b. Pulse and respiration increase.
c. Stress, tension, and anxiety increase.
d. Body functions speed up.

34. Which of the following is not a measure used to promote sleep?
a. Drinking alcoholic beverages at bedtime.
b. Following bedtime rituals.
c. Eating a bedtime snack.
d. Reducing noise.

35. Distraction means to:
a. Be free of mental and physical stress.
b. Focus on a pleasant scene.
c. Change the person's center of attention.
d. Control pain with drugs.

150

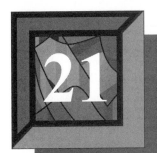

Body Mechanics

Instructor's Preparation

I. Read Chapter 21 in the textbook. Carefully review chapter objectives, key terms, and review questions.

II. Read the outline in Chapter 21 of the instructor's guide. Carefully review the classroom activities, the student assignment, and the quiz.

III. If you are using the accompanying student workbook, review the activities for Chapter 21.

IV. Review the appropriate sections of video #1, video #2, and video #3 in Mosby's Nursing Assisting Video Series.

V. Gather all necessary supplies and equipment for classroom activities and student assignments.

   A. Prepare appropriate flip charts

   B. Gather correct videos

   C. Gather the following transparencies: TA29 through TA33

   D. Gather coloured markers

   E. Gather the equipment and supplies needed to demonstrate and have each student return demonstrate the procedures in this chapter.

   F. Gather any other items that will be needed for classroom activities

   G. Assemble items in the order they will be used

IV. Make sure that the necessary equipment is available and in good working order.

Objectives

- Define the key terms listed in this chapter
- Explain the purpose and rules of using good body mechanics
- Identify comfort and safety measures for lifting, turning, and moving clients in bed
- Explain how to lift and move clients in bed
- Explain why good body alignment and position changes are important for the client
- Identify the comfort and safety measures for positioning persons in bed
- Explain the purpose of a transfer belt
- Describe the safety measures for transferring clients
- Explain how to position a client in the basic bed positions and in a chair
- Learn the procedures described in this chapter

Key Terms

base of support
body alignment
body mechanics
dorsal recumbent position
Fowler's position
friction
gait belt
lateral position
logrolling
posture
prone position
shearing
Sims' position
supine position
transfer
transfer belt

Outline

Body Mechanics

I. INTRODUCTION
  A. Good body mechanics protects you and the person from injury
  B. Review of the structure and function of the musculoskeletal system (see Chapter 13)
II. BODY MECHANICS
  A. Using the body in an efficient and careful way
  B. It involves using good posture and balance, and using the body's strongest and largest muscles for work
  C. Posture is the way body parts are aligned with one another
    1. Good alignment lets the body move and function with strength and efficiency
    2. Figure 21-1, p. 264 in the textbook, shows a person standing in good body alignment
  D. Base of support is the area on which an object rests
    1. When standing, your feet are your base of support
    2. A wider base of support provides more balance
    3. When a person stands with good posture:
      a. Head and neck are erect and straight
      b. Shoulders and hips are parallel to each other
      c. Shoulders are back
      d. Chest is out
      e. Spine is straight
      f. Abdomen is tucked in
      g. Knees are slightly flexed
      h. Arms are hanging comfortably at the side
      i. Feet are about shoulder-width apart
      j. Toes are pointing forward, one foot is slightly forward
    4. Lying down and sitting also require good alignment
    5. Use the strongest and largest muscles to lift and move heavy objects
      a. Shoulders, upper arms, hips, and thighs
    6. Good body mechanics involve:
      a. Bending your knees and squatting to lift heavy objects ; do not bend from the waist (see Figure 21-2, p. 265)
      b. Holding items close to your body and base of support
    7. All activities require good body mechanics
    8. Follow the guidelines in Box 21-1, p. 265

in the textbook, for good body mechanics
III. LIFTING AND MOVING PERSONS IN BED
  A. Comfort and safety
    1. The person's skin is protected during lifting and moving
    2. Friction and shearing injure the skin, causing infection and pressure ulcers
      a. Friction is the rubbing of one surface against another
      b. Shearing is when the skin sticks to a surface and muscles slide in the direction the body is moving (see Figure 21-4, p. 267)
        (1) Occurs when the person slides down or is moved in bed
      c. Reduce friction and shearing by rolling or lifting the person
        (1) Lift sheets are used (see Chapter 24)
    3. Focus on older persons
      a. Skin is fragile and easily torn
      b. Use a lift sheet or turning pad
    4. The following comfort and safety measures are considered before moving persons in bed:
      a. Check with your supervisor, the care plan, and if appropriate, the client, to find out how much help they can give
      b. Decide how to move the person and how much help you will need befre attempting the move
      c. Ask for help before starting the procedure
      d. Communicate directions with your helper, by counting 1-2-3, then move
      e. Move the client in small increments
      f. Cover and screen the person
      g. Protect any tubes or drainage containers
      h. Position clients in good body alignment
      i. Make sure linens are wrinkle-free
  B. Raising the person's head and shoulders
    1. Raise the person's shoulders easily and safely by locking arms with the person (see Figure 21-5, p. 268)
    2. Ask for help with older persons (see Figure 21-6, p. 269)
      a. This protects the client from pain and injury
    3. Raising the Person's Head and Shoulders ▶ p. 276
  C. Moving the person up in bed
    1. When sitting up in bed, the client can

easily slide down (see Figure 21-7, p. 271)

2. Proper alignment and comfort are established

3. If able to help, the client helps you by pushing up with hands or feet (see Figure 21-8, p. 273)

4. May have a trapeze attached to the bed (see Figure 21-9, p. 273)

5. At least two caregivers are needed to move heavy, weak, or very old persons up in bed (see Figure 21-10, p. 273)

6. You can usually move children up in bed alone

7. Moving the Person Up in Bed ▶ p. 272

D. Moving the person up in bed with a lift sheet

1. A co-worker helps
   a. Sometimes possible to do by yourself (see Figure 21-11, p. 275)

2. Friction and shearing are reduced

3. The person is lifted more evenly

4. Use lift sheets for persons who are unconscious, paralyzed, or recovering from spinal cord surgery or who have spinal cord injuries

5. Also used for older persons

6. Moving the Person Up in Bed with a Lift Sheet ▶ p. 274

E. Moving the person to the side of the bed

1. Required for repositioning and care procedures

2. One method involves moving the client in segments (see Figure 21-12, p. 277)

3. Some clients cannot be moved in segments (e.g. older adults, spinal injuries)

4. Check with your supervisor for the correct procedure to use with each client

5. Moving the Person to the Side of the Bed ▶ p. 276

F. Turning persons

1. Turning persons onto their sides helps prevent complications from bedrest (see Figures 21-13 and 21-14, p. 279)

2. Certain medical and nursing procedures require the side-lying position

3. Many clients have conditions that make turning painful for them
   a. It is best to logroll using a turning sheet

4. Turning the Person ▶ p. 278

G. Logrolling

1. Turning the person as a unit, in alignment, with one motion (see Figure 21-15, p. 281)

a. The spine is kept straight

2. Used to turn:
   a. Older persons with arthritic spines or knees
   b. Persons recovering from hip fractures
   c. Persons with spinal cord injuries
   d. Persons recovering from spinal surgery

3. Two or three staff members are needed

4. Sometimes a turning sheet is used

5. Logrolling the Person ▶ p. 280

IV. SITTING ON THE SIDE OF THE BED

A. Persons sit on the side of the bed (dangle) for many reasons (see Figure 21-16, p. 283)

1. To increase activity in stages

2. Surgical patients
   a. To cough and deep breathe
   b. To move their legs and to stimulate circulation

3. Is part of preparing a person to walk or transfer

4. Two staff members may be needed

5. Focus on older persons
   a. Circulatory changes can cause persons to become dizzy or faint
   b. Support the person to prevent falling and other injuries

6. Report and record the following:
   a. Pulse and respiration (if instructed)
   b. Pale or bluish skin colour
   c. Complaints of dizziness, light-headedness, or difficulty breathing
   d. How well the activity was tolerated
   e. The length of time the person dangled
   f. The amount of help needed
   g. Other observations or complaints

B. Helping the Person Sit on the Side of the Bed (Dangle) ▶ p. 282

V. POSITIONING

A. The person must be properly positioned at all times

B. Regular position changes and good alignment:
   1. Promotes comfort and well-being
   2. Makes breathing easier
   3. Promotes circulation
   4. Prevents pressure ulcers (see Chapter 41) and contractures (see Chapter 22)

C. Follow the person's care plan

D. Follow these guidelines to safely position a person:
   1. Check with your supervisor and with the care plan about position changes
   2. Know how often to turn a person and to what positions

3. Use good body mechanics
4. Ask for help before beginning, if necessary
5. Explain the procedure to the person
6. Be gentle when moving the person
7. Provide privacy
8. Place the signal light within reach after positioning
9. Leave the client in good body alignment; consult the care plan if pillows are used
10. Make sure linens are wrinkle-free

E. Fowler's position (see Figure 21-17, p. 285)
1. Raising the head of bed 45 to 60 degrees
2. Keep the spine straight, support the head with a small pillow; support the arms with pillows

F. Supine position—dorsal recumbent (see Figure 21-18, p. 285)
1. The back-lying position
2. The bed is flat
3. The head and shoulders are supported on a pillow
4. Arms and hands are at the person's sides
5. Pillows may be used to support the arms and hands
6. Often, a small pillow is under the thighs or ankles
7. A rolled towel may be placed under the lower back

G. Prone position (see Figure 21-20, p. 286)
1. The person lies on the abdomen with the head turned to one side
2. Small pillows are placed under the head, abdomen, and lower legs
3. Arms are flexed at the elbows with the hands near the head
4. Many persons cannot tolerate the prone position
5. Use the prone position only if it is called for in the care plan
6. To place a client in prone position
   a. Bed should be flat
   b. Remove pillows and turn person on the side and then abdomen
   c. Turn the person's head to one side
   d. Bend the arms at the elbows and place the hands near the head
   e. Place small pillows under the person's head, abdomen and lower legs (see Figure 21-19, p. 285)
   f. If feet hang over end of bed do not place pillow under lower legs (see Figure 21-20, p. 286)

H. Lateral position—side-lying (see Figure 21-

21, p. 286)
1. The person lies on one side or the other
2. A pillow is under the head and neck
3. The upper leg is placed in front of the lower leg
4. The upper leg and thigh are supported with pillows
5. The upper hand and arm and the back are supported by pillows

I. Sims' position (see Figure 21-22, p. 286)
1. A left side-lying position
2. The upper leg is sharply flexed; the lower leg is not lying under the upper leg
3. The lower arm is behind the person
4. Pillows are used to support the head and shoulders, the upper leg, and the upper arm and hand
5. Check with the nurse before positioning an older person in the Sims' position

J. Sitting position
1. The person must hold the upper body and head erect (see Figure 21-23, p. 287)
2. The back and buttocks are against the back of the chair
3. The feet are flat on the floor or on wheelchair footrests
4. The backs of the knees and calves are slightly away from the edge of the seat
5. The care plan will tell you if a pillow is to be used behind the person's back
   a. Do not use a pillow if restraints are used (see Chapter 17)
6. Paralyzed arms are supported on pillows (see Figure 21-25, p. 288)
7. Ask your supervisor about the proper use of special positioners
8. Some people require special postural supports (see Figure 21-24, p. 287)
   a. The person's safety, dignity, and function are considered

K. Repositioning in a chair or wheelchair
1. Clients can slide down and need to be repositioned so that their back and buttocks are against the back of the chair
2. If the client can help:
   a. Lock the wheelchair wheels
   b. Stand in front of the client and block their knees and feet with yours
   c. Figure 21-26, p. 288 in the textbook, shows proper use of a transfer belt
   d. If you are not using a transfer belt put your arms under the clients arms and place your hands around the client's shoulder blade

e. Ask the client to push with feet and arms on count of 1-2-3

f. Lift the client as they push

g. If the client cannot help you, ask someone else to help (see Figure 21-27, p. 288)

VI. TRANSFERRING PERSONS

A. Moving persons from beds to chairs, wheelchairs, or stretchers

1. The rules of body mechanics apply

2. Safety and comfort measures for lifting and moving persons apply

3. Some clients need only minimal help while others require two or three people to help

4. Your supervisor and the care plan will tell you how much help the person requires and if one side is weaker than the other

5. Report and record the following after transferring a client:

a. Pulse rate (if requested) before and after

b. Complaints of lightheadedness, pain, discomfort, difficulty breathing, weakness or fatigue

c. Amount of help needed

d. How client helped

B. Applying transfer belts

1. A transfer belt (gait belt or safety belt) is used to transfer unsteady and disabled persons

2. The belt goes around the person's waist

3. You grasp the belt to support the person during the transfer (see Figure 21-28, p. 290)

4. The belt is called a gait belt when used for walking with a person

5. Applying a Transfer Belt ▶ p. 290

C. Transferring the person to a chair or wheelchair (see Figure 21-30, p. 294)

1. Safety is important

2. You must prevent falls

3. The person wears shoes or slippers with non-skid soles

4. The chair or wheelchair must support the person's weight

5. The number of staff members needed for transfer depends on the person's physical capabilities, condition, and size

6. If the client cannot assist with a transfer, a mechanical lift is used

7. The person is helped out of bed on his or her strong side

a. The strong side moves first and pulls

the weak side along

8. Ask about proper use of equipment and placement of special cushions

9. Some long-term care facilities require the use of a transfer belt (see Figure 21-29, p. 293)

10. Transferring the Person to a Chair or Wheelchair ▶ p. 291

11. Transferring the Person to a Wheelchair with Assistance ▶ p. 295

D. Using a mechanical lift

1. Mechanical lifts are used for transfers to chairs, stretchers, tubs, shower chairs, toilets, whirlpools, or cars (see Figure 21-33, p. 301)

2. There are manual and electric lifts

3. Before using a lift:

a. Make sure you are trained

b. Make sure it works

c. Compare the person's weight and the lift's weight limit

4. At least two staff members are usually needed

a. Follow the manufacturer's instructions

5. Transferring a Person Using a Mechanical Lift ▶ p. 300

E. Moving the person to a stretcher

1. Stretchers are used to transport persons to other areas

2. Used for persons who:

a. Cannot sit up

b. Must stay in a lying position

c. Are seriously ill

3. With your supervisor's permission, raise the head of the stretcher for comfort

4. Safety straps are used when the person is on the stretcher

5. Stretcher side rails are kept up during transport

6. Move the person feet first

a. The person at the head watches the person's breathing and colour

b. Never leave a person on a stretcher unattended

7. At least three staff members are needed for a safe transfer

8. Transferring a Person to a Stretcher ▶ p. 302

Classroom Activities

1. Review the structure and function of the musculoskeletal system with students.

a. See Chapter 13.

2. Write the following terms on the chalkboard or flip chart:
   a. Body mechanics
   b. Posture
   c. Base of support
   Call on students to define these terms. Write in the correct answers.

3. Show the following section of video #1 of Mosby's Nursing Assisting Video Series:
   a. Body mechanics
   Allow time for discussion and questions.

4. Place a box on the floor in front of the classroom. Call on a student to demonstrate how to pick up the box using good body mechanics.
   a. Ask the other students to observe, evaluate, and provide feedback.

5. Place a box on the desk or a table in front of the classroom. Call on a student to demonstrate how to move and pick up the box using good body mechanics.
   a. Ask the other students to observe, evaluate, and provide feedback.

6. Call on students to define: "friction and shearing."

7. Divide students into groups of three. Provide each group with several sheets of notebook paper. Ask each group to list what comfort and safety measures are considered before moving a person.
   a. Allow 10 minutes for discussion.
   b. Call on a student from one group to report to the class. Ask other students to give input as appropriate.

8. Show the following sections of video #2 in Mosby's Nursing Assisting Video Series:
   a. Positioning patient in bed with and without assistance
   b. Positioning patient in bed with a turning sheet
   c. Move a patient to side of the bed without assistance
   d. Move a patient onto his side
   e. Perform the logrolling turning procedure
   f. Position a patient in Fowler's position
   g. Position a patient in Sims' position

9. Show the following sections of video #3 in Mosby's Nursing Assisting Video Series:
   a. Move a patient from bed to wheelchair with

   and without a safety belt
   b. Move a patient from bed to stretcher or portable bath tub

10. Use the procedure checklist provided.
    a. Demonstrate each procedure.
    b. Have each student practice and return demonstrate each procedure. Ask each student to assume the role of the patient/resident.
       (1) When practicing and demonstrating the procedures, ask the students to discuss their experience.

11. Ask students why regular position changes and good alignment are important when providing care to patients or residents.
    a. Write correct answers on the chalkboard. Clarify any wrong answers.

12. Divide students into three groups. Provide each group with several sheets of notebook paper. Ask each group to list the guidelines for safely positioning a person.
    a. Allow 10 minutes for discussion.
    b. Call on a student from one group to report to the class. Ask other students to provide input as appropriate.

13. Ask students to demonstrate each bed position and the sitting position. Then, have each student assume one position for 15 minutes. Have students discuss their experience.
    a. Were they comfortable? If not, what factors caused discomfort? How could the discomfort be relieved?
    b. How will their experience help them provide better care?

Homework Assignments

Ask students to answer the questions at the end of Chapter 21 in the textbook. Tell students the date and time that this assignment must be completed and turned in.

If the accompanying student workbook is being used, assign the Chapter 21 workbook exercises. Tell students the date and time that this assignment must be completed and turned in.

Chapter 21 Student Assignment

Name _____

Date _____

Body Mechanics

Matching

Match the terms with the correct definitions.

a. Body mechanics
b. Friction
c. Logrolling
d. Shearing
e. Base of support
f. Body alignment
g. Sims' position
h. Transfer belt
j. Prone position

1. _____ A belt used to hold onto a person during a transfer or when walking with the person; a gait belt or safety belt

2. _____ A side-lying position in which the upper leg is sharply flexed so that it is not on the lower leg and the lower arm is behind the person

3. _____ When skin sticks to a surface and muscles slide in the direction the body is moving

4. _____ Lying on the abdomen with the head turned to one side

5. _____ Turning the person as a unit, in alignment, with one motion

6. _____ The rubbing of one surface against another

7. _____ A semi-sitting position; the head of the bed is elevated 45 to 60 degrees

8. _____ Using the body in an efficient and careful way

9. _____ The way in which body parts are aligned with one another; posture

10. _____ The area on which an object rests

Fill in the Blanks

Write your answers in the spaces provided.

11. Keep your body in good alignment with a

_____

base of support.

12. Keep objects _____
to your body when you lift, move, or carry them.

13. _____

your work area. This prevents unnecessary

_____.

14. _____,

_____,

or _____
heavy objects whenever you can.

15. Bend your _____

and _____
to lift heavy objects from the floor.

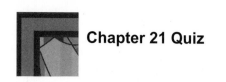

Chapter 21 Quiz

Name _____

Date _____

Body Mechanics

True or False

Mark **T** *for true or* **F** *for false.*

1. _____ The muscles in the lower back are used to lift heavy objects from the floor.

2. _____ The bed is in the lowest horizontal position when you are giving a person care.

3. _____ Using a lift sheet to move a person up in bed reduces shearing and friction.

4. _____ When transferring a person, you move the weak side first.

5. _____ Proper positioning helps prevent many complications.

Multiple Choice

Circle the BEST answer.

6. The back-lying position is the:
   a. Sims' position.
   b. Semi-Fowler's position.
   c. Dorsal recumbent position.
   d. Prone position.

7. You are helping Mr. Jones transfer from the bed to the chair. Which is incorrect?
   a. Mr. Jones wears shoes or slippers with non-skid soles.
   b. Mr. Jones is helped out of bed on his strong side.
   c. The bed is in the highest horizontal position.
   d. Help him to dangle. Make sure his feet touch the floor.

8. When logrolling a person, you must:
   a. Make sure the bed is in the Fowler's position.
   b. Lower the bed to the lowest position.
   c. Lower both bed rails.
   d. Turn the person as a unit, in alignment, with one motion.

9. You and a co-worker are transporting a resident on a stretcher. Which is incorrect?
   a. The side rails are kept up during transport.
   b. The resident is moved head first.
   c. Safety straps are applied when the resident is on the stretcher.
   d. The resident is not left unattended.

10. A person is positioned in a chair. Which is correct?
    a. The back and buttocks are against the chair.
    b. Feet are 3 to 4 inches off the floor.
    c. The back of the legs and calves fit snugly against the edge of the seat.
    d. A pillow is used behind the back if restraints are used.

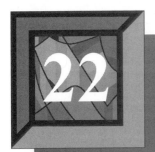

Exercise and Activity

Instructor's Preparation

I. Read Chapter 22 in the textbook. Carefully review chapter objectives, key terms, and review questions.

II. Read the outline in Chapter 22 of the instructor's guide. Carefully review the classroom activities, the student assignment, and the quiz.

III. If you are using the accompanying student workbook, review the activities for Chapter 22.

IV. Review video #2 (Lifting, Moving, & Positioning) and video #3 (Transfer Techniques/Ambulation) in Mosby's Nursing Assisting Video Series.

V. Gather all necessary supplies and equipment for classroom activities and student assignments.

A. Prepare overhead transparencies

B. Gather the correct videos

C. Gather the necessary equipment and supplies needed to demonstrate and have each student return demonstrate the procedures in this chapter

D. Gather any other items that will be needed for classroom activities

E. Assemble items in the order they will be used

VI. Make sure that the necessary equipment is available and in good working order

VII. Contact guest speakers to confirm the day, date, time, and location that they are expected

A. Ask the speakers if they require any special equipment or supplies; make sure these are available.

Objectives	Key Terms
• Define the key terms listed in this chapter	abduction
• Describe bedrest	adduction
• Describe the complications of bedrest and how to prevent them	ambulation
• Describe the devices used to support and maintain body alignment	atrophy
• Explain the purpose of a trapeze	brac
• Describe range-of-motion exercises	contracture
• Explain how to help a falling person	deconditioning
• Describe four walking aids	dorsiflexion
• Perform the procedures described in this chapter	extension
	external rotation
	flexion

footdrop
hyperextension
internal rotation
orthosis
orthostatic hypotension
plantar flexion
postural hypotension
pronation
range-of-motion (ROM)
rotation
supination
syncope

Outline

Exercise and Activity

I. INTRODUCTION
  A. Being active is important for physical and mental well-being
  B. Illness, surgery, injuries, chronic illness, pain, and aging can cause weakness and limit activity
  C. Some disorders are progressive, causing a decrease in activity (see Chapter 31)
  D. Deconditioning is the loss of muscle strength from inactivity
  E. Can affect older adults quickly
  F. Use encouragement and consult the care plan about the client's activity level
  G. To assist in promoting exercise and activity, you need to understand:
    1. Bedrest
    2. How to prevent complications from bedrest
    3. How to help persons exercise
II. BEDREST
  A. Ordered by the doctor to:
    1. Reduce physical activity
    2. Reduce pain
    3. Encourage rest
    4. Regain strength
    5. Promote healing
  B. Common types of bedrest:
    1. Bed rest—the person stays in bed; some ADL are allowed
    2. Strict bedrest—everything is done for the person; no ADL are allowed
    3. Bedrest with commode privileges—the person can use the bedside commode for elimination
    4. Bedrest with bathroom privileges—the person can use the bathroom for elimina-

tion needs
  C. The nursing care plan and your assignment sheet tell you the activities for each person
  D. Complications of bedrest
    1. Every body system is affected; the following can occur
      a. Pressure ulcers
      b. Constipation and fecal impaction
      c. Urinary tract infection and renal calculi
      d. Pneumonia
      e. Contractures and muscle atrophy (see Figures 22-1 and 22-2, p. 308)
        (1) A contracture is the lack of joint mobility caused by abnormal shortening of a muscle
        (2) Muscle atrophy is a decrease in the size of a muscle
      f. Orthostatic hypotension is a drop in blood pressure when the person stands
        (1) Box 22-1, p. 309 in the textbook, lists measures that prevent orthostatic hypotension
      g. Blood clots
      h. Syncope is a brief loss of consciousness (faintness)
    2. Complications from bedrest are prevented by good nursing care
      a. Positioning in good body alignment
      b. Range-of-motion exercises
  E. Positioning
    1. Supportive devices are often used to support and maintain the person in a certain position
      a. Bed boards are placed under the mattress to prevent it from sagging (see Figure 22-3, p. 309)
      b. Footboards are placed at the foot of the mattress (see Figure 22-4, p. 309)
        (1) Prevent plantar flexion (foot drop)
        (2) Keep top linen off the feet
      c. Trochanter rolls prevent the hips and legs from turning outward—external rotation (see Figure 22-5, p. 310)
      d. Hip abduction wedges keep the hips abducted; placed between the client's legs (see Figure 22-6, p. 310)
      e. Hand rolls or hand grips prevent contractures of the thumb, fingers, and wrist (see Figure 22-7, p. 311)
        (1) Foam rubber balls, sponges, and finger cushions are also used (see

Figure 22-8, p. 311)
   f. Splints keep the elbows, wrists, thumbs, fingers, ankles, and knees in normal position (see Figure 22-9, p. 311)
F. Exercise
   1. Helps prevent contractures, muscle atrophy, and other complications
   2. A trapeze is used for exercises to strengthen arm muscles (see Figure 22-10, p. 312)
      a. Also used to move up and turn in bed (see Chapter 21)
   3. Range-of-motion (ROM) exercises
      a. The movement of a joint to the extent possible without causing pain
      b. Usually done at least twice a day
      c. Active ROM exercises are done by the person
      d. Passive ROM exercises involve having another person move the joints through their range of motion
      e. Active-assistance range-of-motion is when the person does the exercises with some help
      f. ROM exercises occur naturally during activities of daily living
      g. Persons on bedrest have little activity; ROM exercises are done
      h. Your supervisor and the care plan tells you which joints to exercise and the type of ROM exercises to be done
      i. Box 220-2, p. 312 in the textbook, describes movements involved in ROM exercises
      j. Injury can occur if not done properly
      k. The rules in Box 22-3, p. 313 in the textbook are practiced when performing or assisting with ROM exercises
      l. Focus on children (see Focus on Children box, p. 312)
         (1) Depending on a child's activity limits, almost any play activity promotes range of motion
         (2) Always check with your supervisor and the care plan for the child's activity limits
      m. Focus on long-term care (see Focus on Long-Term Care box, p. 313)
      n. Range of motion exercises can cause injury if not done properly
         (1) Follow guidelines in Box 22-3, p. 313

         (2) Report and record the following after performing ROM
            (a) Time performed
            (b) Joints exercised
            (c) Number of time exercise performed on each joint
            (d) Complaints of pain or stiffness or spasm
            (e) Degree of client participation
      o. Performing Range-of-Motion Exercises ▶ pp. 314-318
III. AMBULATION
   A. For most persons on bedrest, activity is increased slowly and in steps
      1. First the person dangles (sits on the side of the bed)
      2. Walking about the room and in the hallway are the next steps
   B. Ambulation is the act of walking
      1. Some patients and residents are weak and unsteady from bedrest, illness, surgery, or injury
         a. You need to help these persons walk
            (1) Use a gait belt if the person is weak or unsteady (see Chapter 21)
      2. For additional support, the client uses hand rails
      3. Always check the client for orthostatic hypotension
      4. Personal choice in walking should be encouraged.
      5. Client may prefer to walk outside, in morning, or afternoon, or wait for a visitor to arrive or leave.
      6. Report and record the following after helping with ambulating
         a. How well tolerated
         b. Complaints of pain or discomfort
         c. Distance walked
      7. Helping the Person to Walk ▶ p. 319
   C. Falls
      1. Clients may:
         a. Be weak, lightheaded, or dizzy
         b. Faint
         c. Slip or slide on spills, waxed floors, throw rugs, or improper shoes (see Chapter 16)
      2. Trying to prevent a fall could cause greater harm
      3. If a person starts to fall, ease him or her to the floor

a. Protect the person's head
4. If working in the home, you will likely be alone (see Focus on Home Care box, p. 321)
5. Do not move or allow the person to get up after the fall
   a. The nurse must check the person for injuries
6. Complete an incident report as required by agency policy
7. Helping the Falling Person ▶ p. 322
D. Walking aids
1. Walking aids support the body
2. Ordered by a physician, RN, or physical therapist
3. Crutches
   a. Used when the person cannot use one leg
   b. Used when one or both legs need to gain strength
   c. Some persons with permanent weakness can use crutches
   d. They usually use Lofstrand crutches (see Figure 22-25, p. 323) which are made of metal and have a metal band that fits around the forearm
   e. Axillary crutches extend from the axilla to the ground (Figure 22- 26, p. 323); they are made of metal or wood
   f. The person learns to crutch walk, climb up and down stairs, and sit and stand
   g. The following safety measures are followed:
      (1) The crutches must fit
      (2) Crutch tips must be attached to the crutches; replace worn crutch tips; dry wet tips
      (3) Crutches are checked for flaws
      (4) Street shoes are worn; should be flat with non-skid soles
      (5) Clothes must fit well; no loose clothing
      (6) Safety rules to prevent falls are followed (see Chapter 16)
      (7) Crutches are kept where the person can reach them
3. Canes
   a. For weakness on one side of the body
   b. Help provide balance and support
   c. Single-tipped or four-point (quad) canes (see Figure 22-27, p. 324)
   d. A cane is held on the strong side of the

body
   e. The cane tip is about 6 to 10 inches to the side of the foot and about 6 to 10 inches in front of the foot on the strong side
   f. The grip is level with the hip
   g. The person walks as follows:
      (1) The cane is moved forward 15-25 centimetres (see Figure 22-28A, p. 324)
      (2) The weak leg is moved forward even with the cane (see Figure 22-28B, p. 324)
      (3) The strong leg is brought forward and ahead of the cane and the weak leg (see Figure 22-28C, p. 324)
4. Walkers
   a. A four-point walking aid (see Figure 22-29, p. 325)
   b. Gives more support than a cane
   c. The standard walker is picked up and moved forward 15-20 centimetres in front of the person, then the person moves forward (see Figure 22-29 and Figure 22-30, p. 325)
   d. The wheeled walker has wheels on the front legs and rubber tips on the back legs (see Figure 22-31, p. 325)
   e. Baskets, pouches, and trays are attached to walkers and used to carry needed items
5. Helping clients with walkers to sit and stand (see Box 22-4, p. 326)
6. Braces (orthosis)
   a. Support weak body parts
   b. Used to prevent or correct deformities
   c. Used to prevent joint movement
   d. Metal, plastic, or leather are used
   e. A brace is applied over the ankle, knee, or back (see Figure 22-32, p. 326)
   f. An ankle-foot orthosis is positioned in the shoe (see Figure 22-33, p. 326)
   g. Bony points under braces are protected
      (1) The skin is kept clean and dry
      (2) Report any signs of redness or skin breakdown (See Chapter 41)
      (3) Report complaints of pain or discomfort
   h. The care plan tells you when to apply and remove a brace

Classroom Activities

1. Call on students to discuss the importance of physical activity and exercise in their daily lives.
   a. What are some of the factors that affect their activity level?

2. Write the following on the chalkboard: " Bedrest is ordered by the doctor to:"
   a. Call on students to give reasons why bedrest is ordered. Write the correct answers on the chalkboard.

3. Display an overhead transparency showing a list of the complications of bedrest.
   a. Review and discuss each item on the list.
   b. Allow time for questions.
   c. Call on students to describe the measures that prevent the complications of bedrest.

4. Arrange for a representative from a medical supply company to bring the following supportive devices to show the class: Bed boards, Foot boards, Trochanter rolls, Hip abduction wedges, Hand rolls, Hand grips, Splints, and Bed cradles. He or she should demonstrate how each device is used.
   a. Allow students to handle and work with each item.
   b. Allow time for discussion.

5. Show the following sections of video #2 (Lifting Moving, & Positioning) in Mosby's Nursing Assisting Video Series:
   a. Range-of-motion exercises
   b. Make and use a trochanter roll

   Stop the video after each section to ask questions.

6. Display the information in Figures 22-1 to 22-18 (movements involved in ROM exercises), pp. 316-17 in the textbook, on an overhead transparency.
   a. Demonstrate each joint movement.

7. Display the guidelines listed on pp. 314-15 in the textbook on an overhead transparency. Review the rules with students. It is important that they understand these rules before they begin to practice active and passive ROM exercises.
   a. Ask students to practice each joint movement by doing active ROM exercises.
   b. Divide students into pairs. Ask students to practice each joint movement by performing passive ROM exercises on one another.

8. Show the following sections of video #3 (Transfer Techniques/Ambulation) in Mosby's Nursing Assisting Video Series:
   a. Assist a patient to walk
   b. Help a patient who is falling
   c. Identify proper use of a cane or walker

   Stop the video after each section. Encourage students to ask questions

9. Use the procedure checklists provided.
   a. Demonstrate the procedures in this chapter.
   b. Have each student practice and return demonstrate the procedures in this chapter. Have each student assume the role of the patient/resident when practicing and return demonstrating a procedure.

10. Arrange for a physical therapist as a guest speaker. He or she should discuss and demonstrate the correct use of the following equipment:
    a. Crutches
       (1) Four-point alternating gait
       (2) Three-point alternating gait
       (3) Two-point alternating gait
       (4) Swing-to gait
       (5) Swing-through gait
    b. Canes
       (1) Single-tipped
       (2) Four-point
    c. Walkers
       (1) Standard
       (2) Wheeled
    d. Braces

    Ask students to write down key points in a notebook.

    Allow time for questions and discussion. Students should be allowed to handle the equipment.

Homework Assignments

Ask students to answer the questions at the end of Chapter 22 in the textbook. Tell students the date and time that this assignment must be completed and turned in.

If the accompanying student workbook is being used, assign the Chapter 22 workbook exercises. Tell students the date and time that this assignment must be completed and turned in.

Chapter 22 Student Assignment

Name _____

Date _____

Exercise and Activity

1. Fill in the blanks. Identify the joint movements described below.

a. _____ Bending a body part

b. _____ Turning the joint outward

c. _____ Turning upward

d. _____ Moving a body part toward the body

e. _____ Straightening a body part

f. _____ Turning downward

g. _____ Bending backward

h. _____ Turning the joint inward

i. _____ Excessive straightening of a body part

j. _____ Moving a body part away from the body

k. _____ Turning the joint

2. List the rules for performing range-of-motion exercises.

a. _____

_____

b. _____

_____

c. _____

_____

d. _____

_____

e. _____

_____

f. _____

_____

g. _____

_____

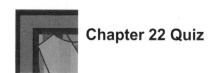

Name _____

Date _____

Exercise and Activity

True or False

Mark **T** *for true or* **F** *for false.*

1. _____ The person with a contracture is permanently deformed and disabled.

2. _____ Moving from a sitting to a standing position quickly prevents postural hypotension.

3. _____ Trochanter rolls prevent the hips from turning inward.

4. _____ If a person starts to fall, ease him or her to the floor.

5. _____ A cane is held on the weak side of the body.

Multiple Choice

Circle the BEST answer.

6. Muscle atrophy is:
   a. The abnormal shortening of a muscle.
   b. Bending backward.
   c. A decrease in the size or a wasting away of the muscle tissue.
   d. Excessive straightening of a body part.

7. Mr. Jones is on bedrest. Which is correct?
   a. No activity is allowed.
   b. Good body alignment is important.
   c. He can use the bathroom for elimination.
   d. He has orthostatic hypotension.

8. Bed cradles are used to:
   a. Keep the weight of top linens off the feet.
   b. Keep the hips abducted.
   c. Prevent plantar flexion.
   d. Prevent the mattress from sagging.

9. Which statement about range-of-motion (ROM) exercises is incorrect?
   a. ROM exercises can cause injury if not done correctly.
   b. The nurse tells you which joints to exercise.
   c. The joint is moved past the point of pain.
   d. The joint is moved slowly, smoothly, and gently.

10. Mrs. Adams uses crutches to walk. Which does not promote safety?
    a. A physical therapist measures and fits her with crutches.
    b. Crutch tips are attached to the crutches.
    c. Clothes must fit well.
    d. Comfortable bedroom slippers are worn.

11. Braces are used to:
    a. Support weak body parts.
    b. Prevent or correct deformations.
    c. Prevent joint movement.
    d. All of the above.

12. Mr. Brown has an ankle brace. You notice a reddened area on the ankle bone when you remove the brace. You should:
    a. Put a bandage on the reddened area.
    b. Massage the reddened area.
    c. Report your observation to the nurse.
    d. All of the above.

Home Management

Instructor's Preparation

I. Read Chapter 23 in the textbook. Carefully review chapter objectives, key terms, and review questions.

II. Read the outline in Chapter 23 of the instructor's guide. Carefully review the classroom activities, the student assignment, and the quiz.

III. If you are using the accompanying student workbook, review the activities for Chapter 23.

IV. Gather all necessary supplies and equipment for classroom activities and student assignments.
   A. Prepare appropriate flip charts
   B. Gather correct videos
   C. Gather the following transparencies: TA29 through TA33
   D. Gather colored markers
   E. Gather the equipment and supplies needed to demonstrate and have each student return demonstrate the procedures in this chapter.
   F. Gather any other items that will be needed for classroom activities
   G. Assemble items in the order they will be used

V. Make sure that the necessary equipment is available and in good working order.

Objectives

- Define the key terms listed in this chapter
- Explain why home management is important
- Explain your role in home management
- Explain how to use cleaning supplies safely
- Describe how to clean bedrooms, living rooms, bathrooms, and kitchens
- Explain how to do laundry

Key Terms

home management
laundry symbols

Outline

Home Management

I. INTRODUCTION
   A. Home management is the cleaning and organizing of a home
   B. Your role in home management involves light housekeeping tasks such as vacuuming, dusting, and making beds or laundry
   C. You may do basic housekeeping tasks in a facility, but they are usually done by housekeeping staff
   D. This chapter will address home management in community care settings

II. YOUR ROLE IN HOME MANAGEMENT
   A. A clean and orderly setting is important for health and safety

B. Dust, dirt and damp areas promote growth of microbes and clutter could cause falls

C. The client, family and case manager decide what tasks are required

D. Listed on care plan and should be completed; however if your client needs personal care that need takes priority

E. See Providing Compassionate Care Box.

F. You may deal with conflicting demands if your client wants something done one way but due to time restraints you can not do that way. (see Support Workers Solving Problems box, p. 330)

III. GETTING ORGANIZED

A. You are usually assigned home management tasks in addition to personal care

B. The key to completing all of your tasks is to use your time wisely

C. Review time management skills in Chapter 8 and follow the guidelines in Box 23-1, p. 330 in the etxbook, and these general points:

  1. Set priorities
  2. Set a routine
  3. Use your time well
  4. Finish tasks, and put items away
  5. Set time limits for each task
  6. Focus on the task
  7. Put the client's needs first

IV. EQUIPMENT AND SUPPLIES—ITEMS NEEDED FOR CLEANING.

A. Equipment

  1. Clean rags, sponges, cloths, or paper towels
  2. Broom, dustpan and brush
  3. Mop and bucket
  4. Toilet brush
  5. Utility gloves
  6. Vacuum cleaner
  7. Dish washing materials.

B. Supplies

  1. Detergents
  2. All-purpose cleaners
  3. Glass cleaners
  4. Special cleaners
  5. Cleansers and scouring powders
  6. Disinfectants
  7. Baking soda
  8. White vinegar
  9. If supplies are not on hand use problem-solving skills (see Support Workers Solving Problem box, p. 331)

C. Using Cleaning Products Safely

  1. Cleaning products can be harmful so re-member the following points:

    a. Read all labels carefully, follow in-structions and be familiar with WHMIS labels
    b. Never mix cleaning products
    c. Wear utility gloves
    d. Never use products in unlabelled con-tainers
    e. Store products in their original con-tainers
    f. Keep cleaning products away from food
    g. Keep products out of reach of children and adults with dementia
    h. Use products only for their intended purpose
    i. Keep aerosol cans away from heat sources
    j. Ask the client if they object before using a strong cleaner on a surface
    k. Rinse strong, abrasive cleaners imme-diately after use
    l. Do no scrub vigorously

V. CLEANING BEDROOMS

A. Some clients spend little time in bed but some spend most or all of their time in bed, and eat their meals in their bedrooms

B. The bedroom should be clean, orderly, and comfortable (see Box 23-2, p.332)

C. You need to:

  1. Make the bed
  2. Straighten bedding as needed
  3. Change the linens as needed

VI. CLEANING LIVING ROOMS

A. Some people seldom use their living room, some use it all the time and in some cases it is turned into the bedroom.

B. It should be kept clean and comfortable (see Box 23-3, p. 333)

VII. CLEANING BATHROOMS

A. Need special attention as microbes grow easily and spread in damp places (see Box 23-4, p. 334)

B. Toilets must be cleaned thoroughly with a dis-infectant or toilet bowl cleaner

C. Use utility gloves and special toilet brushes

D. Some cleaners scratch surfaces, so use special bathroom cleaners, or laundry detergent or vinegar and water solutions

E. Practice the hygienic measures listed on p. 334 in the textbook

F. Some clients, such as those on chemotherapy, are at high risk for infection so their bathrooms must be kept very clean; the care plan will list the extra measures you need to take

VIII. CLEANING KITCHENS
  A. A clean kitchen is critical to preventing the spread of foodborne illnesses (see Chapter 25)
  B. Box 23-5, p. 335 in the textbook, describes how to clean the kitchen
  C. Remember the following:
    1. Do not pour dirty or contaminated liquids down the sink; flush down the toilet
    2. Use one cloth for counters another for wiping floors and another for dishes
    3. Use paper towels to dry your hands
    4. Change cloths daily or as needed
    5. Clean microwave after every use
    6. Do not put soiled diapers in kitchen garbage

IX. DOING LAUNDRY
  A. Your goal is to clean items without causing damage
  B. Ask your client or family about which detergent, bleach, and fabric softener to use, as well as any special laundry instructions
  C. Box 23-6, p. 337 in the textbook, describes how to do laundry
  D. Most garments have laundry symbols on labels (see Figure 23-3, p. 339), follow these instructions carefully
  E. Follow employer policy and Standard Precautions (see Chapter 18) when handling laundry soiled with blood, body fluids, secretions, or excretions
  F. When removing stains, handle chemicals carefully (see Box 23-7, p. 338)
  G. Follow instructions carefully and if possible treat stains immediately before they become set in the fabric

Classroom Activities

1. Write the following words on the board:
   a. Bedrooms
   b. Living Rooms
   c. Kitchens
   d. Bathrooms
   e. Laundry
   Divide the class into small groups (3-4) and ask each group to make a list of the cleaning products they use to clean each room. Have a person from each group report back to the class and write the variety of products on the board.

2. On a transparency draw ten of the laundry symbols from p. 339 in the textbook and ask the class to identify what each means.

3. Ask the class to list the ways they get rid of stains on clothing and linens and compare to the list in Box 23-7, p. 338 in the textbook.

4. Write "Cleaning Kitchens" on the board and ask students to list the top ten things in the kitchen that they should clean, which supplies they would use, and what equipment they would use.

5. Ask the students to identify the hygienic measures they should use when cleaning the bathrooms and compare with the list on p. 334 in the textbook.

Homework Assignments

Ask students to answer the questions at the end of Chapter 23 in the textbook. Tell students the date and time that this assignment must be completed and turned in.

If the accompanying student workbook is being used, assign the Chapter 23 workbook exercises. Tell students the date and time that this assignment must be completed and turned in.

Name _____

Date _____

Home Management

Fill in the Blanks

Write your answers in the spaces provided.

1. Which time management skills will help you get organized when performing household management tasks?

   a. _____

   b. _____

   c. _____

   d. _____

   e. _____

   f. _____

2. What points should you remember when using cleaning products?

   a. _____

   b. _____

   c. _____

   d. _____

   e. _____

   f. _____

   g. _____

3. What is the process for cleaning kitchen surfaces (counters, stovetop, and table)?

   a. _____

   b. _____

   c. _____

   d. _____

Name _____

Date _____

Home Management

4. What guidelines should you follow when using a dryer?

a. _____

b. _____

c. _____

d. _____

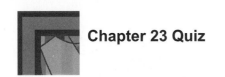

Chapter 23 Quiz

Name _____

Date _____

Home Management

<table>
<tr>
<td>

True or False

*Mark **T** for true or **F** for false.*

1. _____ It is okay to use products in unlabelled containers if your client says it is okay.

2. _____ Vinegar will disinfect a toilet.

3. _____ You must look after your client's personal needs before housekeeping tasks.

4. _____ Change linens daily even if not needed.

5. _____ As long as you rinse your cloth, you can use the same cloth to wipe counters and floors.

6. _____ Bloodstains can be removed in hot water.

7. _____ The circle symbol means that a garment needs to be dry cleaned.

</td>
<td>

Multiple Choice

Circle the BEST answer.

8. Which is not a cleaning guideline:
   a. work from higher to lower
   b. work from dry to wet
   c. work from near to far
   d. rinse and dry washed surfaces

9. Which household product will remove stains?
   a. disinfectant
   b. baking soda
   c. vinegar
   d. boiling water

10. Which is not part of your responsibilities when cleaning bedrooms?
    a. change the linens
    b. straighten the bed
    c. make the bed
    d. organize the client's dresser drawers.

11. Which steps will help you organize your time?
    a. Set priorities
    b. Set time limits for each task
    c. Focus on the task
    d. All of the above

</td>
</tr>
</table>

Beds and Bedmaking

24

Instructor's Preparation

   I. Read Chapter 24 in the textbook. Carefully review chapter objectives, key terms, and review questions.

  II. Read the outline in Chapter 24 of the instructor's guide. Carefully review the classroom activities, the student assignment, and the quiz.

 III. If you are using the accompanying student workbook, review the activities for Chapter 24.

 IV. Gather all necessary supplies and equipment for classroom activities and student assignments.

    A. Prepare appropriate flip charts

    B. Prepare overhead transparencies

    C. Prepare situation/index cards

    D. Gather correct video

    E. Gather the following transparency: TA35

    F. Gather coloured markers

    G. Gather supplies and equipment needed to demonstrate and have each student in turn demonstrate the procedures in this chapter

    H. Gather any other items that will be needed for classroom activities

    I. Assemble items in the order they will be used

  V. Make sure that the necessary equipment is available and in good working order.

Objectives

- Define the key terms listed in this chapter
- Know the basic bed positions
- Describe how to handle linens according to the rules of medical asepsis
- Explain the purposes of plastic drawsheets and cotton drawsheets
- Describe general rules for bedmaking
- Describe the differences between open, closed, occupied, and surgical beds
- Perform the procedures described in this chapter

Key Terms

drawsheet
plastic drawsheet

Outline

Beds and Bedmaking

  I. INTRODUCTION

    A. Many clients spend a great deal of time in bed because of illness, disability, surgery, or injury; others are on ordered bed rest (see Chapter 41)

    B. Bedmaking is an important function

      1. A clean, dry, and wrinkle-free bed helps the person's comfort

      2. Clean, neat, dry, wrinkle-free beds help prevent skin breakdown and pressure ulcers (see Chapter 41)

      3. Beds are usually made in the morning after baths

      4. People like their beds made and rooms

clean before visitors arrive

5. Straighten linens whenever loose or wrinkled and at bedtime

6. Change linens whenever they are wet, soiled, or damp

7. Follow Standard Precautions

II. THE BED

A. Many home care clients use their regular beds or may require a hospital bed; long-term facilities and hospitals use hospital beds

B. Regular beds

1. Come in all sizes from twin to king, waterbeds to cots

2. Cannot be raised so the lower the bed the more you need to bend when giving care or making the bed

3. Use good body mechanics (see Chapter 21)

C. Hospital beds

1. Have electrical or manual controls to raise and lower

2. The lowest position helps the client get out of bed (see Figure 24-1, p. 342)

3. Most beds are electric and the client is instructed on how to use the controls (see Figure 24-2, p. 343)

4. Most electric beds can be locked into position to protect the client from potentially dangerous positions, or prevent the client from changing an ordered position

5. Manually operated beds are still in use in some facilities (see Figure 24-3, p. 343)

6. A hospital bed can be easily moved on its wheels, which can also be locked to prevent the bed from moving (see Figure 24-4, p. 343)

D. Bed positions

1. Flat—usual sleeping position

2. Fowler's position—a semi-sitting position

a. The head of the bed is raised 45 to 60 degrees (see Figure 24-5, p. 344)

b. Reasons for positioning are described in Chapter 21 in the textbook

3. Semi-Fowler's position

a. The head of the bed is raised 45 degrees and knee position is raised 15 degrees (see Figure 24-6, p. 344)

b. Comfortable position that prevents clients from sliding down in bed

c. Check with care plan and your supervisor before positioning a client in the semi-Fowler's position

d. Employers may differ in their defini-

tion of this position, so be sure you know your policy (see Focus on Home Care box, p. 344)

4. Trendelenburg's position

a. The head of the bed is lowered and the foot of the bed is raised (see Figure 24-7, p. 344)

b. This position requires a physician's order

5. Reverse Trendelenburg's position

a. The head of the bed is raised and the foot is lowered (see Figure 24-8, p. 344)

b. This position requires a physician's order

III. LINENS

A. When handling linens, follow the rules of medical asepsis

B. Always hold linens away from your body and uniform (see Figure 24-10, p. 345)

C. Never shake linens in the air (this spreads microbes)

D. Place clean linen on a clean surface

E. Never put clean linens or dirty linen on the floor

F. Collect clean linens in the order of use

1. The item you will use first is at the bottom

a. Mattress pad

b. Bottom sheet (flat or fitted)

c. Plastic drawsheet or disposable bed protector

d. Cotton drawsheet

e. Top sheet (flat sheet)

f. Blanket

g. Bedspread

h. Pillowcase

i. Bath towel

j. Hand towel

k. Washcloth

l. Clean pyjamas or hospital gown (if needed)

m. Bath blanket

2. Use one arm to hold the linens and the other hand to pick them up

a. You need the mattress pad first

b. To get it into place, turn the stack over onto your arm (see Figure 24-11, p. 346)

G. Follow Standard Precautions when removing linen; used linen is considered dirty (contaminated with microbes)

H. Wear gloves if the linens are soiled with blood, body fluids, secretions, or excretions

I. Check linens for misplaced personal belongings and watch for stray needles in the linen
J. Remove each piece separately and roll the linen away from you
K. The side that touched the client will be inside the roll (see Figure 24-12, p. 346)
L. Place linens in a laundry container or special linen bag
M. Follow employer policy for soiled linen (see Chapter 18)
N. Table 24-1, p. 347 in the textbook, shows different settings for how often linen is changed
O. Follow the care plan and employer policy
P. In all settings, linens are changed when wet, damp, or soiled
Q. Focus on home care
   1. Linens are usually changed weekly
   2. Follow the person's routine
   3. Contact the RN if the person refuses to have linens changed
R. A drawsheet is a small sheet placed over the middle of the bottom sheet
   1. A plastic drawsheet is waterproof
     a. Placed between the bottom sheet and the cotton drawsheet
   2. Many agencies use waterproof pads instead of plastic drawsheets
   3. Plastic-covered mattresses cause some persons to perspire
     a. This increases discomfort
   4. A cotton drawsheet reduces heat retention and absorbs moisture
   5. Cotton drawsheets are often used as lifting or turning sheets (see Chapter 21)
   6. Focus on home care (see Focus on Home Care box, p. 347)
     a. A flat sheet folded in half or a twin-sized sheet can be used as a drawsheet
     b. Your supervisor and the care plan tell you what to use
     c. Do not use plastic trash bags or dry cleaning bags
       (1) The danger of suffocation is high

IV. GUIDELINES FOR BEDMAKING
A. Box 13-1, p. 297 in the textbook, lists the rules for bedmaking
B. Your job description will include making beds
C. Safety and medical asepsis are important
D. Standard precautions and the Bloodborne Pathogen Standard are followed
E. Focus on home care (see Focus on Home Care box, p. 347)

F. Focus on children
   1. Cribs and crib linens present safety hazards
   2. Mattresses, linens, and bumper pads can lead to suffocation and strangulation
   3. Follow the safety rules for cribs and crib linens listed on p. 348 in the textbook
   4. Report any safety hazards to the nurse
   5. See Focus on Children box, p. 348 in the textbook

V. THE CLOSED BED
A. Made after a person is discharged
   1. Made after the frame and mattress are cleaned
B. Focus on long-term care
   1. Made if the resident will be out of bed for most of the day
   2. Clean linens are used as needed
C. Focus on home care
   1. A closed bed means linens are not folded back
   2. Clean linens are used as needed
D. Making a Closed Bed ▶ p. 349

VI. THE OPEN BED
A. A closed bed becomes an open bed by folding the top linens back (see Figure 24-21, p. 354)
B. Made when the client is out of bed for a short time and allows the client to easily get into bed
C. The person is out of bed when the bed is being made
D. Making an Open Bed ▶ p. 354

VII. THE OCCUPIED BED
A. Made when the person cannot be out of bed because of illness or injury (see Figure 24-22, p. 355)
   1. Keep the person in good body alignment
   2. Know about restrictions or limits in the person's movement or positioning
   3. Explain each step of the procedure to the person before it is done
     a. Important, even if the person does not respond
   4. Making an Occupied Bed ▶ p. 355

VIII. THE SURGICAL BED
A. Recovery bed, postoperative bed, or anesthetic bed
B. A form of the open bed
C. Made so the person can be transferred from a stretcher to the bed (see Figure 24-27, p. 359)
D. If the bed is made for a postoperative patient, a complete linen change is done
E. Making a Surgical Bed ▶ p. 359

Classroom Activities

1. Write the following terms on the chalkboard:
   a. Closed bed
   b. Open bed
   c. Occupied bed
   d. Surgical bed
   Call on students to define each term. Write the correct answer beneath each term on the chalkboard.

2. Show the following section of video #4 in Mosby's Nursing Assisting Video Series.
   a. Efficiently collect linen

3. Display the guidelines for bedmaking listed in Box 24-1, p. 347 in the textbook, on an overhead transparency. Use this as a basis for discussion.

4. Ask students to discuss the safety rules for cribs and crib linens.
   a. Stress the importance of following all safety rules.

5. Show the remaining sections of video #4 in Mosby's Nursing Assisting Video Series.
   a. Allow time for discussion and questions.

6. Use the procedure checklists provided.
   a. Demonstrate each procedure. Have each student practice and in turn demonstrate each procedure. Have each student assume the role of the patient or resident for the occupied bed.

Homework Assignments

Ask students to answer the questions at the end of Chapter 24 in the textbook. Tell students the date and time that this assignment must be completed and turned in.

If the accompanying workbook is being used, assign the Chapter 24 workbook exercises. Tell students the date and time that this assignment must be completed and turned in.

Chapter 24 Student Assignment

Name _____

Date _____

Beds and Bedmaking

Write your answers in the spaces provided.

1. You are collecting linens to make a bed.
   List the linens you will collect in the correct order.

   a. _____

   b. _____

   c. _____

   d. _____

   e. _____

   f. _____

   g. _____

   h. _____

   i. _____

   j. _____

   k. _____

   l. _____

   m. _____

2. Your uniform is considered
   _____. Therefore, you al-
   ways hold linens _____
   _____ your body and uniform.

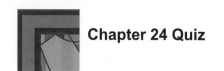 **Chapter 24 Quiz**

Name _____

Date _____

Beds and Bedmaking

True or False	Multiple Choice

*Mark **T** for true or **F** for false.*

1. _____ When removing dirty linens, roll the linens toward you.

2. _____ Wash your hands before handling clean linens and after handling dirty linens.

3. _____ Linens are changed when they are loose or wrinkled.

4. _____ Soiled linen is placed on the floor in the person's room until you finish making the bed.

5. _____ When making an occupied bed, you must keep the person in good body alignment.

6. _____ Wet, damp, and soiled linens are changed at the end of your shift.

7. _____ Residents of long-term care facilities are allowed to bring pillows and bedspreads from home.

8. _____ Plastic bags or dry cleaning bags can be used in the home to protect the mattress.

9. _____ Pillows are used to position babies in cribs.

10. _____ The space between the mattress and crib sides should be no more than 2 inches.

Circle the BEST answer.

11. A bed that is ready for a new patient or resident is:
    a. An open bed.
    b. An occupied bed.
    c. A surgical bed.
    d. A closed bed.

12. You are making an occupied bed. Which is incorrect?
    a. Keep the person in good body alignment.
    b. Raise the bed for good body mechanics.
    c. Cover the person with the bedspread.
    d. Lower the bed rail nearest you.

13. Which is correct when handling linens?
    a. Shake linens in the air to remove wrinkles.
    b. Place dirty linen on the floor.
    c. Collect linens in the order of use.
    d. Return unused linen to the linen closet.

14. The type of bed used for a person arriving on a stretcher is:
    a. A closed bed.
    b. A surgical bed.
    c. An open bed.
    d. An occupied bed.

15. A cotton drawsheet:
    a. Is always used when a plastic drawsheet is used.
    b. Must completely cover the plastic drawsheet.
    c. Keeps the mattress and bottom sheet clean and dry.
    d. All of the above.

178

25

Basic Nutrition and Fluids

Instructor's Preparation

I. Read Chapter 25 in the textbook. Carefully review chapter objectives, key terms, and review questions.

II. Read the outline in Chapter 25 of the instructor's guide. Carefully review the classroom activities, the student assignment, and the quiz.

III. If you are using the accompanying student workbook, review the activities for Chapter 25.

IV. Review the appropriate sections of videos #7 and #11 in Mosby's Nursing Assisting Video Series.

V. Gather all necessary supplies and equipment for classroom activities and student assignments.

   A. Prepare the correct number of handouts

   B. Prepare appropriate flip charts

   C. Prepare overhead transparencies

   D. Gather correct video

   E. Gather coloured markers

   F. Gather anatomical models

   G. Gather simulators

   H. Gather supplies and equipment needed to demonstrate and have each student in turn demonstrate the procedures in this chapter

   I. Gather any other items that will be needed for classroom activities

   J. Assemble items in the order they will be used

VI. Make sure that the necessary equipment is available and in good working order.

VII. Contact guest speakers to confirm the day, date, time, and location that they are expected.

   A. Ask the speakers if they require any special equipment or supplies.

Objectives

- Define the key terms listed in this chapter
- Describe the functions and major sources of protein, carbohydrates, fats, vitamins, minerals, and water
- Explain the principles of *Canada's Food Guide to Healthy Eating*
- Explain the purpose of food labels
- Explain how nutrient requirements change throughout the life cycle
- Describe factors that affect eating and nutrition
- Explain your role in meal planning and preparation
- Explain why food safety is important
- Describe special diets
- Explain your role in assisting clients to eat
- Explain how to feed clients
- Describe adult fluid requirements and the common causes of edema and dehydration
- Describe three common special fluid orders
- Explain the purpose of intake and output records
- Learn the procedures described in this chapter

Outline

Basic Nutrition and Fluids

I. INTRODUCTION
   A. The need for food and water is a basic physical need necessary for life and health
   B. The amount and quality of foods are important
   C. Poor diet and eating habits increase a person's risk for infection and acute or chronic illness, healing problems, and abnormal physical and mental function
   D. Eating and drinking provide pleasure; they are a part of social activities (see Figure 25-1, p. 363)
   E. Review of the structure and function of the digestive system in the textbook (see Chapter 13)

II. BASIC NUTRITION
   A. Nutrition is the many processes involved in the ingestion, digestion, absorption, and use of foods and fluids by the body
      1. Good nutrition is needed for growth, healing, and maintaining body functions
   B. Select foods to provide a well-balanced diet and correct calorie intake
      1. High fat, high calories = weight gain
      2. Not enough calories = weight loss
   C. Foods and fluids contain nutrients
      1. A nutrient is a substance that is ingested, digested, absorbed, and used by the body
      2. Nutrients are grouped into fats, proteins, carbohydrates, vitamins, and minerals
      3. Fats, proteins, and carbohydrates give the body fuel for energy
      4. A calorie is the amount of energy produced from burning of food by the body

   a. 1 gram of fat supplies 9 calories
   b. 1 gram of protein supplies 4 calories
   c. 1 gram of carbohydrate supplies 4 calories
   D. Nutrients
      1. A well-balanced diet ensures adequate intake of essential nutrients
      2. Protein
         a. The most important nutrient
         b. Is needed for tissue growth and repair
         c. Sources include meat, fish, poultry, eggs, milk products, cereals, beans, peas, and nuts
      3. Carbohydrates
         a. Provide energy and fiber for bowel elimination
         b. Found in fruits, vegetables, breads, cereals, and sugar
         c. There are three main types
            (1) Simple sugars—fruits
            (2) Starches—bread, etc.
            (3) Fibre—bran, nuts, cannot be digested so passes through intestines undigested
            (4) Most are broken down to sugars and absorbed into blood stream
      4. Fats
         a. Provide energy, add flavor to food, and help the body use certain vitamins
         b. Sources include meats, lard, butter, shortening, salad and vegetable oils, milk, cheese, egg yolks, and nuts
         c. Three main types of dietary fats
            (1) Saturated fat is in animal and dairy products
            (2) Unsaturated fat in fish and vegetable oil
            (3) Trans-fat created when liquid oil is chemically altered to form a more solid substance—found in margarine, shortening, etc.
         d. Unsaturated fats are healthier than saturated and trans-fat
      5. Vitamins
         a. Do not provide calories but are essential nutrients
         b. Vitamin C and B complex vitamins are not stored by the body
            (1) They must be ingested daily
         c. Each vitamin is needed for a certain body function
         d. Table 25-1, p. 365 in the textbook, lists sources and major functions of common vitamins

6. Minerals
   a. Are needed for bone and tooth formation, nerve and muscle function, fluid balance, and other body processes
   b. Table 25-2, p. 365 in the textbook, lists the major functions and dietary sources of common minerals
7. Water
   a. Most important nutrient for life
   b. Body needs it to maintain cell function, regulate body temperature, deliver nutrients, remove waste, etc.
   c. Enters through fluids and foods and exits through urine, feces, skin and lungs.
E. *Canada's Food Guide to Healthy Eating*
   1. Developed by Health Canada to promote wise food choices
   2. Healthy eating is needed to:
      a. Ensure essential nutrients
      b. Promote health
      c. Reduce risk of nutrient-related health problems
   3. Food Guide divides foods into four groups
      a. Grain Products—cereals, pastas etc
      b. Vegetables and Fruits
      c. Milk Products—cheese, milk etc
      d. Meat and Alternatives—meat, eggs, peas, nuts, etc.
   4. Healthy diet contains food from each group (see Figure 25-2, pg. 366)
   5. Rainbow bands are different lengths, which indicates how much of your diet should come from each group
      a. Most food servings should come from the yellow band
   6. Fifth band left off the chart represents foods such as sugars, jams, soft drinks, etc.
      a. It is left off to remind people to use in moderation
   7. Guide for everyone over the age of 4 years
   8. Follow guidelines reduces risk for diseases such as diabetes, heart disease, etc.
   9. Box 25-1, p. 367 in the textbook, lists guidelines for healthy eating
F. Servings from the food groups
   1. Recommended servings
      a. Number of servings depends on age, size, gender, and activity level
      b. Guide gives a range for size and number of servings
      c. Children should choose the lowest; pregnant women, teenage boys, and very active people should choose the highest number (see Figure 25-3, pg. 368)
   2. Grain products
      a. 5 to 12 servings per day recommended
      b. carbohydrates, protein, iron, thiamin, niacin, riboflavin, folic acid, iron and zinc are main nutrients
      c. Whole–grain products are high in fibre
   3. Vegetables and fruits
      a. 5 to 10 servings per day recommended
      b. dark green vegetables are rich in folic acid and iron
      c. orange fruits and vegetables are rich in Vitamin A
      d. vegetables become high in fat if fried or eaten with sauces
      e. fresh vegetables and juices are best
   4. Milk products
      a. Rich in protein, calcium, carbohydrates, fat, riboflavin, and vitamins A and D
      b. Richest source of calcium
      c. 2 to 4 servings per day recommended
      d. Ages 4-9 need 2-3; youths 10-16, pregnant women, and breastfeeding mothers need 3 to 4 servings
      e. Choose lower-fat milk products
   5. Meat and alternatives
      a. Protein, fat, thiamin, vitamin B12, and iron are main nutrients
      b. Recommends 2 to 3 servings
      c. Foods in this group vary in fat content
      d. Processed meats are high in fat
      e. Refer to p. 369 in the textbook for details regarding fat content
G. Food labels
   1. Useful for planning a healthy diet
      a. List ingredients, nutrition facts, and nutrition claims
   2. List of ingredients
      a. Listed in order of most plentiful ingredients
      b. Compare two or more products
   3. Nutrition facts
      a. Figure 25-4, p. 369 in the textbook, contains information on calories and 13 nutrients including fat, carbohydrates,

and protein

b. The Daily Value (DV) shows how a serving fits into the daily diet of an adult

c. Recommended
   (1) 60% carbohydrates
   (2) 10% protein
   (3) 30% (or less) fat
   (4) 10% (or less) saturated fat

4. Nutrition claims
   a. Manufacturers' nutrition claims about foods must meet government requirements
   b. The following diet-related health claims are allowed:
      (1) Healthy diet
      (2) Low in sodium, high in potassium may reduce riskof hypertension
      (3) Adequate in calcium or Vitamin D may reduce risk of osteoporosis
      (4) Low in saturated fat and trans-fat may reduce risk of heart disease
      (5) Rich in vegetables and fruit may reduce risk of some types of cancer

H. Nutrition throughout the life cycle
   1. Infancy and childhood
      a. Infancy is a period of rapid growth and development
      b. Formula provides nutrients, while breast milk provides nutrients and antibodies
      c. At 4–6 months of age, iron-fortified cereals are introduced, followed by pureed foods
      d. At 10 months to 1 year of age finger foods are introduced
      e. After 1 year of age growth rate slows
      f. Fat is needed for brain development
      g. When caring for infants and children, consult the care plan, and take instructions from tour supervisor
   2. Adolescence
      a. Biggest growth stage since infancy
      b. Increased nutrients are needed
      c. Many form unhealthy eating habits such as skipping meals and fast food, which can lead to eating disorders, iron deficiency, and poor health
   3. Young and middle adulthood
      a. Depends on age, gender, activity level, and body size

b. If calorie intake exceeds energy needs, weight is gained

4. Pregnancy
   a. Need about 500 additional calories
   b. If your client doesn't eat meat, they need to discuss diet with a physician
   c. Should increase folic acid, iron, and calcium to avoid risks to fetus (see Chapter 38)

5. Late adulthood
   a. Variation in health and nutrients status: emotional, social, and physical factors can affect these
   b. Don't want to eat alone, can't drive to grocery store, low incomes, no family or friends to help
   c. Loss of hearing, smell, and taste affect appetite and meal preparation
   d. Decrease in saliva may cause dysphagia; decrease in digestive juices may cause nutrients not to be absorbed
   e. Medications can cause side affects
   f. Loss of teeth or ill-fitting dentures makes chewing difficult
   g. Energy levels are lower so fewer calories are needed, but nutritional requirements remain high

III. FACTORS AFFECTING EATING AND NUTRITION
   A. Personal choice—likes and dislikes for foods are a personal matter
      1. Food likes begin in childhood
      2. Body reactions affect food choice
   B. Allergies—sensitivity to a substance that causes body to react
      1. Reactions can range from skin rashes to anaphylactic shock
      2. Nuts and seafood cause the most severe reactions
   C. Food Intolerances
      1. Reaction to food that does not involve the immune system
      2. Common reactions are indigestion and diarrhea
      3. Someone with lactose intolerance, for example, cannot digest milk
   D. Culture—influences dietary practices, food choices, and food preparation (see Respecting Diversity box, p. 371)
   E. Religion—selecting, preparing, and eating food often involves religious practices
      1. You need to respect the person's religious practices
   F. Finances—people on limited incomes often

lack protein and certain vitamins and minerals

G. Appetite—relates to the desire for food
1. Aromas and thoughts of food can stimulate appetite
2. Loss of appetite (anorexia) can occur
a. Causes include illness, drugs, unpleasant thoughts, sights and smells, anxiety, pain, and depression

H. Illness
1. Appetite usually decreases during illness and recovery from injury
2. Nutritional needs increase; the body must fight infection, heal tissue, and replace lost blood cells
3. Nutrients lost through vomiting and diarrhea must be replaced

I. Age affects nutrition
1. Infancy is a period of rapid growth and development
2. During puberty boys and girls have their biggest growth spurt
3. Most adults have lower energy requirements than adolescents
4. Older adults vary greatly in their health and nutritional status, which is affected by emotional, social, and physical factors

IV. MEAL PLANNING AND PREPARATION
A. Your role depends on the care plan and your client's needs.
B. Most home care agencies expect families to provide groceries and main meals.
C. You may be required to make light meal or prepare several meals and freeze them for future use. Occasionally you may plan menus and shop for groceries.
D. When preparing meals consider:
1. Dietary requirements—the care plan or your supervisor will tell you about special diets, mealtime instructions, dietary practices, and food allergies and intolerances
2. Food preferences—follow the client's wishes; never give clients food that they are not allowed, and consult your supervisor if you have concerns
3. Eating habits—some people have large meal at noon, some at supper, others eat several small meals; many varieties so follow your client's wishes and check the care plan
4. If you are expected to shop for groceries, keep a list and ask the client to add items

V. CHECKING EXPIRY DATES
A. By law expiry or best before dates must appear on products with a limited shelf life
B. Sell by—last recommended day of sale
C. Best before—last date manufacturer will guarantee freshness
D. Expiry date—last date product can be safely consumed

VI. HANDLING CLIENT'S MONEY
A. Some clients have grocery accounts; others provide cash for groceries
B. Always keep track of the money and receipts, and return change to client
C. Most agencies have strict policies about handling clients' money; be sure to follow these policies

VII. FOOD SAFETY
A. Foodborne illness is caused by improperly cooked or stored food
B. Can cause diarrhea, nausea, and vomiting, and can also lead to serious illness or death
C. Most at risk are infants, children, older adults, and people with chronic illness and weakened immune systems
D. Many foods naturally have pathogens (e.g. fish, poultry, eggs); if not cooked properly can cause illness
E. Cross-contamination can occur (for example, meat juices drip onto vegetables, or the same cutting surface is used for meat and other foods without proper cleaning)
F. Pathogens can be destroyed by proper cooking and by storing at a temperature below 4 degrees C (see Table 25-4, p. 375)
G. Pathogens thrive at room temperature, so refrigerate foods as soon as possible
H. If you prepare and serve meals to clients, know safe food-handling practices (see Box 25-3 p. 374)

VIII. SPECIAL DIETS
A. Ordered by the doctor for a nutritional deficiency or disease, to eliminate or decrease certain substances in the diet, or for weight control (see Table 25-5, p. 376)
B. Special diets are common before and after surgery
C. Allergies, obesity, and other disorders also require special diets
D. When a special diet is ordered, the RN and dietician work together to meet the person's needs
1. The plan includes personal choice, culture, religion, and food allergies

2. They also plan for any eating problems
E. A special diet is ordered for persons with difficulty swallowing
   1. They often need pureed food
F. Regular diet, general diet, and house diet have no dietary limitations
G. The sodium-restricted diet
   1. The average amount of sodium in the daily diet is 3000 to 5000 mg (the body needs half this amount)
   2. Healthy people excrete excess sodium in the urine
   3. Heart and kidney disease, some drugs, and some complications of pregnancy cause the body to retain sodium
   4. Sodium causes the body to retain water; this places a greater work load on the heart
      a. A sodium-restricted diet is needed
      b. The doctor orders the amount of sodium restriction
         (1) 2000 mg to 3000 mg sodium diet is called a low-salt diet
            (a) All high-sodium foods are omitted
         (2) 1000 mg sodium diet—the sodium restriction is moderate
         (3) 500 mg sodium diet—the sodium restriction is severe
H. Diabetes meal planning
   1. Necessary for persons with diabetes mellitus (see Chapter 31)
      a. Diabetes is usually treated with insulin or drugs, diet, and exercise
   2. The doctor determines the amount of carbohydrates the person should have
   3. The dietician and client develop a consistent-carbohydrate diabetes meal plan
      a. The plan also specifies a certain amount of fat and protein
      b. The person's age, gender, activity, and weight are considered
   4. The person ingests a consistent amount of protein, fat, and carbohydrates each day
      a. Eaten at each breakfast, lunch, and dinner, and as part of each snack
      b. The person must eat only what is allowed and all that is allowed
      c. If all food is not eaten, a between-meal nourishment is needed
      d. Meal and snack times are consistent from day to day
      e. The amount of insulin given depends on the person's daily food intake, ex-

ercise, etc.
IX. ASSISTING THE PERSON WITH EATING
A. Factors that affect a person's appetite and ability to eat
   1. Weakness and illness
   2. Odors
   3. Unpleasant equipment
   4. Uncomfortable position
   5. The need for oral hygiene
   6. The need to eliminate
   7. Pain
B. Getting the person ready for meals
   1. Assist with oral hygiene; make sure dentures are in place
   2. Provide for elimination needs
   3. Change clothing and provide clean linens for incontinent persons
   4. Make sure dentures, eyeglasses and hearing aids are in place
   5. Assist the person with hand washing
   6. Position the person for eating
      a. In bed—raise the person to a comfortable sitting position
      b. In a chair—assist the person to transfer; position the overbed table in front of the person
   7. Assist persons to the dining room
C. Making meals enjoyable
   1. Some people lose interest in eating because of illness or other factors
   2. Small details can help
   3. Check the care plan as some of the following measures may not apply to clients on special diets
      a. Assist with menu choices—long-term facilities help select from menu—if planning and preparing involve the client
      b. Make the setting attractive—in home care, let the client choose table linens and utensils
      c. Serve hot meals immediately
      d. Serve moderate portions—some may lose interest when faced with too much food; ask the client about amounts
      e. Make mealtimes social occasions—encourage long-term residents to dine with others; in home care, keep the client company
D. Assisting clients with eating problems
   1. Changes resulting from aging, illness and disabilities can cause eating problems.
   2. Chewing problems—foods that provide

soft bulk are served
  a. Follow the care plan
  b. To help ease chewing problems, offer plenty of fluids, small mouthfuls, and give the person time to chew
3. Swallowing problems (dysphagia)
  a. Certain medications decrease saliva resulting in dry mouth
  b. If paralysis may have trouble as throat muscles may be affected
  c. Thick, soft, moist foods are best
  d. Care plan may include:
    (1) Client should sit upright, leaning slightly forward
    (2) Ask the client to lower the chin while swallowing
    (3) Offer plenty of fluids
    (4) Give the client time to chew and swallow
    (5) Ask the client to remain sitting for at least 30 minutes after the meal
  e. People with swallowing problems are at risk for choking and aspiration
    (1) A client who cannot talk or cough may be choking
    (2) Call for help immediately
    (3) If no help, follow emergency measures for choking (see Chapter 47)
4. Weakness—some clients are too weak to chew and swallow
  a. May become even weaker
  b. Less energy to eat
  c. Never force a client to eat; inform your supervisor if the client is not eating
  d. Offer frequent, small, high-calorie meals, and soft foods; serve nutritious drinks which may include dietary supplements
  e. Follow the care plan and do the following:
    (1) Let the client rest before and after meals
    (2) Provide a straw (if allowed)
    (3) Provide light weight utensils and dishes
5. Vision loss
  a. Often keenly aware of food aromas, and can identify foods served
  b. Most can eat independently with some guidance

  c. To assist:
    (1) Identify the location of foods and fluids on the table or tray
    (2) Use the numbers on a clock to identify the location of foods and fluids (see Figure 25-6, p. 379)
    (3) If you are feeding the client, describe what you are offering
E. Serving meal trays
  1. Persons may eat in their room, dining rooms, the cafeteria, or lounges
  2. You will serve meal trays after preparing persons for meals
  3. Serve trays promptly
  4. See Focus on Long-Term Care box, p. 379 in the textbook
    a. Long-term care centers have special programs
      (1) Social dining—residents eat in a dining room
        (a) Food is served as in a restaurant
      (2) Family dining food is placed in bowls and/or platters; residents serve themselves
      (3) Assistive dining for residents who need assistance; special tables are used
  5. Serving Meal Trays ▶ p. 380
F. Feeding the person
  1. Provide a relaxed mood so the person does not feel rushed
  2. Provide time and privacy for prayer if the person wishes
  3. Ask the person in what order to offer foods and fluids
  4. Spoons are used for safety
    a. The spoon should be only 1/3 full
  5. Remember to offer fluids
  6. Persons who cannot feed themselves may feel angry, humiliated, or embarrassed
    a. Some are depressed or resentful
    b. Be supportive and encouraging (see Providing Compassionate Care box, p. 381)
  7. Engage the person in pleasant conversation
    a. Give the person enough time to chew and swallow
  8. Sit so that you face the person
    a. Standing may communicate that you are in a hurry
    b. Facing the person allows you to ob-

serve how well the person is eating
and swallowing
  9. Feeding a Person ▶ p. 382
 G. Between-meal nourishments
  1. A part of many special diets
  2. Serve nourishments as soon as they arrive
  3. Provide needed eating utensils, a straw,
and napkin
 H. Calorie counts
  1. A flow sheet is provided for this purpose
  2. Note what the person ate and how much
(e.g., all of the chicken, 1/2 of the pudding)
   a. A nurse or dietician converts these
portions into calories
X. FLUID BALANCE
 A. After oxygen, water is the most important
physical need for survival
 B. Water enters the body through fluids and
foods
 C. Water is lost through urine, feces, perspiration, and expiration
 D. The amount of intake and the amount of
output must be equal
  1. Edema is when fluid intake exceeds
output causing body tissue to swell with
water
   a. Common in people with heart and
kidney disease
  2. Dehydration is a decrease in the amount
of fluid in the tissues; occurs when fluid
output exceeds intake
   a. Common causes are inadequate fluid
intake, diarrhea, vomiting, bleeding,
excessive sweating, and increased
urine production
 E. Normal requirements
  1. Adults need 1500 ml of water daily to
survive
  2. Approximately 2000 ml to 2500 ml of
fluid per day is needed for normal fluid
balance
   a. Water requirements increase with hot
weather, exercise, fever, and illness
  3. See Focus on Children box, p. 383 in the
textbook
   a. Infants and children need more fluids
than do adults
   b. Excessive fluid loss will quickly cause
death
  4. See Focus on Older Adults box, p. 383 in

the textbook
   a. The amount of body water decreases
with age
   b. Older adults are at risk for diseases
that affect fluid balance
 F. Special orders
  1. Special orders are noted in the care plan;
the physician may order the amount of
fluid that a client can have in a 24-hr. period
  2. Encourage fluids—means that the person
drinks increased amounts of fluid
   a. The order may be a general or a specific amount
   b. Records of intake are kept
   c. A variety of fluids are offered
   d. Fluids are within the person's reach
and at the correct temperature
   e. Fluids are offered frequently to persons who cannot feed themselves
  3. Restrict fluids—means fluids are limited
to a certain amount
   a. Fluid is offered in small amounts
   b. The water pitcher is removed from the
room or kept out of sight
   c. Accurate intake records are kept
   d. Frequent oral hygiene is provided
  4. Nothing by mouth (NPO)—means the
person cannot eat or drink anything
   a. NPO may be ordered before and after
surgery, before some laboratory tests
and x-ray procedures, and in treatment
of certain illnesses
   b. An NPO sign is posted above the bed
   c. The water pitcher and glass are removed
   d. Frequent oral hygiene is needed
    (1) The person cannot swallow fluid
 G. Intake and output records (I&O)
  1. The physician or RN may want the
client's intake and output measured
  2. I&O records are used to evaluate fluid
balance and kidney function
  3. Used in planning and evaluating medical
treatment
  4. Kept when the person has special fluid
orders
  5. To measure intake, all fluids are measured
   a. Those taken by mouth
   b. Those given in IV fluids and tube
feedings

6. Output includes urine, vomitus, diarrhea, and wound drainage
7. Measuring intake and output
   a. Measured in milliliters (ml) or cubic centimeters (cc)
      (1) These metric measures are equal in amount
      (2) 30ml = 1oz
          500ml = 1 pt
          1000ml = 1 qt
   b. You need to know the size of bowls, dishes, cups, pitchers, glasses, and other containers used to serve fluids
   c. A graduate is used to measure fluids
      (1) Is like a measuring cup
   d. Plastic urinals and kidney basins often are calibrated
   e. An I&O record is usually kept at the bedside (see Figure 25-12, p. 384)
      (1) Amounts are measured and recorded each time fluid is ingested or output
      (2) Amounts are totaled at the end of the shift
   f. The purpose of I&O is explained to the person
      (1) How the person can take part is also explained
      (2) The toilet is not used
      (3) Toilet paper is not put into the container
   g. Medical asepsis and Standard Precautions are followed
   h. Measuring Intake and Output ▶ p. 385

Classroom Activities

1. Review the structure and function of the digestive system with students (see Box 13-18, p. 141).
   a. Display the overhead transparency showing the digestive system. Use this to reinforce the information.

2. Call on students to identify and discuss the factors that affect nutrition and eating habits.

3. Divide students into groups of three. Provide each group with several sheets of notebook paper. Ask each group to plan a nutritious menu for 1 day using Canada's Food Guide to Healthy Eating. Menus should include three meals and two snacks.
   a. Allow 15 minutes for planning. Then ask each group to share their menu with the class.

(1) Allow time for discussion.

4. Write "Dietary Guidelines for Americans" on the chalkboard. Call on students to list the guidelines. Write the correct answers on the chalkboard.

5. Provide students with cans and boxes of food. Ask students to read the food labels and find the information about serving size, number of calories, amount of fat, amount of saturated fat, cholesterol, sodium, protein, dietary fiber, sugars, vitamins, calcium, and iron.
   a. Discuss how food labels are used to plan a healthy diet and to follow special diets.

6. Arrange for a registered dietician from a long-term care center to speak to the class.
   a. Ask students to write key points in a notebook.
   b. Allow time for questions and discussion.

7. Call on students to discuss how age affects eating habits and appetite.

8. Provide students with diet cards showing special diets (include the following diets: regular, sodium-restricted, low-fat dysphagia, and diabetic). These can be obtained from a hospital or long-term care center.
   a. Allow students to study the diet cards. Encourage questions and comments.
   b. Stress the importance of knowing what type of diet is ordered for each patient or resident.

9. Use the procedure checklists provided.
   a. Demonstrate the procedures in this chapter.
   b. Have each student practice and return demonstrate the procedures in this chapter. Ask each student to assume the role of the patient/resident when practicing and return demonstrating procedures when appropriate. Use a simulator or an anatomical model when appropriate.

10. Call on students to list the important tasks involved in getting a person ready for meals.
    a. Write the correct answers on the chalkboard.
    b. Discuss why each task is important.

11. Show the following sections of video #7 (Nutrition and Oral Hygiene) in Mosby's Nursing Assisting Video Series.
    a. Assisting with eating
    b. Feeding someone who is unable to feed himself
    c. Record amounts of food eaten
    Allow time for questions and discussion.

12. Provide meal trays for students. Divide students into pairs
    a. Ask each to take a turn feeding his or her partner. Then ask each student to take a turn being fed.
    b. Ask students to discuss the experience.
       (1) How did it feel to be fed?
       (2) Were they given appropriate bite sizes?
       (3) Were they given enough time to chew?
       (4) Were liquids offered between bites?
       (5) Were they given a choice of which food they wanted next?
       (6) Were food temperatures appropriate?

13. Write the following terms on the chalkboard:
    a. Dehydration
    b. Edema
    c. Encourage fluids
    d. Restrict fluids
    e. NPO
    f. I&O
       (1) Call on students to provide the definition for each term. Write the correct answers on the chalkboard.
       (2) Discuss the special fluid needs of children and older persons.

14. Show the following section of video #11 (Reporting & Recording Observations) in Mosby's Nursing Assisting Video Series:
    a. Chart fluid intake and output
    Allow time for questions.

15. Make available intake and output records from a hospital and a long-term care center. Provide each student with a copy of an I&O sheet.
    a. Explain how the form is used.
    b. Set up a variety of containers filled with different amounts of liquid. Have each student practice measuring and recording intake.
    c. Set up a variety of fluids as output. Use urinals, emesis basins, and graduates filled to different levels. Have each student practice measuring and recording output.
    d. Stress the importance of accuracy.

Homework Assignments

Ask students to answer the questions at the end of Chapter 25 in the textbook. Tell students the date and time that this assignment must be completed and turned in.

If the accompanying workbook is being used, assign the Chapter 25 workbook exercises. Tell students the date and time that this assignment must be completed and turned in.

Name _____

Date _____

Basic Nutrition and Fluids

Matching

Match each nutrient with its function in the body.

a. Protein
b. Carbohydrates
c. Fats
d. Vitamin A
e. Folic acid
f. Vitamin D
g. Vitamin K
h. Calcium
i. Iron
j. Sodium

1. _____ Allows red blood cells to carry oxygen

2. _____ The most important nutrient; needed for tissue growth and repair

3. _____ Needed for growth; vision; healthy hair, skin, and mucous membranes; resistance to infection

4. _____ Provides energy and fiber for bowel elimination

5. _____ Needed for formation of red blood cells, functioning of the intestines, protein metabolism

6. _____ Provides energy, adds flavor to food, helps the body use certain vitamins

7. _____ Needed for fluid balance; nerve and muscle function

8. _____ Needed for blood clotting

9. _____ Needed for absorption and metabolism of calcium and phosphorus; healthy bones

10. _____ Needed for formation of teeth and bones, blood clotting, muscle contraction, heart function, nerve function

11. Many elderly do not eat properly. List some of the reasons.

a. _____

b. _____

c. _____

d. _____

e. _____

f. _____

g. _____

h. _____

i. _____

j. _____

12. Convert the following amounts of liquids into cc or ml using the scale below:

1 ounce = 30 cc (ml)
1 cup = 240 cc (ml)

a. 6-ounce cup of coffee: _____ cc (ml)
b. 1/2 of a 6-ounce cup of tea: _____ cc (ml)
c. 2 ounces of Ensure: _____ cc (ml)
d. 8-ounce glass of milk: _____ cc (ml)
e. 5 ounces of Jello: _____ cc (ml)
f. 1/2 of an 8-ounce glass of water: _____ cc (ml)
g. 10 ounces of broth: _____ cc (ml)

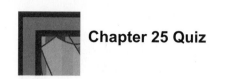

Chapter 25 Quiz

Name _____

Date _____

Basic Nutrition and Fluids

True or False

Mark **T** *for true or* **F** *for false.*

1. _____ Canada's Food Guide encourages a low-fat diet.

2. _____ Canada's Food Guide recommends 2 servings a day from the vegetable group.

3. _____ Skim milk has less fat than whole milk.

4. _____ When preparing meats, roasting, broiling, and baking are better than frying.

5. _____ Nutritional needs decrease during illness.

6. _____ Good oral hygiene and denture care improve the ability to taste.

7. _____ Rice, pasta, breads, and cereals are not allowed on a low-sodium diet.

8. _____ Sodium causes the body to retain water.

9. _____ Infants and children need more fluids than do adults.

10. _____ Stand beside the person to feed him or her.

Multiple Choice

Circle the BEST answer.

11. The breathing of fluid or an object into the lungs is:
    a. Gavage
    b. Dysphagia
    c. Aspiration
    d. Regurgitation

12. Dietary guidelines for Canadians include all of the following except:
    a. Eat a variety of food.
    b. Maintain a healthy weight.
    c. Choose a diet low in fat.
    d. Choose a high-sodium diet.

13. Which foods are high in vitamin C?
    a. Citrus fruits, tomatoes, and green vegetables
    b. Meat and peanuts
    c. Milk, butter, and liver
    d. Pasta, cereal, and oatmeal

14. Which vegetables are not allowed on a 1000 mg sodium diet?
    a. Steamed carrots
    b. Steamed broccoli
    c. Sauerkraut
    d. Lettuce

15. How much water does an adult need daily to survive?
    a. 3000 cc (ml)
    b. 1500 cc (ml)
    c. 1000 cc (ml)
    d. 500 cc (ml)

16. Mrs. Sanchez has an order for NPO. This means that:
    a. Fluids are restricted.
    b. Records are kept of oral intake.
    c. She cannot eat or drink anything.
    d. She is encouraged to drink a variety of fluids.

190

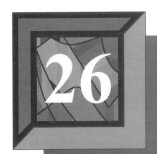

26

Enteral Nutrition and IV Therapy

Instructor's Preparation

I. Read Chapter 26 in the textbook. Carefully review chapter objectives, key terms, and review questions.
II. Read the outline in Chapter 26 of the instructor's guide. Carefully review the classroom activities, the student assignment, and the quiz.
III. If you are using the accompanying student workbook, review the activities for Chapter 26.
IV. Gather all necessary supplies and equipment for classroom activities and student assignments.
   A. Prepare the correct number of handouts
   B. Prepare appropriate flip charts
   C. Prepare overhead transparencies
   D. Gather correct video

   E. Gather coloured markers
   F. Gather anatomical models
   G. Gather simulators
   H. Gather supplies and equipment needed to demonstrate and have each student in turn demonstrate the procedures in this chapter
   I. Gather any other items that will be needed for classroom activities
   J. Assemble items in the order they will be used
V. Make sure that the necessary equipment is available and in good working order.
VI. Contact guest speakers to confirm the day, date, time, and location that they are expected.
   A. Ask the speakers if they require any special equipment or supplies.

Objectives

- Define the key terms listed in this chapter
- Explain the purpose of enteral nutrition and necessary comfort measures
- Explain how to prevent aspiration and regurgitation
- Identify the signs and symptoms of aspiration
- Identify the solutions, equipment, and complications involved in IV therapy
- Explain the safety measures necessary for IV therapy and your role in maintaining the flow rate

Key Terms

aspiration
enteral nutrition
flow rate
gastrostomy tube
gavage
intravenous (IV) therapy
jejunostomy tube
nasogastric (NG) tube
nasointestinal tube
percutaneous endoscopic gastrostomy (PEG) tube
regurgitation

Enteral Nutrition and IV Therapy

I. ENTERAL NUTRITION
  A. Often required by persons who cannot chew or swallow
    1. Enteral nutrition is giving nutrients through the gastrointestinal tract
    2. A nurse gives formula through a feeding tube (gavage is another term for tube feeding)
  B. There are different types of feeding tubes:
    1. A tube is inserted into the stomach or small intestine
    2. A nasogastric tube (NG tube) is inserted through the nose into the stomach (see Figure 26-1, p. 389)
    3. A nasointestinal tube is inserted through the nose into the duodenum or the jejunum of the small intestine (see Figure 26-2, p. 389)
    4. A gastrostomy is a surgically created opening into the stomach (see Figure 26-3, p. 389)
    5. A jejunostomy is a surgically created opening into the middle part of the small intestine (see Figure 26-4, p. 389)
    6. A percutaneous endoscopic gastrostomy (PEG) tube is inserted with an endoscope (see Figure 26-5, p. 390)
      a. An endoscope is a lighted instrument that allows the doctor to see into a body cavity or organ
      b. The tube is inserted through a stab wound
  C. Feeding tubes are used when food cannot pass normally from the mouth into the esophagus and into the stomach
    1. Cancer, trauma, surgery, coma, and dysphagia are causes
    2. Persons with dementia may require tube feedings
    3. The ostomy may be temporary or permanent
  D. Formulas
    1. The doctor orders the type of formula and how much to give
    2. Commercially prepared, or prepared by the dietary department
  E. Scheduled and continuous feedings
    1. Scheduled feedings are usually given 4 times per day with a syringe or feeding bag (see Figure 26-6, p. 390)
    2. Continuous feedings require electronic feeding pumps (see Figure 26-7, p. 391)
      a. Nasointestinal and jejunostomy feedings are always continuous
    3. Formula is given at room temperature
    4. The nurse adds formula to continuous feedings every 3 to 4 hours (see Focus on Home Care box, p. 391)
  F. Preventing aspiration
    1. Aspiration is the breathing of fluid or an object into the lungs
      a. A major complication of nasogastric and nasointestinal tubes
      b. It can cause pneumonia and death
    2. After insertion, an x-ray film is the best way to determine placement
    3. The tube can move after insertion as the result of sneezing, coughing, vomiting, suctioning, and poor positioning
    4. Movement into the respiratory tract can cause aspiration
      a. The RN checks tube placement before every scheduled tube feeding
      b. With continuous feedings, placement is checked every 4 to 8 hours
    5. Aspiration also occurs from regurgitation (backward flow of food from the stomach into the mouth)
    6. To prevent regurgitation:
      a. The person sits or is in a semi-Fowler's position for the feeding
      b. The person remains in this position for at least 1 hour after the feeding
      c. The left side-lying position is avoided
    7. The risk of regurgitation is less with nasointestinal and jejunostomy tubes
    8. Observations
      a. The nurse must be alerted to signs and symptoms of aspiration and other complications
      b. Report the following to the nurse immediately:
        (1) Nausea
        (2) Discomfort during the tube feeding
        (3) Vomiting
        (4) Diarrhea
        (5) Distended abdomen
        (6) Coughing
        (7) Complaints of indigestion or heartburn
        (8) Redness, swelling, drainage, odor, or pain at the ostomy site
        (9) Elevated temperature
        (10) Signs and symptoms of respira-

tory distress (see Chapter 27)
(11) Increased pulse rate
(12) Complaints of flatulence
G. Comfort measures
1. The person is usually NPO (nothing by mouth)
2. Dry mouth, lips, and sore throat are sources of discomfort
a. Some person's are allowed hard candy or gum
b. Frequent oral hygiene, lip lubricants, and mouth rinses are needed
3. The nose and nostrils are cleaned every 4 to 8 hours as directed by the nurse and care plan
4. Tubes can irritate and cause pressure on the nose
a. Securing the tubes helps prevent problems
b. Tube holders are helpful
II. ADMINISTRATION OF FLUIDS INTO A VEIN—IV THERAPY
A. A needle or catheter is inserted into a vein
B. Doctors order IV therapy to:
1. Provide needed fluids
2. Replace minerals and vitamins
3. Provide sugar for energy
4. Administer drugs or blood
5. Provide *hyperalimentation*—a solution highly conecntrated with nutrients
C. RNs are responsible for IV therapy
1. RNs start and maintain the infusion according to the physician's orders
2. They also give IV medications and blood
D. IV therapy is given in hospitals, outpatient, subacute care, long-term care, and home settings
E. Sites
1. Peripheral sites are located away from the center of the body (see Figure 26-9, p. 392)
a. Scalp and dorsal foot veins are peripheral sites for children (see Figure 26-10, p. 393)
2. The subclavian and the internal jugular vein are central venous sites (the cephalic and basilic veins in the arm are also used)
a. These sites are close to the heart (see Figure 26-11, p. 393)
b. The catheter is called a central venous catheter or a central unit
c. Catheters inserted into these sites are

called peripherally inserted central catheters (PICC)
d. Doctors and specially trained RNs insert PICC
F. Focus on home care
1. Patients receive IV therapy in the home
2. The RN teaches the patient and family about giving drugs and managing the catheter
G. Assisting with IV Therapy
1. Support workers meet the hygiene and activity needs of clients with IVs
2. Never responsible for starting or maintaining IV
3. Follow safety measures listed in Box 26-1, p. 394 in the textbook
4. Complications can occur so immediately report any signs and symptoms listed in Box 26-2, p. 394 in the textbook

Classroom Activities

1. Write the following terms on the chalkboard or flip chart. Then call on students to provide the definition for each term. Write the correct answers on the chalkboard or flip chart.
a. Enteral nutrition
b. Nasogastric tube
c. Nasointestinal tube
d. Gastrostomy
e. Jejunostomy
f. Percutaneous endoscopic gastrostomy tube

2. Have available various types of enteral nutrition feeding systems for students to look at and handle.

3. Nursing assistants will care for persons with various types of feeding tubes. Call on students to list what observation they must report to the nurse when caring for persons with enteral feeding tubes.
a. Write the correct answers on the chalkboard.

4. Ask a representative from a medical supply company to demonstrate how IV administration equipment works. Discuss the role of assistive personnel in assisting with IV therapy.
a. Display the signs and symptoms listed in Box 18-7, p. 472 in the textbook on an overhead transparency.
(1) Review the list with students.
(2) Stress the importance of reporting these signs and symptoms to the RN immediately.

Homework Assignments

Ask students to answer the questions at the end of Chapter 26 in the textbook. Tell students the date and time that this assignment must be completed and turned in.

If the accompanying workbook is being used, assign the Chapter 26 workbook exercises. Tell students the date and time that this assignment must be completed and turned in.

Chapter 26 Student Assignment

Name _____

Date _____

Enteral Nutrition and IV Therapy

Write your answers in the spaces provided.

1. Define where the following tubes are inserted:

   a. Nasogastric tube

   _____

   b. Nasointestinal tube

   _____

   c. Gastrostomy tube

   _____

2. What conditions may result in a client's inability to swallow?

   a. _____

   b. _____

   c. _____

   d. _____

   e. _____

   f. _____

   g. _____

   h. _____

3. List comfort measures a support worker can provide to a client who is NPO.

   a. _____

   _____

   b. _____

   _____

   c. _____

   _____

   d. _____

   _____

   e. _____

   _____

4. List reasons a client may need to receive IV therapy.

   a. _____

   _____

   b. _____

   _____

   c. _____

   _____

   d. _____

   _____

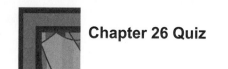

Chapter 26 Quiz

Name _____

Date _____

Enteral Nutrition and IV Therapy

True or False	Multiple Choice

*Mark **T** for true or **F** for false.*

1. _____ The person with a feeding tube is usually allowed liquids by mouth.

2. _____ Support workers are responsible for IV therapy.

3. _____ Support workers regulate IV solution flow rates.

4. _____ Gavage is another term for tube feeding.

5. _____ Feeding tube formulas should be given at room temperature.

6. _____ A support worker should check the placement of the tube by aspirating gastric juices with a syringe.

7. _____ The subclavian vein is usually used in infants for IV therapy.

8. _____ Central venous sites are used to give large amounts of fluids.

9. _____ It is usual for a client to have pain at the IV site.

10. _____ Flow rate is the number of drops per minute.

Circle the BEST answer.

11. The alarm is sounding on an IV infusion pump. You must:
    a. Tell the nurse immediately.
    b. Turn off the pump.
    c. Adjust the controls on the pump.
    d. Unplug the pump.

12. A client with a feeding tube is usually:
    a. NPO
    b. On bed rest
    c. Allowed a regular diet
    d. In a coma

13. Which type of feeding tube can be inserted by an RN?
    a. gastrostomy tube
    b. nasogastric tube
    c. jejunostomy tube
    d. PEG

14. Sites used for IV therapy include:
    a. hand
    b. scalp
    c. jugular vein
    d. all of the above

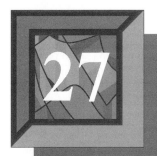

27

Personal Hygiene

Instructor's Preparation

I. Read Chapter 27 in the textbook. Carefully review chapter objectives, key terms, and review questions.
II. Read the outline in Chapter 27 of the instructor's guide. Carefully review the classroom activities, the student assignment, and the quiz.
III. If you are using the accompanying student workbook, review the activities for Chapter 27.
IV. Review videos # 5 and #7 in Mosby's Nursing Assisting Video Series.
V. Gather all necessary supplies and equipment for classroom activities and student assignments.
   A. Prepare appropriate flip charts
   B. Gather correct video
   C. Gather the following transparencies: TA36 through TA40
   D. Gather colored markers
   E. Gather anatomical models
   F. Gather simulators
   G. Gather all equipment and supplies needed to demonstrate and have each student return demonstrate the procedures in this chapter
   H. Gather any other items that will be needed for classroom activities
   I. Assemble items in the order they will be used
VI. Make sure that the necessary equipment is available and in good working order.

Objectives

- Define the key terms listed in this chapter
- Explain the importance of personal hygiene
- Describe oral hygiene and the observations to report
- Describe the guidelines for bathing and the observations to report
- Identify the safety precautions for persons taking tub baths or showers
- Explain the purposes of a back massage
- Identify the purposes of perineal care
- Describe menstrual care
- Learn the procedures described in this chapter

Key Terms

afternoon care
AM care
aspiration
early morning care
evening care
HS care
morning care
oral hygiene
pericare
perineal care
plaque
PM care
tartar

Outline

Personal Hygiene

I. INTRODUCTION
   A. Cleanliness and skin care promote comfort, safety, and health

B. The skin is the body's first line of defense against disease

C. Good hygiene promotes cleanliness, prevents body and breath odor, promotes relaxation, and increases circulation

　1. See Figure 13-4, p. 128 in the textbook for a review of body structures and functions related to this chapter

D. Culture and personal choice affect hygiene

　1. See Respecting Diversity box, p. 397 in the textbook

E. Bathing frequency varies

F. Illness, age, and the changes of aging, affect the ability to practice hygiene

G. Many factors affect hygiene and skin care needs (perspiration, vomiting, urine and bowel elimination, wound drainage, bedrest, and activity)

H. The care plan tells you how to meet the person's hygiene needs

II. DAILY CARE

A. Routine care is given at specific times

B. You assist with personal hygiene whenever necessary (see Focus on Long-Term Care box, p. 398)

C. Before breakfast

　1. Early morning care or AM care (given before breakfast)

D. After breakfast

　1. Morning care (given after breakfast)

　2. Hygiene and skin care measures are more thorough at this time

E. Afternoon care

　1. Routine hygiene is performed after lunch and the evening meal

　2. If done before visiting hours, the person feels more refreshed and can visit without interruption

F. Evening care

　1. Care given at bed time (HS care, evening care, or PM care)

　2. Preformed before the person is ready for sleep

　3. Promotes comfort and relaxation

G. See Providing Compassionate Care box, p. 398 in the textbook, for a review of DIPPS

III. ORAL HYGIENE

A. Keeps the mouth and teeth clean

B. Prevents mouth odors and infection

C. Increases comfort and makes food taste better

D. Cavities (dental caries) are prevented

E. Periodontal disease is prevented

F. Poor oral hygiene allows the build up of plaque and tartar

　1. Plaque and tartar build-up lead to periodontal disease; tooth loss is common

G. Your supervisor and the care plan tell you the type of mouth care and assistance needed

H. Oral hygiene is given on awakening, after each meal, and at bedtime

　1. Many people practice oral hygiene before meals

I. Equipment

　1. Toothbrush, toothpaste, dental floss, and mouthwash are needed

　2. The toothbrush should have soft bristles

　3. Persons with dentures need denture cleaner, a denture cup, and brush

　4. Sponge swabs are used for persons with sore mouths and for unconscious persons

　　a. Always check the foam pad to make sure it is tight on the stick

　5. Wear gloves and follow Standard precautions

J. Observations

　1. Report and record the following if observed while assisting with oral hygiene:

　　a. Dry, cracked, swollen, or blistered lips

　　b. Redness, swelling, irritation, sores, or white patches in the mouth or tongue

　　c. Bleeding, swelling, or redness of the gums

　　d. Loose teeth

　　e. Rough, sharp, or chipped areas on dentures

　　f. Complaints of pain or discomfort

K. Brushing teeth

　1. Many people perform oral hygiene themselves

　2. Others need help with part or all of the process

　3. Focus on children

　　a. Children learn to brush their teeth around age 3

　　b. They may not be thorough

　　c. Older children can do a thorough job

　　　(1) Reminders are necessary

　4. Assisting the Person to Brush the Teeth ▶ p. 400

　5. Brushing the Person's Teeth ▶ p. 401

L. Flossing

　1. A preventive measure; removes plaque and tartar from the teeth

　2. Usually done after brushing

　3. If done only once a day, bedtime is the best time to floss

　4. See Focus on Children box and Focus on Older Adults box, p. 404 in the textbook

5. Flossing the Person's Teeth ▶ p. 403

M. Mouth care for the unconscious person

1. Unconscious persons cannot eat or drink; they breathe with their mouths open and usually receive oxygen (see Chapter 43)

2. The mouth, tongue, and mucous membranes are often dry and crusted

3. Good mouth care is important

4. The care plan tells you what cleaning agent to use

   a. Use sponge swabs to apply the cleaning agent

   b. Apply lubricant to the lips after cleaning

5. Unconscious persons usually cannot swallow

   a. To prevent aspiration, position the person on one side with the head turned well to the side

   b. Use only a small amount of fluid

   c. Sometimes oral suctioning is part of the procedure (see Chapter 43)

6. The person's mouth is kept open with a padded tongue blade (see Figure 27-5, p. 405)

   a. Do not use your fingers

7. Unconscious persons cannot speak or respond to what is happening; however, some can hear

   a. Explain what you are doing step by step

8. Mouth care is given at least every 2 hours

   a. Check with your supervisor and the care plan

   b. Combining mouth care, skin care, and other comfort measures increases comfort and safety

9. Providing Mouth Care for an Unconscious Person ▶ p. 406

N. Denture care

1. Dentures are cleaned for persons who cannot do so themselves

2. Mouth care is given and dentures are cleaned as often as natural teeth; wear gloves when handling dentures

3. Dentures are the person's property; losing or damaging dentures is negligent conduct

4. Dentures are slippery when wet

   a. When cleaning, hold them firmly over a basin of water lined with a paper towel; use gauze or a clean cloth to grasp the dentures

5. Hot water warps dentures; do not use hot water to clean or store dentures

6. If not worn, store dentures in a container of cool water

7. Remind people not to wrap dentures in tissues or napkins; they can be discarded

8. Many people clean their own dentures

   a. They may need some help

9. Providing Denture Care ▶ p. 408

IV. BATHING

A. Cleans the skin

B. Cleans the mucous membranes of the genital and anal areas

C. Is refreshing and relaxing

D. Stimulates circulation

E. Provides exercise

F. Gives you the opportunity to make important observations

G. Gives you time to get to know the person

H. The person gets a complete bath, partial bath, tub bath, or a shower

I. Bathing time and frequency is a personal matter

J. Box 27-1, p. 410 in the textbook, lists guidelines for bathing clients

K. Table 27-1, p. 411 in the textbook, describes common skin care products

L. See Focus on Older Adults box, p. 410 in the textbook

N. Observations

1. Report the following observations to the nurse:

   a. Color of skin, lips, nail beds, and sclera

   b. Location and description of rashes

   c. Dry skin

   d. Bruises or open skin areas

   e. Pale or reddened areas

   f. Drainage or bleeding

   g. Skin temperature

   h. Complaints of pain or discomfort

O. The complete bed bath

1. Involves washing the person's entire body in bed

2. Ask your supervisor about the person's ability to assist with the bath

3. Ask about any activity or position limits

4. Follow standard precautions

5. A bed bath is often a new experience for some people

   a. Some are embarrassed and fear exposure

   b. Explain the procedure

6. Giving a Complete Bed Bath (for adults) ▶ p. 412 ; see Chapter 37 for infants

7. Towel baths—a large bath towel is saturated with a cleaning solution and a quick drying agent so the client's body dries quickly
    a. Clients with dementia often respond well to this type of bath
8. Bag baths—commercially prepared or prepared by the employer
    a. Eight to ten washcloths in a plastic bag
    b. Moistened with cleaning agent that does not require rinsing
    c. Warmed in a microwave
    d. New washcloth for each body part and skin air dries
    e. Check with your supervisor and manufacturer's instruction for proper use
9. Focus on Children
    a. See Chapter 37 for bathing infants
    b. Lower water temperatures are used
    c. Ask the nurse what water temperature to use
P. The partial bath
    1. Involves bathing the face, hands, axillae, back, buttocks, and perineal area
    2. You give partial baths to persons who cannot bathe themselves
    3. Persons who are able, bathe themselves in bed or at the bathroom sink
        a. You assist as needed
        b. Box 27-1, p. 410 in the textbook lists guidelines for partial baths
    4. Giving a Partial Bath ▶ 418
Q. Tub baths and showers
    1. Burns from hot water and falls are risks (see Box 27-2, p. 419)
    2. Only give a tub bath or shower if it is written in the care plan
    3. Box 27-2, p. 419 in the textbook lists safety measures
    4. Tub baths
        a. A tub bath can cause a person to feel faint, weak, or tired
            (1) A bath lasts no longer than 20 minutes
    5. Clean the tub and shower before use
    6. Follow the measures in Box 27-2, p. 419 in the textbook, to prevent slipping, falls, and chills
    7. Some agencies have portable tubs (see Figure 27-17, p. 420)
        a. The sides lower to transfer the person from the bed to the tub
        b. Transport the person to the tub room

    c. Fill the tub and bathe the person in the usual manner
8. Whirlpool tubs (see Figure 27-18, p. 420)
    a. Have hydraulic lifts
    b. The person is transferred to a special wheelchair and taken to the tub room
    c. The chair is attached to the lift and the chair and person are lifted into the tub
    d. The whirlpool action cleans the person's lower body
    e. You wash the upper body
9. Some tubs have special stretchers for persons who cannot sit up (see Figure 27-19, p. 421)
    a. The person is lowered into the tub on the stretcher
10. Remember to cover the person with a blanket during transports and transfers
11. Showers
    a. Some rooms have private baths or showers
        (1) If not, reserve the room
    b. Clean the tub and shower before use
    c. Protect the person from falls and chills
    d. Shower chairs are used to transport some patients and residents (see Figure 27-21, p. 421)
        (1) The wheels are locked during the shower
    e. Some shower rooms may have more than one stall or cabinet
        (1) Always protect the client's privacy
        (2) Properly screen and cover the person
    f. Focus on home care
        (1) Make sure there are safety bars for the person's use
        (2) Assist the person in and out of the shower as needed
        (3) A shower chair can be rented, or a sturdy chair can be used
    g. See Focus on Children box, p. 422 in the textbook
        (1) The RN tells you how much help and supervision to give
12. Assisting with a Tub Bath or Shower ▶ p. 422
R. Dealing with bathing problems
    1. The client refuses the bath
        a. The client has a right to refuse a bath
        b. Some may be too weak, too ill, afraid of falling etc.

c. Listen carefully to learn the reason
d. Talk to your supervisor if the client continues to refuse a bath
2. The client who has dementia—often frightened from not understanding what is happening to them
   a. May resist, become agitated, shout at you, or cry
   b. Check the care plan for help measures
   c. Follow the guidelines in Box 27-1, p. 410 in the textbook
   d. Other measures include
      (1) Do not rush the client
      (2) Use a calm, pleasant voice
      (3) Divert the client's attention (see Chapter 34)
      (4) Calm the client, try the bath later
3. The client who cannot tolerate the bathing position
   a. Because of disease, surgery, or SOB, the client may not be able to sit or lie on their back or side for long
   b. Follow your supervisor's directions and the care plan
   c. You will need to adapt your technique
4. The client who urinates or has a bowel movement
   a. Some people cannot control urination or bowel movements (see Chapters 29 and 30)
   b. If this occurs during a bedbath—put on gloves, clean up the client, put toilet tissue in the bedpan, change linen if necessary, clean the bedpan, remove gloves, and continue after changing the bathwater and washcloths
   c. If this occurs during a tub bath—drain the bath, cover and help the client out of the tub, clean and refill the tub and continue using clean washcloths
5. Hardened secretions or stool on the client's body
   a. To remove, use unscented lotion or petroleum jelly on a clean damp washcloth
   b. Repeat if necessary but do not rub or scratch as it can damage tissue
6. A client has an erection
   a. Privacy is important—in a professional and calm manner, tell him you will give him some time alone
   b. Provide for safety and leave the room but make sure your client can be left alone if in a tub

c. Knock on the door before re-entering and continue with the bath
d. An erection is a normal reaction to physical contact to the genital area
e. Try not to show embarrassment because the client is probably embarrassed as well

V. THE BACK MASSAGE
   A. Relaxes muscles and stimulates circulation
   B. Normally given after the bath and with HS care
      1. It should last 3 to 5 minutes
   C. Observe the skin before starting
   D. Lotion reduces friction when giving the massage
      1. Warm the lotion before applying
   E. The prone position is best; the side-lying position is often used
   F. Some persons should not have a back massage
      1. Check with the nurse and the nursing care plan before giving a back massage to those with heart disease, back injury, back surgery, skin disease, and lung disorders
   G. Giving a Back Massage ▶ p. 425

VI. PERINEAL CARE
   A. Involves cleaning the genital and anal areas
   B. Given to prevent infection and odors and to promote comfort
   C. Done at least daily during the bath
   D. Also done whenever the area is soiled with urine or feces
   E. Given before and after some surgeries and after childbirth
   F. Patients and residents do their own perineal care if able
   G. People may not know the term perineum or perineal
      1. Use terms the person understands (privates, private parts, crotch, genitals, or the area between your legs)
   H. Standard precautions are followed; wear gloves
   I. Work from the cleanest area to the dirtiest area
   J. Use warm water, not hot
   K. Pat dry after rinsing
   L. See Focus on Children box, p. 427 in the textbook
      1. Children of all ages need perineal care
   M. Giving Female Perineal Care ▶ pp. 428-29
   N. Giving Male Perineal Care ▶ pp. 431-32

Classroom Activities

1. Introduce this chapter by explaining that personal hygiene and cleanliness are very personal matters. They must always be respectful and sensitive when providing personal care to others.
   a. Ask students to always think about how they would feel if they were in the patient's or resident's situation.
   b. Review Providing Compassionate Care box, p. 398 in the textbook, with students.

2. Ask students to discuss the importance of cleanliness in their personal lives.
   a. Ask students to write in their notebooks their individual daily routines related to cleanliness. Allow 10 minutes.
      (1) Morning routine
      (2) After meal routine
      (3) Bedtime routine
   b. Call on students to discuss how illness or hospitalization would affect these routines.

3. Write the following on a flip chart or chalkboard. Then call on students to describe the care given at the times listed. Write the correct answers on the chalkboard or flip chart.
   a. Before breakfast
   b. After breakfast
   c. Afternoon care
   d. Evening care

4. Ask students to discuss the importance of oral hygiene. Identify the results of poor oral hygiene.
   a. Call on students to identity what observations to make and what to report to the nurse when giving oral care.

5. Show the following sections of video # 7 (Nutrition & Oral Hygiene) in Mosby's Nursing Assisting Video Series: Use this as a basis for introducing the procedures in this chapter related to oral hygiene
   a. Assist with brushing and flossing teeth
   b. Remove and care for dentures
   c. Provide oral care for the unconscious person
   d. Make a padded tongue blade
      (1) Stop the video after each section to allow time for questions.

6. Discuss with students the importance of perineal care.
   a. Identify dignity issues.
   b. Allow students time to express any feeling and/or concerns they may have about giving baths and perineal care.

7. Show video # 5 (Bed Bath, Perineal Care, & Back Massage) in Mosby's Nursing Assisting Video Series. Use this as a basis for introducing the procedures in this chapter related to bathing, perineal care, and back massage.
   a. Stop the video after each section to allow time for questions.

8. Ask students to share any personal experiences with an illness that had an effect on their ability to meet cleanliness and oral hygiene needs.
   a. How did the experience affect comfort needs?
   b. How will the experience help the student to provide better care?

9. Stress the importance of observation while providing care.
   a. Ask students what observations they should report to the nurse. Write the correct answers on the chalkboard.

10. Use the procedure checklists provided.
    a. Demonstrate the procedures in this chapter.
       (1) Make sure all necessary equipment and supplies are available.
    b. Have each student practice and return demonstrate the procedures in this chapter. Have each student take a turn in the patient/resident role. Use simulators for male and female perineal care.

Homework Assignments

Ask students to answer the questions at the end of Chapter 27 in the textbook. Tell students the date and time time that this assignment must be completed and turned in.

If the accompanying student workbook is being used, assign the Chapter 27 workbook exercises. Tell students the date and time that this assignment must be completed and turned in.

Name _____

Date _____

Personal Hygiene

Write your answers in the blanks provided.

1. The following are reported to your supervisor if observed during oral care:

   a. _____

   b. _____

   c. _____

   d. _____

2. The skin is observed during bathing procedures. You report the following to your supervisor:

   a. _____

   b. _____

   c. _____

   d. _____

   e. _____

   f. _____

   g. _____

   h. _____

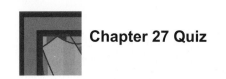

Chapter 27 Quiz

Name _____

Date _____

Personal Hygiene

| **True or False** | **Multiple Choice** |

*Mark **T** for true or **F** for false.*

1. _____ Hot water is used for cleaning dentures.

2. _____ The skin is the body's first line of defense against disease.

3. _____ Follow standard precautions and the Bloodborne Pathogen Standard when giving oral hygiene.

4. _____ You are giving oral care to an unconscious person. The person's mouth is held open with your fingers.

5. _____ A tub bath lasts no longer than 20 minutes.

6. _____ The towel bar can be used for support when the person gets in or out of the tub.

7. _____ Drain the tub before the person gets out of the tub.

8. _____ A back massage is safe for all persons.

9. _____ Young children do not need perineal care.

Circle the BEST answer.

10. Good oral hygiene:
    a. Prevents mouth odor and infection.
    b. Is only done once a day.
    c. Is not important for unconscious persons.
    d. Allows build up of tartar and plaque.

11. You are assisting Mr. Wilson with a tub bath. Which is incorrect?
    a. Place a bath mat in the tub.
    b. Have him use safety bars when getting in and out of the tub.
    c. Use bath oils to soften the skin.
    d. Fill the tub half way with warm water (105° F, 41° C).

12. You are giving Mr. Wilson a back massage. Which is incorrect?
    a. Warm the lotion before applying it.
    b. The massage should last about 1 minute.
    c. Use firm strokes.
    d. Always keep your hands in contact with his skin.

13. Which statement about giving perineal care is correct?
    a. Use hot water.
    b. Clean from the anal area to the urethra.
    c. Pat dry after rinsing.
    d. All of the above.

28

Grooming and Dressing

Instructor's Preparation

I. Read Chapter 28 in the textbook. Carefully review chapter objectives, key terms, and review questions.

II. Read the outline in Chapter 28 of the instructor's guide. Carefully review the classroom activities, the student assignment, and the quiz.

III. If you are using the accompanying student workbook, review the activities for Chapter 28.

IV. Review video # 6 in Mosby's Nursing Assisting Video Series.

V. Gather all necessary supplies and equipment for classroom activities and student assignments.

    A. Prepare overhead transparencies

    B. Gather correct video

    C. Gather the following transparencies: TA41 and TA42

    D. Gather simulators

    E. Gather all equipment and supplies needed to demonstrate and have each student return demonstrate the procedures in this chapter

    F. Gather any other items that will be needed for classroom activities

    G. Assemble items in the order they will be used

VI. Make sure that the necessary equipment is available and in good working order.

Objectives

- Define the key terms listed in this chapter
- Explain the importance of hair care and shaving
- Identify the factors that affect hair care
- Explain how to care for matted and tangled hair
- Describe how to shampoo hair
- Describe how to shave a client
- Explain why nail and foot care are important
- Describe how to dress and undress clients
- Explain the purpose of elastic stockings and bandages, and when you assist with them
- Perform the procedures described in this chapter

Key Terms

alopecia
dandruff
hirsutism
pediculosis (lice)
pediculosis capitis
pediculosis corporis
pediculosis pubis

Outline

Grooming and Dressing

I. INTRODUCTION

    A. Shaving, and beard grooming are important to many men

    B. Many women shave their legs and underarms

II. HAIR CARE

    A. How the hair looks and feels affects mental well-being

    B. The care plan addresses the client's hair care

needs; culture, personal choice, skin and scalp condition, physical and mental health and self-care abilities are considered.

C. Terms common in nursing care plans:
1. Alopecia means hair loss
   a. Hair loss may be complete or partial
   b. It can be a result of heredity, aging, cancer treatment, skin disease, stress, poor nutrition, pregnancy, some drugs, and hormone changes
2. Hirsutism is excessive body hair in women and children
   a. It is due to heredity or abnormal amounts of male hormone
3. Dandruff is excessive amounts of dry, white flakes from the scalp
   a. Itching often occurs
   b. Eyebrows and ear canals can be involved
   c. Medicated shampoos correct the problem
4. Pediculosis means infestation with lice
   a. Pediculosis capitis is infestation of the scalp
   b. Pediculosis pubis is infestation of the pubic hair
   c. Pediculosis corporis is infestation of the body
   d. Lice eggs attach to clothing and furniture
   e. Lice easily spread to other persons through clothing, furniture, bed linen and sexual contact
   f. Medicated shampoos, lotions, and creams are used to treat lice
   g. Thorough bathing is necessary; clothing and linen is washed in hot water
   h. Report any signs of lice to the nurse immediately

D. Brushing and combing hair
1. Part of early morning, morning, and afternoon care
2. Patients and residents are encouraged to do their own hair
3. Assist with or perform hair care as needed
4. Let the person choose how to brush, comb, and style hair (see Focus on Children box, p. 436)
5. Long hair mats and tangles
   a. Daily brushing and combing helps prevent problems
   b. Never cut hair to remove mats or tangles

6. When brushing and combing hair, start at the scalp
7. Place a towel across the client's shoulders to protect their garments
8. Special measures are needed for curly, coarse, or dry hair
   a. Use a wide-toothed comb for curly hair
   b. Start at the neckline and work upward
   c. Wetting the hair or applying a conditioner makes combing easier
9. The person's personal preferences and routines are part of the care plan
10. The person can guide you when giving hair care
11. Report and record the following if observed:
    a. Scalp sores
    b. Flaking
    c. The presence of lice (tiny, white oval-shaped specks in the hair)
    d. Patches of hair loss
    e. Very dry or very oily hair
12. Brushing and Combing Hair ▶ p. 437

E. Shampooing
1. Usually done at least weekly
   a. Many factors affect frequency
2. Shampoo and hair conditioner involve personal choice
3. Clients often need help shampooing
4. Tell the supervisor if a shampoo is requested
5. There are several shampoo methods
   a. The method used depends on the person's condition, safety factors, and personal choice
   b. Your supervisor decides which method to use
   c. Hair is dried and styled as quickly as possible after shampooing
6. The guidelines listed in Box 28-1, p. 437 in the textbook, apply when shampooing
7. Report and record the following observations:
   a. Scalp sores
   b. Hair falling out in patches
   c. How the client tolerated the procedure
   d. The presence of lice
8. Shampooing during the shower or tub bath
   a. A hand held nozzle is used
   b. Assist as necessary
   c. Some people will tip their head back-

wards and some prefer to lean forward.
    d. Support the back of the head if tipping
       backwards or place your one hand on
       their forehead to support if leaning
       forward
  9. Shampooing at the sink—if the person
    faces away from the sink
    a. The chair or wheelchair is placed so
       the person faces away from the sink
    b. The head is tilted back over the edge
       of the sink
    c. A folded towel is placed over the sink
       to protect the neck
    d. A water pitcher or hand-held nozzle is
       used to wet and rinse hair
 10. If the person prefers to lean back over the
    sink
    a. Place the chair or wheelchair so it
       faces away from the sink
    b. Place a folded towel over the sink edge
       to protect the neck
    c. Help the person tilt his or her head
       back over the edge of the sink
    d. Give the person a folded washcloth to
       hold over the eyes
    e. Wet and rinse the hair using a water
       pitcher or hand held nozzle
 11. Shampooing a person on a stretcher
    a. Positioned the stretcher in front of a
       sink
    b. Place a pillow under the head and
       neck
    c. Tilt the head over the edge of the sink
    d. Use a water pitcher or hand-held
       nozzle to wet and rinse hair
    e. Safety measures include locking the
       stretcher wheels, using safety straps,
       and raising the far rail
 12. Shampooing a person in bed
    a. Used for those who cannot be out of
       bed
    b. A rubber or plastic trough is used
    c. The trough drains water into a basin
       placed on a chair by the bed
    d. Use a water pitcher to wet and rinse
       hair
 13. Focus on children
    a. Oil gland secretion increases during
       puberty
       (1) Frequent shampooing is often
          necessary
 14. Focus on long-term care

    a. Oil gland secretion decreases with age
       (1) The client may shampoo less
          often
    b. See Focus on Long-Term Care box, p.
       439 in the textbook
 15. Focus on home care
    a. You can make a trough from a plastic
       shower curtain or table cloth
 16. Shampooing the Person's Hair ▶ p. 440
III. SHAVING
  A. Many men want clean-shaven faces
  B. Many women shave their legs and underarms
  C. Shaving guidelines are listed in Box 28-2, p.
    442 in the textbook
  D. Some people use electric shavers
    1. Shavers are cleaned between each use
    a. Follow safety precautions for using
       electrical equipment
  E. Some people prefer blade shavers (razor
    blade)
    1. Razor blades can cause nicks and cuts
    a. Follow Standard Precautions
    2. Discard used razor blades and disposable
      shavers in a sharps container
    3. Blade shavers are not used for persons
      who are receiving anticoagulant drugs
    a. These drugs prevent or slow blood
       clotting
    4. Before shaving with a blade, soften the
      beard by applying a warm washcloth or
      face towel to the face for a few minutes
    5. Take care not to cut or irritate the skin
      while shaving
    6. Shaving the Person ▶ p.443
  F. Caring for mustaches and beards
    1. Beards and mustaches are washed and
      combed daily
    2. Ask the person how to groom his beard
      or mustache
    3. Never trim or shave a beard or mustache
      without the person's consent
  G. Shaving female legs and underarms
    1. The practice varies among cultures
    2. They are shaved after bathing when the
      skin is soft
    a. Use a kidney basin to rinse the razor
       rather than using bath water
    3. Similar to shaving the face; practice the
      measures in Box 28-2, p. 442 in the text-
      book
IV. CARE OF NAILS AND FEET
  A. Nails and feet need special attention to pre-
    vent infection, injury, and odor

1. Hangnails, ingrown toenails, and nails torn away from the skin cause breaks in the skin
2. Long or broken nails scratch the skin or snag clothing
3. Dirty feet or stockings harbor microbes and cause odors
4. Shoes that fit poorly cause blisters
5. Healing is prolonged in persons with poor circulation
   a. Diabetes mellitus and vascular disease are common causes
   b. Gangrene and amputation are serious complications (see Chapter 31)
6. Check the client's feet every day.
7. Notify your supervisor if you observe any of the following:
   a. Very dry skin
   b. Foot odours
   c. Cracks or breaks in the skin, especially between the toes
   d. Ingrown nails
   e. Loose nails
   f. Reddened, irritated, or calloused areas
   g. Drainage or bleeding
   h. Change in colour or texture of nails
   i. Corns, bunion, or blisters.
8. Trimming and clipping toenails can easily cause injuries; support workers do not cut or trim toenails if the client:
   a. Has diabetes
   b. Has poor circulation to the legs and feet
   c. Takes medications that affect blood clotting
   d. Has very thick or ingrown nails
9. Some employers do not allow support workers to cut or trim toenails under any circumstance--follow employer policy
10. A podiatrist treats corns, bunions, and blisters
11. Fingernails are easier to trim and clean right after they are soaked
12. Nail clippers are used; never use scissors
13. Be careful; you must not damage surrounding tissue
14. Check with your supervisor about water temperature for soaking
B. Focus on home care
   1. Feet are soaked in the tub or in a basin
   2. Fingers are soaked in the sink, a bowl, or basin
C. Giving Nail and Foot Care ▶ p. 446

V. CHANGING CLOTHING AND HOSPITAL GOWNS
A. Hospital gowns or pajamas are changed after the bath and when wet or soiled
B. Persons who wear regular clothes change into hospital gowns or pajamas for bed
C. Incontinent persons may change more often
D. Patients and residents may need help
E. These guidelines are followed (See Box 28-3, p. 448):
   1. Provide for privacy
   2. Encourage the person to do as much as possible
   3. Allow the person to choose what to wear
   4. Remove clothing from the strong or "good" side first (RUF)
   5. Put clothing on the weak side first (DAF)
   6. Support the arm or leg when removing or putting on a garment
F. Changing hospital gowns
   1. If there is injury or paralysis, the gown is removed from the good arm first
      a. Support the weak arm
      b. Put the clean gown on the weak arm first (see Figure 28-17, p. 455)
   2. Special gowns may be used for persons receiving IV infusions
   3. The gowns open along the sleeve and close with ties, snaps, or Velcro
   4. If a standard hospital gown is worn, use the following procedure; if the client as an IV pump do not use the following procedure--the arm with the IV is not put through the sleeve
G. Changing the Gown of a Person with an IV ▶ p. 456
J. Undressing a Person ▶ p. 448
K. Dressing the Person ▶ p. 453
VI. APPLYING ELASTIC STOCKINGS AND BANDAGES
A. Some clients must wear elastic stockings or bandages on their legs as ordered by a physician
B. Helps prevent blood clots (thrombi)
C. Most stockings have an opening used to check circulation and skin colour and temperature
D. Elastic bandages have the same purpose as elastic stockings
E. Applying Elastic Stockings ▶ p. 458
F. Applying Elastic Bandages ▶ p. 460
G. Review Providing Compassionate Care box, p. 462 in the textbook

Classroom Activities

1. Divide students into groups of three. Give each group 10 minutes to discuss how cleanliness and skin care meet basic needs. Then call on one student from each group to report to the class. Allow time for discussion.

2. Ask students to discuss the importance of hair care in promoting mental well-being. Call on students to answer the following questions:
   a. What factors affect hair care?
   b. How does illness and disability affect the person's ability to meet hair care needs?

3. Write the following terms on the chalkboard. Then call on students to provide the definitions. Write the correct answers on the chalkboard after the term.
   a. Alopecia
   b. Hirsutism
   c. Dandruff
   d. Pediculosis
   e. Pediculosis capitis
   f. Pediculosis pubis
   g. Pediculosis corporis

4. Show the following sections of video # 6 (Grooming, Dressing, & Undressing) in Mosby's Nursing Assisting Video Series. Use this as a basis to introduce the procedures related to hair care.
   a. Hair brushing in sections and removing tangles
   b. Washing hair and using a portable shampoo tray
      (1) Allow time after each section for questions.

5. Display the guidelines in Box 28-2 on p. 442 in the textbook on an overhead transparency. Use it as a basis to discuss the importance of safety with students.
   a. Call on students to explain the importance of shaving in promoting comfort and well-being.
      (1) For men
      (2) For women

6. Show the following section of video # 6 (Grooming, Dressing, & Undressing) in Mosby's Nursing Assisting Video Series.
   a. Shaving a man's face
      (1) Allow time for questions after the video.

7. Show the following section of video # 6 (Grooming, Dressing, and Undressing) in Mosby's Nursing Assisting Video Series.
   a. Perform fingernail and toenail care
      (1) Allow time for questions after the video.

8. Call on students to list the rules for changing gowns and clothing. Write correct answers on the chalkboard.
   a. Ask students to discuss how following these rules promotes comfort.

9. Show the following section of video #6 (Grooming, Dressing, & Undressing) in Mosby's Nursing Assisting Video Series.
   a. Assist with dressing and undressing
      (1) Allow time for questions after the video.

10. Use the procedure checklists provided.
   a. Demonstrate the procedures in this chapter.
   b. Have each student practice and return demonstrate the procedures in this chapter. Have each student assume the role of the patient/resident for each procedure. Use a simulator for shaving or find a person willing to be shaved.

Homework Assignments

Ask students to answer the questions at the end of Chapter 28 in the textbook. Tell students the date and time that this assignment must be completed and turned in.

If the accompanying student workbook is being used, assign the Chapter 28 workbook exercises. Tell students the date and time that this assignment must be completed and turned in.

Name _____

Date _____

Grooming and Dressing

Write your answers in the spaces provided.

1. What factors are considered by your supervisor to meet the person's hair care needs?

   a. _____

   b. _____

   c. _____

   d. _____

   e. _____

2. List the rules for shaving.

   a. _____

   b. _____

   c. _____

   d. _____

   e. _____

   f. _____

   g. _____

   h. _____

   i. _____

   j. _____

3. List the rules that are followed when changing clothing or hospital gowns.

   a. _____

   b. _____

   c. _____

   d. _____

   e. _____

   f. _____

Name _____

Date _____

Grooming and Dressing

True or False

Mark **T** *for true or* **F** *for false.*

1. _____ Cut hair to remove matted or tangled hair.

2. _____ You never trim or shave a beard or moustache without the person's consent.

3. _____ Women in long-term care facilities are not interested in shaving their legs or underarms.

4. _____ Do not use a razor blade when shaving a person receiving an anticoagulant drug.

5. _____ Support workers do not cut or trim toenails.

6. _____ Water temperature for soaking feet should be 100° F unless otherwise instructed by your supervisor.

7. _____ When helping a person to dress, put clothing on the strong side first.

Multiple Choice

Circle the BEST answer.

8. The infestation of the body with lice is:
   a. Pediculosis corporis.
   b. Dandruff.
   c. Pediculosis pubis.
   d. Pediculosis capitis.

9. Hair loss is:
   a. Hirsutism.
   b. Pediculosis.
   c. Alopecia.
   d. Decubitus.

10. You assist Mr. Gomez with shaving. Which is incorrect?
    a. Soften the skin before shaving.
    b. Hold the skin taut as necessary.
    c. Shave away from the direction of hair growth.
    d. Report nicks or cuts to the nurse immediately.

11. Which of the following statements about foot care is incorrect?
    a. Feet are easily infected and injured.
    b. Support workers use scissors to cut toenails.
    c. Dirty feet and socks harbor microbes.
    d. Cleaning toenails is easier after soaking.

12. You are assisting Mrs. Bowman to change her hospital gown. Her right arm is injured. Which is correct?
    a. Support the right arm while removing the gown.
    b. Remove the gown from the right arm first.
    c. Put the clean gown on the left arm first.
    d. The person is exposed during the procedure.

29

Urinary Elimination

Instructor's Preparation

I. Read Chapter 29 in the textbook. Carefully review chapter objectives, key terms, and review questions.

II. Read the outline in Chapter 29 of the instructor's guide. Carefully review the classroom activities, the student assignment, and the quiz.

III. If you are using the accompanying student workbook, review the activities for Chapter 29.

IV. Review video # 8 in Mosby's Nursing Assisting Video Series.

V. Gather all necessary supplies and equipment for classroom activities and student assignments.

A. Prepare appropriate flip charts

B. Prepare overhead transparencies

C. Gather correct video

D. Gather the following transparencies: TA43 through TA48

E. Gather coloured markers

F. Gather anatomical models

G. Gather simulators

H. Gather all equipment and supplies needed to demonstrate and have each student return demonstrate the procedures in this chapter

I. Gather any other items that will be needed for classroom activities

J. Assemble items in the order they will be used

Objectives

- Define the key terms listed in this chapter
- Identify the characteristics of normal urine
- Describe the guidelines for maintaining normal urinary elimination
- List the observations to make about urine
- Describe urinary incontinence and the care required
- Explain why catheters are used
- Explain the differences between straight, indwelling, suprapubic, and condom catheters
- Describe the guidelines for caring for clients with indwelling catheters
- Describe two methods of bladder training
- Describe the guidelines for collecting urine specimens
- Explain how to care for a client with an eureterostomy
- Learn the procedures described in this chapter

Key Terms

acetone
catheter
catheterization
condom catherer
dysuria
Foley catheter
functional incontinence
glucosuria
glycosuria
hematuria
indwelling catheter
ketone body
micturition
nocturia
oliguria

ostomy
overflow incontinence
polyuria
reflex incontinence
retention catheter
stoma
straight catheter
stress incontinence
suprapubic catherer
ureterostomy
urge incontinence
urinary frequency
urinary incontinence
urinary urgency
urination
voiding

Outline

Urinary Elimination

I. INTRODUCTION
  A. The urinary system removes waste from the blood and maintains the body's water balance
    1. See Chapter 13 for a review of the structure and function of the urinary system
II. NORMAL URINATION
  A. The healthy adult excretes about 1500 ml (3 pints) of urine per day
  B. Factors that affect urine production include age, disease, amount and kinds of fluids ingested, dietary salt, and drugs
  C. Urination, micturition, and voiding mean the process of emptying urine from the bladder
  D. Urination patterns depend on many factors:
    1. Amount of fluid intake
    2. Personal habits
    3. Availability of toilet facilities
    4. Activity, work, and illness
III. MAINTAINING NORMAL URINATION
  A. Some persons need help getting to the bathroom
  B. Others use bedpans, urinals, or commodes
  C. Follow the rules in Box 29-2, p. 466 in the textbook, to help maintain normal elimination
  D. Observations
    1. Urine is normally pale yellow and clear, with no particles
    2. A faint odor is normal
    3. Some foods affect the color of urine
    4. Observe urine for color, clarity, odor, amount, and particles
    5. Ask the nurse to observe any urine that looks or smells abnormal
    6. Report complaints of urgency, burning on urination, or dysuria
    7. Report problems described in Table 29-1, p. 467 in the textbook
  E. Follow the guidelines in Box 29-1, p. 466 in the textbook, for Infection Control Precaution
  F. Bedpans
    1. Used when persons cannot get out of bed
    2. Men use them only for bowel movements
    3. Made of plastic or stainless steel
      a. Stainless steel bedpans are often cold; they are warmed with water and dried before use
    4. Fracture pans
      a. Have a thinner rim and are only about 1/2 inch deep at one end
      b. Used for persons in traction, or with casts, limited back motion, fragile bones, or painful joints
      c. Focus on older persons
        (1) Fracture pans are often more comfortable for older persons
    5. Follow medical asepsis and Standard Precautions when handling bedpans and their contents
    6. Giving the Bedpan ▶ p. 468
  G. Urinals
    1. Men use urinals to void
    2. The urinal hooks to the bed rail within the man's reach
    3. Plastic urinals have caps at th etop and hook type handles
    4. The man stands, if possible; he may also sit on the side of the bed or lay in bed
    5. You may have to place and hold the urinal for some men
    6. Remind men not to place urinals on the overbed table and bedside stand
      a. These are eating and work surfaces and must not be contaminated with urine
    7. Follow medical asepsis, Standard Precautions, and the Bloodborne Pathogen Standard when handling urinals and their contents
    8. Empty urinals promptly
      a. Prevents spilling, odors, and spread of microbes
    9. Urinals are cleaned like bedpans
    10. Giving the Urinal ▶ p. 472
  H. Commodes
    1. A bedside commode is a portable chair or wheelchair with an opening for a bedpan or container
    2. It allows a normal position for elimination
    3. The container is cleaned after use like a

regular bedpan

    4. Some commodes are wheeled to the bathroom

        a. Make sure the wheels are locked and the commode is positioned over the toilet

    5. Helping the Person to the Commode ▶

        p. 473

IV. URINARY INCONTINENCE

  A. The involuntary loss of urine from the bladder

  B. May be temporary or permanent

  C. Different types:

    1. Stress incontinence is the loss of small amounts of urine with exercise and certain movements

        a. Often called dribbling

        b. Occurs with laughing, sneezing, coughing, lifting, and other activities

        c. More common in women

        d. Pelvic muscles weaken after multiple pregnancies and with age

    2. Urge incontinence is the involuntary loss of urine after feeling a strong need to void

        a. The person cannot stop urinating and cannot get to the bathroom in time

        b. Frequency, urgency, and nighttime voidings are common

        c. Causes include urinary tract infection, decreased bladder capacity, alcohol, caffeine, and increased fluid intake

    3. Overflow incontinence is the loss of urine when the bladder is too full

        a. The person feels like the bladder is never completely empty

        b. Nocturia is common

        c. Causes include fecal impaction, diabetes, and spinal cord injuries; also caused by prostate enlargement in men

    4. Functional incontinence is the involuntary, unpredictable loss of urine

        a. Immobility, restraints, unanswered signal lights, not having signal lights within reach, and not knowing where to find the bathroom are causes

        b. Difficulty removing clothing, confusion, and disorientation are other causes

    5. Reflex incontinence is the loss of urine at predictable intervals

        a. Urine is lost when the bladder is full

        b. The person doesn't know the bladder is full and has no urge to void

        c. Central nervous system disorders and injuries are common causes

    6. Mixed incontinence is a combination of urge and stress incontinence

        a. More common in older women

  D. Incontinence is embarrassing

  E. Clothing and linens get wet and odors develop

  F. There is physical discomfort

  G. Skin irritation, infection, and pressure ulcers can occur

  H. Falling is a risk

  I. The person's pride, dignity, and self-esteem are affected

  J. Check with your supervisor and consult the care plan for the best ways to meet the client's needs

  K. The person's care plan may include some of the measures listed in Box 29-3, p. 475 in the textbook

    1. Good skin care and dry clothing and linens are always essential

  L. Following the rules for maintaining normal elimination prevents incontinence in some people

  M. Some people need bladder retraining programs

  N. A variety of incontinence products are available

  O. Sometimes catheters are ordered

  P. Some people wear garment protectors or incontinence pads

  Q. Incontinence drawsheets help keep people dry

    1. Fluid passes through the first layer and is absorbed by the lower layer

  R. Incontinence is a link to abuse, mistreatment, and neglect

    1. Caring for these persons is stressful

    2. Do not lose patience

    3. The incontinence is beyond the person's control

        a. Kindness, empathy, understanding, and patience are very important

V. CATHETERS

  A. A catheter is a tube used to drain or inject fluid through a body opening

  B. A urinary catheter is inserted through the urethra into the bladder; it drains urine

    1. A straight catheter drains the bladder and is removed

    2. An indwelling catheter (retention or Foley catheter) is left in the bladder so urine drains constantly into a drainage

bag
  a. A balloon at the tip is inflated after insertion
    (1) This prevents the catheter from slipping out of the bladder (see Figure 29-9, p. 476)
  3. A suprapubic catheter is surgically inserted into the bladder through the abdomen
    a. Indwelling, and is attached to a drainage bag
    b. May be used by people needing long-term catheterization or after some surgeries
    c. The insertion site and the tubing must be cleaned daily
    d. Follow the care plan
C. Catheters are used before, during, and after surgery
D. They allow hourly urinary output measurements in critically ill persons
E. They are a last resort for incontinence
  1. Do not treat the cause of incontinence and the risk of infection is high
  2. Can protect wounds and pressure ulcers from urine
F. Can promote comfort for persons who are too weak or disabled to use the bedpan, commode, or toilet
G. They are also inserted for diagnostic purposes and to collect urine specimens
H. The guidelines in Box 29-4, p. 477 in the textbook, promote comfort and safety for persons with indwelling catheters
I. Giving Catheter Care ▶ p. 478
J. Drainage Systems
  1. A closed drainage system is used for indwelling catheters
    a. Nothing can enter the system
  2. The drainage system consists of a tubing and a drainage bag
    a. The bag hangs from the bed frame, chair, or wheelchair; it must not touch the floor
    b. Some people wear leg bags (see Figure 29-17, p. 485)
  3. The bag is kept lower than the bladder to prevent urine from flowing back into the bladder (see Figure 29-10, p. 477)
  4. Sometimes a catheter is disconnected accidentally
    a. Do not touch the ends of the catheter or tubing

    b. Do the following:
      (1) Wash your hands and put on gloves
      (2) Wipe the end of the tube and the catheter with antiseptic wipes
      (3) Do not put the ends down
      (4) Connect the tubing to the catheter
      (5) Discard the wipes into a biohazard plastic bag
  5. Leg bags are switched to drainage bags when the person is in bed
  6. Drainage bags are emptied at the end of each shift
    a. They are also emptied when changing from a leg bag to a drainage bag and vice versa
    b. Always measure the contents and note colour, clarity, odour, or particles in the urine
K. Changing a Leg Bag to a Drainage Bag ▶ p. 481
L. Emptying a Urinary Drainage Bag ▶ p. 483
M. The condom catheter
  1. External catheter; urinary sheath
  2. Often used for incontinent men
  3. Is a soft, rubber sheath that slides over the penis
    a. Tubing connects the catheter to the drainage bag (see Figure 29-17, p. 485)
  4. A new condom catheter is usually applied daily
    a. Follow the care plan
  5. The penis is cleaned and dried before applying the catheter
  6. Elastic tape secures the catheter in place
    a. Never use adhesive tape, it does not expand; blood flow to the penis is cut off, injuring the penis
  7. Follow medical asepsis and Standard Precautions
  8. Report and record the following
    a. Reddened or open areas on the penis
    b. Swelling of the penis
    c. Colour, clarity and odour of urine
    d. Particles in the urine
  9. Removing and Applying a Condom Catheter ▶ p. 485
VI. BLADDER TRAINING
  A. Programs are developed for persons with urinary incontinence
  B. Voluntary control of urination is the goal

C. The bladder training program is part of the nursing care plan
   1. You assist with bladder training as directed by the nurse
D. Two basic methods:
   1. The client uses the toilet, commode, bedpan, or urinal at scheduled times
      a. The rules for maintaining normal urination are followed
      b. Privacy is important
   2. The second method is used with catheters
      a. A clamping schedule is used before the catheter is removed
      b. When the catheter is removed, urination is encouraged every 3 to 4 hours

VII. COLLECTING URINE SPECIMENS
A. Urine specimens are collected for urine tests
   1. Test results are used to make a diagnosis or evaluate treatments
B. Each specimen sent to the laboratory needs a requisition slip
C. Box 29-5, p. 487 in the textbook, lists the rules to follow when collecting specimens
D. Focus on children
   1. For infants and toddlers who are not toilet trained, a collection bag is applied to the genital area
   2. Urine specimens may embarrass older children and adolescents
E. The random urine specimen
   1. Collected for a urinalysis
   2. No special measures are needed
   3. Collected at any time
   4. Collecting a Random Urine Specimen ▶ p. 488
F. The midstream specimen
   1. Also called a clean-voided specimen or a clean-catch specimen
   2. The perineal area is cleaned before collecting the specimen
   3. Collecting a Midstream Specimen ▶ p. 489
G. The 24-hour urine specimen
   1. All urine voided during a 24-hour period is collected
   2. The urine is chilled during the collection period to prevent the growth of microbes
   3. The person voids to begin the test; this voiding is discarded
   4. The rules for collecting urine specimens are followed
   5. Collecting a 24-hour Urine Specimen ▶ p. 491

H. Collecting a specimen from an infant or child
   1. A collection bag is applied over the urethra
   2. A parent or another staff member assists if the child is agitated
   3. Collecting a Urine Specimen from an Infant or Child ▶ p. 493

VIII. TESTING URINE
A. You must be accurate and promptly report the results to the nurse
B. Testing for pH
   1. Measures if urine is acidic or alkaline
   2. Normal pH54.6 to 8.0
   3. Changes occur from illness, foods, and drugs
   4. Use reagent strips
   5. A routine urine specimen is needed
C. Testing for glucose and ketones
   1. Persons with diabetes mellitus may have glucosuria (sugar in the urine) and ketones in the urine
   2. The doctor orders the type and frequency of urine tests
      a. Test results are used to regulate the person's medication and diet
   3. Double-voided specimens are best
   4. Reagent strips are used for testing
D. Testing for blood
   1. Normal urine is free of blood
   2. Hematuria is blood in the urine
      a. Is caused by injury and disease
   3. Unseen blood is called occult blood
      a. Use reagent strips to test for occult blood
      b. A routine urine specimen is needed
E. Using reagent strips
   1. Strips have different sections that change color when they react with urine
      a. Compare the strip to the color chart
   2. Read the manufacturers instructions before you begin
   3. Testing Urine with Reagent Strips ▶ p. 495
F. Straining urine
   1. Stones (calculi) can develop in the kidneys, ureters, or bladder
   2. Stones vary in size from pinhead to the size of an orange
   3. Some stones require surgical removal
   4. Some stones exit the body through urine
      a. All the person's urine is strained
      b. Passed stones are sent to the laboratory for examination
   5. Straining Urine ▶ p. 496

Classroom Activities

1. Review the structure and function of the urinary system. See p. 376 in the textbook.
   a. Display the overhead transparency showing the urinary system. Use this as a basis for discussion.

2. Divide students into groups of three. Provide each group with several sheets of notebook paper.
   a. Ask students to identify and discuss the factors that affect normal elimination. Allow 10 minutes. Then call on one student from each group to report to the class.

3. Display the guidelines in Box 29-2, p. 466 in the textbook, on an overhead transparency. Review each guideline with the students.

4. Show the following sections of video # 8 (Assisting with Elimination) in Mosby's Nursing Assisting Video Series.
   a. Identify normal and abnormal urine
   b. Help prevent incontinence
   c. Help maintain normal voiding pattern
   d. Assist with bedside commode, urinal, and bedpan
      (1) Stop the video after each section to allow time for discussion.

5. Write the following terms on a flip chart. Use a different colored marker for each term. Leave space after each term for the definition.
   a. Urge incontinence
   b. Stress incontinence
   c. Mixed incontinence
   d. Overflow incontinence
   e. Functional incontinence

6. Divide students into groups of three. Provide each group with several sheets of notebook paper.
   a. Ask students to identify and discuss the physical and psychological effects of incontinence. They should also identify the measures needed to meet the needs of persons with incontinence.
      (1) Allow 15 minutes for discussion. Then call on one student from each group to report to the class.

7. Show the following section of video # 8 (Assisting with Elimination) in Mosby's Nursing Assisting Video Series. Use this as a basis to discuss care for persons with catheters.
   a. Care for a person with a catheter
      (1) Allow time for discussion.

8. Display the guidelines in Box 29-4, p. 477 in the textbook, on an overhead transparency. Review each rule with the students.

9. Call on students to identify and define the two basic methods of bladder training.

10. Display the guidelines for collecting specimens listed in Box 29-5, p. 487 in the textbook, on an overhead transparency. Review each rule with students. Encourage questions and discussion.

11. Write the following terms on a flip chart. Use a different color marker for each term. Leave space after each term.
    a. The random urine specimen
    b. The midstream specimen
    c. The 24-hour urine specimen
       (1) Call on students to describe the purpose of each specimen and how each specimen is collected.
       (2) Write the correct answers on the flip chart. Clarify any wrong answers.

12. Use the procedure checklists provided.
    a. Demonstrate the procedures in this chapter.
    b. Have each student practice and return demonstrate the procedures in this chapter. Have each student assume the role of the patient/resident for procedures when appropriate. Use simulators and anatomical models when appropriate
       (1) Make sure all necessary equipment and supplies are available

13. Have each student take a turn at being placed on the bedpan. Each student should remain on the bedpan for at least 10 minutes.
    a. Ask each student to describe his or her experience. Discuss level of comfort and any concerns. How will the student's experience affect the care they provide?

Homework Assignments

Ask students to answer the questions at the end of Chapter 29 in the textbook. Tell students the date and time that this assignment must be completed and turned in.

If the accompanying student workbook is being used, assign the Chapter 29 workbook exercises. Tell students the date and time that this assignment must be completed and turned in.

Name _____

Date _____

Urinary Elimination

Match each term with the correct definition.

a. Catheter
b. Dysuria
c. Glucosuria
d. Hematuria
e. Micturition
f. Oliguria
g. Polyuria

1. _____ The process of emptying urine from the bladder

2. _____ Painful or difficult urination

3. _____ The production of abnormally large amounts of urine

4. _____ A tube used to drain or inject fluid through a body opening

5. _____ Scant amount of urine

6. _____ Sugar in the urine

7. _____ Blood in the urine

8. List and define the 6 types of urinary incontinence.

a. _____

_____

b. _____

_____

c. _____

_____

d. _____

_____

e. _____

_____

f. _____

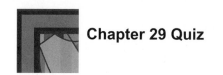

Chapter 29 Quiz

Name _____

Date _____

Urinary Elimination

True or False

Mark **T** *for true or* **F** *for false.*

1. _____ The healthy adult excretes about 1500 ml of urine per day.

2. _____ When using a fracture pan, the larger end is placed under the buttocks.

3. _____ Urinals are placed on the overbed table.

4. _____ Urinary incontinence may be temporary or permanent.

5. _____ Catheters treat the cause of urinary incontinence.

6. _____ The normal pH of urine is from 4.6 to 8.0.

7. _____ Catheterization increases the risk of urinary tract infection.

8. _____ Adhesive tape is used to secure condom catheters.

9. _____ Follow medical asepsis, Standard Precautions, and the Bloodborne Pathogen Standard when handling bedpans and their contents.

10. _____ The goal of bladder training programs is voluntary control of urination.

11. _____ Urine is strained to check for occult blood.

Multiple Choice

Circle the BEST answer.

12. Frequent urination at night is:
    a. Polyuria.
    b. Nocturia.
    c. Dysuria.
    d. Urgency.

13. The involuntary loss of urine after feeling a strong urge to void is called:
    a. Overflow incontinence.
    b. Mixed incontinence.
    c. Functional incontinence.
    d. Urge incontinence.

14. Which is correct when applying a condom catheter?
    a. A new catheter is applied weekly.
    b. Elastic tape secures the catheter in place.
    c. Apply tape completely around the penis.
    d. All of the above.

15. Mrs. Andrews has an indwelling catheter. Which is incorrect?
    a. Attach the drainage bag to the bed rail.
    b. She should not lie on the tubing.
    c. Keep the drainage bag below the bladder.
    d. Provide perineal care daily and after bowel movements.

Copyright © 2004 Mosby, Inc. All rights reserved.

30

Bowel Elimination

Instructor's Preparation

I. Read Chapter 30 in the textbook. Carefully review chapter objectives, key terms, and review questions.

II. Read the outline in Chapter 30 of the instructor's guide. Carefully review the classroom activities, the student assignment, and the quiz.

III. If you are using the accompanying student workbook, review the activities for Chapter 30.

IV. Review video #8 (Assisting with Elimination) in Mosby's Nursing Assisting Video Series.

V. Gather all necessary supplies and equipment for classroom activities and student assignments.
   A. Prepare overhead transparencies
   B. Prepare situation/index cards
   C. Gather correct video
   D. Gather anatomical models
   E. Gather simulators
   F. Gather all equipment and supplies needed to demonstrate and have each student return demonstrate the procedures in this chapter.
   G. Gather any other items that will be needed for classroom activities.
   H. Assemble items in the order they will be used.

VI. Make sure that the necessary equipment is available and in good working order.

Objectives

- Define the key terms listed in this chapter
- Describe normal stools and the normal pattern and frequency of bowel movements
- List the observations to make about bowel movements
- Identify the factors that affect bowel elimination
- Describe common bowel elimination problems
- Describe the measures that promote comfort and safety during defecation
- Describe bowel training
- Explain why enemas are given
- Know the common enema solutions
- Describe the comfort and safety measures for giving enemas
- Explain the purpose of rectal tubes
- Describe how to care for a person with an ostomy pouch
- Explain why stool specimens are collected
- Learn the procedures described in this chapter

Key Terms

anal incontinence
colostomy
constipation
defecation
dehydration
diarrhea
enema
fecal impaction
fecal incontinence
feces
flatulence
flatus

ileostomy
melena
ostomy
peristalsis
stoma
stool
suppository

Outline

Bowel Elimination

I. INTRODUCTION
   A. Bowel elimination is a basic need
   B. Factors that affect bowel elimination:
       1. Privacy, personal habits, age, diet, exercise and activity, fluids, and drugs
   C. See Chapter 13 in the textbook for a review of the gastrointestinal (GI) tract
   D. Bowel elimination problems and treatments may be uncomfortable, frustrating, embarrassing, and humiliating for the client
   E. Be sensitive and offer emotional support (see Providing Compassionate Care box, p. 501)
   F. Follow Standard Precautions and the infection control guidelines listed in Box 29-1, p. 466 in the textbook

II. NORMAL BOWEL MOVEMENTS
   A. Frequency of bowel movements varies from person to person
   B. Stools are normally brown in color
       1. Diet, disease, and infection affect the color of stools
   C. Stools are normally soft, formed, moist, and shaped like the rectum
       1. They have a characteristic odor caused by bacterial action
   D. Observations
       1. Your observations are important for the nursing process
       2. Stools are carefully observed before disposal
       3. Report to your supervisor: color, amount, consistency, odor, shape, size, frequency of defecation, and complaints of pain

III. FACTORS AFFECTING BOWEL ELIMINATION
   A. Normal regular defecaion is affected by many factors:
       1. Privacy—lack of privacy prevents many people from defecating despite having the urge
           a. Ignoring the urge to defecate can lead to constipation
       2. Personal habits—defecation is easier when a person is relaxed and follows a routine
       3. Diet—a well-balance diet and bulk are needed
           a. Foods cause diarrhea, constipation, and gas
       4. Fluids—feces contain water; drinking six to eight glasses of water every day promotes normal bowel elimination
           a. Warm fluids increase peristalsis
       5. Activity and exercise maintain muscle tone and stimulate peristalsis
           a. Irregular elimination and constipation result from inactivity and bedrest
       6. Medications—drugs can prevent constipation or control diarrhea
           a. Drugs also have diarrhea or constipation as side effects
       7. Age
           a. Focus on children
               (1) Bowel training is learned between 2 and 3 years of age
           b. Focus on older persons
               (1) As people age, feces pass through the intestines at a slower rate
               (2) Some older persons loose control over defecation
               (3) Older persons are at a higher risk for intestinal tumors and disorders
               (4) Older persons do not always completely empty the rectum
                   (a) They may need to use the bathroom again

IV. COMFORT AND SAFETY
   A. See Box 30-1, p. 506 in the textbook for Comfort and Safety During Bowel Elimination

V. COMMON PROBLEMS
   A. Constipation
       1. The passage of hard, dry stool
       2. The person strains to have a bowel movement
       3. Large stools can cause pain as they pass
       4. Common causes include:
           a. Low-fiber diet
           b. Ignoring the urge to defecate
           c. Decreased fluid intake
           d. Inactivity
           e. Drugs
           f. Aging
           g. Certain diseases

B. Fecal impaction
   1. The prolonged retention and accumulation of feces in the rectum
      a. It results if constipation is not relieved
      b. The person cannot defecate
      c. Liquid seeping from the anus is a sign of fecal impaction
      d. Abdominal discomfort, cramping, and rectal pain are common
      e. A digital examination is done to check for impaction by a physician or nurse
         (1) Often produces the urge to defecate
      f. The doctor may order drugs and enemas
      g. Often it is necessary to remove the fecal mass with a lubricated, gloved finger; done by a physician or nurse
         (1) A doctor's order is required
         (2) Digital removal of an impaction is uncomfortable and embarrassing

C. Diarrhea
   1. The frequent passage of liquid stools
      a. Feces move through the intestines rapidly
   2. The need to defecate is urgent
   3. Abdominal cramping, nausea, and vomiting may also occur
   4. Causes include infections, certain drugs, irritating foods, and microbes in food and water
   5. Nursing measures:
      a. Promptly assisting the person to the bathroom, commode, or bedpan
      b. Prompt disposal of stools
      c. Good skin care
   6. Fluid lost is replaced to prevent dehydration (excessive loss of water from tissues)
   7. Signs and symptoms of dehydration:
      a. Pale or flushed skin
      b. Dry skin
      c. Coated tongue
      d. Oliguria (scant amount of urine)
      e. Thirst
      f. Weakness
      g. Dizziness
      h. Confusion
      i. Falling blood pressure and increased pulse and respirations are serious signs
   8. IV therapy may be necessary in severe cases
   9. Diarrhea is often caused by microbes

   10. Always practice Standard Precautions
   11. Focus on children
      a. Children are at risk for dehydration
      b. Death can occur quickly
      c. Report liquid or watery stools to the nurse immediately
      d. Note the number of wet diapers
   12. Focus on older persons
      a. They are at risk for dehydration
      b. Report signs of diarrhea to the nurse immediately
      c. Death is a risk

D. Fecal incontinence
   1. The inability to control the passage of feces and gas through the anus
   2. Causes include:
      a. Intestinal diseases
      b. Nervous system disease and injury
      c. Fecal impaction
      d. Diarrhea
      e. Some drugs
      f. Persons with mental health problems or cognitive disorders may not recognize the need to defecate (see Chapters 23 and 24)
      g. Unanswered signal lights when the person needs to use the bathroom, commode, or bedpan

E. Flatulence
   1. Gas and air are normally found in the stomach and intestines
   2. Expelled through the mouth (belching, eructating)
   3. Expelled through the anus (flatus)
   4. Flatulence is the excessive formation of gas in the stomach and intestines
   5. Common causes are:
      a. Swallowing air while eating and drinking
      b. Bacterial action in the intestines
      c. Gas-forming foods
      d. Constipation
      e. Bowel and abdominal surgeries
      f. Drugs that decrease peristalsis
   6. If flatus is not expelled, the intestines distend
      a. Abdominal cramping or pain, shortness of breath, and a swollen abdomen occur
   7. Walking and the left side-lying position often produce flatus
      a. Enemas, medications, or rectal tubes may be ordered

VI. BOWEL TRAINING
    A. Has two goals:
        1. To gain control of bowel movements
        2. To develop a regular pattern of elimination
    B. Fecal impaction, constipation, and fecal incontinence are prevented
    C. The urge to defecate is usually felt after a meal
        1. Encourage use of the toilet, commode, or bedpan at this time
    D. Follow the nursing care plan and the bowel training program
    E. These include:
        1. High-fibre diet
        2. Increased fluids
        3. Warm fluids
        4. Activity
        5. Privacy
    F. The doctor may order suppositories or enemas to stimulate defecation
        1. A rectal suppository is a cone-shaped, solid medication inserted into the rectum by a nurse—assist as needed (see Chapter 39)

VII. ENEMAS
    A. The introduction of fluid into the rectum and lower colon
    B. Ordered by doctors
    C. Given to remove feces and relieve constipation or fecal impaction
    D. Also performed to clean the bowel of feces before certain surgeries, x-ray procedures, and childbirth
    E. Sometimes ordered to relieve flatus and intestinal distention
    F. Bowel training programs can involve enemas
    G. Enemas are usually safe procedures
        1. Considered dangerous for older persons and those with certain heart and kidney diseases, therefore, giving an enema is a delegated task (see Chapter 5)
    H. Comfort and safety measures are practiced
        1. The guidelines listed in Box 30-2, p. 508 in the textbook, are followed
    I. Before giving an enema, make sure that:
        1. Your provincial or territorial laws and your employer allow you to perform the procedure
        2. The procedure is in your job description
        3. You have had the necessary education and training
        4. You review the procedure with a nurse
        5. A nurse is available to answer questions and to supervise you

        6. Comfort and safety measures are practised (see Box 30-2, p. 508)
    J. Enema solutions
        1. The solution depends on the purpose of the enema
            a. Tap water enemas (obtained from a faucet)
            b. Soap suds enema (SSE)—add 3-5mL ($1/2$ to 1 teaspoon) castile soap to 500-1000 mL tap water
            c. Saline enema—add 5-10 mL (1-2 teaspoons) table salt to 500-1000 mL tap water
            d. Oil-retention enema—mineral oil or commercial oil-retention
            e. Commercial enema—contains about 120 mL (4 ounces) of solution
    K. Consult your supervisor and use the agency procedure manual to safely prepare and give uncommon enemas
    L. Do not administer enemas that contain drugs
    M. The cleansing enema
        1. Cleans the bowel of feces and flatus
        2. Sometimes given before surgery, x-ray procedures, and childbirth
        3. The doctor may order enemas until clean
            a. Enemas are given until the return solution is clear and free of fecal material
               (1) Ask your supervisor how many to give
        4. Tap water enemas can be dangerous; they can cause fluid imbalance
            a. Only one is given; do not repeat
            b. Takes effect in 15-20 minutes
        5. Soap suds enemas are very irritating to the bowel's mucous lining
            a. Repeated enemas can damage the bowel
            b. Using more than 3-5 mL of castile soap or using stronger soaps can damage the bowel
            c. Takes effect in 10-15 minutes
        6. The saline enema is similar to body fluid
            a. Excess absorption of salt can cause fluid imbalance
            b. Takes effect in 15-20 minutes
        7. Focus on children
            a. Only saline enemas are used for children
            b. The amount of solution varies for infants and children
            c. If you are delegated to give an enema

to a child, your supervisor will give you the necessary instructions

    8. Giving a Cleansing Enema to an Adult ▶ p. 509

N. The commercial enema

    1. Causes defecation by irritating and distending the rectum

    2. Often ordered for constipation or when complete cleansing of the bowel is not needed

    3. Manufacturers prepare and package commercial enemas; ready for use

    4. Usually given at room temperature

    5. Insert the commercial enema tip 5 centimetres (2 inches) into the rectum (see Figure 30-3, p. 513)

    6. The plastic bottle is squeezed and rolled up from the bottom

       a. Do not release pressure on the bottle

    7. Encourage the person to retain the solution until feeling the urge to defecate

    8. The person assumes the Sims' or side-lying position (see Figure 30-2, p. 511)

    9. Giving a Commercial Enema to an Adult ▶ p. 512

VIII. RECTAL TUBES

  A. Inserted into the rectum to relieve flatus and intestinal distention

    1. Inserted by a nurse 4 inches into the adult rectum

  B. Left in place 20 to 30 minutes

  C. Can be reinserted every 2 to 3 hours

  D. Rectal tubes are not used after rectal surgery

  E. The tube may be connected to a flatus bag or a container of water

  F. Feces may be expelled along with flatus

    1. If a flatus bag is not used, place the open end in a folded waterproof pad

IX. THE PERSON WITH AN OSTOMY

  A. Sometimes surgical removal of part of the intestines is necessary

    1. Cancer, diseases of the bowel, and trauma are common reasons

  B. An ostomy is sometimes necessary (the surgical creation of an artificial opening)

    1. The opening is called a stoma

    2. The person wears a pouch over the stoma to collect feces and flatus

    3. Stomas do not have nerve endings and are not painful

  C. Colostomy

    1. The surgical creation of an artificial opening between the colon and abdominal wall

    2. Part of the colon is brought out onto the abdominal wall and a stoma is made

       a. They can be permanent or temporary

    3. The site depends on the site of colon disease or injury (see Figure 30-5, p. 514)

       a. Stools are liquid or formed

    4. Feces irritate the skin

       a. Skin care prevents skin breakdown around the stoma

       b. Skin is washed and dried when the pouch is removed

       c. Skin barrier is applied around the stoma (may be part of the pouch or a separate device)

D. Ileostomy

    1. The surgical creation of an artificial opening between the ilium and the abdominal wall

    2. Part of the ilium is brought out onto the abdominal wall and a stoma is made

    3. The entire large intestine is removed (see Figure 30-6, p. 515)

    4. Liquid feces drain constantly from an ileostomy

    5. Digestive juices are irritating to the skin

       a. The pouch must fit well to prevent leakage

       b. Good skin care is essential

    6. Ostomy pouches

       a. The pouch has an adhesive backing that is applied to the skin

       b. Sometimes belts are used to secure pouches

       c. Many pouches have a drain at the bottom that is closed with a clip, clamp, or wire closure

         (1) The drain is opened to empty the pouch

       d. The pouch is emptied when $1/3$ to $1/2$ full

       e. The pouch is changed every 3 to 7 days

       f. Many people handle their ostomies without help

       g. Odors are prevented

       h. Good hygiene is essential

       i. Empty the pouch when feces are present

       j. Avoid gas-forming foods

       k. Special deodorants may be used (ask your supervisor)

       l. Showers and baths are delayed 1 to 2

hours after applying a new pouch
m. Do not flush pouches down the toilet
  (1) Follow agency policy for disposal
n. Focus on children
  (1) Children of all ages can have ostomies
  (2) The nurse will give you necessary instructions
o. Changing an Ostomy Pouch ▶ p. 516

X. STOOL SPECIMENS
A. When internal bleeding is suspected, feces are checked for blood
B. Stools are also studied for fat, microbes, worms, and other abnormal contents
C. The guidelines for collecting urine specimens apply (see Chapter 29)
D. Follow Standard Precautions
E. The stool specimen must not be contaminated with urine
F. A warm specimen is required for some tests
  1. Take to the laboratory immediately
G. Collecting a Stool Specimen ▶ p. 518
H. Testing stools for blood
  1. Causes of blood in stools include ulcers, colon cancer, hemorrhoids
  2. Melena is a black, tarry stool (bleeding in the stomach or upper GI tract)
  3. Bleeding in small amounts is difficult to detect
    a. Stools are checked for occult (hidden or unseen) blood
  4. There are many types of tests; follow manufacturers instructions
  5. Follow Standard Precautions and the Bloodborne Pathogen Standard
  6. Factors that affect results include eating red meat, bleeding from hemorrhoids, and menstrual periods
  7. Testing a Stool Specimen for Blood ▶ p. 520

Classroom Activities

1. Review the structure and function of the GI tract with students

2. Use Divide students into groups of three. Provide each group with several sheets of notebook paper. Ask students to identify and discuss the factors that affect bowel elimination. They should also identify measures needed to meet elimination needs.
a. Allow 15 minutes for discussion. Then call on

one student from each group to report to the class.
b. Allow time for questions and discussion.

3. Show the following section of video # 8 (Assisting with Elimination) in Mosby's Nursing Assisting Video Series.
a. Assist with normal bowel elimination
  (1) Allow time for questions and discussion.

4. Write the following terms on the chalkboard. Then call on students to provide the definition for each term. Write the correct answer on the chalkboard after the appropriate term.
a. Constipation
b. Fecal impaction
c. Diarrhea
d. Fecal incontinence
e. Flatulence

5. Divide students into pairs or groups of three. Write these terms on separate index cards: Constipation, Fecal impaction, Diarrhea, Fecal incontinence, and Flatulence. Ask one student from each pair or group to pick one index card.
a. Allow each pair or group 15 minutes to identify the signs and symptoms, the causes, and the nursing interventions for the condition written on their index card.
b. Ask one student from each pair or group to report to the class.
  (1) Allow time for questions.

6. Call on students to identify the two goals of bowel training.

7. Write the following statement on the chalkboard: "Before performing any procedures described in this chapter make sure that:"
a. _____
b. _____
c. _____
d. _____
e. _____
  (1) Call on students to complete the statement. Write the correct answers on the chalkboard.

8. Use the procedure checklists provided.
   a. Demonstrate the procedures in this chapter.
   b. Have each student practice and return demonstrate the procedures in this chapter. Use a simulator or anatomical model when appropriate.
   c. Stress the need to follow Standard Precautions and the Bloodborne Pathogen Standard.
   d. Review special considerations for children and older persons.

9. Have available various ostomy pouches and supplies for students to manipulate. Encourage students to ask questions.

Homework Assignments

Ask students to answer the questions at the end of Chapter 30 in the textbook. Tell students the date and time that this assignment must be completed and turned in.

If the accompanying student workbook is being used, assign the Chapter 30 workbook exercises. Tell students the date and time that this assignment must be completed and turned in.

Chapter 30 Student Assignment   Name _____

Date _____

Bowel Elimination

Matching

Match each term with the correct definition.

a. Colostomy
b. Constipation
c. Diarrhea
d. Enema
e. Feces
f. Flatus
g. Melena
h. Ostomy
i. Peristalsis
j. Stool

1. _____ The introduction of fluid into the rectum and lower colon

2. _____ Excreted feces

3. _____ Gas or air passed through the anus

4. _____ An artificial opening between the colon and the abdominal wall

5. _____ The frequent passage of liquid stools

6. _____ The surgical creation of an artificial opening

7. _____ The semi-solid mass of waste products in the colon

8. _____ A black, tarry stool

9. _____ The passage of a hard, dry stool

10. _____ The alternating contraction and relaxation of intestinal muscles

11. Name the types of enema solutions described below:

a. _____
obtained from a faucet.

b. _____
add 5 mL of castile soap to 1000 mL of tap water.

c. _____
a solution of salt and water. Add 2 teaspoons of table salt to 1000 mL of tap water.

d. _____
mineral oil or a commercially prepared enema is used.

e. _____
contains about 120mL (4 ounces) of solution prepared and packaged by a manufacturer. Ready to give.

228

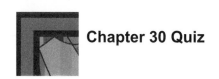

Chapter 30 Quiz

Name _____

Date _____

Bowel Elimination

True or False

*Mark **T** for true or **F** for false.*

1. _____ Ignoring the need to defecate can lead to constipation.

2. _____ Up to three tap water enemas are given to cleanse the bowels.

3. _____ The person is positioned in the right side-lying position for a cleansing enema.

4. _____ A rectal tube is left in place for 1 hour.

5. _____ Stomas do not have nerve endings and are not painful.

6. _____ All colostomies are permanent.

7. _____ Ostomy pouches are flushed down the toilet.

8. _____ Liquid feces drain constantly from an ileostomy.

9. _____ Follow Standard Precautions when collecting stool specimens.

Multiple Choice

Circle the BEST answer.

10. Which is not a cause of constipation?
    a. Decreased fluid intake
    b. High-fiber diet
    c. Some medications
    d. Inactivity

11. Mrs. Harvey complains of abdominal discomfort. Watery stool has been leaking from her rectum. This is probably:
    a. Diarrhea.
    b. Anal incontinence.
    c. A fecal impaction.
    d. Constipation.

12. Mr. Adams has fecal incontinence. You know that:
    a. Good skin care is required.
    b. A bowel training program will cure his incontinence.
    c. The condition is permanent.
    d. He has dementia.

13. You are giving a cleansing enema to a 4-year-old child. Which is correct?
    a. No special precautions are needed.
    b. Give 500 ml of the solution.
    c. Insert the tube 4 inches into the rectum.
    d. The enema solution is given at room temperature.

14. A person has an ileostomy. Which is incorrect?
    a. The stool is formed.
    b. Good skin care is essential.
    c. The entire large intestine has been removed.
    d. The pouch must fit well.

31

Common Diseases and Conditions

Instructor's Preparation

I. Read Chapter 31 in the textbook. Carefully review chapter objectives, key terms, and review questions.

II. Read the outline in Chapter 31 of the instructor's guide. Carefully review the classroom activities, the student assignment, and the quiz.

III. If you are using the accompanying student workbook, review the activities for Chapter 31.

IV. Gather all necessary supplies and equipment for classroom activities and student assignments.
   A. Prepare the correct number of handouts
   B. Prepare appropriate flip charts
   C. Prepare overhead transparencies
   D. Prepare situation/index cards
   E. Gather correct slides
   F. Gather coloured markers
   G. Gather anatomical models
   H. Gather simulators
   I. Gather any other items that will be needed for classroom activities
   J. Assemble items in the order they will be used

V. Make sure that the necessary equipment is available and in good working order.

VI. Contact guest speakers to confirm the day, date, time, and location that they are expected.
   A. Ask the speakers if they require any special equipment or supplies.

Objectives

- Define the key terms listed in this chapter
- Describe cancer and its treatment
- Describe common cardiovascular disorders and the care required
- Describe common respiratory disorders and the care required
- Describe common neurological disorders and the care required
- Identify the causes and effects of brain and spinal cord injuries and the care required
- Describe common musculoskeletal disorders and the care required
- Explain how to care for clients in casts, in traction, and with hip fractures
- Describe the effects of amputation
- Describe common endocrine disorders and the care required
- Describe common digestive disorders and the care required
- Explain what to do when a client vomits
- Describe common urinary disorders and the care required
- Describe common communicable diseases and the care required

Key Terms

acquired brain injury
acquired immunodeficiency syndrome (AIDS)
amputation
amyotrophic lateral sclerosis (ALS)
angina pectoris
arrhythmia
arthritis
arthroplasty

asthma
benign
cancer
cerebral vascular accident (CVA)
chronic obstructive pulmonary disease (COPD)
communicable disease
congestive heart failure (CHF)
coronary artery disease (CAD)
diabetes
diverticulosis
fibromyaliga
fracture
gangrene
heart attack
hemiplegia
hepatitis
Huntington's disease
hypertension
influenza
malignant
metastasis
multiple sclerosis (MS)
myocardial infarction (MI)
osteoporosis
paralysis
paraplegia
Parkinson's disease
pneumonia
quadriplegia
renal calculi
sexually transmitted disease (STD)
stroke
tuberculosis
tumour

Outline

Common Diseases and Conditions

I. INTRODUCTION
  A. Some diseases and conditions are acute, some chronic, some progressive
  B. Some clients may be immobile and confined to bed; others are on a physician's ordered bed rest
  C. Understanding the disease is important when providing care
  D. Your supervisor gives you more information as needed
  E. See Providing Compassionate Care box, p. 524 in the textbook
  F. Review Chapters 13, 33-36, and 38 for descriptions of other health problems
II. CANCER
  A. A tumour is a new growth of abnormal cells

1. Benign tumours grow slowly in a localized area
  a. Usually do not cause death
2. Malignant tumours (cancer) grow rapidly and invade healthy tissue (see Figure 31-1, p. 525)
  a. Death occurs if not treated and controlled
3. Metastasis is the spread of cancer to other body parts (see Figure 31-2, p. 525)
B. Cancer is the second leading cause of death in Canada
  1. Occurs in people of all ages
  2. Leukemia (a type of blood cancer) is the most common cancer in children
C. Factors contributing to development include:
  1. A family history of cancer
  2. Exposure to radiation (including the sun)
  3. Exposure to certain chemicals
  4. Smoking
  5. Alcohol
  6. High-fat, high-calorie diet
  7. Viruses
  8. Hormones
D. Cancer can be treated and controlled with early detection
  1. Box 31-2, p. 526 in the textbook, lists warning signs of cancer
E. Treatment depends on the type of tumour, site, size, and whether or not it has spread
  1. The treatment can be used to cure the cancer, keep cancer from spreading, slow growth of cancer, and/or relieve symptoms caused by the cancer
F. The three major cancer treatments are surgery, radiation therapy, and chemotherapy
  1. Surgery involves removing malignant tissue
    a. Done to cure or control cancer and relieve pain
  2. Radiation therapy destroys living cells
    a. High-energy rays are directed at the tumour or implants are inserted near the tumour.
    b. Cancer cells and normal cells are destroyed
    c. Done to cure or control cancer and relieve pain
    d. Side effects include discomfort, nausea, vomiting, fatigue, anorexia, and diarrhea
    e. Skin breakdown can occur
  3. Chemotherapy involves drugs that kill cells

a. Affects normal cells and cancer cells
b. Done to cure cancer or control the growth rate of cancer cells
c. Side effects include:
  (1) Irritation of the gastrointestinal (GI) tract
    (a) Nausea, vomiting, and diarrhea result
  (2) Stomatitis (inflammation of the mouth) may develop
  (3) Hair loss (alopecia) may occur
  (4) Decreased production of blood cells puts the person at risk for bleeding and infection
4. Persons with cancer have many needs:
a. Pain relief or control
b. Adequate rest and exercise
c. Fluids and nutrition
d. Preventing skin breakdown
e. Preventing bowel elimination problems
f. Dealing with side effects of radiation and chemotherapy
g. Psychological social, sexual, and spiritual needs
  (1) Anger, fear, and depression are strongly felt
    (a) Talk to the person
    (b) Do not avoid the person
    (c) Use touch
    (d) Listen
    (e) Some persons get comfort by talking to a spiritual leader
    (f) Persons are often referred to hospice programs

III. CARDIOVASCULAR DISORDERS
A. Problems occur in the heart or blood vessels
B. Hypertension
1. A condition in which the blood pressure is abnormally high
a. Systolic of 140 mm Hg or higher
b. Diastolic of 90 mm Hg or higher
c. A high reading must occur on two different occasions (see Chapter 40)
2. Risk factors are listed in Box 31-3, p. 527 in the textbook
3. Causes:
a. Narrowed blood vessels
b. Kidney disorders
c. Head injuries
d. Complications of pregnancy
e. Tumours
4. Can damage other body organs
5. May not cause signs and symptoms at

first
6. Signs and symptoms develop as the disorder progresses:
a. Headache
b. Blurred vision
c. Dizziness
7. Complications include stroke, heart attack, kidney failure, and blindness
8. Treatment:
a. Drugs that lower blood pressure
b. Exercise
c. Rest
d. Stop smoking
e. Sodium-restricted diet may be ordered
f. If overweight, a low-calorie diet is ordered
C. Coronary artery disease (CAD)
1. Coronary arteries narrow
2. One or all of the arteries may be affected
3. Heart muscle gets less blood
4. Most common cause is atherosclerosis
a. Fatty material collects on the arterial walls (see Figure 31-3, p. 527)
b. Arteries narrow and obstruct blood flow
c. If arteries are completely occluded (blocked), permanent damage to the heart occurs
5. Risk factors include:
a. Sex (male gender)
b. Age (more common in older persons)
c. Obesity
d. Cigarette smoking
e. Lack of exercise
f. High blood cholesterol
g. Hypertension
h. Family history of CAD
i. Uncontrolled diabetes
6. Treatment:
a. Involves reducing risk factors
D. Angina pectoris
1. Chest pain from reduced blood flow to a part of the heart muscle
2. Occurs when the heart muscle needs more oxygen
a. Physical exertion is the most common trigger, but emotional stress, extreme cold/heat, and heavy meals can also trigger
3. Signs and symptoms:
a. Chest pain, tightness, or discomfort in the left side of the chest
b. Pain may radiate to other sites (see Figure 31-4, p. 528)

c. Person may be pale, feel faint, and perspire

d. Dyspnea is common

4. Rest often relieves symptoms in 3 to 15 minutes

a. Reduces the need for oxygen

5. Nitroglycerin is given to relieve angina

a. The tablet is placed under the tongue

b. Tablets are often kept at the bedside

6. Some people need coronary artery bypass surgery

a. Many people with angina eventually have heart attacks

E. Myocardial infarction (MI)

1. Is caused by lack of blood supply to the heart muscle

2. Atherosclerosis or a thrombus (blood clot) obstructs blood flow through an artery

3. The area of damage may be samll or large (see Figure 31-5, p. 528)

4. Sudden cardiac death (cardiac arrest) can occur (see Chapter 47)

5. The person has one or more signs and symptoms listed in Box 31-4, p. 528 in the textbook

6. MI is an emergency

7. Efforts are directed at:

a. Relieving pain

b. Stabilizing vital signs

c. Giving oxygen

d. Calming the person

8. The person is treated in a coronary care unit (CCU)

9. When stable, the person is transferred

a. Activity is increased gradually

b. Drug therapy and measures to prevent complications continue

c. A cardiac rehabilitation program is planned; the goal is to prevent another heart attack

(1) Life-style changes may be necessary

F. Arrhythmia—abnormal heart rhythms

1. Heart's electrical system malfunctions

2. May skip a beat or have extra beats

3. Usually not life threatening but some arrhythmia's can be serious

4. Pacemakers are medical devices implanted in the body which will monitor heart rate and give small electric shocks to stimulate heartbeat

5. Clients with pacemakers should avoid areas or equipment with strong electric or magnetic fields

G. Congestive heart failure (CHF)

1. Occurs when the heart cannot pump blood normally

a. Blood backs up and causes congestion of tissues

2. Right-sided failure—blood backs up into the venae cavae and into the venous system

a. Feet and ankles swell, neck veins bulge, and the abdomen is congested with fluid

b. Liver congestion causes decreased liver function

c. Signs and symptoms of left-sided failure eventually occur

3. Left-sided heart failure—blood backs up into the lungs

a. Signs and symptoms of respiratory congestion occur

(1) Include dyspnea, increased sputum, cough, and gurgling sounds in the lungs

(2) Signs and symptoms also occur from effects on other organs that do not get enough blood

(3) A severe form of left-sided failure is pulmonary edema; death can occur

4. Heart failure is usually caused by a weakened heart

a. MI, hypertension, and damaged heart valves are causes

5. Can be treated and controlled

a. Medications strengthen the heart and reduce the amount of body fluid

b. A sodium-restricted diet is ordered

c. Oxygen is given

d. Most persons prefer semi-Fowler's or Fowler's position

e. Weigh daily as it can indicate signs of fluid build-up

6. You may be involved in the following aspects of care:

a. Maintain bedrest or limited activity

b. I&O and daily weights

c. Restricted fluids

d. Good skin care

e. ROM exercises

f. Assisting with transfers, ambulation, and self-care activities

g. Maintaining good body alignment

h. Elastic stockings

7. Focus on children (see p. 529)

8. Focus on older persons (see p. 529)
IV. RESPIRATORY DISORDERS
  A. Chronic obstructive pulmonary disease (COPD)
    1. Chronic lung disorder that obstructs the airways making breathing difficult
    2. Caused by smoking, long-term exposure to chemical fumes, or dusts
    3. Cannot be cured but can be controlled
    4. Treatment may include
      a. Medications—delivered by inhalers (see Chapter 39)
      b. Client must quit smoking
      c. Breathing exercises
      d. Oxygen therapy
      e. Fluid intake encouraged to decrease thickness of secretions
  B. These disorders are grouped under COPD
    1. Chronic bronchitis
      a. Chronic inflammation of the bronchi
      b. Large amounts of mucus are produced, is thick and difficult to cough up, so it is not cleared completely and obstructs the airways
      c. Body can't get normal amounts of oxygen
      d. Infection is a risk as mucus provides a growth media for bacteria
      e. Coughing is first and most common symptom but as disease progress client has more and more difficulty breathing
    2. Emphysema—the alveoli enlarge
      a. The walls of the alveoli are less elastic; do not expand and shrink normally with inspiration and expiration
      b. Air is trapped in the alveoli and is not exhaled
      c. As the disease progresses, more alveoli are involved
      d. Normal exchange of oxygen and carbon dioxide cannot occur
      e. Cigarette smoking is the most common cause
      f. Signs and symptoms include:
        (1) Shortness of breath
        (2) Smoker's cough
        (3) Sputum may contain pus
        (4) Barrel chest develops as the disease progresses (see Figure 31-6 p. 530)
        (5) Breathing is easier when the person sits upright and slightly forward

  C. Asthma—the air passages narrow
    a. Dyspnea results
    b. Allergies, exercise, cold air, and emotional stress are common causes
    c. Episodes occur suddenly (asthma attacks)
    d. The person has shortness of breath, wheezing, coughing, rapid pulse, perspiration, and cyanosis
    e. The person is frightened; fear makes the attack worse
    f. Treatment:
      (1) Medications are used to prevent or lessen asthma attacks
      (2) Emergency room treatment may be necessary
      (3) The person and family learn how to prevent attacks
    g. Repeated attacks can damage the respiratory system
  D. Pneumonia
    1. An infection of lung tissue
    2. Alveoli fill with pus, mucus, other liquids; oxygen and carbon dioxide are not exchanged normally
    3. Caused by bacteria, viruses, aspiration, or immobility
    4. The person with pneumonia is very ill
      a. Fever, chills, painful cough, chest pain, and a rapid pulse occur
      b. Cyanosis may be present
      c. Sputum is clear, green, yellowish, or rust colored depending on the cause
    5. Treatment:
      a. Antibiotics to fight the infection and medications for pain, cough
      b. Fluids are encouraged
      c. Oxygen may be necessary
      d. Semi-Fowler's position
    6. Standard Precautions are followed
    7. Isolation Precautions may be necessary
  E. Influenza
    1. Respiratory tract infection caused by a virus
    2. Flu season in Canada is from November to May
    3. Spread by airborne methods as well as indirect (touching contaminated objects, e.g., public telephones, handrails, etc.)
    4. Onset is usually sudden and many different symptoms can occur involving the respiratory and digestive systems
    5. Recovery usually takes 1 to 2 weeks however some people develop serious

and life-threatening complications which include pneumonia
6. Good hygiene, Standard Precautions, washing hands, flu vaccine all reduce chance of infection
7. Your employer may require you to get the yearly flu vaccine as you are working with at-risk people such as the elderly
F. Tuberculosis (TB)
1. A bacterial infection
a. Affects the lungs
b. Can also occur in the kidneys, bones, lymph nodes, urinary and digestive systems
2. Bacteria that cause TB are spread by airborne droplets (see Chapter 18)
a. Spread occurs during coughing, sneezing, speaking, or singing
3. Persons who have close, frequent contact with an infected person are at risk
4. Spread of the disease is more likely to occur in close, crowded areas
5. Persons with HIV infection are also at risk
6. Person may not have symptoms at first
a. TB is found on a routine chest x-ray or when a TB skin test is required for a job
7. Signs and symptoms:
a. Tiredness
b. Loss of appetite and weight loss
c. Fever and night sweats
d. Coughing
(1) Becomes more frequent as the disease progresses
(2) Sputum production increases
e. Chest pain
8. Treatment:
a. Drug therapy for TB
9. Persons with TB
a. Persons with active TB may require hospital care
b. Need to cover the nose and mouth with tissues when coughing or sneezing
c. Tissues are flushed down the toilet or placed in a paper bag and burned
(1) In health care agencies, tissues are disposed of in biohazardous waste containers following agency policy
d. Hand washing after contact with sputum is essential
e. Standard Precautions and airborne pre-

cautions are practiced (see Chapter 18)
V. NEUROLOGICAL DISORDERS
A. Can affect mental and physical functions
1. Physical functions include tasks such as moving, seeing, hearing touching and controlling elimination
2. Cognitive functions include tasks controlled by the mind which include thinking, remembering, reading and problem solving
B. Stroke
1. A cardiovascular disease affecting the blood vessels that supply blood to the brain
a. Blood supply to part of the brain is suddenly interrupted
(1) Brain cells do not get oxygen and nutrients
(2) Brain damage occurs
(3) Functions controlled by the part of the brain involved are lost or impaired
2. A ruptured blood vessel is one cause
3. Blood clots are another cause
4. Stroke is the fourth leading cause of death in Canada
5. Stroke is the leading cause of disability in adults
6. Stroke is a medical emergency
7. Box 31-5, p. 532 in the textbook, lists the warning signs of stroke
a. A transient ischemic attack (TIA) is when blood supply to the brain is interrupted for a short time; warns of a stroke
8. Stroke is more common in persons over age 65
9. Risk factors include high blood pressure, smoking, diabetes, heart disease, high blood cholesterol, lack of exercise, and high alcohol intake
10. If the person survives the stroke, some brain injury is likely
a. Functions lost depend on the area injured
b. Effects of stroke include:
(1) Hemiplegia
(2) Loss of face control
(3) Changing emotions
(4) Dysphagia
(5) Dimmed vision
(6) Slow or slurred speech
(7) Changes in perception
(8) Impaired memory

(9) Urinary frequency, urgency, or incontinence

(10) Depression

(11) Frustration

11. Rehabilitation starts immediately

12. Many stroke survivors return home

13. Home nursing services are often needed

14. Some stroke survivors need long-term care

C. Parkinson's disease

1. A slow, progressive disorder with no cure

2. Degeneration of part of the brain occurs

3. Usually seen in persons over 50 years of age

4. Signs and symptoms become worse over time and may include:

   a. Tremors—pill-rolling movements in fingers, or in legs, jaw, and face

   b. Stiff muscles—in arms, legs, neck, and face

   c. Masklike expression—cannot blink or smile, face has a fixed glare

   d. Slow shuffling movement

   e. Stooped posture and impaired balance which makes falls a risk

   f. Swallowing and chewing problems

   g. Bowel and bladder problems

   h. Sleep problems and depression

   i. Dementia (see Chapter 34)

   j. Slurred, monotone, and soft speech

5. The physician orders drugs specific for Parkinson's disease

6. Exercise and physical therapy are ordered

7. Measures to promote normal elimination are practiced

8. Safety practices are followed to prevent injury

9. Treat the person with dignity and respect—remember mask-like expressions don't show their true feelings

D. Huntington's disease

1. An inherited neurological disorder that destroys brain cells and causes uncontrolled movements, emotional disturbances, and cognitive losses

2. Signs and symptoms usually appear between the age of 20 and 60

3. Begin with twitching, fidgeting, and clumsiness; over time the person's arms and legs constantly move

4. May have difficulty eating and swallowing and performing ADLs

5. As progresses may have slurred speech, depression, cognitive problems

6. Currently, there is no cure or treatment

7. Care plans depend on client's needs; you must keep the client safe

E. Multiple sclerosis (MS)

1. A progressive disease in which:

   a. The myelin sheath, spinal cord, and white matter in the brain are destroyed

   b. Functions are impaired or lost

2. Canadians have one of the highest rates of MS in the world

3. Symptoms usually start between ages 20 and 40

4. Women are affected more than men

5. Common symptoms are:

   a. Blurred vision, double vision, or blindness

   b. Extreme fatigue

   c. Loss of balance, dizziness, difficulty walking, and clumsiness

   d. Muscle weakness and stiffness

   e. Tingling, numbness, or a burning feeling in one area of the body

   f. Sensitivity to heat

   g. Difficulty speaking and swallowing

   h. Bladder and bowel problems

   i. Impotence or diminished sexual arousal

   j. Short-term memory loss

   k. Difficulties concentration

   l. Impaired judgment or reasoning

6. The person becomes totally dependent on others for care

7. There is no known cure

8. Persons are kept as active as possible

9. Nursing care depends on the person's needs and condition

F. Amyotrophic Lateral Sclerosis—Lou Gehrig's Disease

1. ALS is a neurological disorder that results in the loss of all muscle control but does not affect intelligence

2. Commonly occurs between ages 40–70

3. Progressive destruction of brain and spinal cells

4. Starts with gradual difficulty with muscle movements, such as picking up a cup, progresses to difficulty walking and then to all other functions including swallowing, breathing, and moving; ends in death

5. Always remember that even if the person cannot speak they can understand what you are saying

6. The person will eventually be confined to

bed

      7. Follow the care plan and the guidelines for clients confined to bed (see Box 31-1, p. 524)

   G. Acquired brain injuries

      1. Damage to brain tissue caused by disease, medical condition, accident or violence

      2. When the head is subjected to violent force the brain is bashed against the skull which can result in bleeding, swelling, or bruising

      3. Some injuries are temporary; others are permanent

      4. Common causes are MVA, falls, sports or recreational injuries, acts of violence and work-related injuries

      5. Babies who are shaken sometimes acquire brain injury

      6. Some acquired brain injuries are caused by lack of oxygen to the brain and can be caused from anything from birth to any type of accident

      7. Signs and symptoms depend on the severity and location of the injury and can affect every system in the body

      8. Care depends on the client's needs and abilities

   H. Spinal cord injuries

      1. If the spinal cord is injured the nerves cannot send messages between the brain and parts of the body, so partial or total paralysis may occur

      2. Most damage is permanent

      3. The higher up the spinal cord the injury happens the greater the paralysis (see Figure 31-8, p. 535)

      4. May cause paraplegia or quadriplegia

      5. Cervical traction is often necessary (see Figure 31-17 and Figure 31-18, p. 541)

      6. If recent spinal cord injury occurred, will require rehabilitation (see Chapter 32)

      7. Paralyzed clients usually need care (see Box 31-6, p. 535)

VI. MUSCULOSKELETAL DISORDERS

   A. Affect the ability to move about

   B. A result of injury and aging

   C. Arthritis means joint inflammation

      1. The most common joint disease

      2. People with severe arthritis may require arthoplasty (surgical replacement)

      3. Osteoarthritis (OA)

        a. Occurs with aging, joint injury, and obesity

        b. Affects weight-bearing joints such as hips, knees, spine

        c. Cartilage gradually breaks down

        d. Eventually bones may rub together

        e. Pain is often less severe in the morning and worsens during the day

        f. Pain occurs with weight bearing and joint movement

        g. Severe pain can interfere with rest and sleep

        h. Cold weather and dampness seem to increase symptoms

        i. Bony growths called Heberden's nodes are common in the fingers

        j. Osteoarthritis has no cure

        k. Treatment involves relieving pain and stiffness

          (1) Aspirin given for pain

          (2) Local heat or cold applications are used

          (3) Weight loss is stressed for obese persons

            (a) A low-fat, low-calorie diet is often ordered

        l. A cane or walker may be needed

        m. Measures to prevent falls are important

        n. Assistance with daily activities is given as needed

          (1) Elevated toilet seats are helpful

      3. Rheumatoid arthritis (RA)

        a. A chronic disease

        b. Usually affects people between the ages of 25 to 50 but can affect all ages from toddlers to older adults.

        c. See Focus on Children box, p. 536

        d. Occurs at any age; more common in women

        e. Connective tissue throughout the body is affected

          (1) Small joints in the fingers, hands, and feet are affected first

          (2) Also affects the heart, lungs, eyes, kidneys, and skin

        f. Severe inflammation causes very painful and swollen joints

        g. As the disease progresses, more joints become involved; changes in other organs eventually occur

        h. Pain and stiffness are usually worst in the morning and gradually decreases during the day.

i. Scar tissue in the joints will cause deformities (see Figure 31-10, p. 536)
j. Treatment goals are to maintain joint motion, control pain, and prevent deformities
 (1) Rest is balanced with exercise
 (2) If bedrest is needed, turning and repositioning are done every 2 hours (see Box 31-1, p. 524)
 (3) Good body alignment is essential
 (4) Adequate sleep is needed each night (8-10 hours)
 (5) Morning and afternoon rest periods are necessary
 (6) Range-of-motion (ROM) exercises are done
 (7) Walking aids may be needed; also splints
 (8) Safety measures to prevent falls are practiced
 (9) Drugs for pain are ordered
 (10) Local heat or cold applications may help
 (11) Joint replacement surgery may be necessary

D. Fibromyalgia
 1. Condition associated with aching, stiffness and fatigue in muscles, ligaments and tendons
 2. Can affect many areas from the neck to the feet
 3. Persistent fatigue makes even simple tasks difficult
 4. No cure, but heat, cold applications, massage, regular stretching, and ROM are helpful

E. Osteoporosis
 1. A bone disorder in which the bone becomes porous and brittle; bones break easily
  a. Spine, hips, and wrists are affected most often
 2. Common in older persons and in women after menopause
  a. Lack of estrogen results in bone changes
  b. Lack of dietary calcium is also a major cause
 3. Smoking, high alcohol intake, and lack of exercise are risk factors
 4. Bedrest and immobility are other causes
  a. If bones do not bear weight, calcium is not absorbed and bones become porous and brittle
 5. Signs and symptoms include:
  a. Low back pain
  b. Gradual loss of height
  c. Stooped posture
 6. Fractures are a major threat
  a. Turning in bed or getting up from a chair can cause a fracture
  b. Fractures are a great risk if the person falls or has an accident
 7. Prevention is important
  a. Calcium, estrogen replacement therapy, and exercise that involves weight bearing are the key
 8. Protect the person from falls; turn and reposition the person gently
 9. Some people wear a back brace, corset, or use walking aids

F. Fractures
 1. A fracture is a broken bone
  a. Tissues around the fracture are usually injured (muscles, blood vessels, nerves, and tendons)
 2. A closed fracture (simple fracture) means the bone is broken but the skin is intact (see Figure 31-11A, p. 537)
 3. An open fracture (compound fracture) means the broken bone has come through the skin (see Figure 31-11B, p. 537)
 4. Causes include falls, accidents, bone tumours, metastatic cancer, and osteoporosis
 5. Signs and symptoms are:
  a. Limb looks bent or out of position
  b. Pain
  c. Swelling
  d. Limited movement and loss of function
  e. Bruising and color changes in the skin
  f. Bleeding (external or internal)
 6. Healing
  a. The bone ends are brought into normal position (reduction)
  b. Closed reduction—moving the bone back into place; the skin is not opened
  c. Open reduction involves surgery; nails, rods, pins, screws, plates, or wires are used to keep the bone in place (see Figure 31-12, p. 537)
  d. After reduction, the bone is immobilized with a cast or traction
 7. Focus on children
  a. Falls and accidents are common

causes of fractures in children
  b. Fractures in infants may be a sign of child abuse
 8. Cast care
  a. Casts are made of plaster of paris, plastic, or fiberglass (see Figure 31-13, p. 538)
  b. Plastic and fiberglass casts dry quickly
  c. A plaster of paris cast needs 24 to 48 hours to dry
  d. Box 31-7, p. 539 in the textbook, lists guidelines for cast care
 9. Traction
  a. Used to reduce and immobilize fractures
  b. Also used for muscle spasms, to prevent or correct deformities, and for other musculoskeletal injuries
  c. Weights, ropes, and pulleys are used (see Figure 31-17, p. 541)
    (1) With skin traction, bandages and strips of material are applied to the skin
      (a) Weights are attached to the material or bandages
    (2) Skeletal traction is applied directly to the bone (see Figure 31-18, p. 541
  d. Box 31-8, p. 542 in textbook, lists guidelines for caring for a person in traction
 10. Hip fractures
  a. Common in older persons, especially older women
  b. Serious because healing is slower in older persons
  c. Postoperative complications include pneumonia, atelectasis, urinary tract infection, and thrombi in leg veins
  d. Persons are also at risk for pressure ulcers, constipation, and confusion
  e. Open reduction is usually required
    (1) The person needs preoperative and postoperative care (see Chapter 45)
  f. Box 31-9, p. 542 in the textbook, lists ghuidelines for care of persons with a hip fracture
  g. Focus on home care
    (1) The prosthesis can dislocate with adduction, internal rotation, and severe hip flexion
    (2) These movements are avoided for 6 to 8 weeks after surgery

    (3) An occupational therapist helps the person learn activities of daily living (ADL)
    (4) Assistive devices are used as needed (see Chapter 32)
    (5) Muscle strengthening exercises are also needed
      (a) A physical therapist helps the person
    (6) A walker is usually needed for ambulation
  h. Focus on long-term care
    (1) Older persons may require subacute care or long-term care after a hip fracture
 G. Amputation of a limb
  1. An amputation is the removal of all or part of an extremity
  2. A traumatic amputation occurs by accident
  3. A surgical amputation occurs when an extremity has been severely injured or to prevent the spread of disease
  4. Gangrene is a condition in which there is death of tissue
  a. Can result from infection, injuries, and circulatory disorders
  b. Tissue becomes black, cold, and shriveled and eventually falls off (see Figure 31-20, p. 543)
  c. If untreated, gangrene spreads through the body and causes death
  5. All or part of an extremity may be amputated
  a. The person may experience phantom pain (pain in a limb that has been amputated)
  b. A major psychological adjustment is necessary
  c. Appearance, ADL, moving about, and work are some areas affected
  d. Most persons are fitted with a prosthesis—an artificial replacement for a missing body part (see Figure 31-21, p. 544)
    (1) For arm and leg prostheses the stump needs to be conditioned so the prosthesis fits
    (2) An elastic bandage or stocking is used to shrink and shape (see Figure 31-22, p. 544)
    (3) Exercises will strengthen the other limb
  e. Prostheses and skin care

(1) Skin care is very important as skin is confined inside the prostheses and is not exposed to air

(2) If skin becomes moist and hot, infection or blisters can occur

(3) Follow the client's care plan for skin care and care of the prostheses

(4) Care may include daily washing (some need medicated soaps), and application of a skin lotion

(5) Notify your supervisor if the client complains of pain at the prostheses site or if you note any sign of redness, swelling, or drainage at the site

VII. THE ENDOCRINE SYSTEM
  A. Is made up of glands, secrete hormones
  B. Diabetes mellitus
    1. The most common endocrine disorder
    2. The body cannot use sugar properly
    3. The pancreas does not secrete enough insulin
    4. Sugar builds up in the blood; the cells do not have enough sugar for energy
    5. Without sugar cells cannot perform their functions and if diabetes is not treated can lead to long-term complications.
    6. Severe hyperglycemia can lead to life-threatening condition
    7. Occurs in children and adults
    8. Risk factors include obesity and a family history of diabetes
      a. The risk increases after age 40
    9. Three types:
      a. Type 1 diabetes (IDDM)
        (1) Occurs most often in children and young adults
        (2) Pancreas does not produce insulin
        (3) Leads to severe hyperglycemia
        (4) Will require daily insulin injections
      b. Type 2 diabetes (NIDDM)
        (1) Occurs in adults over age 40
        (2) The pancreas secretes insulin; the body cannot use it effectively
        (3) Or the body does not make enough insulin
        (4) Obesity is a risk factor.
        (5) Often diet, exercises, and oral medications will control the symptoms
      c. Gestational diabetes

(1) Develops during pregnancy
(2) Usually disappears after childbirth
  (a) The woman is at risk for type 2 diabetes
    10. Signs and symptoms:
      a. Increased urine production
      b. Increase thirst and hunger
      c. Weight loss
      d. Extreme tiredness
      e. Blurred vision
      f. Frequent infection and slow healing of sores
    11. Blood tests show increased sugar levels
    12. Complications occur if not controlled
      a. Blindness
      b. Renal failure
      c. Nerve damage
      d. Hypertension and circulatory disorders
        (1) Can lead to stroke, heart attack, and slow wound healing
      e. Foot and leg wounds
        (1) Infection and gangrene can occur
    13. Treatment for diabetes:
      a. Type 1 diabetes is treated with daily insulin therapy, diet, and exercise
      b. Type 2 diabetes is treated with diet and exercise; oral drugs may be needed
      c. Some persons need insulin
    14. Both types require glucose monitoring
    15. Good foot care is important
    16. Hypoglycemia occurs with too much insulin
    17. Hyperglycemia occurs if the person does not get enough insulin
    18. Both can lead to death if not corrected
    19. Table 31-1, p. 546 in the textbook, lists causes and signs and symptoms of hypoglycemia and hyperglycemia
VIII. DIGESTIVE DISORDERS
  A. Diverticular disease—many people have small pouches in their colons and do not have problems until they are older and have a low fiber diet
    1. When feces enter these pouches they can become inflamed and infected so the client will have abdominal pain, fever, vomiting, or other digestive problems
    2. A ruptured pouch is rare
    3. A pouch can cause a block in the intestine so that stool can not pass
    4. These conditions need surgery
  B. Vomiting

1. The act of expelling stomach contents through the mouth
2. A sign of illness or injury
3. Vomitus can be aspirated and obstruct the airway
4. Shock can occur if large amounts of blood are vomited
5. The following measures are practiced:
   a. Use Standard Precautions
   b. Turn the person's head well to one side
   c. Place a kidney basin under the person's chin
   d. Remove vomitus from the person's immediate environment
   e. Provide for oral hygiene
   f. Eliminate odors
   g. Change linens as necessary
   h. Observe vomitus for color, odor, and undigested food
   i. Measure or estimate the amount of vomitus (for example, cup full)
   j. Report immediately to your supervisor that the client has vomited

IX. DISORDERS OF THE URINARY SYSTEM
A. Urinary tract infections (UTIs)
   1. Can occur in the bladder or kidney
   2. The urinary system is normally sterile
   3. Microbes can enter the urinary system through the urethra
   4. Causes include:
      a. Catheterization
      b. Urological examinations
      c. Sexual intercourse
      d. Poor perineal hygiene
      e. Poor fluid intake
   5. Women are at greater risk than men
   6. Older men are at risk (an enlarged prostate increases the risk)
   7. Older persons are at risk due to incomplete bladder emptying, fecal incontinence, and poor nutrition
   8. Cystitis is inflammation of the bladder caused by bacteria
      a. Signs and symptoms include:
         (1) Urinary frequency and urgency
         (2) Oliguria
         (3) Dysuria
         (4) Pain or burning during urination
         (5) Foul-smelling urine
         (6) Hematuria and pyuria
         (7) Fever and chills
         (8) Lower back or abdomen pain
      b. Antibiotics are the treatment of choice

   (1) Fluids are encouraged (usually 2000 mL per day
B. Urinary diversion
   1. It is sometimes necessary to surgically remove the urinary bladder
      a. A new pathway is made for the urine to exit the body
         (1) The new pathway is called a urinary diversion
   2. Many types of urinary diversions
      a. Often an ostomy is involved
         (1) Ureterostomy—the surgical creation of an artificial opening between the ureter and the abdomen
   3. You may care for persons who have long-standing ureterostomies
      a. The person wears a pouch
      b. Urine drains into the pouch
      c. Good skin care is essential
      d. Standard Precautions and the Bloodborne Pathogen Standard are followed
C. Renal calculi
   1. Referred to as kidney stones
   2. Risk factors
      a. White men between ages 20 and 40 have high risk
      b. Bedrest and immobility are factors
   3. Stones vary in size
   4. Signs and symptoms include:
      a. Severe cramping, pain in the back and side (can also be in the abdomen, thigh, and urethra)
      b. Nausea and vomiting
      c. Fever and chills
      d. Dysuria
      e. Frequency and urgency
      f. Oliguria
      g. Hematuria
      h. Foul smelling urine
   5. Treatment involves:
      a. Pain relief and encouraging fluids (2000-3000 mL per day)
      b. All urine is strained (see Chapter 29)
      c. Surgical removal of the stone may be necessary
D. Renal failure
   1. The kidneys do not function or are severely impaired
   2. Waste products are not removed from the blood
   3. Fluids are retained
   4. Heart failure and hypertension can result
   5. Acute renal failure

a. Occurs suddenly; involves severe decreased blood flow to the kidneys
b. Causes include:
   (1) Postoperative bleeding
   (2) Bleeding from trauma
   (3) MI
   (4) Severe congestive heart failure
   (5) Burns
   (6) Severe allergic reaction
c. Every system is affected by build-up of waste products; death can occur
d. Occurs in phases—at first oliguria occurs (lasts a few days to 2 weeks) then diuresis occurs
e. Recovery period can take from one month to one year
f. Some do not recover and develop chronic renal failure
g. The physician orders drug therapy, restricted fluids, and diet therapy
h. The care plan is likely to include:
   (1) Measuring and recording urine output every hour
       (a) Output of less than 30 ml per 1 hour is reported to the nurse immediately
   (2) Measuring and recording I&O
   (3) Restricting fluids
   (4) Daily weight with the same scale
   (5) Turning and repositioning at least every 2 hours
   (6) Measures to prevent pressure ulcers
   (7) Frequent oral hygiene
   (8) Measures to prevent infection
6. Chronic renal failure
   a. The kidneys cannot meet the body's needs; nephrons are destroyed over the years
   b. Hypertension and diabetes are the most common causes
   c. Signs and symptoms appear when 80% to 90% of kidney function is lost (e.g., yellow skin, inflammation of mouth, bruises)
   d. Every system is affected by build-up of waste products in the blood
   f. Treatment includes fluid restriction, diet therapy, drugs, and dialysis (the process of removing waste products from the blood)
   g. Some persons have kidney transplants
   h. Box 31-10, p. 548 in the textbook, describes general care

X. COMMUNICABLE DISEASES
   A. Can be transmitted from one person to another
   B. Can be transmitted in the following ways (see Chapter 18):
      1. Direct—from the infected person
      2. Indirect—from dressings, linens, or surfaces
      3. Airborne—from persons through sneezing or coughing
      4. Vehicle—through ingestion of contaminated food, water, drugs, blood, or fluids
      5. Vector—from animals, fleas, and ticks
   C. Table 31-2, p. 549 in the textbook, outlines common childhood communicable diseases
   D. Standard Precautions are followed
   E. Hepatitis
      1. An inflammation of the liver caused by a virus
      2. When first occurs, called acute hepatitis and may or may not cause symptoms recognized by the infected person
      3. Lasts 1 to 2 months
      4. Symptoms can vary from nausea to pain in the abdomen and then after about 2 weeks dark urine and perhaps jaundice
      5. Some have light-coloured stools, muscle pain, irritability, diarrhea and general aching
      6. For mild cases no medication or treatment is available or necessary.
      7. If it lasts longer than 6 months called chronic hepatitis, which causes liver damage over a long period of time.
      8. Normal cells replaced with scar tissue (cirrhosis), can cause complete liver failure
      9. When liver fails person will only survive with a liver transplant
      10. Three major viruses cause hepatitis in Canada, and can be passed from one person to another:
         a. Hepatitis A virus is spread by the fecal-oral route
            (1) Transmitted when feces are ingested usually through food, water and drinking and eating vessels.
            (2) Risk factors include crowded living conditions, poor sanitation and hygiene
            (3) Always wear gloves when assisting with perineal care, cleaning incontinent clients and

handling bedpans

    (4) Confused clients can cause contamination so carefully look for contaminated items and areas

    (5) Good hand washing is essential for everyone so assist the client if necessary

    (6) Hepatitis A does not cause chronic hepatitis

    (7) See Focus on Children

b. Hepatitis B and C viruses—are in an infected person's blood and certain body fluids (semen and vaginal secretions)

    (1) Spread through intercourse or sharing needles, blood transfusions, and childbirth

    (2) Can be spread by needlestick injuries and by direct contact between open skin and infected blood or body fluids (see Chapter 18)

    (3) Follow Standard Precautions

    (4) Transmission-Based Precautions are ordered as necessary

    (5) Both hepatisis B and C can cause chronic hepatitis

F. Acquired Immunodeficiency Syndrome (AIDS)

1. Affects the person's ability to fight infection such as pneumonia and TB

2. They are also at risk for cancers and central nervous system damage, which can among other symptoms cause dementia

3. May be infected with HIV (human immunodeficiency virus) but do not have symptoms of AIDS, and as carriers they can infect others

4. No cure, but medications are available to slow the progress

5. Spread through exchange of bodily fluids during intercourse, needle-sharing, or from HIV mothers at birth or through breast-feeding

6. Also spread when infected body fluids come in contact with broken skin

7. AIDS is the last stage of HIV infection and usually develops 10 years after initial infection

8. Possible warning signs of HIV infection include:

  a. Rapid weight loss

  b. Dry cough

  c. Fever or night sweats

  d. Fatigue

  e. Swollen glands in the armpits, groin or neck

  f. Diarrhea that lasts for more than a week

  g. White spots or unusual blemishes on the tongue, in the mouth or in the throat

  h. Pneumonia

  i. Red, brown, pink or purplish blotches on the skin or inside the mouth, nose or eyelids

  j. Memory loss, confusion or dementia

  k. You may care for a client with AIDS or is an HIV carrier.

  l. Use Standard Precautions as you would with any client.

  m. HIV is not spread by saliva, tears, urine, seat, sneezing, coughing, insects, or casual contact such as hugging, touching, or shaking hands

  n. See Focus on Older Adults box, p. 551

G. Sexually transmitted diseases (STDs)

1. Spread by sexual contact (see Table 31-3, p. 551)

2. Some people are not aware of being infected

  a. Others know, but do not seek treatment

3. May involve the genital areas, rectum, ears, mouth, nipples, throat, tongue, eyes, and nose (see Figure 31-24, p. 552)

4. Most are spread by sexual contact

5. The use of condoms helps prevent the spread of STDs

6. STDs also spread through breaks in the skin, contact with infected body fluids, or by contaminated blood or needles

7. Standard Precautions are followed

Classroom Activities

1. Ask students to use chapter 13 as a resource when they study this chapter.

2. Write the following topics on a flip chart in outline form using a variety of colored markers. Use the flip chart to present information and ask for input from students. Leave space after each item to add information.

  a. Cancer

    (1) Definition

(2) Contributing factors

(3) Seven warning signs

(4) Warning signs in children

(5) Treatment

(6) Special needs of persons with cancer

Call on students to provide information about each topic. Write in the correct answers. Clarify any wrong answers. Allow time for discussion.

3. Write the following terms on the chalkboard:
   a. Malignant tumour
   b. Benign tumour
   c. Metastasis
   d. Chemotherapy
   e. Stomatitis
   f. Alopecia
   Call on students to define each term. Write the correct answers on the chalkboard after the appropriate term.

4. Arrange for a representative from the Canadian Cancer Society to visit the class. Ask the person to bring educational materials and handouts describing their role and the services they provide.
   a. Allow time for questions and discussion.

5. Write each of the following musculoskeletal disorders on a separate index card: Osteoarthritis, Rheumatoid arthritis, Osteoporosis, Fractures, and Loss of a limb.
   a. Divide students into five groups. Distribute one index card to each group. Provide each group with several sheets of notebook paper.
   b. Ask each group to provide the following information about the musculoskeletal disorder on their index card:
      (1) Definition
      (2) Signs and symptoms
      (3) Complications
      (4) Treatment and treatment goals
      (5) Special needs of children and/or older persons
   c. Allow 20 minutes for this exercise. Then call on one student from each group to report to the class.
      (1) Allow time after each presentation for questions and discussion

6. Write the following terms on the chalkboard:
   a. Arthritis
   b. Arthroplasty
   c. Closed fracture
   d. Open fracture

e. Amputation

f. Gangrene

Call on students to define each term. Write the correct answer on the chalkboard after the appropriate term.

7. Display the rules for cast care (see Box 31-7, p. 539) on an overhead transparency.
   a. Carefully review each rule with students. Allow time for questions.

8. Display the rules for care of a person in traction (see Box 31-8, p. 542) on an overhead transparency.
   a. Carefully review each rule with students. Allow time for questions.

9. Display the rules for care of a person with a hip fracture (see Box 31-9, p. 542) on an overhead transparency.
   a. Carefully review each rule with students. Allow time for questions.

10. Arrange for a representative from the Arthritis Foundation to visit the class. Ask the person to bring educational materials and handouts describing their role and the services they provide.
    a. Allow time for questions and discussion.

11. Write each of the following nervous system disorders on a separate index card: Stroke, Parkinson's disease, Multiple sclerosis, Head injuries, and Spinal cord injuries.
    a. Divide students into five groups. Distribute one index card to each group. Provide each group with several sheets of notebook paper.
    b. Ask each group to provide the following information about the nervous system disorder on their index card:
       (1) Definition
       (2) Risk factors
       (3) Signs and symptoms
       (4) Complications
       (5) Treatment and treatment goals
    c. Allow 20 minutes for this exercise. Then call on one student from each group to report to the class.
       (1) Allow time after each presentation for questions and discussion

12. Write the following terms on the chalkboard:
    a. Expressive aphasia
    b. Receptive aphasia

c. Expressive-receptive aphasia
d. Paraplegia
e. Quadriplegia
f. Hemiplegia
Call on students to define each term. Write the correct answer on the chalkboard after the appropriate term.

13. Arrange for a representative from the Multiple Sclerosis Society to visit the class. Ask the person to bring educational materials and handouts describing their role and the services they provide.
   a. Allow time for questions and discussion.

14. Arrange for a representative from a head injury/spinal cord injury rehabilitation facility to visit the class. Ask the person to bring educational materials and handouts describing their role and the services they provide.
   a. Allow time for questions and discussion.

15. Display the overhead transparency showing the respiratory system. Use this as a basis to discuss chronic obstructive pulmonary disease.
   a. Ask students to identify the structures of the respiratory system affected by:
      (1) Chronic bronchitis
      (2) Emphysema
      (3) Asthma
   b. Call on students to define the terms listed above. Write the correct answers on the chalkboard.

16. Stress the importance of smoking as a risk factor for chronic bronchitis and emphysema.
   a. Obtain and show slides of healthy lungs, the lungs of a person who has smoked for 20 years, the lungs of a person with chronic bronchitis, and the lungs of a person with emphysema.

17. Divide students into two groups. Provide each group with a flip chart and colored markers.
   a. Ask one group to provide the following information about pneumonia:
      (1) Definition
      (2) Causes
      (3) Signs and symptoms
      (4) Special precautions taken when providing care
      (5) Treatment
      (6) Persons at risk
   b. Ask one group to provide the following information about tuberculosis:
      (1) Definition
      (2) Causes
      (3) Signs and symptoms
      (4) Special precautions taken when providing care
      (5) Treatment
      (6) Persons at risk
   c. Allow 20 minutes for this exercise. Then call on one student from each group to report to the class.
      (1) Allow time after each presentation for questions and discussion.

18. Write the word "Hypertension" on the chalkboard. Call on students to define hypertension. Write the correct answer on the chalkboard.

19. Write the following topics on a flip chart in outline form using a variety of colored markers. Use the flip chart to present information and ask for input from students. Leave space after each item to add information.
   a. Coronary artery disease
      (1) Definition
      (2) Common causes
      (3) Risk factors
      (4) Complications
      (5) Treatment
Call on students to provide information about each topic. Write in the correct answers on the flip chart. Clarify any wrong answers. Allow time for discussion.

20. Divide students into two groups. Provide each group with a flip chart and colored markers.
   a. Ask one group to provide the following information about angina pectoris:
      (1) Definition
      (2) Causes
      (3) Signs and symptoms
      (4) Treatment
      (5) Persons at risk
   b. Ask one group to provide the following information about myocardial infarction:
      (1) Definition
      (2) Causes
      (3) Signs and symptoms
      (4) Treatment
      (5) Persons at risk
   c. Allow 20 minutes for this exercise. Then call on one student from each group to report to the class.
      (1) Allow time after each presentation for ques-

tions and discussion.

21. Call on students to define heart failure. List its causes and treatments on the chalkboard.

22. Arrange for a representative from the Canadian Heart Association to visit the class. Ask the person to bring educational materials and handouts describing their role and the services they provide.
    a. Allow time for questions and discussion.

23. Write on the chalkboard: "Causes of urinary tract infections include:" Call on students to list the causes. Write the correct answers on the chalkboard.

24. Write the following terms on the chalkboard:
    a. Cystitis
    b. Pyelonephritis
    c. Urinary diversion
    d. Renal calculi
    e. Renal failure
    Call on students to define each term. Write the correct answers on the chalkboard after the appropriate term.

25. Write the following topics on a flip chart in outline form using a variety of colored markers. Use the flip chart to present information and ask for input from students. Leave space after each item to add information.
    a. Diabetes mellitus
       (1) Definition
       (2) Risk factors
       (3) Types
       (4) Signs and symptoms
       (5) Complications
       (6) Treatment
    Call on students to provide information about each topic. Write in the correct answers on the flip chart. Clarify any wrong answers. Allow time for discussion.

26. Display the signs and symptoms of hypoglycemia and hyperglycemia (see Table 31-1, p. 546) on an overhead transparency. Use this as a basis for discussion. Stress the importance of knowing these signs and symptoms when caring for persons with diabetes mellitus.

27. Call on students to define vomiting and to discuss complications on vomiting.

28. Call on students to identify the measures practiced when caring for the person who is vomiting. Write the correct answers on the chalkboard.

29. Write on the flip chart: Communicable diseases can be transmitted in the following ways:
    a. _____
    b. _____
    c. _____
    d. _____
    e. _____
    Call on students to come forward and write in the answers.

30. Arrange for a representative from your local health unit to speak to the class. He or she should cover the following topics: Hepatitis, AIDS, and sexually transmitted diseases.
    a. Mode of transmission and special precautions for each disease should be covered.
    b. Brochures and handouts about each disease can help reinforce the information presented.
    c. Ask students to write key points in a notebook for future reference.
    d. Allow time for questions and discussion.

31. Arrange for a representative from an AIDS support group to visit the class. Ask the person to bring educational materials and handouts describing their role and the services they provide.
    a. Allow time for questions and discussion.

Homework Assignments

Ask students to answer the questions at the end of Chapter 31 in the textbook. Tell students the date and time that this assignment must be completed and turned in.

If the accompanying workbook is being used, assign the Chapter 31 workbook exercises. Tell students the date and time that this assignment must be completed and turned in.

Common Diseases and Conditions

Fill in the Blanks

Write your answers in the spaces provided.

1. List nine factors that contribute to the development of cancer.

    a. _____

    b. _____

    c. _____

    d. _____

    e. _____

    f. _____

    g. _____

    h. _____

    i. _____

2. This type of arthritis occurs with aging. Joint injury and obesity are other causes.

    _____

3. List the causes of osteoporosis.

    a. _____

    b. _____

    c. _____

    d. _____

    e. _____

    f. _____

4. Why is traction used?

    a. _____

    b. _____

    c. _____

    d. _____

5. The common causes of spinal cord injuries include:

    a. _____

    b. _____

    c. _____

    d. _____

    e. _____

6. List the three disorders grouped under chronic obstructive pulmonary disease (COPD).

    a. _____

    b. _____

    c. _____

7. List the five warning signs of stroke.

    a. _____

    b. _____

    c. _____

    d. _____

    e. _____

Common Diseases and Conditions

8. List the risk factors for coronary artery disease (CAD).

   a. _____

   b. _____

   c. _____

   d. _____

   e. _____

   f. _____

   g. _____

   h. _____

   i. _____

9. Heart failure or congestive heart failure occurs when _____.

10. AIDS is transmitted mainly by:

    a. _____

    b. _____

    c. _____

    d. _____

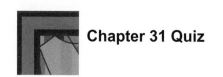

Chapter 31 Quiz

Name _____

Date _____

Common Diseases and Conditions

True or False	Multiple Choice

Mark **T** *for true or* **F** *for false.*

Circle the BEST answer.

1. _____ A malignant tumour grows slowly and does not invade healthy tissue.

2. _____ Radiation destroys cancer cells and normal cells.

3. _____ Chemotherapy affects only cancer cells.

4. _____ Osteoporosis is common in young men.

5. _____ A closed fracture means the bone is broken but the skin is intact.

6. _____ Elevating an arm or a leg in a cast on a pillow reduces swelling.

7. _____ Traction is removed to make the person's bed.

8. _____ Stroke is the leading cause of disability in adults.

9. _____ A common cause of stroke is hypertension.

10. _____ Multiple sclerosis is cured with medications and diet.

11. _____ Quadriplegia is paralysis of the arms, legs, and trunk.

12. _____ Cigarette smoking is the most common cause of emphysema.

13. _____ Angina pectoris means chest pain.

14. _____ Men are at greater risk for urinary tract infection than are women.

15. _____ The use of condoms helps prevent the spread of STDs.

16. The surgical replacement of a joint is called:
   a. Metastasis.
   b. Arthroplasty.
   c. Osteoporosis.
   d. Open reduction.

17. A plaster cast is applied to Mr. Adams' leg. Which is incorrect?
   a. Cover the cast with a blanket.
   b. Use pillows to support the entire length of the cast.
   c. Keep the cast dry.
   d. Turn him as directed by the nurse.

18. Which is incorrect when caring for a person with a hip fracture.
   a. Give good skin care.
   b. Prevent external rotation of the hip.
   c. Perform range-of-motion exercises as directed.
   d. Keep the operated leg adducted at all times.

19. Mrs. Linn has had a stroke. Which is incorrect?
   a. Rehabilitation starts about 1 week after the stroke.
   b. Give emotional support and encouragement.
   c. Give good skin care.
   d. Encourage coughing and deep breathing.

20. Which statement about multiple sclerosis is correct?
   a. The onset is sudden.
   b. Symptoms usually start after age 60.
   c. Men are affected more than women.
   d. Blurred vision and double vision occur first.

21. You are caring for a person with congestive heart failure. Which is not likely to be part of the person's care?
   a. Measuring intake and output
   b. Measuring daily weight
   c. Encouraging fluids to 2000 ml per day
   d. Applying elastic stockings

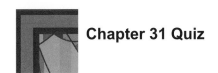

Name _____

Date _____

Common Diseases and Conditions

22. Inflammation of the bladder caused by bacteria is:
    a. Cystitis.
    b. Pyelonephritis.
    c. Renal calculi.
    d. Dialysis.

23. Dialysis is:
    a. Abnormal breathing patterns.
    b. The process of removing waste products from the blood.
    c. Inflammation of the mouth.
    d. A glucose monitoring system.

24. Which statement about type 1 diabetes is incorrect?
    a. The amount of sugar in the diet is limited.
    b. It is treated with diet and exercise only.
    c. The person needs to eat at regular times.
    d. If it is not controlled, complications occur.

25. Mr. Lee has type 1 diabetes. Which is not a cause of hypoglycemia?
    a. Eating too much food
    b. Increased exercise
    c. Too much insulin
    d. Vomiting

26. This type of Hepatitis is spread by the fecal-oral route:
    a. Hepatitis B
    b. Hepatitis D
    c. Hepatitis C
    d. Hepatitis A

27. The HIV virus is spread by:
    a. Sneezing.
    b. Insects.
    c. Unprotected oral sex.
    d. Holding hands.

32

Rehabilitation and Restorative Care

Instructor's Preparation

I. Read Chapter 32 in the textbook. Carefully review chapter objectives, key terms, and review questions.

II. Read the outline in Chapter 32 of the instructor's guide. Carefully review the classroom activities, the student assignment, and the quiz.

III. If you are using the accompanying student workbook, review the activities for Chapter 32.

IV. Gather all necessary supplies and equipment for classroom activities and student assignments.
  A. Prepare the correct number of handouts.
  B. Prepare appropriate flip charts.
  C. Prepare overhead transparencies.
  D. Gather coloured markers.
  E. Gather any other items that will be needed for classroom activities.
  F. Assemble items in the order they will be used.

V. Make sure that the necessary equipment is available and in good working order.

VI. Confirm all plans for the field trip.
  A. Contact the facility to confirm day, date, time, and location.
  B. Prepare an index card for each student with the location, day, date, and time of the field trip; include any special instructions (i.e., Dress code).

Objectives

- Define the key terms listed in this chapter
- Describe the goals of rehabilitation
- Explain how rehabilitation involves the whole person
- Explain the family's role in the rehabilitation process
- Explain the role of therapy and training in rehabilitation
- Describe four rehabilitation settings
- Explain the role of the rehabilitation team in the rehabilitation process

Key Terms

orthosis
prosthesis
rehabilitation
restorative care

Outline

Rehabilitation and Restorative Care

I. INTRODUCTION
  A. Rehabilitation is the process of restoring the person to the highest possible level of physical, psychological, social, and economic functioning
    1. The focus is on improving the persons's abilities
    2. If improvement is not possible, the focus is on maintaining the highest level of function possible and preventing further disability
  B. Restorative care helps a person regain health, strength, and independence
  C. Often begins during rehabilitation

D. Involves measures that promote:
1. Self-care
2. Elimination
3. Positioning
4. Mobility
5. Communication
6. Cognitive function

II. GOALS OF REHABILITATION
   A. Goals depend on the client's condition and circumstances
   B. The following goals are common:
      1. Restore function to former levels
      2. Improve functional abilities
      3. Learn new skills
      4. Prevent further disability and illness

III. THE REHABILITATION PROCESS
   A. May be a short process (e.g., person with a shoulder injury may only need exercises), or it may be a long process
   B. Box 32-1, p. 557 in the textbook, shows the process for a client with a serious brain injury
   C. The rehabilitation team
      1. Members of the team may vary depending of client's needs
      2. Usually involve the client, family, physicians, nurses, occupational and/or physiotherapists, support workers, and others
      3. Meet often to discuss progress and make changes in the plan
      4. Restorative care usually involves the client and family, nurses and support workers; others are consulted as needed
   D. Emphasis on the whole person
      1. Rehabilitation treats all dimensions of health
         a. Physical health
            (1) Physical condition and ability to perform ADLs are assessed
            (2) Complications prevented
            (3) ROM exercises are done
            (4) The client learns or relearns self-care and mobility skills
         b. Emotional and social health are assessed
            (1) Work skills are also assessed
            (2) Family counseling and assistance reentering the community and workplace are provided as needed
         c. Intellectual health
            (1) Thinking, speech, memory, and organization are assessed
            (2) Measures to improve cognitive functioning are planned

d. Spiritual health
   (1) Counselling from spiritual advisers is provided as needed
e. All aspects are connected
   (1) The rehabilitation team encourages the client to control as many aspects of care as possible
   (2) Being a key member gives the client some control

E. The role of the family
   1. Families learn about the condition and how to care for their loved one
   2. May involve helping the person learn new skills, or the family learning new skills (e.g., how to communicate with someone who cannot speak or how to dress someone with a disability)
   3. Counselling is provided, if necessary, to cope with changes

F. Therapy and training
   1. Professionals, or the rehabilitation team, choose the therapy and training needed to meet goals
   2. The client is taught how to improve or perform skills
   3. The client practices alone or with caregiver or family
   4. You may help clients practice (see Chapter 12)
   5. May involve learning how to use self-help devices
   6. Equipment is ordered to meet their needs
      a. Prostheses—artificial replacements for missing body parts
         (1) Goal is to imitate the missing body part in function and/or appearance
         (2) Most are powered by the person's muscles in the stump or by other nearby muscles
         (3) Physiotherapist works with the client to strengthen muscles
         (4) You may work with client to assist or with skin care or with wearing (see Chapter 31)
      b. Orthoses—apparatus worn to support, align, prevent, or correct problems with the musculoskeletal system (e.g., splints, braces, foot supports)
         (1) You might help client putting them on or practicing using the orthosis (see Chapter 22)
      c. Eating and drinking devices—include glass holders, plate guards, etc. (see

Chapter 22)

d. Self-care devices—include electronic toothbrushes, long-handled brushes (Figure 32-1, p. 558)

(1) Also devices to help with dressing (Figure 32-2, p. 559)

e. Devices to aid mobility—include crutches, canes, walkers, and braces

(1) Some need wheelchairs and learn how to transfer to and from the wheelchair (Figure 32-3, p. 560)

f. Other equipment—some clients need feeding tubes (see Chapter 26) or mechanical ventilation (see Chapter 43)

(1) Some are weaned from the ventilator while others adapt to life-long ventilation

IV. REHABILITATION SETTINGS

A. Many common health problems require rehabilitation (see Box 32-2, p. 561)

B. Services can be found in:

1. Hospitals—most have rehabilitation units for inpatients and outpatients

a. Some focus on brain injury and tumours, spinal cord injury and stroke, and cardiac and respiratory rehabilitation

2. Specialized facilities—some facilities focus on specific problems such as mental illness and substance abuse/addiction

3. Long-term care facilities—most provide services similar to hospitals

4. Community care—home care services (see Focus on Home Care box, p. 561) and adult day programs are examples

V. ASSISTING WITH REHABILITATION AND RESTORATIVE CARE

A. You will be working with many clients undergoing some form of rehabilitation or restorative care

1. Some are facing overwhelming changes

2. Can be slow and frustrating before progress is noted

3. You must be patient, supportive, and empathic (see Providing Compassionate Care box, p. 561)

Classroom Activities

1. Write the word "Rehabilitation" on the chalkboard. Call on students to define rehabilitation. Write the correct answer on the chalkboard.

a. Discuss the importance and the focus of rehabilitation.

2. Divide students into two groups. Provide each group with a flip chart and colored markers.

a. Ask one group to identify and list the physical aspects of rehabilitation. They should include any special needs of children and older persons.

b. Ask one group to identify and list the psychological and social aspects of rehabilitation. They should include any special needs of children and older persons.

Allow 15 minutes for this exercise. Then call on one student from each group to report to the class. Allow time for questions and discussion after each presentation.

3. Discuss the importance of the rehabilitation process.

a. Call on students to identify and discuss the role of each member of the rehabilitation team.

b. Call on students to identify and discuss the roles of various health care agencies involved in the rehabilitation process.

(1) Distribute brochures from agencies in your community that provide rehabilitation services. Allow 5 minutes for students to review the brochures. Then call on students to discuss:

(a) What services are provided.

(b) Where the facility is located.

(c) What population is served.

4. Arrange for students to tour a rehabilitation department in a hospital or subacute care center.

a. Ask the physical therapist, occupational therapist, and speech/language pathologist to explain his or her role in rehabilitation. Also, ask them to explain the equipment they use.

b. What is the role of assistive personnel?

Allow time after the tour for discussion and questions.

5. Provide students with a variety of prostheses and self-help devices used in the rehabilitation process. Ask them to handle and manipulate these items. Discuss how each item is used.

Homework Assignments

Ask students to answer the questions at the end of Chapter 32 in the textbook. Tell students the date and time that this assignment must be completed and turned in.

If the accompanying workbook is being used, assign the Chapter 32 workbook exercises. Tell students the date and time that this assignment must be completed and turned in.

Chapter 32 Student Assignment   Name _____

Date _____

Rehabilitation and Restorative Care

Fill in the blanks in the spaces provided.

1. Rehabilitation begins when _____.

2. During rehabilitation, the person must focus on _____.

3. Rehabilitation is the process of restoring the person to the highest possible level of

    _____, _____,

    _____, and _____ functioning.

4. Who are the members of the rehabilitation team?

    a. _____

    b. _____

    c. _____

    d. _____

    e. _____

5. List six agencies that provide rehabilitation services.

    a. _____

    b. _____

    c. _____

    d. _____

    e. _____

    f. _____

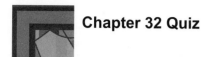

Chapter 32 Quiz

Name _____

Date _____

Rehabilitation and Restorative Care

True or False

*Mark **T** for true or **F** for false.*

1. _____ Rehabilitation focuses on the person's disabilities.

2. _____ Self-care is a major goal of rehabilitation.

3. _____ Rehabilitation often takes longer in older persons than in other age groups.

4. _____ Persons with both legs amputated cannot learn self-care.

5. _____ A disability often affects self-esteem and relationships.

Multiple Choice

Circle the BEST answer.

6. Rehabilitation begins when:
   a. The person leaves the hospital.
   b. The person enters a subacute rehabilitation program.
   c. The person seeks health care.
   d. The person goes home with home health care

7. Rehabilitation focuses on:
   a. The physical aspects of care.
   b. The psychological aspects of care.
   c. Goals set by the physical therapist.
   d. The whole person.

8. You prevent pressure ulcers by:
   a. Providing good skin care.
   b. Turning and repositioning the person as directed.
   c. Performing range-of-motion exercises as directed.
   d. All of the above.

9. Mr. Juarez does not feel that he is making progress. He is angry. You should:
   a. Tell him that being angry will only make things worse.
   b. Try to understand his feelings. Offer support.
   c. Offer sympathy.
   d. Call his doctor.

10. You promote the person's quality of life by:
    a. Providing privacy when the person is practicing new skills.
    b. Making choices for the person.
    c. Discussing the person's program with co-workers in the hallway.
    d. Doing as much for the person as possible.

11. You are caring for Mr. Clark. You are feeling frustrated by his slow progress. You should:
    a. Tell him that you are frustrated.
    b. Be firm. Tell him that he must work harder.
    c. Discuss your feelings with the nurse.
    d. Ask a co-worker to care for Mr. Clark.

258

Mental Health Disorders

Instructor's Preparation

I. Read Chapter 33 in the textbook. Carefully review chapter objectives, key terms, and review questions.

II. Read the outline in Chapter 33 of the instructor's guide. Carefully review the classroom activities, the student assignment, and the quiz.

III. If you are using the accompanying student workbook, review the activities for Chapter 33.

IV. Gather all necessary supplies and equipment for classroom activities and student assignments.
   A. Prepare overhead transparencies
   B. Prepare situation/index cards
   C. Gather any other items that will be needed for classroom activities
   D. Assemble items in the order they will be used

V. Make sure that the necessary equipment is available and in good working order.

VI. Contact guest speakers to confirm the day, date, time, and location that they are expected.
   A. Ask the speakers if they require any special equipment or supplies.

Objectives

- Define the key terms listed in this chapter
- Describe the effects of mental health disorders on everyday life
- List factors that may contribute to mental health disorders
- Describe the major mental health disorders
- Describe the stigma experienced by people with mental health disorders
- Describe the effect of mental health disorders on families
- Explain how to support clients with mental health disorders
- List the warning signals for suicide intent

Key Terms

affective disorders
anxiety disorders
bipolar disorder
clinical depression
delusions
eating disorders
emotional illness
hallucination
major depression
mental disorder
mental health
mental health disorder
mental illness

paranoia
personality disorder
psychosis
psychiatric disorder
psychotherapy
schizophrenia
stigma

Outline

Mental Health Disorders

I. INTRODUCTION
  A. Mental health disorders affect the person physically, psychologically, socially, and spiritually
  B. Sometimes mental and physical health problems are not related, but sometimes mental health problems can cause physical problems, and physical problems can cause mental health problems
II. MENTAL HEALTH AND MENTAL ILLNESS
  A. Mental health is a state of mind in which a person copes with and adjusts to the stresses of everyday living in socially acceptable ways
    1. They express and control their emotions appropriately
    2. Everyone feels anxiety, sadness, grief, and loneliness at times
  B. Mental illness is a disturbance in a person's ability to cope with or adjust to stress
    1. Thinking, mood, or behaviours are affected
    2. Mental illness is also known as mental disorder, mental health disorder, emotional illness, and psychiatric disorders
    3. People with this illness usually feel high levels of distress and fear and often have trouble coping with everyday life
    4. Mental illness and its symptoms range from mild to severe
      a. The Canadian Mental Health Association (CMHA) estimates that one in five Canadian adults will experience a mental health disorder at some time during their lives
  C. Causes of mental health disorders
    1. Biological factors—chemical imbalances in the body
      a. Some disorders run in families
    2. Childhood experience—childhood trauma or conflict, particularly when repressed can cause mental health disorders

  a. Repression means to keep unpleasant or painful thoughts form the conscious mind
    3. Social and cultural factors—poverty, discrimination, social isolation
    4. Stressful live events—family situations, workplace pressures, change (see Chapter 8), loss of loved ones
    5. Poor physical health or disability—seriously ill, injured, or disabled people are at risk of some mental health disorders
  D. Treating mental health disorders
    1. Until the 1960s many patients lived in psychiatric facilities
    2. Today some live in facilities or group homes, but most are living in the community; some are homeless
    3. Treatment is usually a team approach, which may include a family physician, nurse, social worker, support worker, and one or more specialists:
      a. psychiatrist—physician who specialized and can prescribe medication
      b. psychologist and psychotherapist—health care professional educated to treat mental health disorders but cannot prescribe medication
    4. Psychotherapy—the patient explores his or her thoughts, feelings, and behaviors with a mental health specialist
      a. Various forms include:
        (1) Psychoanalysis—explores unconscious conflicts and underlying reasons behind the problems
        (2) Behaviour therapy—attempts to change behaviour
        (3) Group therapy—group discusses problems under guidance of a specialist
        (4) Family therapy—family meets regularly with a specialist to discuss problems
    5. Occupational therapists can help a person learn or relearn skills
    6. Social workers may help a client resolve employment problems
    7. Medication can help in many disorders
    8. Care planning process used to address needs of clients
III. COMMON MENTAL HEALTH DISORDERS
  A. Anxiety disorders
    1. Anxiety is a vague, uneasy feeling in re-

sponse to stress
  a. People with anxiety disorders have excess fears and worries that affect normal functioning
2. Panic disorder
  a. Panic is the highest level of anxiety
    (1) An intense and sudden feeling of fear, anxiety, terror, or dread
    (2) Occurs suddenly with no obvious reason
    (3) The person cannot function
    (4) May experience rapid heart rate, SOB, chest pain
    (5) Panic attacks last a few minutes or for hours
3. Phobic disorder
  a. Phobia means fear, panic, or dread
  b. A phobic disorder involves an intense fear of an object or situation
  c. Common phobias—agoraphobia and claustrophobia
4. Obsessive-compulsive disorder
  a. Obsession—a persistent thought or idea
  b. Compulsion—the uncontrolled performance of an act
  c. The person knows the act is wrong, but has much anxiety if it is not done
    (1) Eating disorders, handwashing, violent acts
B. Affective disorders
  1. Involve feelings, emotions, and moods
    a. Major depression involves intense and prolonged feelings of sadness, hopelessness, and worthlessness
    b. Has physical and emotional effects
    c. Sleep, eating, work, study, and other activities are affected
    d. May think about or attempt suicide
    e. May occur just once as a result of a stressful event or for some people it occurs throughout life
    f. Occurs at any age, common among older adults (see Focus on Older Adults, p. 567)
    g. Learn the signs and symptoms (see Box 33-1, p. 567)
  2. Bipolar disorder (formerly called manic-depressive illness)
    a. The person has extreme mood swings
      (1) Depression is at one extreme; mania (elation) at the other extreme

  b. The person may:
    (1) Be more depressed than manic
    (2) Be more manic than depressed
    (3) Alternate between depression and mania
  c. When depressed, the person is very sad, self-esteem is low; may be suicidal
  d. In the manic phase, the person is excited, has much energy, is very busy, and cannot sleep
    (1) Delusions of grandeur are common
3. Major depression
  a. Involves intense and prolonged feelings of sadness, hopelessness, and worthlessness
  b. Has physical and emotional effects
  c. Sleep, eating, work, study and other activities are affected
  d. May think about or attempt suicide
  e. May occur just once as a result of a stressful event or for some people it occurs throughout life
  f. Occurs at any age; common among older adults (see Focus on Older Adults box, p. 567)
  g. Learn the signs and symptoms (Box 33-1, p. 567)
C. Schizophrenia
  1. A mental health disorder in which thinking and behaviour are disturbed
    a. Affects a person's ability to function in all aspects of life including work, school, social life, family relationships, and self-care
    b. The term means "split mind" which refers to the person's feelings of being "split off" from reality
  2. The following terms will help you understand schizophrenia
    a. Psychosis—a mental disorder in which perception of reality is impaired
    b. Delusion—false beliefs
      (1) Delusions of grandeur—an exaggerated belief about one's own importance, wealth, power, or talents
      (2) Delusion of persecution—the false belief that one is being mistreated, abused, or harassed
    c. Hallucination—seeing, hearing, or feeling something that is not real

d. Paranoia—a disorder of the mind
   (1) The person has false beliefs and is suspicious about a person or situation
3. Without treatment a person with schizophrenia has a severe mental impairment
   a. Has problems relating to others
   b. Responses are inappropriate
   c. May ramble or repeat what others say and their speech may be hard to understand
   d. Some people have one severe psychotic episode which others suffer throughout life but have periods of remission
   e. In cases of severe schizophrenia people may withdraw from others and the world
D. Personality disorders
   1. Group of disorders involving rigid and socially unacceptable behaviours
   2. Have problems relating to others; may be demanding, hostile, and manipulative
   3. Personality disorders include:
      a. Abusive personality—the person copes with anxiety by abusing others
      b. Paranoid personality—the person is very suspicious and distrusts others
      c. Antisocial personality—the person has poor judgement, lacks responsibility, and is hostile
         (1) Has no loyalty to any person or group
         (2) Morals and ethics are lacking
         (3) The person has no guilt and does not learn from past experience or punishment
         (4) Is often in trouble with the law
E. Eating disorders
   1. Involve disturbances in eating behaviors
   2. Anorexia nervosa
      a. Occurs when a person has an abnormal fear of weight gain and obesity
      b. The person refuses to eat or eats only small amounts
      c. Most common in adolescent girls—intense exercise and vomiting are common
      d. Sleep problems, depression, and amenorrhea occur
      e. Some abuse laxatives, enemas, and diuretics
      f. Depression and suicidal thoughts

occur
   g. The person can be emaciated
3. Bulimia
   a. The person craves food
   b. Constant eating or binge eating can occur
   c. After eating, the person induces vomiting
   d. Some persons fast or take diuretics, laxatives, enemas
   e. Intense exercise is sometimes used
F. Substance-related disorders
   1. The deliberate misuse of medications, illegal drugs, alcohol, or other substances.
      a. Often develop relationship and work problems
      b. Abused substances affect the central nervous system
      c. Some have calming or depressing effects while other have a stimulating effect; all affect thinking and the mind
      d. May cause the person to be happy, self-confident, relaxed, aggressive, or to have hallucinations
      e. May have substance dependence disorder, which means they show evidence of tolerance and withdrawal
      f. Withdrawal symptoms can be mild to severe
      g. Common causes of death are overdoses, suicide, and diseases from contaminated needles
      h. Treatment depends on substance; most involve psychotherapy
      i. Detoxification may be needed, and is usually done in hospital
      j. Alcohol abuse:
         (1) Most abused substance
         (2) Signs and symptoms include intoxication, memory problems, difficulty concentrating, tremors and loss of interest in family and friends
         (3) Liver, pancreas, and heart problems can occur
         (4) Fetal alcohol syndrome can occur (see Chapter 37)
         (5) The person may also be addicted to nicotine
         (6) May be emotional, aggressive, and abusive
         (7) May drink every day or binge drink

(8) Main treatment is to stop drinking; main source of treatment is Alcoholics Anonymous

IV. THE STIGMA OF MENTAL HEALTH DISORDERS
   A. A stigma is a characteristic that marks a person as different or flawed
   B. People sometimes discriminate against those with mental health disorders because of fear, not understanding mental health disorders, don't know what to expect or may believe they are dangerous.
   C. This can cause them to avoid or exclude the person
   D. The person themselves may feel ashamed, rejected and isolated.
   E. The Canadian Alliance for Mental Illness and Mental Health (CAMIMH) represents professionals and individuals concerned with mental health
      1. Their main goal is to prevent stigma and discrimination through educational programs

V. CARING FOR CLIENTS AND THEIR FAMILIES
   A. Mental health disorders affect people in different ways
      1. Those with mild disorders have few problems
   B. Severe illness almost always causes distress for individuals and their families
      1. The person in unable to function and their behaviour may be disruptive
   C. Family members must make difficult decisions abut care, treatment, and housing
   D. There may be financial burdens and the family may blame themselves for the illness
   E. Stress is significant and they are at risk of depression
   F. Family members may also feel the stigma as friends may tend to avoid contact
   G. Be sensitive to the feelings of your clients and their family
   H. Examine your own attitudes about mental health and mental illness
   I. To provide compassionate care you must be self-aware (see Providing Compassionate Care box, p. 571)
   J. Follow the guidelines listed in Box 33-2, p. 570 in the textbook, and follow the care-plan

VI. THE RISK OF SUICIDE
   A. Common cause of death from adolescence through middle age
   B. Men commit suicide more often than women, use more violent means, and attempts are often fatal
   C. Women use less violent means and may survive
   D. Sign of serious mental health problems and in need of professional care
   E. Risk factors include:
      1. Mental illness, especially depression, bipolar disorder, and schizophrenia
      2. A history of abuse
      3. A family history of suicide
      4. The suicide of a friend
      5. A prior suicide attempt
      6. A major crisis such as the loss of a relationship, family problems, loss of position in society and work, money or legal problems
      7. Pressure to succeed
      8. Isolation
      9. Early losses in life
      10. Sexual identity issues
      11. Feelings of deep hopelessness and helplessness
      12. Recent diagnosis of a life-threatening illness
      13. Substance abuse
   F. See Focus on Older Adults box, p. 571
   G. Common warning signals of suicide are listed in Box 33-3, p. 571
   H. If your client talks about suicide take it seriously and inform your supervisor immediately
      1. Don't leave them alone, and encourage them to talk
   I. Be a good listener
   J. In a home care setting stay with the client until help arrives
   K. Your supervisor may send a nurse, case manager, or emergency personnel to help the person

Classroom Activities

1. Write the terms mental health and mental illness on the chalkboard.
   a. Call on students to define each term. Write the correct answers on the chalkboard.
   b. Call on students to identify the causes of mental health disorders.

2. Display the signs and symptoms of depression in older persons (see Box 33-1, p. 567) on an over-

head transparency.
  a. Carefully review each item with students.
  b. Allow time for questions and discussion.

3. Ask students to share some stressors in their lives that lead to anxiety.
  a. Ask them to identify the defense mechanisms they use to relieve anxiety.

4. Have students share any feelings and fears that they may have about caring for persons with mental health disorders.
  a. Discuss ways to handle their fears so that they are able to meet the person's needs.

5. Invite a psychiatric nurse to talk to the class about approaches to care and treatment options for persons with mental health disorders.

Homework Assignments

Ask students to answer the questions at the end of Chapter 33 in the textbook. Tell students the date and time that this assignment must be completed and turned in.

If the accompanying workbook is being used, assign the Chapter 33 workbook exercises. Tell students the date and time that this assignment must be completed and turned in.

Mental Health Disorders

Write your answers in the spaces provided.

1. List four signs or symptoms of depression.

    a. _____

    b. _____

    c. _____

    d. _____

2. Define the following terms:

    a. psychosis

    _____

    _____

    b. delusion

    _____

    _____

c. hallucination

_____

_____

d. anorexia nervosa

_____

_____

e. stigma

_____

_____

3. Why are older adults at risk of suicide?

    a. _____

    b. _____

    c. _____

    d. _____

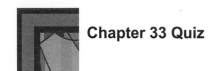

Chapter 33 Quiz

Name _____

Date _____

Mental Health Disorders

True or False

Mark **T** *for true or* **F** *for false.*

1. _____ Unmet needs at any age affect personality development.

2. _____ Anxiety is seen in all mental health disorders.

3. _____ Only illegal drugs are abused.

4. _____ Communication is important when caring for persons with mental health disorders.

5. _____ Panic is the highest level of anxiety.

6. _____ Depression is uncommon in older persons.

Multiple Choice

Circle the BEST answer.

7. A vague, uneasy feeling that occurs in response to stress is:
   a. Obsession.
   b. Delusion.
   c. Anxiety.
   d. Mental disorder.

8. The set of attitudes, values, behaviors, and traits of a particular person is:
   a. Phobia.
   b. Personality.
   c. Affect.
   d. Id.

9. Which statement about defense mechanisms is incorrect?
   a. They are used to relieve anxiety.
   b. They are a symptom of mental illness.
   c. They are used to block unpleasant feelings.
   d. They are unconscious reactions.

10. The person with this disorder has severe mood swings:
    a. Paranoia
    b. Major depression
    c. Bipolar disorder
    d. Psychosis

11. Mr. Jansen is 75 years old. His daughter notices that he is agitated, has poor grooming, complains of not sleeping and feeling tired all the time. These are signs and symptoms of:
    a. Aging
    b. A phobia
    c. Abusive personality
    d. Depression

12. The most abused substance is:
    a. Marijuana.
    b. Cocaine.
    c. Heroin.
    d. Alcohol.

13. The person with bulemia:
    a. Refuses to eat.
    b. Craves food.
    c. Is very suspicious.
    d. Has violent behavior.

266

34

Confusion and Dementia

Instructor's Preparation

I. Read Chapter 34 in the textbook. Carefully review chapter objectives, key terms, and review questions.

II. Read the outline in Chapter 34 of the instructor's guide. Carefully review the classroom activities, the student assignment, and the quiz.

III. If you are using the accompanying student workbook, review the activities for Chapter 34.

IV. Review the following Mosby videos: Caring for Persons with Dementia and Dealing with Difficult Behaviors.

V. Gather all necessary supplies and equipment for classroom activities and student assignments.

   A. Prepare appropriate flip charts

   B. Prepare overhead transparencies

   C. Prepare situation/index cards

   D. Gather correct videos

   E. Gather coloured markers

   F. Gather any other items that will be needed for classroom activities

   G. Assemble items in the order they will be used

VI. Make sure that the necessary equipment is available and in good working order.

VII. Contact guest speakers to confirm the day, date, time, and location that they are expected.

   A. Ask the speakers if they require any special equipment or supplies. Ensure these are available.

VIII. Confirm all plans for the field trip.

   A. Contact the agency to confirm location, day, date, and time

   B. Prepare an index card for each student with the location day, date, and time of the field trip; include special instructions (i.e., dress code)

Objectives

- Define the key terms listed in this chapter
- Describe confusion and delirium and their causes
- List the measures that help clients who are confused
- Describe dementia and its signs and symptoms
- List different forms and causes of dementia
- Describe the common stages of dementia

- Describe the care required by a client with dementia
- List examples of challenging behaviours and possible causes
- Describe how primary caregivers may be affected by caring for family members with dementia

Alzheimer's Disease
confusion
delirium
delusion
dementia
hallucination
sundowning

Outline

Confusion and Dementia

I. INTRODUCTION
  A. Some changes in the brain and nervous system occur normally with aging (see Box 34-1, p. 574)
  B. Certain diseases also affect cognitive function
    1. Cognitive function relates to memory, thinking, reasoning, ability to understand, judgement, and behaviour

II. CONFUSION
  A. Mental state—person disorientated to person, time, or place
  B. Memory and ability to make good judgements impaired or lost
  C. Behaviour changes common—may include anger, restlessness, depression, anxiety, tremors, hallucinations, delusions
    1. Refer to p. 582 in the textbook for descriptions
  D. Delirium—sudden onset of confusion, usually temporary
    1. Could be caused by medications, infection, poor nutrition, dehydration, food poisoning or other illness.
    2. Is an emergency
    3. Often first or only sign of physical illness in older adults and in people with dementia
    4. Report any sudden occurrence to your supervisor at once
  E. Confusion caused by physical changes cannot be cured
    1. Some measures help improve the person's functioning (see Box 34-2, p. 575)

III. DEMENTIA
  A. A term used to describe the loss of cognitive function caused by changes in the brain
    1. Starts slowly and progresses gradually
      a. Refer to p. 575 in the textbook for affected functions

  B. Is not a normal part of aging
  C. Only a small number of older adults affected
  D. Can affect people 40s and 50s; more common after age of 65
  E. Early warning signs
    1. Memory loss affecting daily activities
    2. Confusion
    3. Problems with language
    4. Poor judgment
    5. Changes in mood, behaviour, or personality
    6. Loss of interest in activities or hobbies
  F. Starts affecting complex tasks (e.g., working, managing money, etc.)
    1. Over time problems occur with simple tasks.
    2. Refer to Box 34-3, p. 576 in the textbook, for other signs
  G. Forms and causes of dementia
    1. Dementia can be reversed or caused by:
      a. Brain injury—if bleeding in skull, surgery can correct it
      b. Brain tumour—depending on location and type, surgery or chemotherapy may correct it
      c. Alcohol—long term abuse can cause it; stopping drinking may reverse it
      d. Thyroid deficiency—underactive thyroid can produce dementia and/or delirium
    2. Most forms cannot be reversed
      a. No prevention or cure
      b. Eventually interferes with all ADL and leads to death

IV. ALZHEIMER'S DISEASE (AD)
  A. Brain cells that control intellectual function are damaged
    1. Memory, thinking, judgement, and behavior are affected
  B. Onset is gradual; the disease progresses over 3 to 20 years and gets worse and worse
  C. More common in older persons; can occur in younger people
  D. Risk increases after age 65
  E. Cause is unknown
    1. Family history of AD and Down syndrome are risk factors
    2. Vascular Dementia (multi-infarct dementia)—caused by small strokes which cause tissues of brain to die
    3. Lewy body dementia (progressive)—abnormal structures in brain cells—more rapid than AD

4. Pick's disease—rare brain disorder affecting people 45–65
   a. Destroys or damages brain cells first in frontal and temporal areas of brain
5. Creutzfeldt-Jacob disease (CJD)—brain tissue slowly dies causing holes in the brain
6. Many other conditions can sometimes cause dementia (see Chapter 31)

F. Stages of dementia
1. Dementia generally has three stages
   a. Box 34-4, p. 577 in the textbook, describes common characteristics of each stage
   b. In early stages, dementia can present itself quite differently, but it becomes similar as stages progress
2. Death occurs when the brain shuts down all body systems

V. CARE OF CLIENTS WITH DEMENTIA
A. Introduction—each client has unique care needs
1. Needs depend on the form of dementia
2. See Box 34-5, p. 578-79 in the textbook, for general guidelines
3. The care plan and your supervisor provide specific instructions

B. Clients with early stage dementia
1. Usually cared for at home by primary caregiver who may be a spouse, adult child, other family member, or friend
2. Some live alone with support
3. Relief for the caregiver can be provided by other caregivers, respite care, adult daycare, or home care
4. Need to feel useful and active, which is one of a focus in adult day care programs
5. In community settings, clients can still make some decisions but may need help to organize, solve simple problems, and remember appointments and medications
6. May need help with tasks, frequent cues, and reminders of facts and conversations
7. Safety is a concern
   a. Follow the care plan (see Providing Compassionate Care box, p. 581)

C. Clients with middle to late stage dementia
1. As disease progresses, needs increase
2. Client cannot be cared for at home
3. Long-term care is needed when at least one of these occurs:
   a. Caregivers cannot meet person's needs
   b. Family members have health problems

c. Person's behaviour is a danger to others or themselves
d. No longer recognizes the caregiver
4. Many facilities have special care units
   a. Family and friends usually continue to be involved in the person's care and are an important part of the team

D. Challenging behaviours
1. People with dementia can display challenging behaviours to caregivers
2. It is important for caregivers to know that dementia, not the client, is to blame
3. Do not to take the behaviour personally
4. Do not become upset or angry or blame yourself
5. Can be a response to illness, infection, or discomfort
6. Your supervisor may be able to determine the cause
7. The following behaviours are common.
   a. Wandering
      (1) Persons are disoriented to person, time, and place
      (2) They may wander away from home or the facility
      (3) They cannot tell what is safe or dangerous
      (4) If not properly dressed, exposure is a risk
      (5) May have no cause or may look for someone or some place
      (6) Caused by pain, medications, stress, anxiety, or restlessness
      (7) Alzheimer's Society of Canada has a national wandering registry that, for a small fee, provides the person with an ID card and bracelet identifying the person, and enabling the police to call a family member or caregiver
   b. Sundowning
      (1) As daylight ends and darkness occurs, confusion, restlessness, and other symptoms increase
      (2) The person's behavior is worse after the sun goes down
      (3) May relate to fatigue or hunger
      (4) In poor light and shadows, the person may see things that are not actually there
      (5) Person may be afraid of the dark
   c. Hallucinations
      (1) Seeing, hearing, or feeling some-

thing that is not really there
d. Delusions
(1) False beliefs
(2) The person may believe the caregiver is someone else
(a) Many other false beliefs can occur
(3) Catastrophic reactions
(4) Extreme responses; the person reacts as if a disaster or tragedy has occurred
(a) The person may scream, cry, be agitated, or combative
(5) Often occurs when there is too much stimuli
e. Agitation and restlessness
(1) The person may pace, hit, or yell
(2) May be due to pain, discomfort, anxiety, lack of sleep, too much or too little stimuli, hunger, or need to eliminate
(3) A calm, quiet setting and meeting basic needs may calm the person
(4) Rushing the person or being impatient may cause agitation; so can giving mixed verbal and non-verbal messages
f. Aggression and combativeness
(1) May result from agitation and restlessness
(2) Examples include hitting, biting pinching, grabbing, or swearing
(3) These behaviors are frightening to caregivers, others in the home, and to patients and residents
(4) Sometimes these behaviors are part of the person's personality
(a) See Chapter 12 for dealing with the angry person
(b) See Chapter 19 for workplace violence
g. Screaming
(1) Related to communication problems
(a) Problems with communication increase as the disease progresses
(2) The person may scream to communicate
(3) Possible causes include:
(a) Hearing and vision problems
(b) Pain or discomfort
(c) Fear

(d) Fatigue
(e) Too much or not enough stimuli
(f) Reactions to a caregiver or family members
(4) Measures that may help:
(a) A calm, quiet setting
(b) Soft music
(c) Make sure hearing aids and glasses are worn (if it is safe for the person)
(d) Family members or favorite caregivers can have a calming effect
(e) Touch may calm some persons
h. Abnormal sexual behaviors
(1) Persons with AD are disoriented to person, time, and place
(a) Sexual behaviors may involve the wrong person, place, and time
(2) The person has lost the ability to control behavior
(3) The person often mistakes someone else for a sexual partner
(4) May mean that the person's sexual needs are not being met
(5) Touching the genitals can signal infection, pain, or discomfort
(a) Poor hygiene is another cause
(6) The nurse encourages the person's sexual partner to show affection
(7) When a person masturbates in public, provide privacy and safety
(8) If the person urinates or has a bowel movement, do not let the person stay wet or soiled
(9) A health professional assesses the person for urinary or reproductive system problems
i. Repetitive behaviors
(1) Persons with AD repeat the same motions over and over
(2) Such behavior is harmless
(a) Can annoy the caregiver and the family
(3) The person is allowed to continue harmless acts
(4) Music, TV, and walks can help

distract the person
E. Meeting basic needs
1. Over time, people with dementia depend on others for all aspects of their care
2. Follow the care plan (see Box 34-5, p. 578)
3. Safety
   a. Fail to recognize safety hazards and may be at risk of falling
   b. If they fall, they may not understand why it is unsafe to move
   c. Talk to them in a quiet and soothing voice, but never use force to hold them down
   d. Always explain what you are doing and be repeat it if necessary
4. Hygiene, grooming, and dressing
   a. People with moderate and severe dementia do not understand the need for personal hygiene
   b. Assist the client with hand washing:
      (1) After elimination
      (2) After coughing, sneezing, or blowing their nose
      (3) Before or after handling food
      (4) Any time hands are soiled
   c. May resist efforts to keep them clean which could cause skin breakdown
   d. Could become agitated, combative, or violent
   e. Skin tears can occur with sudden movements
   f. If the client resists, contact your supervisor and consult the care plan
      (1) Refer to page 583 in the textbook for measures that may work
   g. During care, look for signs or symptoms that may be causing pain
5. Elimination needs
   a. With moderate or severe dementia the client may urinate in the wrong places
   b. They may smear stool
   c. Offer assistance with elimination needs often
   d. Provide perineal care after elimination
   e. Consult your supervisor if the client resists
   f. Never restrict fluids in an effort to control elimination
F. Nutrition
1. May become distracted during meals or unable to sit long enough
2. In late dementia, they may forget how to use utensils
3. May have trouble swallowing
4. May have to be fed, and may resist
5. A quiet and calm dining area is helpful
G. Fluids
1. May not recognize thirst and can risk dehydration
2. Encourage drinking and offer fluids whenever nearby
H. Exercise
1. Inactivity and immobility are risk factors for pneumonia and pressure ulcers
   a. May resist, but it is important to encourage exercise
   b. Do not force activity, and check with the care plan and your supervisor
I. Health problems
1. May not recognize pain, fever, constipation, or other signs or symptoms
2. Changes in usual behaviour may signal pain or discomfort
3. Report any changes to your supervisor
J. Comfort
1. Ensure the client is physically comfortable
2. A quiet environment helps
3. Massage therapy, soothing touch, music, and a calm voice can all help
4. Clothing should be comfortable
K. Therapy and activities
1. Need to feel worthwhile as long as able and need to be active
2. Long-term care facilities and community adult daycare have therapy and activities, which will meet the client's needs
L. Secured units
1. Some long-term care residents may wander or try to leave the facility
2. These residents are moved to a locked unit, which will provide a safe setting
3. A form of environmental restraint requiring dementia diagnosis and a physician's order
4. Resident's rights must be protected
5. In the advanced stage, the resident is in bed and can be moved to another unit
6. Legislation has standards of care for special care units, including special training for staff, and programs that promote dignity, personal freedom, and safety
M. Caregivers needs
1. Being a primary caregiver can be very stressful

2. There are physical, emotional, social, and financial stresses
3. Many adult children are responsible for two families and their work
4. Caregivers can suffer from anger, anxiety, sleeplessness, and depression
5. Abuse can occur because of the stress
6. Caregivers are vulnerable to health problems because of the demands and stress
7. Caregivers need much support and encouragement; Alzheimer's Society of Canada has support groups
8. Caregivers often feel helpless, as nothing can stop the progression
   a. Guilt feelings are common because they know the person does not choose to have dementia, but can be very difficult to deal with
9. You play a very important role in caregiver relief
   a. You may be assisting the caregiver or providing care when they are not there
   b. You must provide competent care so the caregiver has confidence in leaving their loved one in your care
10. You need to observe and report to your supervisor and signs of caregiver stress or abuse of the client (see Support Workers Solving Problems box, p. 585)

Classroom Activities

1. Display an overhead transparency listing the changes in the nervous system with aging (see Box 34-1, p. 574).
   a. Review each item on the list with students. Allow time for questions.

2. Write the following topics on a flip chart in outline form using a variety of coloured markers. Use the flip chart to present information and ask for input from students. Leave space after each item to add information.
   a. Confusion
   (1) Definition
   (2) Causes
   (3) Signs and symptoms
   (4) Causes and characteristics of acute confusion
   (5) Measures to help improve functioning

Call on students to provide information about each topic. Write in the correct answers on the flip chart. Clarify any wrong answers.

Allow time for discussion.

3. Ask students what the most common cause of dementia is. Write Alzheimer's Disease on the chalkboard.
   a. Call on students to write other types and causes on the chalkboard.
   b. Discuss treatable causes.

4. Display the early warning signs of Alzheimer's disease and the signs and symptoms of depression on an overhead transparency. Use this as a basis to discuss the similarities between the two.
   a. Allow time for questions.

5. Display the stages of Alzheimer's disease on an overhead transparency (see Box 34-4, p. 577).
   a. Carefully review each stage with students. Allow time for questions and discussion.

6. Show the following Mosby videos: Caring for Persons with Dementia, and Dealing with Difficult Behaviors.
   a. Allow time after each video for questions and discussion.

7. Write each of the following terms associated with Alzheimer's disease on separate index cards: Wandering, Sundowning, Hallucinations, Delusions, Catastrophic reactions, Agitation and Restlessness, Aggression and Combativeness, Screaming, Abnormal sexual behavior, and Repetitive behaviors.
   a. Call on students to pick a card. Ask the student for the following information about the term on his or her card:
   (1) The definition
   (2) The behaviors involved
   (3) Care measures that might help

All students may provide input as appropriate.

8. Arrange for the class to tour an Alzheimer's unit. Ask the RN in charge to speak to the class about:
   a. How the physical environment of the unit is designed to meet the residents' needs.
   b. Special nursing care approaches and programs designed to meet the needs of the residents on the unit.
   c. How families are involved with the care of the residents on the unit.

Ask students to write key points in a notebook for future reference. Allow time for questions and discussions

9. Arrange for one or more representative(s) from an Alzheimer's support group to talk to the class.
   a. Ask the representative(s) to discuss how the disease has affected the person and the family.
      (1) What life-style changes have occurred?
      (2) What is the financial impact of the disease?
      (3) What support systems are in place?
   b. Allow time for informal social time. Provide a healthy snack.

Homework Assignments

Ask students to answer the questions at the end of Chapter 34 in the textbook. Tell students the date and time that this assignment must be completed and turned in.

If the accompanying student workbook is being used, assign the Chapter 34 workbook exercises. Tell students the date and time that this assignment must be completed and turned in.

Name _____

Date _____

Confusion and Dementia

Write your answers in the spaces provided.

1. Persons with signs and symptoms of dementia need to see a doctor to determine the cause. Treatable causes include:

   a. _____

   b. _____

   c. _____

   d. _____

   e. _____

   f. _____

   g. _____

   h. _____

   i. _____

2. List the early signs and symptoms of Alzheimer's disease.

   a. _____

   b. _____

   c. _____

   d. _____

   e. _____

   f. _____

   g. _____

   h. _____

3. Persons with Alzheimer's disease are usually cared for in the home. The decision for long-term care is usually made when:

   a. _____

   _____

   b. _____

   _____

   c. _____

   _____

   d. _____

   _____

   e. _____

   _____

274

Name _____

Date _____

Confusion and Dementia

True or False	**Multiple Choice**

Mark **T** *for true or* **F** *for false.*

Circle the BEST answer.

1. _____ Acute confusion is usually permanent.

2. _____ When caring for the confused person, you should give clear and simple answers to questions.

3. _____ Dementia is a normal part of aging.

4. _____ Mr. Lewis has Alzheimer's disease. He wants to leave the facility. You must restrain him.

5. _____ Mrs. Adams has Alzheimer's disease. You promote her safety by explaining the safety rules to her.

6. _____ Approach the person with Alzheimer's disease in a calm, quiet manner.

7. _____ The person with Alzheimer's disease may scream to communicate.

8. _____ Persons with Alzheimer's disease choose to be agitated and rude.

9. _____ Quality of life is important for all persons with confusion and dementia.

10. _____ Confused and demented persons do not have the right to personal choice.

11. _____ Caring for persons with Alzheimer's disease can be frustrating.

12. _____ Restraints can make confusion and dementia worse.

13. The most common type of dementia is:
    a. Multi-infarct dementia.
    b. Alzheimer's disease.
    c. Stroke.
    d. Syphilis.

14. The most common mental health problem in older persons is:
    a. Delirium.
    b. Alcoholism.
    c. Depression.
    d. Anxiety.

15. Catastrophic reactions involve:
    a. False beliefs.
    b. Restless behavior.
    c. Seeing something that is not there.
    d. Extreme responses.

16. Agitated and restless behavior may be the result of:
    a. Pain or discomfort.
    b. Too much stimuli.
    c. Lack of sleep.
    d. All of the above.

17. The person in Stage 1 of Alzheimer's disease:
    a. Has difficulty finishing thoughts.
    b. Is totally incontinent of bowel and bladder.
    c. Cannot swallow.
    d. Has movement and gait disturbances.

18. The person with Alzheimer's disease:
    a. Is restrained to prevent wandering.
    b. Cannot keep and use personal possessions.
    c. Must be kept free from abuse, mistreatment, and neglect.
    d. Does not have the right to privacy and confidentiality.

35

Speech and Language Disorders

Instructor's Preparation

I. Read Chapter 35 in the textbook. Carefully review chapter objectives, key terms, and review questions.

II. Read the outline in Chapter 35 of the instructor's guide. Carefully review the classroom activities, the student assignment, and the quiz.

III. If you are using the accompanying student workbook, review the activities for Chapter 35.

IV. Gather all necessary supplies and equipment for classroom activities and student assignments.

A. Prepare the correct number of handouts
B. Prepare appropriate flip charts
C. Prepare overhead transparencies
D. Prepare situation/index cards
E. Gather correct slides
F. Gather coloured markers
G. Gather anatomical models
H. Gather simulators
I. Gather any other items that will be needed for classroom activities
J. Assemble items in the order they will be used

V. Make sure that the necessary equipment is available and in good working order.

VI. Contact guest speakers to confirm the day, date, time, and location that they are expected.

A. Ask the speakers if they require any special equipment or supplies; ensure these are available.

Objectives	Key Terms

- Define the key terms listed in this chapter
- Describe three types of aphasia
- Describe apraxia of speech
- Describe dysarthria
- Explain how speech and language disorders are treated
- Explain what communication aids are
- Describe the emotional effects of a language disorder
- Describe how to communicate with clients with language disorders

aphasia
apraxia of speech
dysarthria
expressive aphasia
expressive-receptive aphasia
receptive aphasia

Speech and Language Disorders

I. INTRODUCTION
   A. Speech and language disorders can occur at any age
   B. Can be caused by:
      1. Genetic problems or conditions at birth
      2. Brain injury
      3. Disease
      4. Hearing loss
      5. Brain tumours
      6. Problems involving the structures used for speech
   C. Refer to Chapter 12 for recommended communication methods

II. APHASIA
   A. Aphasia is the partial or complete loss of speech and language skills, caused by brain injury
   B. Most people with dementia have aphasia (see Chapter 34)
   C. There are three types of aphasia:
      1. Receptive aphasia
      2. Expressive aphasia
      3. Expressive-receptive aphasia

III. APRAXIA OF SPEECH
   A. Persons with apraxia of speech:
      1. Are unable to move the muscles used to speak
      2. Cannot say the desired sounds and words
      3. Are difficult to understand and their speech is usually slow

IV. DYSARTHRIA
   A. Difficulty in speaking clearly
   B. Caused by weakness or paralysis in the muscles used for speech
   C. Persons with dysarthria:
      1. Usually have slurred, slow, soft speech and speak in flat, harsh, or nasal tones
      2. May have problems forming words

V. EMOTIONAL EFFECTS OF SPEECH AND LANGUAGE DISORDERS
   A. Frustration, depression, and anger are common along with low-esteem, shame, and guilt
   B. Being unable to communicate may cause the person to avoid social situations, and family and friends may avoid the person
   C. Can be very stressful for families as everyday conversations are affected
   D. All areas of daily living can be affected
   E. Emotional reactions vary, so observe and listen to your clients and their family

F. See Box 35-1, p. 589 in the textbook, for comments from people who have had aphasia

VI. TREATMENT FOR SPEECH AND LANGUAGE DISORDERS
   A. Speech therapists help people with the disorder learn to communicate
      1. Also help family members learn new communication techniques
   C. Methods used depend on the disorder, its cause, and severity
   D. Practice and exercises may help
   E. People with speech and language disorders may learn to improve existing skills such as body language and facial expressions
   F. Some people may be helped by communication boards (see Figure 35-1, p. 590) or mechanical and electronic devices (see Figure 35-2, p. 590)

VII. COMMUNICATING WITH CLIENTS
   A. You must be aware of how you communicate
   B. Follow the care plan and your supervisor's instructions
   C. The effort of understanding others and making oneself understood can be exhausting
   D. Spend extra time with these clients and treat them with respect and empathy (see Providing Compassionate Care box, p. 590)
   E. Follow the guidelines listed in Box 35-2, p. 591 in the textbook

---

Classroom Activities

1. Contact a speech therapist to speak to the class about ways to help clients with aphasia.

2. On the board, write "receptive aphasia", "expressive aphasia", and "expressive-receptive aphasia." Divide the class into small groups and ask them to write down examples of each type of aphasia. Then ask them to suggest ways to help communication with a client who has each type of aphasia. Allow 20 minutes, then have each group share their ideas.

3. Ask the students to list ways they can provide compassionate care for clients who have speech and language disorders.

Homework Assignments

Ask students to answer the questions at the end of Chapter 35 in the textbook. Tell students the date and time that this assignment must be completed and turned in.

If the accompanying workbook is being used, assign the Chapter 35 workbook exercises. Tell students the date and time that this assignment must be completed and turned in.

Chapter 35 Student Assignment   Name _____

Date _____

Speech and Language Disorders

Write your answers in the spaces provided.

1. List three possible causes of speech and language disorders..

   a. _____

   b. _____

   c. _____

2. For communication to occur, a message must be sent, received, and interpreted. What process is affected in each of these conditions?

   a. receptive aphasia

   _____

   b. expressive aphasia

   _____

   c. expressive-receptive aphasia

   _____

3. What emotional effects can a client have who has a language or speech disorder?

   a. _____

   b. _____

   c. _____

   d. _____

4. How can you communicate effectively with a client with speech or language disorders?

   a. _____

   b. _____

   c. _____

   d. _____

   e. _____

Chapter 35 Quiz

Name _____

Date _____

Speech and Language Disorders

True or False	Multiple Choice

Mark **T** *for true or* **F** *for false.*

1. _____ Most people with dementia have aphasia.

2. _____ People with receptive aphasia have difficulty speaking.

3. _____ Apraxia means difficulty speaking.

4. _____ Cerebral palsy can cause dysarthria.

5. _____ Aphasia means partial or complete loss of speech.

6. _____ Minimizing distractions can help with communications.

7. _____ Some clients with speech disorders can become withdrawn.

8. _____ A person with dysarthria has a complete loss of speech.

Circle the BEST answer.

9. Apraxia of speech is caused by:
   a. Brain injury
   b. Weakness in the muscles used to speak
   c. Paralysis in the muscles used to speak
   d. Lack of coordination in the muscles used to speak

10. Phasia means:
    a. Speech and language skills
    b. Speaking clearly
    c. Move the muscles used to speak
    d. Loss

11. Treatment for speech and language disorders includes:
    a. Speech therapy
    b. Practice
    c. Exercises
    d. All of the above

36

Hearing and Vision Problems

Instructor's Preparation

I. Read Chapter 36 in the textbook. Carefully review chapter objectives, key terms, and review questions.

II. Read the outline in Chapter 36 of the instructor's guide. Carefully review the classroom activities, the student assignment, and the quiz.

III. If you are using the accompanying student workbook, review the activities for Chapter 36.

IV. Gather all necessary supplies and equipment for classroom activities and student assignments.
   A. Prepare appropriate flip charts
   B. Prepare overhead transparencies
   C. Gather coloured markers
   D. Gather supplies and equipment needed to demonstrate and have each student in turn demonstrate the procedures in this chapter
   E. Gather any other items that will be needed for classroom activities
   F. Assemble items in the order they will be used

V. Make sure that the necessary equipment is available and in good working order.

VI. Contact guest speakers to confirm the day, date, time, and location that they are expected.
   A. Ask the speakers if they require any special equipment or supplies; ensure these are available.

Objectives

- Define the key terms listed in this chapter
- Describe the major ear disorders
- Describe the effects of hearing problems
- Describe aids for clients with hearing problems
- Explain how to care for clients with hearing loss
- Describe the major eye disorders
- Describe aids for clients with vision problems
- Explain how to care for clients with vision loss
- Perform the procedures described in this chapter

Key Terms

age-related macular degeneration (AMD; ARMD)
Braille
cataract
diabetic retinopathy
dominant progressive hearing loss
glaucoma
Ménière's disease
otitis media
otosclerosis
presbycusis
presbyopia
retinal detachment
tinnitus
vertigo

Outline

Hearing and Vision Problems

I. INTRODUCTION
   A. Sight and hearing are valuable senses
      1. They allow communication, learning, and moving about

2. They are important for activities of daily living (ADL)

3. They are important for safety and security needs

B. Hearing and vision problems are common among all age groups
   1. Common causes are:
      a. Birth defects
      b. Accidents
      c. Infections
      d. Diseases
      e. Aging

II. EAR DISORDERS AND HEARING PROBLEMS

A. The ear is important for hearing and balance
   1. See Figure 36-1, p. 595 in the textbook, for a review of the structures and functions of the ear

B. Otitis media—common in infants and children
   1. An infection of the middle ear
   2. Chronic otitis media can damage the tympanic membrane or the ossicles
      a. Permanent hearing loss can occur
   3. Fluid build up occurs in the ear
   4. Signs and symptoms include pain, hearing loss, fever, and tinnitus
   5. Antibiotics are usually ordered

C. Otosclerosis
   1. Hardening of ossicles in middle ear
   2. Hereditary condition that is a common cause of hearing loss in adults
   3. Gradual and progressive hearing loss and tinnitus
   4. Surgery can be helpful

D. Ménière's disease
   1. Involves increased fluid in the inner ear
   2. There are three symptoms:
      a. Vertigo or dizziness (the major symptom)
         (1) Can cause nausea and vomiting
      b. Tinnitus (ringing in the ears)
      c. Hearing loss

E. Dominant progressive hearing loss
   1. Impairment of nerves used to hear
   2. Hearing loss is progressive
   3. Can start in early childhood, but usually starts in early or middle adulthood

F. Presbycusis
   1. Gradual hearing loss that occurs with aging
   2. Occurs after 50
   3. No cure but hearing aids and speech reading can be helpful

G. Temporary hearing loss
   1. Blockage of ear with ear wax
   2. Common in older adults
   3. Hearing improves when wax is removed by a physician or nurse

H. The effects of hearing problems
   1. Hearing losses range from slight hearing impairment to complete deafness
   2. Clear speech, responding to others, safety, and awareness of surroundings require hearing
   3. Temporary hearing loss can occur when the ear canal is blocked with ear wax
   4. Effects on the person
      a. A person may be unaware of gradual hearing loss
      b. Changes in behavior and attitude may occur
      c. Signs of hearing impairment:
         (1) Speaking too loudly
         (2) Leaning forward to hear
         (3) Turning and cupping the better ear toward the speaker
         (4) Answering questions or responding inappropriately
         (5) Asking for words to be repeated
      d. Psychological and social effects
         (1) Avoiding social situations
         (2) Loneliness, boredom, and feeling left out
         (3) Some may become suspicious
         (4) Some control the conversation to avoid responding
         (5) It can cause speech problems
            (a) Slurred speech and improper pronunciation
            (b) Monotone speech
            (c) Dropping word endings
      e. Review Chapter 35 for communicating with clients who have speech problems.
   5. Aids for people with hearing loss
      a. Fits in the ear and makes sounds louder (see Figure 36-2, p. 596)
      b. It does not correct or cure hearing problems
      c. If a hearing aid does not seem to work properly:
         (1) Check if the hearing aid is on
         (2) Check the battery position
         (3) Insert a new battery if needed
         (4) Clean the earmold if necessary
      d. Hearing aids are expensive; handle and care for them properly

(1) Report lost or damaged hearing aids to your supervisor immediately

(2) Follow manufacturer's instructions for proper care and use

e. The battery is removed at night

f. When not in use, the hearing aid is turned off

g. Special telephone systems

(1) TTYs (once called telephone teletypes) are machines that allow the users to type messages back and forth

(2) Amplified telephone handsets make the caller's voice louder

(3) Extension bells make the telephone ring more loudly

h. Signaling devices

(1) Attached to telephones, doorbells and smoke alarms

(2) When the device makes a sound, a light flashes to alert the person

(3) Some devices include a vibrating option

6. Communication with the person

a. Persons may wear hearing aids or read lips

b. They also watch facial expressions, gestures, and body language

c. Some people learn sign language (see Figure 36-3, p. 597)

d. Some have hearing dogs

e. Follow the guidelines in Box 36-1, p. 598 in the textbook, for clients with hearing loss

III. EYE DISORDERS AND VISION PROBLEMS

A. Vision problems occur at all ages

B. Problems range from mild vision loss to complete blindness

C. Vision loss is sudden or gradual

D. One or both eyes are affected

E. Surgery, eyeglasses, or contact lenses are often necessary

F. See Figure 13-12, p. 136 in the textbook, for a review of the function of the eye

G. See Figure 36-4, p. 599 in the textbook, for a review of the structures of the eye

H. Glaucoma

1. Pressure within the eye is increased

a. This damages the optic nerve

2. Can be gradual or sudden in onset

3. Signs and symptoms include tunnel vision, blurred vision, blue-green halos

around lights, eye discomfort, and aching

4. Treatment involves drug therapy and possible surgery

a. The goal is to prevent optic nerve damage

I. Age-related macular degeneration (AMD; ARMD)

1. Breakdown of the macula

2. Most common cause of blindness in people over 50

3. Onset can be slow or sudden

4. Central vision becomes fuzzy or shadowy; vision becomes worse

5. Some go completely blind; others may retain peripheral vision

6. No cure for AMD

7. Can also affect young adults and children

J. Retinal detachment

1. Separation of the retina from its supporting tissue

2. Permanent blindness can result

3. If reattached by surgery vision may be saved

K. Diabetic retinopathy

1. Caused by diabetes

2. Blood vessels in retina damaged

3. Blood can leak from vessels.

4. New blood vessels grow over retina creating scar tissue which pulls retina away from the back of the eye

5. Retinal detachment and blindness may result

L. Presbyopia

1. Gradual inability to focus

2. Most people experience this after age 40

3. Glasses or contact lens help the problem

M. Cataract

1. The lens becomes cloudy, which prevents light from entering the eye

2. Gradual blurring and dimming of vision occur

3. The person is sensitive to light and glares

4. Can occur in one or both eyes

5. Aging is the most common cause

a. Persons age 60 or older are at risk

6. Surgery is the only treatment

a. The cloudy lens is removed; a plastic lens is implanted

b. Vision returns to normal

IV. THE EFFECTS OF VISION PROBLEMS

A. Severe vision loss affects all aspects of a person's well being

B. Although process is long and hard, many

people can learn to lead independent lives, new reading methods, and complete ADLs
C. Some people use guide dogs or white canes with a red tip
D. Corrective lenses
 1. Eyeglasses and contact lenses are prescribed to correct vision problems
 2. Eyeglasses
  a. Lenses are made of hardened glass or plastic
  b. Protect the person's glasses from breakage or other damage
   (1) Put them in their case when not worn
   (2) Put the case in the drawer of the bedside stand
  c. Caring for Eyeglasses ▶ p. 600
 3. Contact lenses
  a. Fit directly on the eye
  b. Two types: hard and soft contact lenses
  c. Contact lenses are removed and cleaned following manufacturer's instructions and care plan
  d. Report any redness, drainage, and complaints of eye pain or blurred vision to your supervisor
 4. Aids for reading
  a. Many people learn to read Braille, a system of raised dots representing each letter (see Figure 36-6, p. 601)
  b. Person uses fingers to feel arrangements of dots (see Figure 36-7, p. 601)
  c. Some books, magazines, newspapers, and keyboards are available in Braille
  d. Other aids include large print books, books on audiotape or CD, and magnifiers
  e. Some magnifiers contain reading lamps
 5. Communication aids
  a. List includes calendars in Braille, large-print clocks that also announce the time, large print or Braille playing cards, large print or Braille bingo cards, etc.
  b. Medical devices:
   (1) Pillboxes that allow the person to use touch to detect if the pill has been taken
   (2) "Talking prescription devices" that describe how to take medications

V. Artificial eyes
 A. Removal of an eye may be necessary because of injury or disease
  1. The person is then fitted with an artificial eye
 B. Made of glass or plastic (see Figure 36-8, p. 602)
 A. May be a permanent implant or removable
  1. If removable, the person is taught to remove, clean, and insert the prosthesis
 C. The artificial eye is the person's property; it is protected from loss or damage
  1. Follow the measures listed on p. 602 in the textbook if the artificial eye is removed and will not be reinserted
 D. The person is blind on the side of the artificial eye
  1. Vision in the other eye may be normal or impaired
VI. CARING FOR CLIENTS WITH VISION PROBLEMS
 A. People with vision loss often have highly developed other senses
 B. They are very sensitive to the tone of your voice
 C. Communicate warmth and respect
 D. Box 36-2, p. 603 in the textbook, lists guidelines for caring for clients with vision loss

Classroom Activities

1. Write on the chalkboard: "Common causes of hearing and vision problems are:"
 a. Call on students to list the causes. Write the correct answers on the chalkboard.

2. Review the structures and functions of the ear (see Chapter 13).
 a. Display the overhead transparency showing the structures of the ear. Use this as a basis for discussion.

3. Write the following terms on the chalkboard. Then call on students to come forward and write in the definition of each term. Clarify any wrong answers.
 a. Otitis media
 b. Tinnitus
 c. Vertigo
 d. Ménière's disease

4. Divide students into two groups. Provide each group with a flip chart and colored markers.

a. Ask one group to list the signs of hearing impairment on the flip chart.
b. Ask one group to list the psychological and social effects of hearing impairment on the flip chart.

Allow 10 minutes for this exercise. Then call on one student from each group to report to the class. Allow time after each presentation for questions and discussion.

5. Invite a professional who works with hearing impaired children and adults to speak to the class.
   a. Ask the person to bring educational materials and handouts to enhance the learning experience
   b. Ask the person to demonstrate different types of hearing aids. Explain the advantages and disadvantages of each.
   c. Ask the person to share communication techniques.
   d. Ask the person to discuss safety issues in the home and in health care agencies.
   e. Ask students to write key points in a notebook for future reference.
   f. Encourage students to ask questions.

6. Review the structures and function of the eye (see p. 136 in the textbook).
   a. Display the overhead transparency showing the structures of the eye. Use this as a basis for discussion.

7. Divide students into two groups. Provide each group with a flip chart and colored markers.
   a. Ask one group to define glaucoma. They should also list signs and symptoms, persons at risk, causes, and treatments.
   b. Ask one group to define cataract. They should also list signs and symptoms, persons at risk, causes, and treatments.
   Allow 15 minutes for this exercise. Then call on one student from each group to report to the class. Allow time after each presentation for questions and discussion.

8. Invite a professional who works with visually impaired children and adults to speak to the class.
   a. Ask the person to bring educational materials and handouts to enhance the learning experience.
   b. Ask the person to share communication techniques.
   c. Ask the person to discuss safety issues in the home and in health care agencies.
   d. Ask students to write key points in a notebook for future reference.
   e. Encourage students to ask questions.

9. Simulate vision and hearing impaired situations with students. Allow time after each activity for them to discuss the experience. Did they feel frustrated, angry, or left out? How will the experience affect the care they provide?
   a. Provide several pairs of glasses for students to use. Put petroleum jelly on the lenses. Have students wear the glasses for 5 minutes.
   b. Cover one eye with an eye patch. Then have students participate in classroom learning activities.
   c. Cover both eyes with an eye patch. Then have students participate in classroom learning activities.
   d. Provide disposable ear plugs. Ask students to place them in their ears. Then have students participate in classroom learning activities.

10. Use the procedure checklist provided. Demonstrate the procedure in this chapter. Have each student return demonstrate the procedure.

Homework Assignments

Ask students to answer the questions at the end of Chapter 36 in the textbook. Tell students the date and time that this assignment must be completed and turned in.

If the accompanying workbook is being used, assign the Chapter 36 workbook exercises. Tell students the date and time that this assignment must be completed and turned in.

Name _____

Date _____

Hearing and Vision Problems

Fill in the Blanks

Write your answers in the spaces provided.

1. The ear is important for _____ and

   _____ .

2. List the obvious signs of hearing impairment in children and adults.

   a. _____

   b. _____

   c. _____

   d. _____

   e. _____

3. With glaucoma, pressure in the eye is increased. This damages _____

   _____ .

4. Treat the blind person with _____ and

   _____ ; not with _____ .

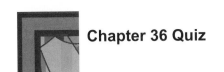

Chapter 36 Quiz

Name _____

Date _____

Hearing and Vision Problems

<table>
<tr><td>

True or False

*Mark **T** for true or **F** for false.*

1. _____ Ménière's disease involves acute infection of the middle ear.

2. _____ A person may be unaware of gradual hearing loss.

3. _____ Hearing loss may cause speech problems.

4. _____ Mr. Alan has a speech problem. You should pretend to understand what he says to avoid embarrassment.

5. _____ Speak in a very loud voice when communicating with the hearing impaired person.

6. _____ Surgery is the only treatment for cataracts.

7. _____ Glaucoma is always sudden in onset.

8. _____ Eyeglasses are kept on the overbed table at night.

</td><td>

Multiple Choice

Circle the BEST answer.

9. Which statement about hearing aids is correct?
   a. Hearing aids amplify sounds.
   b. Hearing aids correct the hearing problem.
   c. The entire hearing aid is washed daily in soapy water.
   d. The battery is left in the hearing aid at night.

10. Cataract is an eye disorder in which:
    a. The optic nerve is damaged.
    b. Pressure within the eye is increased.
    c. The lens becomes cloudy.
    d. Severe eye pain is common.

11. When caring for the blind person, do all of the following except:
    a. Face the person when speaking.
    b. Use a normal tone of voice.
    c. Avoid using the words "see," "look," or "read."
    d. Identify yourself when you enter the room.

12. To communicate with the speech impaired person, you should:
    a. Listen and give the person your full attention.
    b. Ask the person to repeat or rephrase, if necessary.
    c. Watch the persons lips move.
    d. All of the above.

13. To communicate with the hearing impaired person, you should:
    a. Approach the person from behind.
    b. Speak very loudly or shout to be heard.
    c. Speak clearly, distinctly, and slowly.
    d. All of the above.

14. Postoperative care after cataract surgery includes all of the following except:
    a. Remind the person not to rub the eye.
    b. Shower the person the day after surgery.
    c. Take care not to bump the eye.
    d. Keep the eye shield in place as directed.

</td></tr>
</table>

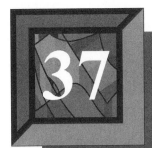

Caring for Mothers, Infants, and Children

Instructor's Preparation

I. Read Chapter 37 in the textbook. Carefully review chapter objectives, key terms, and review questions.

II. Read the outline in Chapter 37 of the instructor's guide. Carefully review the classroom activities, the student assignment, and the quiz.

III. If you are using the accompanying student workbook, review the activities for Chapter 37.

IV. Gather all necessary supplies and equipment for classroom activities and student assignments.

A. Prepare overhead transparencies.

B. Gather anatomical models.

C. Gather simulators.

D. Gather the necessary equipment and supplies needed to demonstrate and have each student in turn demonstrate the procedures in this chapter.

E. Gather any other items that will be needed for classroom activities.

F. Assemble items in the order they will be used.

V. Make sure that the necessary equipment is available and in good working order.

Objectives

- Define the key terms listed in this chapter
- List physical and emotional changes a new mother may experience
- Identify the signs and symptoms of postpartum complications
- Identify the signs and symptoms of illness in infants
- Describe how to hold and comfort infants
- List precautions that reduce the risk of sudden infant death syndrome (SIDS)
- Explain how to help mothers with breastfeeding and bottle-feeding
- Explain how to burp and diaper an infant
- Describe how to give cord and circumcision care
- Explain how to bathe infants
- Explain why infants are weighed
- Describe your role in providing childcare
- Learn the procedures described in this chapter

Key Terms

circumcision
episiotomy
lactation
lochia
mastitis
postpartum
postpartum blues
postpartum depression
postpartum psychosis
sudden infant death syndrome (SIDS)
umbilical cord

Outline

Caring for Mothers, Infants, and Children

I. INTRODUCTION
  A. Mothers and newborns usually stay in the hospital for only a short while
  B. When assisting a new mother, you usually do one or more of the following:
    1. Provide physical care for the mother
    2. Provide care for the newborn
    3. Help with childcare when other young children are in the home
    4. Help with home management tasks like meal preparation or housekeeping
  C. Some need home care
    1. Common reasons for home care include:
      a. Complications in the mother before or after childbirth
      b. Younger children in the home
      c. Multiple births
      d. Help with meals and housekeeping
      e. Physical or mental disability
  D. Babies are helpless; they depend on others for their basic needs
    1. A review of growth and development will help you care for newborns and infants (see Chapter 14)
II. CARE FOR NEW MOTHERS
  A. The postpartum period begins with the birth of the baby
    1. Ends 6 weeks later
    2. Mother's body returns to its normal state
    3. Mother adjusts physically and emotionally to childbirth
    4. Uterus returns almost to its prepregnant size
    5. If the mother does not breast-feed, menstruation starts within 3 to 8 weeks
      a. She can get pregnant again unless practicing birth control
  B. Because of the many changes the mother needs rest and recovery
    1. Encourage her to rest or nap when the baby is sleeping
    2. Encourage her to take time for herself and her partner
    3. She also has nutritional needs (see Chapter 25)
    4. Postpartum hemorrhage, infection, or other complications are possible
      a. Inform your supervisor immediately if you notice any of the signs or symp-

toms listed in Box 37-1, p. 607 in the textbook
  C. A vaginal discharge occurs during postpartum; it is called lochia
    1. Lochia changes color and decreases in amount
      a. Lochia rubra is a dark or bright-red discharge seen during the first 3 to 4 days
      b. Lochia serosa is a pinkish brown discharge that lasts until about 10 days after birth
      c. Lochia alba is a whitish drainage that continues for 2 to 6 weeks after birth
    2. Lochia increases with breast-feeding and activity
    3. Normally, it smells like menstrual flow
      a. Foul-smelling lochia is a sign of infection
  D. Perineal Care
    1. An episiotomy is an incision into the perineum
      a. The doctor performs this procedure to increase the size of the vaginal opening for delivery of the baby
    2. The doctor may order sitz baths or cold packs for comfort and hygiene (See Chapter 42)
      a. Practice Standard Precautions
    3. Complications can develop; infection and dehiscence
      a. Tell your supervisor if the mother complains of pain, discomfort, or discharge
  E. Care of abdominal incision
    1. The baby is delivered through an abdominal incision
    2. This is done when:
      a. The baby must be delivered to save the baby's or mother's life
      b. The baby is too large to pass through the birth canal
      c. The mother has a vaginal infection that could be transmitted to the baby
      d. A normal vaginal delivery would be difficult for the baby or mother
    3. The C-section incision needs to heal (see Chapter 41 for wound healing and wound care)
    4. Tell your supervisor if the mother complains of pain around the incision site
      a. Also report any bleeding, redness, swelling, or drainage from the incision

F. Breast care
1. Lactation (process of producing and secreting milk) usually begins around the third day after childbirth
2. The breasts may become engorged (overfilled); they become swollen, hard, and painful
3. Once breastfeeding is established or the milk dries up (if the mother chooses not to breastfeed), the engorgement decreases
4. Cold packs, warm showers, and a good nursing bra all help with comfort
5. Follow the care plan
6. Sometimes a milk duct can become plugged causing a tender lump
   a. If untreated a breast infection can occur
   b. Treatment usually involves:
      (1) Encouraging frequent nursing
      (2) Keeping pressure off the clogged duct—make sure clothing and bra are not too tight
      (3) Applying warm washcloths to the affected area or having warm showers to promote drainage
7. Mastitis (breast infection) occurs when bacteria enters a milk duct through a cracked nipple
8. Usually painful; early treatment is essential
9. Tell you supervisor as soon as signs and symptoms appear (see Box 37-2, p. 607)
10. Medications may be ordered and the mother will need bed rest
11. Breastfeeding is encouraged even from the affected breast

G. Postpartum blues, depression, and psychosis
1. Emotional changes occur during the postpartum period and can affect the mother's moods
   a. Other factors affecting moods can be:
      (1) Lack of sleep
      (2) More responsibilities
      (3) Isolation
      (4) Poor body image
      (5) Lack of support from spouse or partner
2. May contribute to feelings of sadness or mild depression during the first two weeks after childbirth
3. Common symptoms can include:
   a. Insomnia
   b. Mood changes
   c. Weepiness
   d. Fatigue
   e. Headaches
   f. Poor concentration
   g. Feelings of sadness, anger or anxiety.
4. Health Canada estimates up to 80% of women are affected
5. Symptoms usually disappear without treatment after 1 or 2 weeks
6. Some women (10–20%) suffer postpartum depression
   a. Major depression, which can occur any time within the first year after childbirth
   b. Professional care is needed, as it can become worse
7. Postpartum psychosis is a rare severe form of depression, which affects 1% of women
   a. Mother loses touch with reality
8. She has delusions, hallucinations or suicidal thoughts (see Chapter 33)
9. She could harm or neglect her child
10. Tell your supervisor immediately if the mother shows any of the signs or symptoms listed in Box 37-3, p. 608 in the textbook

III. CARING FOR INFANTS
A. Babies cannot protect themselves
B. They need to feel safe and secure
C. Babies cry to communicate
1. When wet, hungry, hot or cold, tired, uncomfortable, or in pain
2. Responding to their cries promotes safety and security (see Box 37-5, p. 610)
D. Infant safety is discussed in Chapter 16 in the textbook
E. Signs and symptoms of illness
1. Your observations are important; babies can become ill quickly
2. Box 37-4, p. 608 in the textbook, lists the signs and symptoms to report to your supervisor immediately
   a. Tell your supervisor when a sign or symptom begins
3. You may need to take vital signs
   a. Axillary temperatures are taken on infants (see Chapter 40)
   b. Your supervisor tells you the method to use for a child younger than 5 years of age
      (1) Tympanic or axillary
   c. Apical pulses are taken on infants and

young children
F. Holding an infant
   1. Use both hands to lift a newborn
   2. Always handle the baby with gentle, smooth movements
   3. Avoid sudden or jerking movements as they may startle or upset the baby
   4. For the first 3 months, always support the head and neck when lifting and holding babies as they have weak neck muscles
   5. Also support the whole body
   6. Figure 37-1, p. 607 in the textbook, shows how to hold a baby
G. Comforting a crying infant
   1. Infants cry to communicate when they are wet, hot, cold, tired, uncomfortable, in pain, over stimulated, or lonely
   2. Responding to their cries helps them feel safe and secure
   3. Ask the mother how she soothes the baby
   4. Follow the guidelines listed in Box 37-5, p. 610 in the textbook
   5. Tell your supervisor if the baby cannot be comforted.
H. Laying the infant down
   1. Safety precautions must be taken to lower the risk of sudden infant death syndrome (SIDS) which is the sudden, unexplained death of an apparently healthy infant under the age of 1 year
      a. Usually occurs while the infant is sleeping
      b. Always remember the following:
         (1) Always lay babies on their backs for sleep
         (2) If the infant has a medical condition requiring them to sleep on their stomach check with your supervisor and the care plan
         (3) Do not lay the baby on soft bedding products such as pillows, quilts, or fluffy or plush products
            (a) Can cause pools or carbon dioxide around baby's head and cause SIDS
            (b) Soft bedding can also cause suffocation
         (4) Make sure the baby is warm but never hot
            (a) Overheating may cause SIDS
            (b) Use a lightweight blanket that can be added or removed depending on temperature

      (c) Check if the baby is too hot; place your hand on the back of the neck; if it is sweaty, the baby is too warm
IV. HELPING MOTHERS BREAST-FEED
   A. Breast-fed babies are fed on demand (when hungry), not on a schedule
      1. They usually nurse every 2 or 3 hours
   B. At first, babies nurse for a short time; eventually for up to 30 minutes
   C. Nurses help new mothers learn to breast feed
      1. They also teach breast care
   D. If the mother or the baby is having a problem, you must tell the nurse
   E. You may help get the mother ready for breast-feeding
   F. You may bring the baby to the mother
      1. When you leave the room, make sure the signal light is within reach
   G. Some mothers want privacy; others want you to stay; ask their preference
   H. Box 37-6, p. 610 in the textbook, describes how you can help with breast-feeding
V. HELPING MOTHERS BOTTLE-FEED
   A. Formula is given to babies who are not breast-fed
      1. It provides essential nutrients needed by the infant
      2. Formula comes in three forms:
         a. Ready-to-feed (see Figure 37-3, p. 611)
         b. Powdered formula
         c. Concentrated formula
            (1) Follow container directions
   B. Bottles are prepared one at a time or in batches for the whole day
      1. Extra bottles are capped and stored in the refrigerator (to be used within 24 hours)
   C. Babies must be protected from infection
      1. Bottles, caps, and nipples must be as clean as possible
      2. Disposable equipment is used in the hospital
      3. Reusable equipment may be used in the home
         a. Must be washed in hot, soapy water or in a dishwasher
            (1) Complete rinsing is needed
      4. Some mothers use disposable plastic liners
         a. They are used once and discarded
   D. Bottle-Feeding Equipment ▶ p. 611
   E. Feeding the baby

1. Babies want to be fed every 3 to 4 hours
2. The amount of formula increases as the baby grows older
3. The baby stops sucking and turns away from the bottle when satisfied
4. Babies are not given cold formula
   a. Warm the bottle in a pan of warm water
   b. Test the temperature on the inside of your wrist (see Figure 37-7, p. 612)
   c. Do not set bottles out to warm at room temperature (microbes grow)
   d. Do not heat formula in microwave ovens; they can heat unevenly and burn the baby's mouth
5. Follow the guidelines in Box 37-7, p. 612 in the textbook, for help in bottle-feeding babies

VI. BURPING THE BABY
   A. Babies take in air when they nurse
      1. Air in the stomach and intestines causes cramping and discomfort
      2. Burps help get rid of air
   B. There are two positions for burping (see Figure 37-10, p. 613):
      1. Hold the infant over your shoulder
         a. Place a clean diaper or towel on your shoulder to protect clothing from spit-ups
      2. Support the baby in a sitting position on your lap
         a. Hold the towel or diaper in front of the baby
   C. Gently pat or rub the baby's back with circular motions for 2 to 3 minutes

VII. DIAPERING
   A. Babies urinate several times a day
   B. Breast-fed babies usually have bowel movements after feedings
      1. Bottle-fed babies may have three bowel movements per day
   C. Stools are usually soft and unformed
      1. Report hard, formed stools to the nurse immediately
      2. Watery, diarrhea stools are also reported to your supervisor immediately
         a. Diarrhea is very serious in infants
         b. Their water balance can be upset quickly (see Chapter 25)
   D. Diapers are changed when wet or soiled; cloth and disposable diapers are available
      1. Cloth diapers are washed daily or every 2 days with laundry detergent made espe-

cially for babies
      2. If possible, hang diapers outside to dry
      3. Cloth diapers are available with Velcro fasteners; this avoids pin sticks
      4. Disposable diapers are placed in the trash
         a. Do not flush down the toilet
   E. Changing diapers often helps prevent diaper rash
      1. Make sure the baby is clean and dry before applying a clean diaper
      2. If a diaper rash develops, tell the nurse immediately
   F. Diapering a Baby ▶ 614

VIII. CARE OF THE UMBILICAL CORD
   A. The umbilical cord connects the mother and fetus (see Figure 37-14, p. 617)
      1. It carries blood, oxygen, and nutrients from the mother to the fetus
      2. It is not needed after birth; the doctor cuts the cord; a stump is left
         a. The stump dries up and falls off in 7 to 10 days
   B. The cord provides an area for growth of microbes
      1. You need to keep it clean and dry
   C. Cord care is done with each diaper change; continue for 1 to 2 days after the cord falls off
   D. Care consists of the following:
      1. Keep the stump dry
      2. Wipe the base of the stump with a cotton ball moistened with warm water (see Figure 37-15, p. 617)
      3. Keep the diaper below the cord (see Figure 37-13, p. 616)
      4. Report any signs of infection
      5. Give sponge baths until the cord falls off
      6. Do not pull the cord off

IX. CIRCUMCISION
   A. Boys are born with foreskin on the penis
      1. The surgical removal of the foreskin is called circumcision
   B. The procedure allows for good hygiene and is thought to prevent cancer of the penis
   C. Usually done in the hospital before the baby goes home
   D. It is a religious ceremony in the Jewish faith
   E. After circumcision, check carefully for signs of bleeding or infection
   F. The area should completely heal in 10 to 14 days
   G. Care involves the following:
      1. The penis is thoroughly cleaned at each

diaper change
   a. Mild soap and water or commercial
      wipes are used
2. The diaper is loosely applied
3. Some doctors advise applying petroleum
   jelly to the penis (see Figure 37-16, p.
   617)
   a. Use a cotton swab to apply
4. Your supervisor tells you if other measures are needed

X. BATHING AN INFANT
   A. Important for cleanliness
   B. Baths comfort and relax
   C. Baths provide time to hold, touch, and talk to
      babies
      1. Helps babies learn safety, security, love,
         and belonging
   D. Planning is an important part of the bath
      1. You cannot leave the baby alone
      2. You need to gather equipment and sup-
         plies before you start
      3. Everything you need must be within your
         reach
   E. Safety measures:
      1. Never leave the baby alone
      2. Always keep one hand on the baby
      3. Hold the baby securely throughout the
         bath
      4. Room temperature should be 24°-27° C
         for the bath
      5. Water temperature needs special attention
         a. Bath water should be 37.7°-40.5° C
            (100°-105° F)
         b. If a thermometer is not available, test
            the temperature with the inside of your
            wrist; the water should feel warm and
            comfortable
   F. Giving a Baby a Sponge Bath ▶ p. 619
      1. Sponge baths are given until the cord
         falls off; the cord must not get wet
   G. Giving a Baby a Tub Bath ▶ p. 621

XI. NAIL CARE
   A. The baby's fingernails and toenails are kept
      short
      1. This prevents the baby from scratching
   B. Nails are best cut when the baby is sleeping
      1. The baby is quiet and will not squirm and
         fuss
   C. Use nail clippers or file with an emery board
      1. Clip nails straight across (see Figure 28-
         7, p. 447)

XII. WEIGHING INFANTS
   A. Infants are weighed at birth

1. Provides a baseline for measuring the infant's growth
B. Your supervisor tells you when to weigh the
   baby
C. You must meet the baby's safety needs
   1. Protect the baby from chills
   2. Keep the room warm and free of drafts
   3. Always keep a hand over the baby to pre-
      vent falls
D. Weighing an Infant ▶ p.622

XIII. CARING FOR CHILDREN
   A. Support workers sometimes care for children,
      help parents of newborns care for other chil-
      dren in the home, or care for sick or disabled
      children
      1. Review stages of growth and develop-
         ment in Chapter 14.
      2. Remember that children have rights too
      3. See Providing Compassionalte Care box,
         p. 623
   B. Discipline
      1. Discipline is the system of rules that gov-
         erns how we act
      2. Positive way of teaching behaviour
      3. Sets limits and provides guidelines
      4. Should be consistent
      5. Recognize the child's efforts when he or
         she tries to follow rules
      6. Be positive
      7. Your role in disciplining the child is to:
         a. Know the rules of acceptable behav-
            iour
         b. Ask an appropriate family member to
            clarify if unsure
         c. Reinforce existing rules
         d. Be consistent
         e. Praise the child's efforts
   C. Punishment
      1. A harsh response that occurs when a dis-
         cipline rule is broken
      2. Punishing a child is *not* your responsi-
         bility
      3. If asked by a family member to carry out
         punishment, explain it is not your
         agency's policy to do so
      4. Contact your supervisor if necessary and
         record the information
   D. Your role
      1. To provide a stable, secure, and safe at-
         mosphere
      2. Your responsibilities vary; usually in-
         clude the following:
         a. Developing positive relationship with

all family members
  b. Maintaining the existing rules of behaviour
  c. Maintaining daily routines
  d. Being alert to situations that may cause harm (see Box 37-8, p. 624)
  3. Box 37-9, p. 624 in the textbook, lists guidelines for caring for children in the home

Classroom Activities

1. Review growth and development of newborns and infants (see Chapter 14).

2. Using the round table discussion format, ask students to share any personal experience caring for newborns and infants.
  a. Ask students what new information they received by reading this chapter.

3. Write on the chalkboard: "Babies can become ill quickly." Then ask students what signs and symptoms to report to the nurse immediately.
  a. Write the correct answers on the chalkboard.

4. Display the information in Box 37-6, p. 610 in the textbook, on an overhead transparency. Use this as a basis to discuss how students will help with breast-feeding.
  a. Allow time for questions and discussion.

5. Provide the equipment and supplies needed for bottle-feeding babies. Have students handle and manipulate these items.

6. Provide concentrated and powdered formulas. Have each student practice preparing these for bottle-feeding.

7. Using an anatomically correct doll, demonstrate care of the umbilical cord and care of the circumcision. Have each student practice cord care and circumcision care.

8. Write on the chalkboard: "Safety Measures for Bathing an Infant:"
  a. Call on students to identify the safety measures. Write the correct answers on the chalkboard.

9. Call on students to discuss the safety measures used when providing nail care to infants.

10. Use the procedure checklists provided.
  a. Demonstrate each procedure in this chapter.
  b. Have each student practice and return demonstrate each procedure in this chapter. Use simulators and anatomical models when appropriate.

11. Discuss the importance of using Standard Precautions when providing perineal to the mother.

12. Write on the chalkboard: "The mother has emotional reactions after childbirth." Then call on students to come forward and write the causes of mood swings on the chalkboard.
  a. Allow time for discussion.

13. Ask students to share any personal experiences with childbirth and caring for newborns.
  a. They can discuss changes in life-style for the mother, father, and any siblings.
  b. How were the basic needs of the mother and the infant met?
  c. What support systems were in place.

Homework Assignments

Ask students to answer the questions at the end of Chapter 37 in the textbook. Tell students the date and time that this assignment must be completed and turned in.

If the accompanying workbook is being used, assign the Chapter 37 workbook exercises. Tell students the date and time that this assignment must be completed and turned in.

Name _____

Date _____

Caring for Mothers, Infants, and Children

Write your answers in the spaces provided.

1. Babies become ill quickly. You must report to your supervisor immediately if the baby:

   a. _____

   b. _____

   c. _____

   d. _____

   e. _____

   f. _____

   g. _____

   h. _____

   i. _____

   j. _____

   k. _____

   l. _____

   m. _____

   n. _____

   o. _____

   p. _____

2. What are the signs and symptoms of postpartum complications?

   a. _____

   b. _____

   c. _____

   d. _____

   e. _____

   f. _____

   g. _____

   h. _____

   i. _____

   j. _____

   k. _____

3. A cesarean section is done when:

   a. _____

   _____

   b. _____

   _____

   c. _____

   _____

   d. _____

   _____

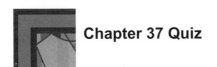
Name _____

Date _____

Caring for Mothers, Infants, and Children

True or False

*Mark **T** for true or **F** for false.*

1. _____ Responding to a baby's cries spoils the baby.

2. _____ Babies feel secure when wrapped and held snugly.

3. _____ Radial pulses are taken on infants and young children.

4. _____ Use both hands to lift a newborn.

5. _____ Do not leave a baby unattended on a table, bed, sofa, high chair, or other high surface.

6. _____ Put pillows, quilts, and soft toys in cribs for comfort.

7. _____ Notify your supervisor immediately if a baby is flushed, pale, or perspiring.

8. _____ Breast-fed babies are fed on an every-two-hour schedule.

9. _____ You have finished bottle feeding a baby. The formula remaining in the bottle is stored in the refrigerator.

10. _____ To burp the baby, gently pat or rub the baby's back with circular motions.

11. _____ Tell your supervisor immediately if you suspect that the baby has diarrhea.

12. _____ Changing diapers often helps prevent diaper rash.

13. _____ Water temperature for giving the baby a bath should be 105° F to 108° F.

14. _____ A sponge bath is given until the cord stump falls off.

15. _____ Use a cuticle scissors to cut the baby's fingernails.

16. _____ When weighing infants, keep the room warm and free of drafts.

17. _____ Postpartum means after childbirth.

18. _____ A vaginal discharge during the postpartum period is a sign of infection.

19. _____ The mother has emotional reactions to childbirth.

20. _____ You should give advice about parenting to the new mother.

Multiple Choice

Circle the BEST answer.

21. Which action does not promote infant safety?
    a. Holding the baby using the football hold
    b. Shaking powder directly over the baby
    c. Using safety straps for the baby's infant seat
    d. Laying babies on their backs or in the side-lying position for sleep

22. If a mother is having problems breast-feeding, you must:
    a. Reassure the mother that everything will be okay.
    b. Take the baby away and have the mother try later.
    c. Call your supervisor.
    d. Do nothing. The baby will eat when he or she is hungry.

23. Which action is correct when bottle feeding the baby?
    a. Hold the baby close to you and relax.
    b. Prop the bottle and lay the baby down.
    c. Leave the baby alone with the bottle.
    d. Burp the baby every 10 minutes.

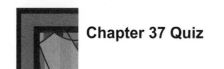

Name _____

Date _____

Caring for Mothers, Infants, and Children

24. Which is incorrect when giving cord care?
    a. Keep the diaper below the cord.
    b. Keep the stump moist.
    c. Report any signs of infection.
    d. Give a sponge bath until the stump falls off.

25. A pinkish-brown vaginal drainage that lasts for about 10 days after birth is called:
    a. Lochia serosa.
    b. Cesarean.
    c. Lochia rubra.
    d. Lochia alba.

Developmental Disabilities

Instructor's Preparation

I. Read Chapter 38 in the textbook. Carefully review chapter objectives, key terms, and review questions.

II. Read the outline in Chapter 38 of the instructor's guide. Carefully review the classroom activities, the student assignment, and the quiz.

III. If you are using the accompanying student workbook, review the activities for Chapter 38.

IV. Gather all necessary supplies and equipment for classroom activities and student assignments.
   A. Prepare the correct number of handouts
   B. Prepare situation/index cards
   C. Gather any other items that will be needed for classroom activities
   D. Assemble items in the order they will be used

V. Make sure that the necessary equipment is available and in good working order.

VI. Contact guest speakers to confirm the day, date, time, and location that they are expected.
   A. Ask the speakers if they require any special equipment or supplies; ensure these are available.

Objectives

- Define the key terms listed in this chapter
- Identify the areas of function limited by a developmental disability
- Explain how a developmental disability affects the child and family across the life span
- Explain when developmental disabilities occur and their causes
- Explain how various developmental disabilities affect functioning

Key Terms

autism
cerebral palsy (CP)
cognitive disability
congenital
convulsion
developmental disability
diplegia
down syndrome
epilepsy
fetal alcohol effect (FAE)
fetal alcohol syndrome (FAS)
intellectual disability
seizure
spastic
spina bifida
tonic-clonic seizure

Outline

Developmental Disabilities

I. INTRODUCTION
   A. A developmental disability occurs before birth, at birth, or during childhood or adolescence.
      1. It impairs the child's development
      2. It is often severe and is always permanent, so people of all ages can have developmental disabilities
      3. The person's ability to function is limited in at least three of the following areas:
         a. Self-care
         b. Understanding and expressing language
         c. Learning
         d. Mobility
         e. Self-direction
         f. The ability to live independently
         g. Economic self-sufficiency
      4. The person needs lifelong assistance, support, and special services
II. DEVELOPMENTAL DISABILITIES AND THE FAMILY
   A. Some families may be adjusting to the news of a child's disability and may still be working out new roles and routines while others may already have routines
      1. Remember, every family situation is different and can cause stress
   B. Primary caregivers require great amounts of time, energy, and work
      1. Need to balance other responsibilities
      2. May experience stigma associated with the child's disability
      3. Are unable to spend time alone with other family members
      4. May be unable to leave the child alone
   C. The caregiver can become physically and emotionally exhausted which could lead to burnout (see Chapter 8)
   D. Home care and other community agencies often provide support and services
   E. Support workers work closely with the family and may provide direct care to the child, help with household chores so parents can care for the child, accompany the child to school (see Figure 38-1, p. 628), or work with the child in school
   F. As child and parents age, it becomes more difficult for caregiver to continue, but the person still needs care
   G. Some adolescents and adults live in community, residential settings, own home, group homes, or specialty licensed long-term care facilities
   H. Staff need special training to care for these clients
   I. Family will, in most cases, still be involved in care
      1. Remember, they know the person's condition and have cared for them most of their lives
III. TYPES OF DEVELOPMENTAL DISABILITIES
   A. Conditions that commonly involve developmental disabilities include:
      1. Intellectual disability
      2. Down syndrome
      3. Cerebral palsy
      4. Autism
      5. Epilepsy
      6. Spina bifida
      7. Fetal alcohol syndrome
      8. Other conditions (see Box 38-1, p. 629)
   B. Intellectual disability
      1. Is an impaired ability to learning
         a. Person can learn but at a slower rate
         b. Often have difficulties with communication, self-care, and social interaction
         c. Once called mental retardation, the term is no longer used in Canada
      2. Can be caused by any genetic abnormality, injury, or disease that impairs development of the brain
      3. See Box 38-1, p. 630 in the textbook, for common causes
      4. May also have other disabilities
      5. Range from mild to severe
         a. Average person's IQ ranges 90 – 100
         b. People with IQ between 70 and 55 are mildly disabled; may be slow to learn and can function in society with some support
         c. People with IQ below 55 are moderately disabled and need daily support at home or work
         d. People with IQ below 25 are severely disabled and need constant support in all areas
      6. The Canadian Association for Community Living is a national organization dedicated to people with intellectual disabilities and their families

a. Their goal is to ensure that people with intellectual disabilities have opportunities to live meaningful, dignified lives

b. Should be allowed to participate in all aspects of community living

c. Should live in families and be integrated into regular schools whenever possible

d. Should play with others with and without disabilities

e. Adults should have the right to control their lives to the fullest extent possible

f. Remember, they have sexual, emotional and social needs and desires, and have the right to privacy and to love and be loved

g. Some adults have life partners; others marry and have children

h. Most can control sexual urges, but some cannot (see Chapter 19 for information on dealing with sexually aggressive clients)

i. Are vulnerable to sexual abuse; report signs immediately (see Chapter 19)

j. Children need to learn about sexual abuse, safe sex, and other sexuality issues

C. Down syndrome

1. Most commonly caused by an extra 21st chromosome
2. In Canada, 14 out of 10 000 births have DS
3. Causes some degree of intellectual disability
4. The child has certain physical characteristics (see Figure 38-2, p. 630)
   a. Oval-shaped eyes slanted upward
   b. Short, wide neck
   c. Large tongue
   d. Wide, flat nose
   e. Small ears
   f. Short stature
   g. Short, wide hands with stubby fingers
   h. Small head
   i. Flat face
   j. Weak muscle tone
5. Many children with Down syndrome have heart defects
   a. They tend to have vision and hearing problems
   b. They are at risk for other health problems

6. Children and adults need speech/language, physical, and occupational therapies
   a. Most can learn self-care skills
7. They need health and sex education
8. A well-balanced diet and exercise are needed

D. Cerebral palsy (CP)

1. Disorder affecting muscle control
2. Depending on which area of the brain is affected one or more of the following may occur:
   a. Involuntary movements
   b. Poor coordination and posture
   c. Muscle weakness
   d. Difficulty or inability to walk
   e. Difficulty or inability to speak
3. Caused by a defect in the motor region of the brain
   a. Results from brain damage that occurs before, during, or shortly after birth
   b. Lack of oxygen to the brain is the usual cause
4. Infants at risk include:
   a. Premature infants
   b. Low-birth weight infants
   c. Infants who do not cry in the first 5 minutes after delivery
   d. Infants who require mechanical ventilation
   e. Infants who have bleeding in the brain
   f. Infants with congenital heart, kidney, or spinal cord defects
   g. Infants with seizure activity
   h. Have blood problems
5. Acquired brain injury in infancy and early childhood also can result in CP (see Table 38-1, p. 629)
6. CP affects body movements and body parts
   a. Types:
      (1) Spastic—uncontrolled contractions of skeletal muscles (most common)
         (a) The muscles cannot relax
         (b) Posture, balance, and movement are affected
         (c) Hand skills are also affected
      (2) Athetoid—the person cannot control muscle movements
         (a) The person has continuous slow, weaving, or writhing motions of the trunk, arms,

and legs
            (i) Tongue, face, and neck
                muscles may be involved
        (3) Ataxic cerebral palsy—weak
            muscle tone and difficulties in
            coordination and movement
            (a) Person appears unsteady and
                shaky and may have trouble
                balancing
            (b) May be very unsteady when
                walking
    b. Terms used to describe the body parts
       involved (see Chapter 31)
        (1) Hemiplegia—affects one side of
            the body; the other side functions
            normally
        (2) Diplegia—affects corresponding
            parts; in most cases, both legs are
            affected and the upper body is
            normal
        (3) Quadriplegia—affects all four
            limbs; the person can't walk or
            use their arms, and may have dif-
            ficulty moving the face and trunk
7. The person with CP can have other im-
   pairments including:
    a. Intellectual disability
    b. Learning disabilities
    c. Hearing and vision impairments
    d. Drooling
    e. Constipation
    f. siezures
    g. Dysphagia
    h. Speech impairments
    i. Attention deficit hyperactivity dis-
       order
    j. Bladder and bowel impairments
    k. Breathing problems from poor posture
    l. Pressure ulcers from immobility
E. Autism
    1. A brain disorder that impairs communica-
       tion, social skills, and behaviour
    2. Extreme difficulties relating to others
    3. In Canada, about 1 in 200 children are af-
       fected
    4. Most common brain disorder affecting
       children; affects boys more than girls
    5. Begins in early childhood—between 18
       months and 3 years of age
    6. Brain function is affected
        a. Reasoning, social interactions, verbal
           and nonverbal communication skills,
           and play activities are impaired

7. The following behaviors are common:
    a. Slow language development
    b. Repeats words, phrases, and/or body
       movements
    c. Does not like to cuddle
    d. Short attention span
    e. Spends time alone
    f. Little or no eye contact
    g. Overreacts to touch and noise
    h. Little reaction to pain
    i. Frequent tantrums
    j. Strong attachment to a single item,
       idea, activity, or person
    k. Needs routines
    l. No fear of danger
    m. Does not respond to others
    n. Very active or very quiet
    o. Aggressive or violent behavior (may
       injure self)
8. Has no cure
    a. Many therapies are used to help the
       person
        (1) Behaviour modification—posi-
            tive behaviours are rewarded and
            negative behaviours are corrected
        (2) Speech and language therapy
        (3) Music, auditory, recreation, and
            sensory therapies
        (4) Occupational therapy
        (5) Medication therapy
        (6) Diet therapy
9. Some adults work and live independently,
   others continue to need support and assistance, and some live in group homes or
   residential care centers
10. Persons with autism may have other dis-
    orders and disabilities
    a. Intellectual disability and epilepsy are
       common
    b. Strict routines are important to chil-
       dren and adults with autism
    c. Follow the routines whenever possible
       as they can become upset if changed
    d. Always warn the person if routine
       must be changed
    e. Children require constant supervision;
       never leave them unattended
    f. Follow the care plan
F. Epilepsy
    1. A condition characterized by recurrent
       seizures (a brief disturbance in the brain's
       normal electrical function) that affects
       awareness, movement, and/or sensation

2. Several types of seizures:
   a. Generalized—affect the whole brain, reactions vary according to which part of the brain is affected
   b. Partial seizures—affect only one part of the brain
   c. Tonic-clonic seizures involve convulsions:
      (1) A violent and sudden contractions or tremors of muscle groups
      (2) Person loses consciousness and falls to the floor
      (3) All muscle groups contract and relax causing jerking and twitching movements
      (4) Urinary and bowel incontinence may occur
      (5) Usually lasts 1 – 7 minutes
3. A single seizure does not mean a person has epilepsy
4. Often the cause is not known
   a. See Box 38-1, p. 630 in the textbook, for known causes
5. Children and young adults are commonly affected
   a. It can develop at any time
6. It often occurs with other problems affecting the brain (i.e., ABI, tumors)
7. It has no known cure
8. Drugs are available to control or prevent seizures
9. When controlled, epilepsy usually does not interfere with learning and activities of daily living (ADL)
10. In severe cases, persons may have activity and job limits
11. Persons with epilepsy have an increased risk of death
    a. They have higher rates for suicide, sudden unexplained death syndrome, and accidental death
    b. See Chapter 47 for emergency care of persons having a seizure
G. Spina bifida
   1. A congenital defect of the spinal column
      a. These are congenital conditions that involve the incomplete development of the brain, spinal cord and protective coverings for these organs.
         (1) Neural tube defects occur during the first few months of pregnancy
         (2) Consuming sufficient folic acid before conception and during early pregnancy reduces the risk of having a baby with neural tube defects (see Chapter 25)
      b. The bones of the vertebrae do not form properly
         (1) A split in the vertebrae leaves the spinal cord unprotected
         (2) Only membrane covers the spinal cord
         (3) Nerve damage occurs; the affected body part does not function properly
         (4) Paralysis can occur
         (5) Bowel and bladder problems are common
         (6) Infection is a threat
      c. The lower back is the most common site
   2. Different types include:
      a. Spina bifida occulta—the vertebrae are closed; there is a defect in the vertebrae closure
         (1) The spinal cord and nerves are normal
         (2) Often the person has no symptoms
         (3) Foot weakness and bowel and bladder problems can occur
         (4) Person may have dimple or tuft of hair on back (see Figure 38-3, p. 633)
      b. Spina bifida cystica—part of the spinal column is contained in a pouch or sac
         (1) A membrane or thin layer of skin covers the sac
         (2) The pouch is easily injured
         (3) Infection is a threat
         (4) Two types (see Figure 38-4, p. 633):
            (a) Meningocele—the sac contains meninges and cerebrospinal fluid
               (i) The sac does not contain nerve tissue
               (ii) Spinal cord and nerves are usually normal
               (iii) The defect is corrected with surgery
               (iv) The sac protrudes from spine (see Figure 38-4 A and Figure 38-5, p. 633)

(b) Myelomeningocele—the pouch contains nerves and spinal cord, meninges, and cerebrospinal fluid (see Figure 38-4 B, p. 633)

    (i) Nerve damage occurs

    (ii) Loss of function occurs below the level of nerve damage

    (iii) The defect is closed with surgery

    (iv) Some children learn to walk with braces or crutches; others use a wheelchair

c. Many have other problems or conditions (e.g., learning problems, attention, language, reading, and math)

d. They are at risk for obesity, GI disorders, mobility problems, skin breakdown, depression, and social, emotional, and sexual issues

e. Hydrocephalus often occurs with certain types of spina bifida (see Table 38-1 pg. 629)

H. Fetal alcohol syndrome

1. A group of physical and mental abnormalities in a child as a result of alcohol consumption by the mother during pregnancy

a. In Canada, one child is born with FAS every day

b. Most common preventable developmental disability

2. The child/person may have any or all of the following problems:

a. Low birth weight, weak muscle tone, and poor weight gain

b. Heart problems, hearing loss, and abnormalities of the spine and joints

c. Characteristic facial features, including an abnormally small head, small eye openings, thin upper lip, and a small chin

d. Usually has intellectual disability

e. May have behaviour, leaning, and emotional problems

f. Older children and adults often have memory problems, poor judgement, daily living skills, poor social skills, or trouble handling anger

g. Many adolescents drop out of school and commit criminal acts

h. Fetal alcohol effect (FAE) is a milder form with similar symptoms but to a lesser degree

IV. CARING FOR CLIENTS WITH DEVELOPMENTAL DISABILITIES

A. Clients often have complicated care needs especially if the disability is severe

B. You must be familiar with special equipment and self-care devices and follow the care plan

1. Check with your supervisor if you have any questions

C. Remember to consider the person before the disability

D. People with developmental disabilities have the same right and needs as everyone else

1. Each person is unique

2. Effects of the disability vary

3. Your supervisor and the care plan tell you how to best meet each client's needs

4. See Providing Compassionate Care box, p. 635 in the textbook

Classroom Activities

1. Call on students to define the term "developmental disability".

a. Ask students to discuss any feelings they have about caring for persons with developmental disabilities. Discuss how their feelings can impact the care they provide.

2. Write each of the following terms on a separate index card: Intellectual Disability, Down syndrome, Cerebral palsy, Autism, Epilepsy, Spina bifida, and Fetal Alcohol Syndrome.

a. Divide students into pairs or groups of three. Provide each pair or group with several sheets of notebook paper

b. Distribute one index card to each pair or group. Ask students to provide the following information about the term on their index card:

    (1) Definition

    (2) Causes of the disability

    (3) Characteristics of the disability

    (4) Special needs

    (5) Agencies that protect persons' rights

Allow 20 minutes for this exercise. Then call on one student from each pair or group to report to the class. Allow time after presentation for questions and discussion.

3. Provide information and brochures to students about programs and services available for persons

with developmental disabilities in their community.
a. Use a round table discussion format to share and discuss the programs and services.

4. Identify facilities in your community that provide care to persons with developmental disabilities. Arrange for a member of the health care team to visit the class. The presentation should include:
a. What special training is required for staff.
b. What special programs, activities, and services are provided.
c. How the family is involved in the person's care.

Ask students to write key points in a notebook for future reference. Allow time for questions and discussion.

5. Arrange for a representative from the school system to talk to the class about any special programs within the school system designed to meet the needs of developmentally disabled persons.
a. Provide brochures and handouts to enhance the learning experience.
b. Allow time for questions and discussion.

Homework Assignments

Ask students to answer the questions at the end of Chapter 38 in the textbook. Tell students the date and time that this assignment must be completed and turned in.

If the accompanying student workbook is being used, assign the Chapter 38 workbook exercises. Tell students the date and time that this assignment must be completed and turned in.

Chapter 38 Student Assignment   Name _____

Date _____

Developmental Disabilities

Write your answers in the blanks provided.

1. Conditions that commonly involve developmental disabilities include:

   a. _____

   b. _____

   c. _____

   d. _____

   e. _____

   f. _____

2. Causes of intellectual disability after birth include:

   a. _____

   b. _____

   c. _____

   d. _____

   e. _____

   f. _____

   g. _____

3. a. Persons with developmental disabilities have the same rights as _____
   _____

308

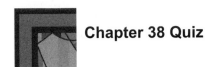

Name _____

Date _____

Developmental Disabilities

<table>
<tr><td>

True or False

Mark **T** *for true or* **F** *for false.*

1. _____ Some facilities admit developmentally disabled children and adults.

2. _____ Intellectual disabilities are always severe. Persons need constant support.

3. _____ Persons with intellectual disabilities do not have sexual urges.

4. _____ Persons with Down syndrome need speech/language, physical, and occupational therapies.

5. _____ Cerebral palsy affects body movements and body parts.

6. _____ Meningitis is the inflammation of the brain.

7. _____ Autism begins in early childhood.

8. _____ Epilepsy cannot be controlled. It always interferes with learning.

</td><td>

Multiple Choice

Circle the BEST answer.

9. A congenital defect of the spinal column is:
   a. A convulsion.
   b. Spina bifida.
   c. Hydrocephalus.
   d. Paralysis.

10. Spastic means:
    a. The person has intellectual disability.
    b. Continuous writhing motions of the trunk, arms, and legs.
    c. Uncontrolled contractions of the skeletal muscles.
    d. Paralysis of both arms and legs.

11. Which statement about autism is incorrect?
    a. Communication skills and play activities are impaired.
    b. Autism has no cure.
    c. Therapies are not effective to help the person control behaviors.
    d. The child with autism has difficulty relating to people.

12. A condition in which cerebrospinal fluid collects in and around the brain is called:
    a. Spina bifida occulta.
    b. Meningocele.
    c. Epilepsy.
    d. Hydrocephalus.

</td></tr>
</table>

39

Assisting with Medications

Instructor's Preparation

I. Read Chapter 39 in the textbook. Carefully review chapter objectives, key terms, and review questions.

II. Read the outline in Chapter 39 of the instructor's guide. Carefully review the classroom activities, the student assignment, and the quiz.

III. If you are using the accompanying student workbook, review the activities for Chapter 39.

IV. Gather all necessary supplies and equipment for classroom activities and student assignments.

A. Prepare the correct number of handouts

B. Prepare appropriate flip charts

C. Prepare overhead transparencies

D. Prepare situation/index cards

E. Gather correct slides

F. Gather coloured markers

G. Gather anatomical models

H. Gather simulators

I. Gather any other items that will be needed for classroom activities

J. Assemble items in the order they will be used

V. Make sure that the necessary equipment is available and in good working order.

VI. Contact guest speakers to confirm the day, date, time, and location that they are expected.

A. Ask the speakers if they require any special equipment or supplies; ensure these are available.

Objectives

- Define the key terms listed in this chapter
- Explain the difference between assisting with medications and administering medications
- Describe the different forms of medications
- Describe your role in assisting with medications
- List the five "rights" of assisting with medications
- Describe guidelines to follow when assisting with medications
- Learn the procedures described in this chapter

Key Terms

alternative remedies
medication
over-the-counter (OTC) medication
prescription (Rx) medication
side effect

Outline

Assisting with Medications

I. INTRODUCTION
  A. Medications are drugs and other substances used to prevent or treat disease or illness
  B. In community care, clients take their medications independently (self-directed medication management)
  C. Some clients will need assistance opening bottles or reading labels

II. ASSISTING VERSUS ADMINISTERING
  A. "Assist" means to help; "administer" means to give
  B. Assisting means helping clients self-medicate such as opening bottles
    1. Strictly a mechanical function where you assume the place of their hands or feet in order for them to obtain their medication
  C. Administering medication means to measure the medication and get it into the client
    1. This requires special judgement and knowledge
    2. This is beyond your scope of practice so NEVER assume this responsibility
  D. Some provinces and territories allow support workers to administer some forms of medication under certain conditions, but be sure this function is in your job description and that you have obtained the proper training and supervision
  E. A minor mistake with medication can cause serious harm to a client

III. TYPES OF MEDICATION
  A. Medications come in many forms (see Table 39-1, p. 639)
  B. Client's may take:
    1. Over-the-counter (OTC) medications
    2. Alternative remedies
    3. Prescription (Rx) medications
  C. You only assist with medications listed on the care plan
  D. If a client asks you to assist with medication not in the care plan, politely refuse
  E. If you are aware that your client is taking alternative medications inform your supervisor,
    1. Certain medications and alternative remedies can cause serious harm if mixed

IV. YOUR ROLE
  A. Your role in assisting with medication depends on your province or territory, your employer's policy, and your training and education

B. May involve one or more of the following:
  1. Reminding the client to take medication
  2. Bringing medication containers to the client
  3. Bringing pre-poured medications, pre-filled syringes, or pill boxes to the client
  4. Reading prescription labels to the client
  5. Loosening or removing container lids
  6. Checking dosage
  7. Providing water or other fluids
  8. Supervising the client pouring medication into hands, measuring spoon, or cup
  9. Steading the client's hand while pouring medication or administering eye drops

C. You are not responsible for monitoring the outcome of the drug therapy, but you must be observant and report any changes in the client's condition or behaviour

D. There might be side-effects (unwanted response to a medication)

E. The nurse or pharmacist will teach the client about their medication, desired effect, possible side effects, how and when to take medications, and other required instructions

F. Some clients store their medication in a pill box (see Figure 39-1, p. 640)

G. It is not your responsibility to fill the box; a nurse or family member does it

H. Documentation
  1. The client's medications and your responsibilities will be on the care plan
  2. A Medication Administration Record (MAR) lists the client's medications and serves as a record for actions taken (see Figure 39-2, p.642)
  3. In facilities, a nurse is responsible for signing the MAR sheets
  4. In the community, a MAR sheet is not always required
  5. If required, the MAR sheet is kept in the home
    a. Whoever administers the medications signs the sheet
    b. If the client takes the medication, they should sign; if unable to write, it may be your responsibility to sign for them
  6. Always follow your employer's policies and procedures

I. Understanding abbreviations
  1. Physicians, nurses, and pharmacists use many abbreviations
  2. The MAR sheets should present information as clearly as possible
  3. Table 39-2, p. 643 in the textbook, lists a

few common abbreviations (see Chapter 48 for more)
   4. If you are unsure of an abbreviation, make sure you check with your supervisor and never guess as this could result in serious harm to your client
V. THE FIVE "RIGHTS" OF ASSISTING WITH MEDICATIONS
   A. The right medication
      1. Read the label to ensure it is the right medication (see Figure 39-3, p. 643)
   B. The right person—follow your employer's policy
   C. The right dose—check the label for correct dose and make sure your client measures liquid medication the correct way
   D. The right route—oral, sublingual, topical, inhalant, parental
   E. The right time—the prescription label states how often the medication should be taken and any special instructions such as "on an empty stomach"
   F. If your client becomes confused about their medication, inform your supervisor, as the client may need a "refresher" on taking their medication
VI. ASSISTING WITH MEDICATIONS
   A. When assisting with medications, follow the guidelines listed in Box 39-2, p. 644 in the textbook, and check the care plan to see how much assistance is required
   B. Assisting with Medications ▶ p. 645

Classroom Activities

1. Write on the board OTC medications, alternative remedies, and Rx medications. Ask the class to list some examples of each type.

2. Collect MAR sheets from a variety of agencies and facilities. Distribute to the class and have them compare the differences.

3. On a transparency write the five "Rights" of assisting with medications. Expand on each of the rights.

4. Write the most common abbreviations on the board and ask the students the meaning of each.

5. If possible, collect examples of the different types of medications so that the students will become familiar with each type.

6. Ask the students to list examples of how they might assist clients with their medication.

Homework Assignments

Ask students to answer the questions at the end of Chapter 39 in the textbook. Tell students the date and time that this assignment must be completed and turned in.

If the accompanying workbook is being used, assign the Chapter 39 workbook exercises. Tell students the date and time that this assignment must be completed and turned in.

Name _____

Date _____

Assisting with Medications

Write your answers in the spaces provided.

1. List the five "Rights" of assisting with medications:

   a. _____

   b. _____

   c. _____

   d. _____

   e. _____

2. Drugs come in many forms. List five.

   a. _____

   b. _____

   c. _____

   d. _____

   e. _____

3. What information is always on a prescription label?

   a. _____

   b. _____

   c. _____

   d. _____

   e. _____

   f. _____

4. List the three things that are always listed on a MAR sheet.

   a. _____

   b. _____

   c. _____

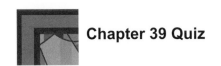

Chapter 39 Quiz

Name _____

Date _____

Assisting with Medications

True or False

Mark **T** *for true or* **F** *for false.*

1. _____ Oral medications should be taken with a small sip of water

2. _____ Read the label on the medication container once before administering the medication

3. _____ When one dose of medication is forgotten or omitted, it is OK for the client to take a double dose the next time.

4. _____ Pull the ear of the infant up and back when administering ear drops

5. _____ Clients place sublingual medication in their cheek

6. _____ When administering eye drops, place the drop in the lower conjunctival sac.

7. _____ The person who takes insulin needs to rotate the sites of injection.

Multiple Choice

Circle the BEST answer.

8. The five rights of assisting with medication does not include:
   a. route
   b. doctor
   c. dose
   d. person

9. The MAR sheet includes the following information
   a. expiration date
   b. pharmacy name
   c. file number
   d. client's name

10. A medication should be stored
    a. opened at the bedside
    b. in a warm, humid are
    c. with other family members' or residents' medication
    d. in its original labeled container

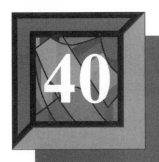

40

Measuring Height, Weight, and Vital Signs

Instructor's Preparation

I. Read Chapter 40 in the textbook. Carefully review chapter objectives, key terms, and review questions.

II. Read the outline in Chapter 40 of the instructor's guide. Carefully review the classroom activities, the student assignment, and the quiz.

III. If you are using the accompanying student workbook, review the activities for Chapter 40.

IV. Review video #9 (Measuring Temperature, Pulse, and Respirations) and video #10 (Measuring Blood Pressure) in Mosby's Nursing Assisting Video Series.

V. Gather all necessary supplies and equipment for classroom activities and student assignments.

   A. Prepare the correct number of handouts

   B. Prepare appropriate flip charts

   C. Prepare overhead transparencies

   D. Prepare situation/index cards

   E. Gather the correct videos

   F. Gather the following transparencies: TA49 through TA51

   G. Gather coloured markers

   H. Gather anatomical models

   I. Gather simulators

   J. Gather the necessary equipment and supplies needed to demonstrate and have each student return demonstrate the procedures in this chapter

   K. Gather any other items that will be needed for classroom activities

   L. Assemble items in the order they will be used

VI. Make sure that the necessary equipment is available and in good working order

Objectives

- Define the key terms listed in this chapter
- Explain how to measure height and weight
- Explain why vital signs are measured
- List the factors affecting vital signs
- Identify the normal ranges for the temperature sites
- Know when to use each temperature site
- Identify the sites for taking a pulse
- Describe normal respirations
- Describe the factors affecting blood pressure
- Describe the practices that are followed when measuring blood pressure
- Know the vital sign ranges for different age groups
- Learn the procedures described in this chapter

Key Terms

---

apical-radial pulse
blood pressure
body temperature
bradycardia
diastole
diastolic pressure
dysrythmia
hypertension
hypotension
pulse
pulse deficit
pulse rate
respiration
sphygmomanometer
stethoscope
systole
systolic pressure
tachycardia
vital signs

Outline

Measuring Height, Weight, and Vital Signs

I. INTRODUCTION
   A. The four vital signs of body function are temperature, pulse, respirations, and blood pressure

II. MEASURING HEIGHT AND WEIGHT
   A. Height and weight are measurured on admission to a facility
      1. Some clients are weighed daily, weekly, or monthly to monitor weight gain or loss
   B. Weigh client same time of day usually before breakfast
   C. Client wears only a gown or pajamas, no shoes or slippers, and should void before weighing to get an accurate weight
   D. See Figure 40-1, p. 653 in the textbook, for different types of scales
      1. Follow employer policy and manufacturer's instructions when using scales
   E. See Figure 40-2, p. 653 in the textbook, for guidelines on using mechanical scales
   F. Refer to Focus on Children box, p. 653 in the textbook
   G. Measuring Height and Weight ▶ p. 654

III. MEASURING AND REPORTING VITAL SIGNS
   A. Vital signs vary within certain limits during any 24-hour period
   B. Factors affecting vital signs include sleep, activity, eating, weather, noise, exercise, drugs,

anger, fear, anxiety and illness
   C. Vital signs
      1. Detect changes in normal body function
      2. Tell about a person's response to treatment
      3. Signal life-threatening events
      4. Are part of the assessment step of the nursing process
   D. Vital signs are measured:
      1. During physical examinations
      2. When a person is admitted to a health care agency
      3. Several times a day for hospital and subacute care patients
      4. Before and after surgery
      5. Before and after complex diagnostic procedures and tests
      6. After some nursing procedures
      7. When certain drugs are taken
      8. When the person complains of pain, fainting, shortness of breath, rapid heart rate, or not feeling well
      9. After a fall or injury
      10. As often as required by the client's condition
      11. As required by the care plan
   E. Vital signs show even minor changes in a person's condition
      1. Accuracy is essential in measuring, recording, and reporting
   F. Unless otherwise ordered, take vital signs with the person lying or sitting
   G. Immediately report to the nurse:
      1. Any vital sign that is a change from a previous measurement
      2. Vital signs above the normal range
      3. Vital signs below the normal range
   H. Follow agency policy for recording vital signs

IV. BODY TEMPERATURE
   A. The amount of heat in the body
      1. A balance between the amount of heat produced and the amount of heat lost
   B. Body temperature remains fairly stable
   C. Factors affecting body temperature include age, weather, exercise, pregnancy, the menstrual cycle, emotion, stress, and illness
   D. Normal body temperature
      1. Temperature is measured using the Fahrenheit (F) and Centigrade or Celsius (C) scales
      2. Common sites are the mouth, axilla, and ear
         a. Body temperature can also be measure in the rectum. Rarely used and if re-

quired it is done by a nurse or other regulated health care provider. Involves inserting an instrument into a body cavity which is not in your scope of practice; if you are delegated this procedure you need to be properly trained and supervised

   b. Normal temperature depends on the site (see Table 40-1, p. 658)

3. Thermometers are used to measure temperature

   a. Types include glass, disposable, electronic, and tympanic

4. Focus on older persons

   a. Older persons generally have lower body temperatures than younger adults

5. Focus on children

   a. Pacifier, thermometers are available

     (1) Used for children under age 5

     (2) Temperature is measured in about 5 minutes

     (3) See Focus On Children box, p. 661 in the textbook

E. Taking oral temperatures

1. Usually taken in older children and adults

2. Do not take an oral temperature if the person:

   a. Is unconscious

   b. Has had surgery or injury to the face, neck, nose, or mouth

   c. Is receiving oxygen

   d. Has a nasogastric tube

   e. Is delirious, restless, confused, or disoriented

   f. Has a sore mouth

   g. Has a history of convulsive disorders

3. Certain activities may temporarily affect oral temperatures, including:

   a. Eating hot or cold foods

   b. Drinking hot or cold fluids

   c. Smoking

   d. Chewing gum

4. Wait for 20 minutes if client has done any of these activities

5. Place thermometer under the client's tongue (see Figure 40-5, p. 658)

6. Tip of thermometer should be at the base of the tongue

7. Client should close lips around thermometer to hold in place

8. Remind the client not to bite down or talk

F. Tympanic membrane thermometers--special thermometers used for the ear (see Figure 40-6, p. 659)

1. Measure temperature at the tympanic membrane in the ear

2. The covered probe is gently inserted into the ear

3. Temperature is measured in 1 to 3 seconds

4. Battery operated and use disposable probes

   a. Must be kept charged

5. Comfortable for the person and are not invasive

6. Useful for children because of speed and comfort (see Focus on Children box, p. 659)

7. Risk of spreading infection is reduced

   a. Fewer microbes in the ear than in the mouth or rectum

8. Not used if there is drainage from the ear

9. Taking a tympanic membrane temperature (see Figure 40-7, p. 659)

G. Taking axillary temperatures

1. Less reliable than oral, rectal, or tympanic membrane temperatures

2. Used when other routes cannot be used

3. The axilla must be dry

4. The thermometer is held in place to maintain proper position (see Figure 40-8, p. 660)

H. Electronic thermometers

1. Battery operated

2. Measure temperature in a few seconds

3. The temperature is displayed on the front of the instrument

4. Have oral and rectal probes

   a. A disposable cover (sheath) covers the probe (see Figure 40-9, p. 660)

   b. Probe covers are used once and discarded; helps prevent the spread of microbes and infection

   c. Medical asepsis and standard precautions are followed

5. Taking a Temperature with an Electronic Thermometer ▶ p. 662

I. Dot matrix thermometers

1. Small chemical dots change color when heated by the body

2. Used only once

3. Measure temperature in 3 minutes

J. Glass thermometers

1. Glass thermometers are considered safety hazards and are now rarely used in any setting

2. The glass thermometer is a hollow tube with a mercury-filled bulb

   a. When heated, mercury expands and

rises in the tube; it contracts and
moves down when cooled
3. Glass thermometers are reusable
4. Disadvantages
   a. They take a long time to register—up
      to 10 minutes
   b. They break easily (mercury is a haz-
      ardous substance and could cause poi-
      soning)
5. How to read a glass thermometer
   a. Centigrade thermometer
      (1) Each long line represents one de-
          gree from 34° C to 42° C
      (2) Each short line represents 0.1
          (one-tenth) of a degree (see
          Figure 40-14, p. 664)
   b. Fahrenheit thermometers
      (1) Every other long line is marked
          in an even degree from 94° F to
          108° F
      (2) The short lines indicate 0.2 (two-
          tenths) of a degree (see Figure
          40-14, p. 664)
   c. To read a glass thermometer, do the
      following:
      (1) Hold the thermometer at the
          stem; bring it to eye level
      (2) Rotate the thermometer until you
          see the numbers and the long and
          short lines
      (3) Turn the thermometer back and
          forth slowly until you see the
          mercury line
      (4) Read the thermometer to the
          nearest degree and tenth of a de-
          gree
6. Using a glass thermometer
   a. Each person has a thermometer to pre-
      vent spread of microbes and infection
   b. Practice the following measures:
      (1) Use only the person's ther-
          mometer
      (2) Clean before use according to
          employer policy
      (3) Check the thermometer for
          breaks and chips
      (4) Shake the thermometer so that
          the mercury is below the lines
          and numbers (see Figure 40-15,
          p. 664)
          (a) Hold at the stem
          (b) Stand away from walls, ta-
              bles, and hard surfaces
          (c) Flex and snap your wrist
      (5) Clean and store the thermometer
          following agency policy
          (a) Wipe with tissue
          (b) Do not use hot water for
              cleaning
      (6) Use plastic covers following
          agency policy
          (a) A cover is used once and dis-
              carded
          (b) The thermometer is inserted
              into a cover and the tempera-
              ture is taken
          (c) The cover is removed to read
              the thermometer
          (d) The thermometer never
              touches the person
      (7) Practice medical asepsis and
          standard precautions
K. Temperature-sensitive tape
   1. Changes color in response to body heat
   2. Applied to the forehead or abdomen
   3. Shows if temperature is normal or above
      normal
      a. Exact temperature is not measured
   4. Color change takes about 15 seconds
V. PULSE
   A. See Chapter 13 for a review of the structure
      and function of the heart and blood vessels
   B. The beat of the heart felt at an artery as a
      wave of blood passes through the artery
   C. Sites for taking a pulse
      1. The temporal, carotid, brachial, radial,
         femoral, popliteal, and dorsalis pedis
         pulses are on both sides of the body (see
         Figure 40-16, p. 663)
      2. The radial site is used most often
         a. It is easy to reach and find
         b. You do not have to disturb or expose
            the person
      3. The carotid site is used during cardiopul-
         monary resuscitation (CPR) and other
         emergencies (see Chapter 47)
      4. The apical pulse is felt over the apex of
         the heart
         a. Taken with a stethoscope
   D. Pulse rate
      1. The number of heart beats or pulses felt
         in 1 minute
      2. The rate varies for different age groups
         (see Table 40-2, p. 665)
      3. Affected by many factors, such as ele-
         vated temperature, exercise, fear, anger,

anxiety, excitement, heat, position, pain, and some drugs

4. The adult rate is between 60 and 100 beats per minute
   a. Tachycardia—a rapid heart rate, over 100 beats per minute
   b. Bradycardia—a slow heart rate, less than 60 beats per minute
   c. You need to know the cklient's normal pulse rate
   d. Report abnormal rates to the nurse immediately

E. Rhythm and force of the pulse
   1. The pulse should be regular and felt in a pattern
      a. The same time interval should occur between beats
      b. An abnormal rhythm is called dysrhythmia and must be reported immediately
   2. The force of the pulse relates to its strength
      a. Forceful—easy to feel; described as strong, full, or bounding
      b. Hard-to-feel pulses are described as weak, thready, or feeble
   3. Electronic blood pressure equipment can count pulses
      a. The pulse rate is displayed along with the blood pressure
      b. No information is given about rhythm or force; you still need to feel the pulse

F. Taking a radial pulse
   1. Used for routine vital signs
   2. Place the first three fingers of one hand against the radial artery (see Figure 40-17, p. 666)
      a. Do not use your thumb; it has a pulse of its own
   3. Count the pulse for 30 seconds, multiply by two to get the number of beats per minute
      a. If the pulse is irregular, count for one full minute
      b. Follow agency policy
      c. Report and record the following:
         (1) Pulse rate
         (2) If pulse rate is less than 60 or more than 100 beats/minute—REPORT THIS AT ONCE
         (3) If pulse rate is higher or lower than normal for the client—RE-

PORT THIS AT ONCE.
         (4) If the pulse is regular or irregular
         (5) Pulse force--strong, full, bounding, weak, thready, or feeble
   4. Taking a Radial Pulse ▶ p. 666

G. Taking an apical pulse
   1. Taken with a stethoscope
   2. Taken on the left side of the chest, slightly below the nipple
   3. Counted for one full minute
   4. Heart beat normally sounds like a "lub-dub"
      a. Each lub-dub is one beat

H. Taking an apical-radial pulse
   1. Apical and radial pulses rates should be equal
   2. Heart contractions may not be strong enough to create a radial pulse
      a. The radial pulse may be less than the apical pulse
   3. Apical and radial pulses are taken by two staff members at the same time to check differences in pulse rates; a nurse takes the apical
      a. The pulse deficit is the difference; subtract the radial from the apical rate
      b. The apical pulse rate is never less than the radial rate
   4. Taking an apical-radial pulse (see Figure 40-18, p. 667)

VI. RESPIRATIONS
A. The act of breathing air into the lungs (inhalation) and out of the lungs (exhalation)
   1. The chest rises during inhalation and falls during exhalation
   2. See Chapter 13 for a review of the respiratory system
B. Healthy adults have 12 to 20 respirations per minute
C. The respiratory rate is affected by the same factors that affect temperature and pulse
D. Normally quiet, effortless, and regular
   1. Both sides of the chest rise and fall equally
E. Respirations are counted when the person is at rest
F. Depth and rate of breathing can be voluntarily controlled
   1. The person should be unaware that you are counting respirations
   2. Counted right after taking a pulse
G. Count respirations by watching the rise and

fall of the chest
  1. Count them for 30 seconds and multiply by two
  2. If an abnormal pattern is noted, count for one full minute
H. Report and record the following
  1. Respiratory rate
  2. Equality and depth of respirations (shallow, normal, or deep)
  3. If regular or irregular
  4. If client has pain or difficulty breathing
  5. Any respiratory noises
  6. Any abnormal respiratory patterns (see Chapter 43)
 I. Counting Respirations ▶ p. 668
VII. BLOOD PRESSURE
  A. The amount of force exerted against the walls of an artery by the blood
  B. Controlled by:
    1. The force of heart contractions
    2. The amount of blood pumped with each heartbeat
    3. How easily the blood flows through the blood vessels
  C. Systole is the period of heart muscle contraction
  D. Diastole is the period of heart muscle relaxation
  E. Systolic pressure is the higher pressure
  F. Diastolic pressure is the lower pressure
  G. Blood pressure is measured in millimeters (mm) of mercury (Hg)
    1. The systolic is recorded over the diastolic
  H. The average adult has a systolic pressure of 120 mm Hg and a diastolic pressure of 80 mm Hg.
    1. Written as 120/80
   I. Factors affecting blood pressure
    1. Blood pressure can change from minute to minute
    2. Box 40-1, p. 669 in the textbook, lists factors affecting blood pressure
    3. Blood pressure has normal ranges
      a. Systolic pressures between 100 mm Hg and 140 mm Hg are considered normal
      b. Diastolic pressures between 60 mm Hg and 90 mm Hg are considered normal
    4. Hypertension is persistent measurements above normal ranges
      a. Report to the nurse immediately systolic pressures greater than 140 mm Hg and diastolic pressures greater than 90 mm Hg
    5. Hypotension is persistent measurements

below normal ranges
      a. Systolic pressures less than 100 mm Hg and diastolic pressures less than 60 mm Hg
    6. Focus on children
      a. Infants and children have lower blood pressures than adults
      b. A newborn's pressure is about 70/55 mm Hg
      c. At one year, the blood pressure increases to 90/55mm Hg
      d. Adult levels are reached between 14 and 18 years of age
    7. See Focus on Older Adults box, p. 669
      a. Both systolic and diastolic pressures are higher in older persons
  J. Equipment
    1. A stethoscope and sphygmomanometer are used
    2. Using a stethoscope
      a. An instrument used to listen to the sounds produced by the heart, lungs, and other body organs
      b. Used to take the apical pulse and to measure blood pressure
      c. Amplifies sounds for easy hearing
      d. Infection control is important
      e. The earpieces and diaphragm are cleaned before and after use
    3. The following measures are practiced
      a. Wipe the earpiece and diaphragm with alcohol wipes between each use
      b. Warm the diaphragm in your hand
      c. Place the earpiece tips in your ears so the bend of the tips points forward
        (1) Should fit snugly
        (2) Should not cause pain
      d. Place the diaphragm over the artery; hold it in place
      e. Prevent noise; nothing should touch the tubing; the person is silent
      f. Wipe the earpiece tips and diaphragm with alcohol after the procedure
    4. The sphygmomanometer consists of a cuff and a measuring device
      a. Three types
        (1) The aneroid type has a round dial and needle that points to the calibrations
        (2) The mercury type has a column of mercury within a calibrated tube
          (a) More accurate than the aneroid type

(3) The electronic sphygmomanometer displays the systolic
and diastolic pressures on the
front of the instrument
  (a) The pulse is usually displayed
  (b) Follow the manufacturer's
  instructions
b. The cuff is wrapped around the upper
arm
  (1) Tubing connects the cuff to the
  manometer
c. A valve on the bulb is turned so the
cuff inflates as the bulb is squeezed
  (1) The inflated cuff causes pressure
  over the brachial artery
d. The valve is turned the other way for
cuff deflation
  (1) Blood pressure is measured as
  the cuff is deflated
e. Sounds are produced as the blood
flows through arteries
  (1) The stethoscope is used to listen
  to the sounds
f. Focus on children
  (1) Pediatric blood pressure cuffs are
  used for children
  (2) Infant and child sizes are also
  available
5. Measuring blood pressure
a. Normally measured in the brachial artery
b. Box 40-4, p. 672 in the textbook lists
the guidelines for measuring blood
pressure
c. Measuring Blood Pressure ▶ p.672

Classroom Activities

1. Write on the chalkboard: "The four vital signs of
the body are:"
  a. Call on students to provide the answers. Write
  the correct answer on the chalkboard.

2. Write on the chalkboard: "Many factors affect
vital signs:"
  a. Call on students to list the factors that affect
  vital signs. Write the correct answers on the
  chalkboard.

3. Write the following terms on separate index cards:
Temperature, Pulse, Respirations, and Blood pressure.

a. Divide students into four groups. Ask each
group to choose one index card.
b. Allow 15 minutes for each group to provide the
following about the term on their card.
  (1) The definition of the term
  (2) How the vital sign is measured (This
  should include the equipment used and the
  site[s] for measuring it)
  (3) The normal range of the measurement
c. Call on one student from each group to report
to the class
  (1) Allow time after each presentation for
  questions and discussion.

4. Show video #9 (Measuring Temperature, Pulse,
and Respirations) in Mosby's Nursing Assisting
Video Series.
  a. Allow time after each section for questions.

5. Show video #10 (Measuring Blood Pressure) in
Mosby's Nursing Assisting Video Series.
  a. Allow time after each section for questions.

6. Write the following on the top of one sheet of a
flip chart: "Oral temperatures are not taken if the
person:" On top of another sheet write: "Rectal
temperatures are not taken if the person:"
  a. Call on students to complete a list of reasons
  for each statement. Write the correct answers
  under each statement.

7. Write the following terms on the chalkboard:
  a. Tachycardia
  b. Bradycardia
  c. Systole
  d. Diastole
  e. Hypertension
  f. Hypotension

Call on students to define each term. Write the
correct definitions after each term.

8. Obtain graphic sheets and other documentation
forms used to record vital signs from a local hospital or long-term care center.
  a. Distribute copies to each student.
  b. Display a copy on an overhead transparency.
  (1) Explain and demonstrate how the documents are used.
  (2) Allow time for questions.

9. Use the procedure checklists provided.
  a. Demonstrate the procedures in this chapter.

b. Have each student practice and return demonstrate the procedures in this chapter. Have each student assume the role of the patient/resident when practicing and return demonstrating each procedure when appropriate.

c. Use a simulator or anatomical model for any invasive procedure.

d. Ask students to report and record vital signs (use the forms provided in exercise #8 above). Stress the importance of accuracy and timeliness.

Homework Assignments

Ask students to answer the questions at the end of Chapter 40 in the textbook. Tell students the date and time that this assignment must be completed and turned in.

If the accompanying student workbook is being used, assign the Chapter 40 workbook exercises. Tell students the date and time that this assignment must be completed and turned in.

Name _____

Date _____

Measuring Height, Weight, and Vital Signs

1. Read and record the temperature on each thermometer

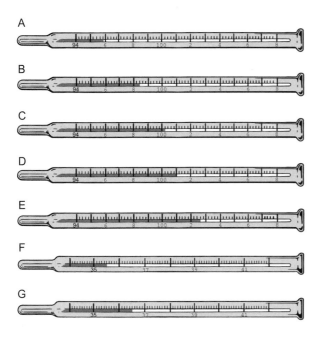

   a. _____ °F

   b. _____ °F

   c. _____ °F

   d. _____ °F

   e. _____ °C

   f. _____ °C

   g. _____ °C

2. List the normal pulse rate ranges for the age groups listed below.

Age	Rate per minute
a. Birth to 4 weeks	_____
b. 4 weeks to 1 year	_____
c. 1 to 2 years	_____
d. 2 to 6 years	_____
e. 6 to 12 years	_____
f. 12 years and older	_____

3. List the normal respiratory rates for the age groups listed below.

Age	Respirations per minute
a. Newborn	_____
b. 1 to 11 months	_____
c. 2 years	_____
d. 4 years	_____
e. 6 years	_____
f. 8 years	_____
g. 10 years	_____
h. 14 years	_____
i. 18 years	_____

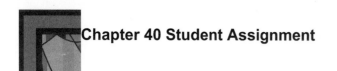

Name _____

Date _____

Measuring Height, Weight, and Vital Signs

4. Read and record the blood pressure that the mercury column shows.

Systolic   **Diastolic**

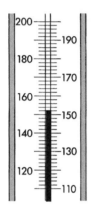   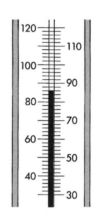

a. _____   b. _____

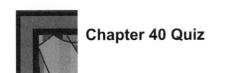

Chapter 40 Quiz

Name _____

Date _____

Measuring Height, Weight, and Vital Signs

<table>
<tr><td align="center">True or False</td><td align="center">Multiple Choice</td></tr>
</table>

*Mark **T** for true or **F** for false.*

1. _____ Unless otherwise ordered, take vital signs with the person standing.

2. _____ A glass thermometer is rinsed under warm running water before use.

3. _____ An oral temperature is not taken if a person is receiving oxygen.

4. _____ Axillary temperatures are more reliable than oral temperatures.

5. _____ To use a tympanic membrane thermometer, the covered probe is inserted gently into the ear.

6. _____ The brachial artery is used most often for taking a pulse.

7. _____ Before using a stethoscope, wipe the earpieces and diaphragm with alcohol wipes.

8. _____ A stethoscope is used to take an apical pulse.

9. _____ An apical pulse is counted for 30 seconds.

10. _____ Respirations are counted right after taking a pulse. The person should be unaware that you are counting respirations.

11. _____ Blood pressure is normally measured in the brachial artery.

12. _____ The blood pressure cuff is applied over clothing.

13. _____ Notify the nurse immediately if you cannot detect a blood pressure.

Circle the BEST answer.

14. The difference between the apical and radial pulse rates is called the:
    a. Apical-radial pulse.
    b. Pulse deficit.
    c. Pulse rate.
    d. Pulse pressure.

15. A person with a persistent blood pressure measurement above 140/90 has:
    a. Tachycardia.
    b. Hypertension.
    c. Hypotension.
    d. Anxiety.

16. The period of heart muscle relaxation is called:
    a. Diastole.
    b. Systole.
    c. Blood pressure.
    d. Hypotension.

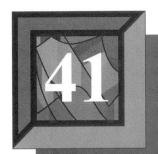

41

Wound Care

Instructor's Preparation

I. Read Chapter 41 in the textbook. Carefully review chapter objectives, key terms, and review questions.

II. Read the outline in Chapter 41 of the instructor's guide. Carefully review the classroom activities, the student assignment, and the quiz.

III. If you are using the accompanying student workbook, review the activities for Chapter 41.

IV. Gather all necessary supplies and equipment for classroom activities and student assignments.
   A. Prepare appropriate flip charts
   B. Prepare overhead transparencies
   C. Prepare situation/index cards
   D. Gather the following transparencies: TA52 through TA54
   E. Gather coloured markers
   F. Gather the necessary equipment and supplies needed to demonstrate and have each student return demonstrate the procedure in this chapter
   G. Gather any other items that will be needed for classroom activities
   H. Assemble items in the order they will be used

V. Make sure that the necessary equipment is available and in good working order.

VI. Contact guest speaker(s) to confirm the day, date, time, and location that he or she is expected.
   A. Ask the speaker if he or she requires any special equipment or supplies. Make sure these are available.

Objectives

- Define the key terms listed in this chapter
- List the clients at risk for skin tears and pressure ulcers
- Describe the causes of skin tears and how to prevent them
- Describe the signs, symptoms, and causes of pressure ulcers and how to prevent them
- Identify the pressure points in the basic bed and sitting positions
- Describe the causes of leg and foot ulcers and how to prevent them

- Describe the process, types, and complications of wound healing
- Describe the observations to make about a wound and wound drainage
- Explain how to secure dressings
- Explain the guidelines for applying dressings
- Explain the purpose of binders and guidelines for applying them
- Describe how to meet the basic needs of clients with wounds
- Learn the procedures described in this chapter

329

abrasion
arterial ulcer
bedsore
bruise
chronic wound
circulatory ulcer
clean wound
clean-contaminated wound
closed wound
contaminated wound
contusion
decubitus ulcer
dehiscence
dirty wound
edema
evisceration
full-thickness wound
hematoma
hemorrhage
incision
infected wound
intentional wound
laceration
open wound
partial-thickness wound
penetrating wound
pressure sore
pressure ulcer
puncture wound
shock
skin tear
stasis ulcer
trauma
unintentional wound
vascular ulcer
venous ulcer
wound

Outline

Wound Care

I. INTRODUCTION
   A. Since the skin is the body's first line of defense, you must do everything possible to keep the skin intact
   B. Infants, children, and older or disabled clients are at risk since their skin is easily injured
      1. See Box 41-1, p. 677 in the textbook, lists the common causes of skin breakdown
   C. A wound is a break in the skin or mucous membrane

   1. Causes include:
      a. Surgical incisions
      b. Trauma
         (1) An accident or violent act can injure the skin, mucous membrane, bones, or internal organs
      c. Pressure
         (1) Poor skin care and immobility can cause wounds at pressure points
      d. Poor circulation
         (1) A decrease in blood flow through arteries and veins can cause circulatory ulcers
   D. A wound is a portal of entry for microbes; infection is a threat
   E. Wound care involves preventing infection and further injury
      1. Preventing blood loss and pain are important
   F. Your role in wound care depends on your provincial or territorial laws, your job description, and the person's condition
II. TYPES OF WOUNDS
   A. See Box 41-2, p. 679 in the textbook
   B. Intentional wounds created for therapy
      1. Surgical wounds and venipuncture are examples
   C. Unintentional wounds resulting from trauma
      1. Falls, accidents, gunshots, stabbings, and other violent acts are sources
   D. An open wound is when the skin or mucous membrane is broken
   E. A closed wound is when tissues are injured, but the skin is not broken
      1. Bruises, twists, and sprains are examples
   F. A clean wound is not infected, and microbes have not entered the wound
      1. Closed wounds and intentional wounds are usually clean wounds
      2. The urinary, respiratory, and gastrointestinal systems are not entered
   G. A clean-contaminated wound occurs from surgical entry of the reproductive, respiratory, and gastrointestinal systems
   H. A contaminated wound has a high risk of infection (unintentional wounds are generally contaminated)
      1. Occurs also from breaks in surgical asepsis and spillage of intestinal contents
   I. An infected wound (dirty wound) contains large amounts of bacteria; shows signs of infection
   J. A chronic wound is one that does not heal easily
      1. Pressure ulcers and circulatory ulcers are

examples

K. A partial-thickness wound is when the dermis and epidermis of the skin are broken

L. A full-thickness wound is when the dermis, epidermis, and subcutaneous tissue are penetrated

    1. Muscle and bone may be involved

M. Wounds also are described by cause:

    1. An abrasion is caused by scraping away or rubbing away of the skin

    2. A contusion is a closed wound caused by a blow to the body

    3. An incision is an open wound with clean straight edges

    4. A laceration is an open wound with torn tissues and jagged edges

    5. A penetrating wound is when the skin and underlying tissue are pierced

    6. A puncture wound is an open wound made by a sharp object

N. Skin tears

    1. Older persons have thin and fragile skin; they are at risk for skin tears

    2. A skin tear is a break or rip in the skin that separates the epidermis from the underlying tissue (see Figure 13-4, p.129)

      a. Hands, arms, and lower legs are common sites

    3. Causes include:

      a. Shearing, pulling, or pressure on the skin (see Chapter 21)

        (1) Skin tears are painful

        (2) Wound complications can develop

        (3) Notify the nurse immediately if you cause or find a skin tear

    4. See Box 41-3, p. 679 in the textbook for guidelines to prevent skin tears

III. PRESSURE ULCERS (decubitus ulcer, bedsore, pressure sore)

A. Any injury caused by unrelieved pressure (see Figure 41-2, p.680)

    1. Usually occurs over a bony prominence (shoulder blades, elbows, hip bones, sacrum, knees, ankles, heels, and toes)

B. Bony prominences are called pressure points because they bear the wight of the body in ceratin prositions (see Figure 41-1, p. 678)

C. Causes:

    1. Pressure, friction, and shearing are common causes

    2. Other factors include breaks in the skin, poor circulation, moisture, dry skin, and irritation by urine or feces

    3. Pressure occurs when the skin over a bony prominence is squeezed between hard surfaces

      a. This prevents blood flow, causing skin and tissues to die (see Figure 41-2, p. 680)

    4. Friction scrapes the skin

      a. The open area is a portal for microbes

        (1) A good blood supply is needed for healing

        (2) Infection is prevented

    5. Shearing is when the skin sticks to a surface and deeper tissues move downward

      a. Blood flow to the area is reduced

D. Persons at risk are those who:

    1. Are confined to bed or chair

    2. Are unable to move

    3. Have loss of bowel or bladder control

    4. Have poor nutrition

    5. Have altered mental awareness

    6. Have problems sensing pain or pressure

    7. Have circulatory problems

    8. Are older, obese, very thin, or malnourished

E. Signs of pressure ulcers

    1. The first sign is pale skin or a reddened area

    2. There may be pain, burning, or tingling in the area

      a. Some people do not feel anything unusual

    3. Box 41-4, p. 680 in the textbook, describes the four stages of pressure ulcer development

    4. Check your client's skin every time you provide care, and immediately notify your supervisor of any signs of pressure sores

F. Sites

    1. Pressure ulcers occur over bony areas

      a. Called pressure points

      b. Pressure from body weight can reduce the blood supply to the area

      c. See Figure 41-1, p. 678 in the textbook

    2. In obese people, pressure ulcers can develop in areas where skin has contact with skin

      a. Between abdominal folds, the legs, the buttocks, and under the breasts

G. Prevention

    1. Is easier than trying to heal the ulcers

    2. Good nursing care, cleanliness, and skin care are essential

3. The measures listed in Box 41-5, p. 682 in the textbook, help prevent skin breakdown and pressure ulcers
   a. Follow the person's care plan

H. Treatment
  1. Directed by the doctor
  2. Wound care products, drugs, treatments, and special equipment are ordered to promote healing
    a. Your supervisor and the care plan tell you about a person's treatment
  3. The following protective devices are often ordered:
    a. Bed cradle (see Figure 41-5, p. 683)
     (1) A metal frame placed on the bed and over the person
     (2) Focus on home care
      (a) A cardboard box is useful as a bed cradle (see Figure 41-6, p. 683)
    b. Elbow protectors (see Figure 41-7, p. 683)
     (1) Made of foam rubber or sheepskin
     (2) Fit the shape of the elbow
     (3) Friction is prevented
    c. Heel elevators (see Figure 41-8, p. 684)
     (1) Pillows or special cushions used to raise the heels off the bed
     (2) Special braces and splints also are used
    d. Flotation pads (see Figure 41-9, p. 684)
     (1) Like water beds; made of a gel-like substance
    e. Eggcrate mattress (see Figure 41-10, p. 684)
     (1) A foam pad that looks like an egg carton
     (2) Placed on top of the regular mattress
      (a) Covered with the bottom sheet
    f. Special beds (see Figure 41-11, p. 684)
     (1) Some beds have air flowing through the mattress; the person floats on the mattress
     (2) Some beds allow repositioning without moving the person
      (a) Pressure points change as the position changes
      (b) Some beds rotate constantly from side to side
    g. Other equipment

     (1) Trochanter rolls and footboards also are used
      (a) Described in Chapter 22

IV. CIRCULATORY ULCERS (vascular ulcers)
  A. Caused by decrease in the blood flow through arteries or veins
    1. Causes pain, open wounds, and edema
    2. Infection and gangrene (death of tissue) can result (See Chapter 31)
  B. These wounds on the legs and feet are often painful and hard to heal
  C. Stasis ulcers (venous ulcers)
    1. Open wounds caused by poor blood return to the heart from the legs and feet (see Figure 41-12, p. 685)
     a. Valves in the leg veins do not close efficiently
     b. Blood and fluid collect in the legs and feet
     c. The skin is brown, dry, leathery, and hard
      (1) Itching is common
     d. The heals and inner aspect of the ankles are common sites
     e. Ulcers can occur from skin injury
      (1) Scratching itching skin is a common cause of injury
     f. Ulcers can occur spontaneously
     g. Ulcers are painful and make walking difficult
      (1) Healing is slow and infection is a great risk
    2. Preventing skin breakdown is important
     a. Good skin care and positioning are important
     b. The person should avoid wearing tight clothing
     c. Avoid injury to feet and legs
     d. The doctor may order elastic stockings or elastic bandages (see Chapter 28)
     e. Professional foot care is important
    3. See Box 41-6, p.685 in the textbook, for guidelines for preventing statis ulcers
  D. Arterial ulcers
    1. Open wounds on the legs and feet caused by poor blood flow through the arteries
    2. The leg and foot may feel cold and look blue and shiny
    3. The ulcer is often painful at rest
     a. Usually worse at night
    4. Causes include:
     a. Diseases or injuries that decrease arterial blood flow to the legs and feet
      (1) High blood pressure and diabetes are common causes

b. Some narrowing of arteries occurs with age

c. Smoking is a risk factor

5. Arterial ulcers are found between the toes, on top of the toes, and on the outer side of the ankle

a. Heels are common sites of these ulcers for persons on bedrest

b. These ulcers can occur in pressure sites from shoes that fit poorly

6. The doctor directs treatment

a. The disease causing the ulcer is treated

b. Drugs, wound care, and a walking program are ordered

c. Professional foot care is important

d. Follow the care plan and prevent injury

e. See Box 41-7, p. 686 in the textbook, for guidelines for preventing arterial ulcers

V. WOUND HEALING

A. The process has three phases:

1. Inflammatory phase (3 days)

a. Bleeding stops and a scab forms

b. Signs and symptoms of inflammation appear

c. Loss of function may occur

2. Proliferative phase (day 3 to day 21)

a. Tissue cells multiply to repair the wound

3. Maturation phase (day 21 to 1 or 2 years)

a. Scar gains strength

B. Types of wound healing

1. Primary intention (first intention, primary closure) is when the wound edges are brought together; this closes the wound

a. Sutures, staples, clips, or adhesive strips are used

2. Secondary intention (second intention) is when wounds are cleaned and dead tissue removed; wound edges are not brought together; healing occurs naturally

a. Used for contaminated and infected wounds

b. Healing takes longer

3. Tertiary intention (third intention, delayed intention) involves leaving a wound open and closing it later

a. Infection and poor circulation are common reasons

C. Complications of wound healing

1. Factors that affect the healing process and increase the risk of complications:

a. The type of wound

b. The person's age and general health

c. Nutrition and life-style

d. Circulation

e. Certain drugs

f. Immune system changes

2. Hemorrhage

a. The excessive loss of blood in a short period of time (see Chapter 47)

b. May be internal or external

c. Internal hemorrhage cannot be seen

(1) A hematoma (collection of blood under the skin) may form

(2) Shock, vomiting blood, coughing up blood, and loss of consciousness are signs of internal hemorrhage

d. You can see external bleeding

(1) Bloody drainage and dressings soaked with blood are common signs

(2) Always check under the body part for pooling of blood

(3) Shock can occur

e. Shock results when there is not enough blood supply to organs and tissues (see Chapter 47)

(1) Signs and symptoms include:

(a) Low or falling blood pressure

(b) Rapid and weak pulse

(c) Rapid respirations

(d) Skin is cold, moist, and pale

(e) The person is restless and may complain of thirst

(f) Confusion and loss of consciousness occur as shock worsens

f. Hemorrhage and shock are emergencies

(1) Practice Standard Precautions when in contact with blood

(a) Gloves are always worn

(b) Gowns, masks, and eye protection are used if blood splashes are likely

3. Infection

a. Wound contamination can occur during or after the injury

b. An infected wound appears inflamed and has drainage

c. The wound is painful and tender

d. The person has a fever

4. Dehiscence

a. The separation of the wound layers (see Figure 41-13, p. 687)

(1) May involve the skin layer or un-

derlying tissues
  b. Abdominal wounds are most commonly affected
  c. Causes include coughing, vomiting, and abdominal distention
  d. Is a surgical emergency
  5. Evisceration
    a. Separation of the wound along with the protrusion of abdominal organs (see Figure 41-14, p. 687)
    b. A surgical emergency
    c. Cover the wound with large sterile dressings saturated with sterile saline
    d. Notify the nurse immediately
  D. Wound appearance
    1. Report observations to your supervisor and record them according to agency policy
    2. Box 41-8, p. 687 in the textbook, lists questions to consider when observing wounds
  E. Wound drainage
    1. Major types are:
      a. Serous drainage—a clear, watery fluid (see Figure 41-15A, p. 688)
      b. Sanguineous drainage—bloody drainage (see Figure 41-15B, p. 688)
        (1) Amount and color are important to note
          (a) Large amount, hemorrhage is suspected
          (b) Bright drainage indicates fresh bleeding
          (c) Darker drainage indicates older bleeding
      c. Serosanguineous drainage—thin, watery drainage that is blood-tinged (see Figure 41-15C, p. 688)
      d. Purulent drainage—thick drainage that is green, yellow, or brown(see Figure 41-15D, p. 688)
    2. Drainage must leave the wound for healing to occur
      a. Drainage trapped in a wound can lead to infection and other complications
    3. When a large amount of drainage is expected, the doctor inserts a drain
      a. A Penrose drain is a rubber tube that drains onto a dressing (see Figure 41-16, p. 688)
        (1) An open drain is a portal of entry for microbes
      b. A closed drainage system is a drainage tube placed in the wound that is attached to suction
        (1) Prevents microbes from entering the wound
        (2) The Hemovac and the Jackson-Pratt drainage systems are used (see Figures 41-17 and 41-18, p. 688)
    4. DA nurse measures grainage in three ways:
      a. Noting the number and size of dressings with drainage
        (1) Describe the amount and kind of drainage on dressings
      b. Weighing dressings before applying them
        (1) Note the weight of each dressing
        (2) Dressings are weighed after removal
        (3) Subtract and note the difference
      c. Measuring the amount of drainage in the collecting receptacle if closed drainage is used

VI. DRESSINGS
  A. Have many functions:
    1. Protect wounds from injury and microbes
    2. Drainage is absorbed and removed along with dead tissue
    3. Promote comfort and cover wounds
    4. Provide a moist environment for wound healing
    5. Pressure dressings help control bleeding
  B. Type and size depend on:
    1. Type, size, and location of the wound
    2. Amount of drainage
    3. Presence or absence of infection
    4. Function of the dressing
    5. Frequency of dressing changes
    6. Doctor and nurse will choose the best type of dressing
  C. Types of dressings:
    1. Gauze—comes in squares, rectangles, pads, or rolls; absorbs moisture (see Figure 41-19, p. 689)
    2. Nonadherent gauze—a gauze dressing with a non-stick back
    3. Transparent adhesive film—prevents fluids and bacteria from entering the wound but allows air into the wound
      a. Drainage is not absorbed; allows for wound observation
  D. Some dressings contain special agents to promote healing
  E. Application methods:
    1. Dry-to-dry dressing—a gauze dressing placed over the wound
      a. Drainage is absorbed by the dressing

and removed with the dressing
    (1) Can stick to the wound
  b. Removed carefully to prevent tissue injury and discomfort
2. Wet-to-dry dressing—a gauze dressing saturated with solution is applied over the wound; the solution softens dead tissue in the wound
  a. Dead tissue is absorbed by the dressing and removed with the dressing
  b. Dressings are removed when dry
3. Wet-to-wet dressing—a gauze dressing saturated with solution is placed in the wound
  a. Dressings are kept moist
F. Securing dressings
  1. Tape
    a. Adhesive, paper, plastic, and elastic tapes are available
      (1) Adhesive:
        (a) Sticks well to skin
        (b) Adhesive part can stay on the skin and is hard to remove
        (c) Can irritate skin
      (2) Paper and plastic tapes are nonallergenic
      (3) Elastic tape allows movement of the body part
    b. Tape is applied to secure top, middle, and bottom of dressing (see Figure 41-20, p. 690)
    c. Tape must not encircle the entire body part
      (1) If swelling occurs, circulation to the part is impaired
  2. Montgomery ties (see Figure 41-21, p. 690)
    a. Used for large dressings and when frequent dressing changes are needed
    b. Consists of an adhesive strip and a cloth tie
      (1) Adhesive strips are placed on both sides of the dressing (two or three on each side)
      (2) Cloth ties are secured over the dressing
      (3) Cloth ties are undone for dressing changes
      (4) Adhesive strips are not removed unless soiled
  3. Focus on children
    a. When changing dressings on a child, let the parent or caregiver hold the

child if possible
    b. Letting the child hold or play with a toy is often comforting
  4. Focus on older persons
    a. Extreme care is needed when removing tape
G. Applying dressings
  1. Some employers allow support workers to apply simple, nonsterile dressings; you may assist the nurse with complex wounds
  3. Box 41-9, p. 690 in the textbook, lists the guidelines for applying dressings
  4. Focus on home care
    a. Make sure you have the necessary supplies
    b. You may be asked to telephone a report to the nurse
  5. Applying a Dry Nonsterile Dressing ▶ p. 692
VII. BINDERS
A. Applied to the abdomen, chest, or perineal areas
B. Promote healing because they:
  1. Support wounds and hold dressings in place
  2. Reduce or prevent swelling
  3. Promote comfort
  4. Prevent injury
C. Usually a nurse applies binders
D. You may provide care for clients with these binders
  1. Straight abdominal binders provide abdominal support and hold dressings in place (see Figure 41-22, p. 693)
  2. Breast binders support the breasts after breast surgery and childbirth (see Figure 41-23, p. 693)
  3. T binders are used to secure dressings in place after rectal and perineal surgeries
    a. Single T binders for women (see Figure 41-24A, p. 693)
    b. Double T binders for men (see Figure 41-24B, p. 693)
VIII. HEAT AND COLD APPLICATIONS
A. Ordered by the doctor to promote healing, promote comfort, and reduce tissue swelling
B. Discussed in Chapter 42 in the textbook
IX. THE PERSON'S BASIC NEEDS
A. Remember that it is the person who has the wound
  1. The person is recovering from surgery or trauma
  2. The wound is a source of pain and dis-

comfort
3. The wound and pain may interfere with breathing and moving
B. Turning, repositioning, and ambulating may be painful
1. Handle the person gently
2. Allow pain medication to take effect before giving care
C. Good nutrition is needed for healing
1. Pain can affect appetite
2. Odors can affect appetite
3. If the person has a taste for certain foods or beverages, report this to the nurse
D. Infection is always a threat
1. Follow Standard Precautions
2. Observe the wound and the person for signs and symptoms of infection (See Chapter 18)
E. Delayed healing and infection are risks for:
1. Older persons
2. Obese persons
3. Persons with poor nutrition
4. Persons with poor circulation and diabetes
F. Fears affect a person's sense of safety and security; fears include:
1. Scarring, disfigurement, delayed healing, and infection
2. Wound "popping" open
3. Costly medical bills
4. Continued hospital care, home care, and long-term care
G. Victims of violence have other concerns
1. Future attacks
2. Finding and convicting the attacker
3. Fear for a family member
H. The location, size, appearance, and odor of the wound affect the person
I. Some wounds affect sex and sexuality
J. Some wounds affect function, vision, appetite, and elimination
K. Whatever the location or size of the wound, physical function and body image are affected
1. The person's sense of love, belonging, and self-esteem are affected
L. You must be sensitive to the person's feelings
1. Be kind, give thoughtful care, and practice good communication
M. Other health team members may be involved in the person's care
1. Social worker, psychiatrist, clergy

Classroom Activities

1. Write on a flip chart:
   a. A wound is:
   b. Wounds are caused by:

   (1) _____

   (2) _____

   (3) _____

   (4) _____

   Call on students to provide the definition and causes of wounds. Write the correct answers on the flip chart.

2. Write each of the following types of wounds on separate index cards: Intentional Wounds, Unintentional Wounds, Open Wound, Closed Wound, Clean Wound, Clean-Contaminated Wound, Infected Wound, Chronic Wound, Partial-Thickness Wound, and Full-Thickness Wound.
   a. Call on individual students to pick one index card and define the term on the card. Clarify any wrong answers. Allow time for input from all students.

3. Write the following terms on the chalkboard or flip chart. Then call on students to define each term. Write the correct answers after the appropriate term.
   a. Abrasion
   b. Contusion
   c. Incision
   d. Laceration
   e. Penetrating wound
   f. Puncture wound

4. Divide students into two groups.
   a. Ask one group to define, list the causes, list the preventive measures, and describe those at risk for skin tears.
   b. Ask one group to define, list the causes, list the preventive measures, and describe those at risk for pressure ulcers.

   Allow 15 minutes to complete this exercise. Then call on one student from each group to report to the class. Allow time after each presentation for questions and discussion.

5. Display Box 41-4, p. 681 in the textbook (The four stages of pressure ulcer development) on an overhead transparency. Review the stages with students.

6. Display Fig.41-1, p. 678 in the textbook on an overhead transparency. Use this as a basis to discuss pressure points and the importance of frequent position changes.

7. Have available the following protective devices: bed cradle, elbow protectors, heel elevators, flotation pads, eggcrate-like mattress, trochanter rolls, footboards. Discuss the use and application of each device. Allow students to manipulate each device.
   a. If possible arrange for a representative from a specialty bed company to display and demonstrate a specialty bed used for pressure relief.

8. Ask each student to assume the positions illustrated on p. 678 in the textbook for 15 to 20 minutes. Then ask students to discuss their experience.
   a. Did they feel areas of increased pressure, numbness, or pain?
   b. Discuss the importance of frequent position changes.

9. Divide students into two groups. Provide each group with a flip chart and colored markers.
   a. Ask one group to write the following information about venous ulcers on the flip chart: Definition, Causes, Location, and Preventive Measures.
   b. Ask one group to write the following information about arterial ulcers on the flip chart: Definition, Causes, Location, and Preventive Measures.

   Allow 15 minutes for this exercise. Then call on one student from each group to report to the class. Allow time after each presentation for questions.

10. Call on students to describe the three phases of wound healing.

11. Write the following terms on the chalkboard:
    a. Primary intention
    b. Secondary intention
    c. Tertiary intention

    Call on students to define each term. Write the correct answers on the chalkboard after the appropriate term.

12. Invite an RN who specializes in wound care to visit the class. Ask her to:
    a. Show slides of various types of wounds.
    b. Discuss the complications of wound healing.
    c. Describe the major types of wound drainage.
    d. Provide and explain the use of a variety of wound dressings.
    e. Provide various types of binders for students to manipulate.

    Ask students to write key points in a notebook for future reference.

    Allow time for questions and discussion.

13. Use the procedure checklist provided.
    a. Demonstrate the procedure in this chapter.
    b. Have each student practice and return demonstrate the procedure in this chapter. Ask each student to assume the patient/resident role when practicing and return demonstrating the procedure.

14. Call on students to discuss the psychosocial needs of persons with wounds. Encourage students to share any personal experiences with wounds.

Homework Assignments

Ask students to answer the questions at the end of Chapter 41 in the textbook. Tell students the date and time that this assignment must be completed and turned in.

If the accompanying student workbook is being used, assign the Chapter 41 workbook exercises. Tell students the date and time that this assignment must be completed and turned in.

Name _____

Date _____

Wound Care

1. Persons at risk for pressure ulcers are those who:

   a. _____

   b. _____

   c. _____

   d. _____

   e. _____

   f. _____

   g. _____

   h. _____

2. Describe the stages of pressure ulcers:

   a. _____

   _____

   b. _____

   _____

   c. _____

   _____

   d. _____

   _____

3. Define the following types of wound healing:

   a. Primary intention: _____

   _____

   b. Secondary intention: _____

   _____

   c. Tertiary intention: _____

   _____

4. List and define four complications of wound healing.

   a. _____

   _____

   b. _____

   _____

   c. _____

   _____

   d. _____

   _____

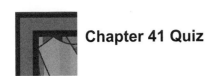

Chapter 41 Quiz

Name _____

Date _____

Wound Care

True or False	**Multiple Choice**

Mark **T** *for true or* **F** *for false.*

1. _____ A wound is a break in the skin or mucous membrane.

2. _____ Wound care involves preventing infection and preventing further injury.

3. _____ Skin tears provide a portal of entry for microbes.

4. _____ A bed cradle is used to keep linen off the feet.

5. _____ Circulatory ulcers are found primarily on the arms.

6. _____ Infants and children are at risk for pressure ulcers.

7. _____ Internal hemorrhage can be seen.

8. _____ Tape is used to secure a dressing. Tape should encircle the entire body part.

9. _____ Incorrect application of binders can cause severe discomfort, skin irritation, and circulatory and respiratory problems.

Circle the BEST answer.

10. Mrs. Smith has cut herself with a knife while cutting meat. Which is correct?
    a. She has an unintentional wound.
    b. She has a clean wound.
    c. She has an infected wound.
    d. She has a chronic wound.

11. A laceration is:
    a. A closed wound caused by a blow to the body.
    b. A partial-thickness wound caused by the scraping away of skin.
    c. An open wound with torn tissue and jagged edges.
    d. The collection of blood under the skin and tissue.

12. An open wound on the lower legs and feet caused by poor return blood flow from veins is called:
    a. A stasis ulcer.
    b. An arterial ulcer.
    c. A pressure ulcer.
    d. A thrombus.

13. Which drainage is green, yellow, or brown?
    a. Serous drainage
    b. Sanguineous drainage
    c. Serosanguineous drainage
    d. Purulent drainage

14. You are changing a nonsterile dressing. Before you begin:
    a. Review the procedure with the nurse.
    b. Allow pain medications time to take effect.
    c. Collect all needed equipment and supplies.
    d. Do all of the above.

15. Binders promote healing because they:
    a. Hold dressings in place.
    b. Reduce or prevent swelling by promoting circulation.
    c. Prevent injury.
    d. All of the above.

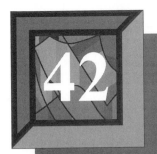

42

Heat and Cold Applications

Instructor's Preparation

I. Read Chapter 42 in the textbook. Carefully review chapter objectives, key terms, and review questions.

II. Read the outline in Chapter 42 of the instructor's guide. Carefully review the classroom activities, the student assignment, and the quiz.

III. If you are using the accompanying student workbook, review the activities for Chapter 42.

IV. Gather all necessary supplies and equipment for classroom activities and student assignments.

   A. Prepare appropriate flip charts

   B. Prepare overhead transparencies

   C. Prepare situation/index cards

   D. Gather coloured markers

   E. Gather the necessary equipment and supplies needed to demonstrate and have each student return demonstrate the procedures in this chapter

   F. Gather any other items that will be needed for classroom activities

   G. Assemble items in the order they will be used

V. Make sure that the necessary equipment is available and in good working order.

Objectives

- Define the key terms listed in this chapter
- Identify the purposes, effects, and complications of heat and cold applications
- List clients at risk for complications from heat and cold applications
- Describe the guidelines for the application of heat and cold
- Learn the procedures described in this chapter

Key Terms

compress
constrict
cyanosis
dilate
pack

Outline

Heat and Cold Applications

I. INTRODUCTION
   A. Physicians, nurses, and physical therapists order heat and cold application to reduce tissue swelling and promote healing and comfort
   B. Heat and cold have opposite effects
     1. Heat increases blood flow
     2. Cold slows blood flow
     3. Risks are involved with both applications and severe injuries can occur if done improperly
   C. You must thoroughly understand the purposes, effects, and complications of heat and cold applications
   D. Before you perform these procedures, make sure that:
     1. Your provincial or territorial laws and employer policies allow you to perform the procedure
     2. The procedure is in your job description
     3. You have the necessary training
     4. You are familiar with the equipment
     5. You review the procedure with a nurse
     6. A nurse is available to answer questions and to supervise you

II. HEAT APPLICATIONS
   A. Can be applied to almost any body part
   B. Used to:
     1. Relieve pain
     2. Relax muscles
     3. Promote healing
     4. Reduce tissue swelling
     5. Decrease joint stiffness
   C. Effects
     1. Blood vessels in the area dilate—expand; open wider (see Figure 42-1B, p. 697
       a. More blood flows through the vessels
       b. Tissues have more oxygen and nutrients for healing
       c. Excess fluid is removed from the area faster
       d. The skin is reddened and feels warm
   D. Complications
     1. High temperatures can cause burns
       a. Pain, excessive redness, and blisters are danger signs
     2. Remove the application and report these signs immediately
     3. Observe for pale skin
       a. When heat is applied too long, blood vessels constrict; blood flow decreases
       b. Tissue damage occurs
     3. Persons at risk (see Box 42-1, p. 698)
       a. People with thin, delicate or fragile skin
       b. People with decreased sensation
       c. People with dementia or confusion
       d. People with metal implants
         (1) Pacemakers and joint replacements are made of metal
         (2) Heat is not applied in the area of the implant
   E. Moist and dry applications
     1. Moist heat applications
       a. The water is in contact with the skin
       b. The effects are greater and occur faster than from dry heat
       c. Heat penetrates deeper
       d. Moist heat applications have lower temperatures to prevent injury
     2. Dry heat applications
       a. Water is not in contact with the skin
       b. Advantages:
         (1) It stays at the desired temperature longer
         (2) It does not penetrate as deeply as moist heat
       c. Dry heat needs higher temperatures to achieve the desired effect (burns are a risk)
     3. Practice the guidelines in Box 42-2, p. 698 in the textbook, to prevent burns and other complications
   F. Hot compresses and packs
     1. Are moist heat applications
     2. Consist of a washcloth, small towel, or gauze dressing
       a. A compress is applied to a small area
       b. Packs are applied to a large area
     3. The application is left in place for 20 minutes
     4. Applying Hot Compresses ▶ p. 699
     5. Commercial compresses
       a. Premoistened and packaged in foil
       b. An infrared lamp is used to heat the compress (follow manufacturers instructions)
   G. Hot soaks
     1. A hot soak involves putting the body part into water
     2. Promotes circulation and muscle relaxation
     3. Can be used for smaller parts such as feet (see Figure 42-3, p. 700)
     4. A tub is used for larger areas (arms, legs, or torso

5. Remember to check water temperature before soaking the body part
6. Soaks last 15 to 20 minutes
7. The person's comfort and body alignment are maintained
8. The Hot Soak ⅛ p. 708

H. The sitz bath
1. Involves immersing the perineal and rectal areas in warm or hot water for 20 minutes
2. Used to clean perineal or anal wounds
3. Used to promote healing, relieve pain and soreness, increase circulation, or stimulate voiding
4. Commonly used:
   a. After rectal or female pelvic surgery
   b. For relief from hemorrhoids
   c. After childbirth
5. Are disposable or built-in (see Figures 42-4 and 42-5, p. 702)
6. The person may become weak, feel faint, become drowsy, or fee lcilled
   a. Observe the person carefully
7. Protect the person from injury
   a. Check the person every 5 minutes
   b. Keep the signal light within reach
8. Assisting the Person to Take a Sitz Bath ▶ p. 702

I. Hot Packs
1. A pack is a treatment that involves wrapping a body part with a wet or dry application
2. Can be hot or cold, single-use or reusable commercial packs
3. Manufacturer's instructions will tell you how to activate (see Figure 42-6, p. 704); always remember to read warning labels and follow the instructions
4. Reusable packs are cleaned after use; they are either wiped with alcohol or washed with soap and water
5. Follow employer policy and the manufacturer's instructions

III. COLD APPLICATIONS
A. Often used to treat sprains and fractures
   1. They reduce pain, prevent swelling, and decrease bleeding
B. They cool the body when fever is present
C. Effects
   1. Has the opposite effect of heat
   2. Blood vessels constrict; decreased blood flow results; less oxygen and nutrients are carried to tissue (see Figure 42-1, p. 697)
   3. Useful right after injury

a. Decreased circulation reduces the amount of bleeding
b. The amount of fluid collecting in tissues is reduced
c. The numbing effect reduces or relieves pain

D. Complications
1. Pain, burns, blisters, and cyanosis occur:
   a. From intense cold
   b. When cold is applied directly to the skin
   c. When cold is applied for a long time, blood vessels dilate, and blood flow increases, which may increase bleeding and swelling

E. Moist and dry applications
1. Cold applications are moist or dry
   a. Dry cold–ice bags, ice collar, and ice glove
   b. Moist cold–cold compress
   c. Moist or dry–cold packs
2. Moist cold applications penetrate deeper than dry ones
3. Temperatures of moist applications are not as cold as dry applications

F. Ice bags, ice collars, and disposable cold packs
1. An ice bag and ice collar are dry cold applications
   a. Filled with crushed ice and placed in a cover
   b. If the cover becomes moist, change it
2. Commercial ice bags are kept frozen until needed
   a. Covers are needed
3. Disposable cold packs are used once and discarded
   a. Come in many sizes
   b. Some have an outer cover; otherwise, a cover is used
4. Focus on home care
   a. Disposable ice packs are common
   b. Plastic bags filled with ice are useful
   c. Plastic bags of frozen fruits and vegetables may be used
      (1) Wrap in a towel, dish cloth, or pillow case
5. Applying an Ice Bag, Ice Collar, or Disposable Cold Pack ▶ p. 706

G. Cold compresses
1. A moist application
2. Left in place no longer than 20 minutes
3. Applying Cold Compresses ▶ p. 708

Classroom Activities

1. Write on the chalkboard: "Before you perform the procedures in this chapter, make sure that:"

   a. _____

   b. _____

   c. _____

   d. _____

   e. _____

   f. _____

   Call on students to provide the answers. Write the correct answers on the chalkboard.

2. Divide students into four groups.
   a. Write each of the following questions on a separate index card:
      (1) Why are heat applications used?
      (2) What are the effects of heat applications?
      (3) What are the complications of heat applications?
      (4) Who are the people at risk for complications from heat applications?
   b. Distribute one index card to each group. Allow each group 10 minutes to answer the question on their index card. Then call on one student from each group to report to the class.

   Allow time for questions and discussion after each presentation.

3. Discuss the differences between dry and moist applications.

4. Display the rules in Box 42-1, p. 698 in the textbook, on an overhead transparency. Carefully review each rule with students.
   a. Allow time for questions.

5. Call on students to list the safety measures that are practiced when using an aquathermia pad.
   a. Write the correct answers on the chalkboard.

6. Divide students into four groups.
   a. Write each of the following questions on a separate index card:
      (1) Why are cold applications used?
      (2) What are the effects of cold applications?
      (3) What are the complications of cold applications?
      (4) Who are the people at risk for complications from cold applications?
   b. Distribute one index card to each group. Allow each group 10 minutes to answer the question on their index card. Then call on one student from each group to report to the class.

   Allow time for questions and discussion after each presentation.

7. Use the procedure checklists provided.
   a. Demonstrate the procedures in this chapter.
   b. Have each student practice and return demonstrate the procedures in this chapter. Have each student assume the role of the patient/resident when practicing and return demonstrating a procedure.
   c. Stress the importance of following safety rules.

Homework Assignments

Ask students to answer the questions at the end of Chapter 42 in the textbook. Tell students the date and time that this assignment must be completed and turned in.

If the accompanying student workbook is being used, assign the Chapter 42 workbook exercises. Tell students the date and time that this assignment must be completed and turned in.

Name _____

Date _____

Heat and Cold Applications

1. When applying heat and cold, you observe the skin for signs of complications. What signs and symptoms are reported to the nurse immediately?

    a. _____

    b. _____

    c. _____

    d. _____

    e. _____

    f. _____

2. List the heat and cold ranges for the following temperatures.

Temperature	Fahrenheit range	Centigrade range
Very hot		
Hot		
Warm		
Tepid		
Cool		
Cold		

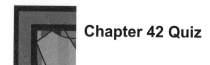

Name _____

Date _____

Heat and Cold Applications

True or False	Multiple Choice

*Mark **T** for true or **F** for false.*

1. _____ When heat is applied to the skin, blood vessels in the area dilate.

2. _____ Fair-skinned people are at great risk for complications from heat applications.

3. _____ Hot compresses and packs are left in place for 30 to 35 minutes.

4. _____ The person's comfort and body alignment are maintained during a hot soak.

5. _____ Burns and blisters tend to occur from intense cold.

6. _____ Moist cold applications penetrate deeper than dry ones.

7. _____ An ice bag is a moist cold application.

8. _____ Before applying an ice bag, place it in a cover.

Circle the BEST answer.

9. Heat applications are used for all of the following except to:
   a. Relieve pain.
   b. Control bleeding.
   c. Relax muscles.
   d. Decrease joint stiffness.

10. You are assisting Mrs. Blake with a sitz bath. Which is incorrect?
    a. Blood flow to the pelvic area decreases.
    b. She may be become weak or feel faint.
    c. Drowsiness can occur.
    d. The signal light is kept within reach.

11. Which is a moist cold application?
    a. An ice collar.
    b. An ice bag.
    c. A disposable cold pack.
    d. A cold compress.

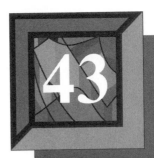

43

Oxygen Needs

Instructor's Preparation

I. Read Chapter 43 in the textbook. Carefully review chapter objectives, key terms, and review questions.
II. Read the outline in Chapter 43 of the instructor's guide. Carefully review the classroom activities, the student assignment, and the quiz.
III. If you are using the accompanying student workbook, review the activities for Chapter 43.
IV. Gather all necessary supplies and equipment for classroom activities and student assignments.
   A. Prepare appropriate flip charts
   B. Prepare overhead transparencies
   C. Prepare situation/index cards
   D. Gather coloured markers
   E. Gather anatomical models

F. Gather simulators
G. Gather necessary equipment and supplies needed to demonstrate and have each student return demonstrate the procedures in this chapter
H. Gather any other items that will be needed for classroom activities.
   I. Assemble items in the order they will be used
V. Make sure that the necessary equipment is available and in good working order.
VI. Contact guest speaker(s) to confirm the day, date, time, and location that he or she is expected.
   A. Ask the speaker if he or she requires any special equipment or supplies. Make sure these are available

Objectives

- Define the key terms listed in this chapter
- Describe the factors affecting oxygen needs
- Identify the signs and symptoms of hypoxia and altered respiratory function
- Describe the tests used to diagnose respiratory problems
- Explain measures that promote oxygenation

- Describe devices used to administer oxygen
- Explain how to safely assist with oxygen therapy
- Describe the safety measures for suctioning
- Explain how to assist in the care of persons with artificial airways, on mechanical ventilation and with chest tubes
- Learn the procedures described in this chapter

Key Terms

apnea
Biot's respirations
bradypnea
Cheyne-Stokes respirations
dyspnea
hemoptysis
hemothorax
hyperventilation
hypoventilation
hypoxemia
hypoxia
intubation
Kussmaul's respirations
mechanical ventilation
orthopnea
orthopneic position
oxygen concentration
pulse oximeter
respiratory arrest
respiratory depression
sputum
suction
tachypnea
tracheostomy

Outline

Oxygen Needs

I. INTRODUCTION
  A. Death occurs within minutes if a person stops breathing
  B. You need to know how to give safe and effective care
    1. See Figure 43-1, p. 712 in the textbook, for a review of the respiratory system
    2. Before giving or assisting with any care described in this chapter, make sure that:
      a. Your province or territory allows you to perform the task
      b. The task is in your job description
      c. You have the necessary training
      d. You know how to use the equipment
      e. You review the task with a nurse
      f. A nurse will supervise you
II. FACTORS AFFECTING OXYGEN NEEDS
  A. Each body system depends on the other
  B. Major factors affecting oxygen needs are:
    1. Respiratory system status
      a. Structures must be intact and functioning
      b. The airway must be open
      c. Alveoli must exchange oxygen and carbon dioxide

2. Cardiovascular system function
  a. Blood must flow freely to and from the heart
  b. Narrowed vessels affect blood flow
  c. Capillaries and cells must exchange oxygen and carbon dioxide
3. Red blood cell count (RBCs)
  a. RBCs contain hemoglobin, which picks up oxygen in the lungs and carries it to the cells
  b. The bone marrow must produce enough RBCs
    (1) Affected by diet, chemotherapy, and leukemia
  c. Blood loss reduces the number of RBCs
4. Intact nervous system
  a. Nervous system disease and injury can affect respiratory muscle function
  b. Brain damage affects respiratory rate, rhythm, and depth
  c. Narcotics and depressant drugs slow respirations
  d. The amount of oxygen and carbon dioxide in the blood affects brain function
5. Aging
  a. Respiratory muscles weaken and lung tissue becomes less elastic
  b. There is decreased strength for coughing; airways may fill with secretions causing pneumonia
  c. There is increased risk of respiratory complications after surgery
6. Exercise
  a. Oxygen needs increase with exercise
  b. Persons with heart and respiratory disease may not be able to meet this increased need for oxygen
7. Fever
  a. Oxygen needs increase
  b. Respiratory rate and depth must increase
8. Pain
  a. Increases the need for oxygen
9. Medications
  a. Some drugs depress the respiratory center in the brain
    (1) Respiratory depression is slow, weak, shallow respirations of fewer than 12 per minute
    (2) Respiratory arrest is when breathing stops
  b. Narcotics must be given in safe amounts
  c. Substance abusers are at risk for respi-

ratory depression and respiratory arrest
   10. Smoking
      a. Causes lung cancer and chronic obstructive pulmonary disease (COPD)
      b. Is a risk factor for coronary artery disease
   11. Allergies
      a. A sensitivity to a substance that causes the body to react with signs and symptoms
      b. Respiratory signs and symptoms include:
         (1) Runny nose, wheezing, and congestion
         (2) Mucous membranes in the upper airway swell (the airway can close)
         (3) Shock and death are risks
      c. Persons with allergies are at risk for chronic bronchitis and asthma
   12. Pollutant exposure
      a. Harmful chemicals or substances in the air or water
      b. They damage the lungs
      c. Exposure occurs at home, work, and in the community settings
   13. Nutrition
      a. Good nutrition is needed for RBC production
      b. RBCs live 3 to 4 months; new ones must replace those that die
      c. The body needs iron and vitamins to produce RBCs
   14. Substance abuse
      a. Alcohol depresses the brain
         (1) Excessive amounts depress the cough reflex and increase the risk of aspiration
            (a) Obstructed airway and pneumonia are risks
      b. Respiratory depression and respiratory arrest are risks when narcotics and depressant drugs are abused
III. ALTERED RESPIRATORY FUNCTION
   A. Respiratory system function involves three processes:
      1. Air moves into and out of the lungs
      2. Oxygen and carbon dioxide are exchanged at the alveoli
      3. Blood transports oxygen to cells and removes carbon dioxide from them
   B. Respiratory function is altered if even one

process is affected
   C. Hypoxia
      1. A deficiency of oxygen in the cells
      2. Caused by any illness, disease, injury, or surgery affecting respiratory function
      3. The brain is very sensitive to lack of oxygen
      4. Report signs and symptoms of hypoxia to the nurse immediately (see Box 43-1, p. 713)
      5. Hypoxia is life-threatening
         a. Oxygen is given; treatment is directed at the cause
   D. Abnormal respirations
      1. The normal rate is 12 to 20 per minute in adults
         a. Infants and children have faster rates
      2. Respirations are normally quiet, effortless, and regular; both sides of the chest rise and fall equally
      3. Abnormal patterns:
         a. Tachypnea is rapid breathing; usually respirations are more than 24 per minute
            (1) Fever, exercise, pain, pregnancy, airway obstruction, and hypoxemia are common causes
               (a) Hypoxemia is a reduced amount of oxygen in the blood
         b. Bradypnea is slow breathing; respirations are fewer than 10 per minute
            (1) Seen with drug overdose and central nervous system disorders
         c. Apnea is the absence of breathing
            (1) Occurs in cardiac arrest and respiratory arrest
         d. Hypoventilation is slow, shallow, irregular respirations
            (1) Causes include lung disorders affecting alveoli, obesity, airway obstruction, drug side effects, nervous system and musculoskeletal disorders affecting respiratory muscles
         e. Hyperventilation is when respirations are rapid and deeper than normal
            (1) Its many causes include asthma, emphysema, infection, fever, central nervous system disorders, hypoxia, anxiety, pain, and some drugs
         f. Dyspnea is difficult, labored, or painful breathing

(1) Heart disease, exercise, and anxiety are common causes

g. Cheyne-Stokes respirations are when respirations gradually increase in rate and depth and then become shallow and slow; breathing may stop for 10 to 20 seconds

(1) Causes are drug overdose, heart failure, renal failure, and brain disorders

(a) Common when death is near

h. Orthopnea is breathing deeply and comfortably only while sitting or standing

(1) Common causes include emphysema, asthma, pneumonia, angina pectoris, and other heart and respiratory disorders

i. Biot's respirations are irregular respirations with periods of apnea

(1) Occur with central nervous system disorders

j. Kussmaul's respirations are very deep and rapid respirations

(1) A sign of diabetic coma

E. Assisting with assessment and diagnostic testing

1. Altered respiratory function may be an acute or chronic problem

2. Report your observations to your supervisor promptly and accurately (see Box 43-2, p. 714)

a. Quick action is necessary to correct the situation and prevent the problem from getting worse

3. Common tests to determine causes of altered respiratory function(see Box 43-3, p. 715):

a. A chest x-ray is used to evaluate changes in the lungs

b. A lung scan is done to see what areas of the lungs are not getting air or blood

(1) The person inhales radioactive gas and is injected with a radioisotope

c. A bronchoscopy is when a scope is passed into the trachea and bronchi

(1) The doctor inspects for bleeding and tumors

(2) Tissue samples (biopsy) may be taken

(3) Mucous plugs and foreign objects can be removed

(4) The person is NPO 6 to 8 hours before the procedure

(5) The person is NPO and watched carefully after the procedure

(6) Preoperative and postoperative care is given as directed by the RN

d. Thoracentesis is when the pleura is punctured and air or fluid is aspirated from it

(1) Air, blood, or fluid in the pleural sac affects respiratory function

(2) Also done to remove fluid for laboratory study or to inject anti-cancer drugs

(3) Post procedure—the person is checked often for shortness of breath, dyspnea, cough, sputum, chest pain, cyanosis, vital sign changes, and other respiratory signs and symptoms

e. Pulmonary function tests measure the amount of air moving into and out of the lungs (volume) and how much air the lungs can hold (capacity)

(1) Used to evaluate the person's risk for lung disease or postoperative pulmonary complications

(2) Also used to measure the progress of lung disease and its treatment

(3) Fatigue is common after the test

f. Arterial blood gasses (ABGs) can be tested when the radial or femoral artery is punctured to obtain arterial blood

(1) Laboratory tests measure the amount of oxygen in the blood

(2) Apply pressure to the artery for at least 5 minutes after the procedure

4. Pulse oximetry measures oxygen concentration in arterial blood

a. The percent of hemoglobin that contains oxygen

b. Normal range is 95% to 100%

c. A sensor is attached to the persons finger, toe, earlobe, nose, or forehead

d. The value and the person's pulse rate are displayed on the monitor

e. An alarm sounds if oxygen concentration is low, the pulse rate is too fast or slow, or other problems occur

f. A good sensor site is needed (see Figure 43-2, p. 715)

(1) Your supervisor tells you what site to use

(2) The site depends on the person's condition

(3) Swollen sites and sites with breaks in the skin are avoided

(4) Finger and toe sites are avoided in persons with poor circulation

g. Nail polish is removed if using a finger site

h. If using a finger site, do not measure blood pressure on that side

i. Report and record measurements accurately

   (1) Abbreviation SpO_2 (S=saturation, p=pulse, O_2=oxygen)

   (2) Date and time

   (3) What the person was doing at the time of measurement

   (4) Oxygen flow rate and the device used

   (5) Reason for measurement

   (6) Other observations

j. Pulse oximetry does not lessen the need for good observation

k. Focus on children

   (1) The earlobe is a good sensor site for children

l. Focus on older persons

   (1) Use the ear, nose, or forehead sites for older persons

m. Focus on home care

   (1) Small hand-held units are available

   (2) Oxygen concentration is often measured with vital signs

n. Using a Pulse Oximeter ▶ p. 716

5. Collecting sputum specimens

a. Respiratory disorders cause lungs, bronchi, and trachea to secrete mucus (called sputum when expectorated through the mouth)

   (1) Different from saliva (the clear liquid produced by the salivary glands in the mouth)

b. Sputum specimens are studied for blood, microbes, and abnormal cells

c. Coughing up sputum is often painful and difficult

   (1) Easier in the morning upon awakening

   (2) Rinse the mouth with water; do not use mouthwash

d. Collecting a sputum specimen can embarrass the person

   (1) Privacy is important

   (2) The specimen container is covered and placed in a bag

e. Always follow Standard Precautions

f. Focus on children

   (1) Breathing treatments and suctioning are often needed to produce a sputum specimen in infants and small children

     (a) The nurse suctions, you assist

g. Focus on older persons

   (1) Older persons may not have the strength to cough up sputum

     (a) Easier after postural drainage

     (b) The nurse or respiratory therapist is responsible for postural drainage (see Figure 43-3, p. 717)

h. Collecting a Sputum Specimen ▶ p. 718

IV. PROMOTING OXYGENATION

A. Air must reach the alveoli for the exchange of oxygen and carbon dioxide

B. Disease and injury can prevent air from reaching the alveoli

C. Pain, immobility, and narcotics interfere with deep breathing and coughing up secretions

D. Secretions collect in the respiratory system and interfere with air movement and alveolar function

E. Secretions provide an environment for microbes; infection is a threat

F. Positioning

1. Breathing is usually easier in the semi-Fowler's and Fowler's positions

2. The orthopneic position is sitting up in bed and leaning forward over the overbed table

   a. Increase comfort by placing a pillow on the overbed table

3. Frequent position changes are important

   a. Usually done at least every 2 hours

   b. Follow the person's care plan

G. Coughing and deep breathing exercises

1. Mucus is removed by coughing

2. Deep breathing promotes air movement into most parts of the lungs

3. Helpful for persons with respiratory disorders

4. Routinely done after surgery and for persons on bedrest

5. The exercises are painful after injury or surgery (see Figure 43-6 and Figure 43-7, p. 721)

6. The exercises help prevent pneumonia and atelectasis (collapse of a portion of the lung)

7. The frequency of coughing and deep breathing varies
   a. Your supervisor tells you how often
   b. You are told how many deep breaths and coughs a person should do
      (1) Follow the client's care plan
8. Assisting with Coughing and Deep Breathing Exercises ▶ p. 720

H. Incentive spirometry
   1. Involves encouraging the person to inhale until reaching a preset volume of air
      a. Balls or bars in the spirometer allow the person to see the movement of air when inhaling (see Figure 43-9, p. 722)
   2. The goal of using a spirometer is to improve lung function and prevent respiratory complications
   3. Air moves deeper into the lungs and secretions become loose
   4. The device is used as follows:
      a. The spirometer is placed upright
      b. The client exhales normally
      c. The client seals his or her lips around a mouthpiece
      d. A slow, deep breath is taken until the balls rises to the desired height
      e. The breath is held for 3 to 6 seconds to keep the balls floating
      f. The client then removes the mouthpiece and exhales slowly, and may cough at this time
      g. After taking some normal breaths, the client uses the device again
   5. You supervisor tells you how often the client needs incentive spirometry and how many breaths they need to take
      a. This information is also on the care plan
   6. Follow agency policy for cleaning and replacing disposable mouthpieces

V. ASSISTING WITH OXYGEN THERAPY
   A. Oxygen is treated as a drug
      1. The doctor orders the amount of oxygen to give and the device to use
   B. Continuous oxygen therapy means the oxygen is never stopped
   C. Intermittent oxygen therapy is for symptom relief
      1. Chest pain and exercise are common reasons for intermittent oxygen
   D. You are not responsible for administering oxygen
      1. The nurse or respiratory therapist starts and maintains oxygen therapy
      2. You assist in providing safe care to persons receiving oxygen
   E. Oxygen sources
      1. Supplied through wall outlets, oxygen tanks, and oxygen concentrators
      2. With the wall outlet, oxygen is piped into each patient or resident unit; connected to a centrally located oxygen supply
      3. The oxygen tank is portable
         a. Small tanks are used for emergencies and transfers
         b. The gauge on the tank tells you how much oxygen is left in the tank
            (1) Tell the nurse if the tank is low
      4. Oxygen concentrators do not need an oxygen source
         a. It removes oxygen from the air
         b. A power source is needed
         c. If the concentrator is not portable, moving about is limited
         d. A portable oxygen tank is needed in case of power failure and for mobility
      5. Liquid oxygen systems also are used
         a. A portable unit is filled from a stationary unit
         b. A liquid content indicator tells when the unit needs refilling
            (1) Tell your supervisor if the tank is low
         c. The portable unit may be worn over the shoulder
         d. Liquid oxygen is very cold; if touched, it can cause the skin to freeze
            (1) Never tamper with the equipment
            (2) Follow agency policies and procedures and the manufacturer's instructions
      6. Focus on home care
         a. Oxygen is supplied by a medical supply company
            (1) Keep the name and phone number near the phone
         b. In the home, the patient and family must practice safety measures where oxygen is used and stored
            (1) The safety measures to prevent fires are practiced (see Box 43-4, p. 724)
            (2) The oxygen source and oxygen tubing are kept away from open flames and heat sources
   F. Devices used to administer oxygen
      1. Nasal cannula—two prongs project from the tubing; the prongs are inserted a short distance into the nostrils (see Figure 43-15, p. 724)

a. The prongs point downward
b. An elastic headband or tubing brought behind the ears keeps the cannula in place
c. Pressure on the ears is possible
2. Simple face mask covers the nose and mouth (see Figure 43-16, p. 724)
  a. Carbon dioxide escapes through small holes in the sides of the mask during exhalation
  b. Room air enters during inhalation
3. Partial-rebreathing mask—a reservoir bag is added to the simple face mask (see Figure 43-17, p. 725)
  a. The bag is for exhaled air
  b. With inhalation, the person inhales oxygen, some exhaled air, and some room air
4. Nonrebreathing face mask prevents exhaled air from entering the reservoir bag (see Figure 43-18, p. 725)
  a. Exhaled air leaves through holes in the mask
  b. With inhalation, oxygen from the reservoir bag is inhaled
5. Venturi mask allows precise amounts of oxygen to be given (see Figure 43-19, p. 725)
  a. Color-coded adapters indicate the amount of oxygen delivered
6. Special care is needed when masks are used
  a. Talking is difficult; listen carefully
  b. Keep the person's face clean and dry
  c. Masks are removed for eating; usually nasal cannulas are used during meals
G. Oxygen flow rates
1. The amount of oxygen given is called the flow rate
2. Measured in liters per minute (L/min)
3. The flow rate is set by the nurse or respiratory therapist
  a. The nurse and the care plan tell you this information
4. When you care for the patient or resident, always check the flow rate
  a. Tell your supervisor immediately if the flow rate is too high or too low
  b. Some employers allow support workers to adjust oxygen flow rates
H. Preparing for oxygen administration
1. Your supervisor may ask you to set up the oxygen administration system
2. The nurse tells you:

a. The person's name, room, and bed number
b. The oxygen administration device ordered
c. If humidification was ordered (see Figure 43-21, p. 726)
3. Oxygen is a dry gas; if not humidified, it dries the mucous membranes
  a. Distilled water is added to the humidifier to create water vapor
  b. Oxygen tubing is attached to the humidifier
  c. Oxygen picks up water vapor as it flows into the system
  d. Bubbling in the humidifier means water vapor is being produced
4. A nurse turns on the oxygen, sets the flow rate, and applies the administration device
5. Setting Up for Oxygen Administration ▶ p. 727
I. Oxygen safety
1. Remember that you assist the nurse with oxygen therapy
  a. You do not adjust flow rates unless allowed by your employer
  b. You must give safe care to persons receiving oxygen
  c. Box 43-5, p. 728 in the textbook lists the rules for assisting with oxygen therapy
VI. ARTIFICIAL AIRWAYS
A. Keep the airway patent (open)
B. Are used when:
1. The person's airway is obstructed from disease, injury, secretions, or aspiration
2. The person is semiconscious or unconscious
3. The person is recovering from anesthesia
4. The person needs mechanical ventilation
C. Intubation is the process of inserting an artificial airway (usually plastic disposable airways are used)
1. Airways come in adult, pediatric, and infant sizes
D. Common types:
1. Oropharyngeal airway—inserted through the mouth into the pharynx (see Figure 43-22A, p. 729)
  a. A nurse or respiratory therapist can insert
2. Nasopharyngeal airway—inserted through a nostril into the pharynx (see Figure 43-22B, p. 729)

a. A nurse or respiratory therapist can insert
3. Endotracheal tube—inserted through the mouth or nose and into the trachea (see Figure 43-22C, p. 729)
  a. A doctor or RN with special training intubates using a lighted scope
  b. A balloon at the end of the tube is inflated to keep the airway in place
4. Tracheostomy tube—inserted through a surgical incision into the trachea (see Figure 43-22D, p. 729)
  a. Some tubes have cuffs that are inflated to keep the tube in place
  b. Inserted by a doctor

E. You assist in caring for persons with artificial airways
1. The person's vital signs are checked often
2. Observe for hypoxia and other respiratory signs and symptoms
3. If an airway comes out or is dislodged, tell your supervisor immediately
4. The person needs frequent oral hygiene; your supervisor tells you when and how to give oral hygiene
  a. This information is also in the care plan

F. Persons with endotracheal tubes cannot speak
1. Use paper and pencil, magic slates, communication boards, or hand signals to communicate

G. Gagging and choking sensations are common
1. The person needs comforting and reassurance
2. Use touch to show you care

H. Tracheostomies
1. Are temporary or permanent
2. Focus on children
  a. Tracheostomies are needed for some congenital defects
  b. Infections can cause airway obstruction
  c. Foreign body aspiration also obstructs airflow
3. Made of plastic or metal
4. A tracheostomy tube has three parts (see Figure 43-23, p. 729)
  a. The outer tube (cannula) is not removed
  b. The inner tube (cannula) is inserted inside the outer cannula and locked in place

    (1) Removed for cleaning and mucus removal
    (2) This keeps the airway patent
  c. Obturator
    (1) Has a rounded end that is used to insert the outer cannula and is removed
    (2) Placed within reach in case the tracheostomy tube falls out and needs to be reinserted
5. Some plastic tracheostomy tubes do not have a inner cannula
  a. Used for persons who are suctioned often
6. The cuffed tracheostomy tube provides a seal between the cannula and the trachea
  a. Used with mechanical ventilation
  b. Prevents air from leaking around the tube
  c. Prevents aspiration
  d. A nurse or respiratory therapist inflates and deflates the cuff
7. Securing tracheostomy tubes in place is important
  a. The tube must not come out
  b. Damage to the airway is possible if the tube is loose and moves up and down in the trachea
8. The tracheostomy tube must remain patent
  a. Some persons cough up secretions
  b. Others require suctioning
  c. Call the nurse if the person shows signs or symptoms of hypoxia or respiratory distress
  d. Call the nurse if the outer cannula comes out
9. Measures are needed to prevent aspiration; nothing can enter the stoma
  a. Patient and family teaching
    (1) Make sure dressings do not have loose gauze or lint
    (2) Keep the stoma or tube covered when outside
    (3) Take tub baths instead of showers
    (4) Be careful when shampooing
    (5) Cover the stoma when shaving
    (6) Do not swim
    (7) Wear a medical alert bracelet; carry a medical alert ID card
10. Tracheostomy care
  a. Involves cleaning the inner cannula,

cleaning the stoma, and applying clean ties or Velcro collar

    (1) Keeps the airway patent

    (2) Prevents skin breakdown and infection

    (3) If the inner cannula is disposable, it is not cleaned; it is discarded and a new one inserted

  b. Your supervisor may ask you to assist with tracheostomy care

    (1) It may be done daily or every 8 to 12 hours

    (2) Done when there are excess secretions, the ties or collar are soiled, or the dressing is soiled or moist

    (3) When the ties are removed, you must hold the outer cannula in place

    (4) The ties or collar must be secure but not tight

  c. Standard Precautions are followed

  d. Focus on children

    (1) When assisting with tracheostomy care for a child, you must hold the child still; position the head so that the neck is slightly extended

VII. SUCTIONING THE AIRWAY

  A. Injury and illness cause secretions to collect in the upper airway

    1. Removing secretions is necessary so air can flow

    2. Hypoxia occurs if secretions are not removed

    3. Usually coughing removes secretions

    4. Sometimes suctioning is necessary

  B. Suctioning is the process of withdrawing or sucking up fluid (secretions)

    1. A tube is connected to a suction source at one end and a suction catheter at the other end; secretions are withdrawn through the catheter

  C. Suctioning routes

    1. Nose, mouth, pharynx are the upper airway

    2. Trachea and bronchi are the lower airway

    3. The oropharyngeal route involves suctioning the mouth and pharynx

    4. The nasopharyngeal route involves suctioning the nose and pharynx

    5. Lower airway suctioning is done through an endotracheal tube or a tracheostomy tube

D. Safety measures

  1. Suctioning can seriously harm the person if not done correctly

    a. Suctioning removes oxygen from the airway

    b. Hypoxia and life-threatening complications can arise (e.g. cardiac arrest, infection, and injury to the airway)

  2. You need to understand the principles and safety measures described in Box 43-6, p. 731 in the textbook

  3. Always make sure needed suction equipment and supplies are at the bedside

  4. Focus on children

    a. Suctioning may frighten children

    b. Clear explanations are needed

    c. You may need to hold the child still

E. Oropharyngeal suctioning

  1. A cycle takes no more than 10 to 15 seconds to complete

    a. Involves inserting the catheter, suctioning, and removing the catheter

  2. Hypoxia is a risk during suctioning

    a. The person's lungs are hyperventilated before suctioning a tracheostomy

    b. A manual resuscitation bag (Ambu bag) is used to hyperventilate; the Ambu bag is attached to an oxygen source

    c. The oxygen delivery device is removed from the tracheostomy tube and the Ambu bag is attached; the Ambu bag is compressed as the person inhales

    d. Three to five breaths are given as directed by the nurse or respiratory therapist

      (1) Remember that oxygen is treated as a drug

      (2) Check on whether your state and agency allow you to use an Ambu bag attached to an oxygen source

  3. Focus on children

    a. For infants and children, suction is applied no longer than 5 seconds

VIII. MECHANICAL VENTILATION

  A. Using a machine to move air into and out of the lungs (see Figure 43-27, p. 732)

  B. Persons on mechanical ventilation have artificial airways

  C. Ventilators have alarms that warn when something is wrong

    1. When any alarm sounds, first check to

see if the client's endotracheal or tracheostomy tube is attached to the ventilator
  a. If it is disconnected, attach it
2. Notify your suoervisor immediately about an alarm
3. Do not reset alarms
D. Persons needing mechanical ventilation are seriously ill
  1. Their reactions to mechanical ventilation are many
E. Mechanical ventilation can be painful for those with chest injuries or chest surgery
F. Tubes and hoses restrict movement
G. Important aspects of the person's care are listed in Box 43-7, p. 733 in the textbook
H. Often the person needs to be weaned from the ventilator
  1. The respiratory therapist and RN plan the weaning process
I. Focus on home care
  1. Home care is often arranged for ventilator-dependent persons
  2. Family members are taught how to assist with the person's care
  3. Make sure that an RN is available by phone
J. Box 43-7, p. 733 in the textbook, lists guidelines for caring for clients receiving mechanical ventilation

IX. CHEST TUBES
A. When the chest is entered, air, blood, or fluid can collect in the pleural space
  1. Occurs with chest surgery or injury
B. Pneumothorax is the collection of air in the pleural space
C. Hemothorax is the collection of blood in the pleural space
D. Pleural effusion is the collection of fluid in the pleural space
E. Pressure caused by the collection of air, blood, or fluid collapses the lungs
  1. Air cannot effectively reach the affected alveoli
  2. Oxygen and carbon dioxide are not exchanged
  3. Respiratory distress and hypoxia result
  4. There is sometimes pressure on the heart
    a. This is a life-threatening problem
F. The doctor inserts chest tubes to remove air, fluid, or blood (See Figure 43-28, p. 733
  1. The sterile procedure is done in surgery, in the emergency room, or at the bedside
    a. A nurse assists

2. Chest tubes are attached to a drainage system
  a. The system must be airtight
  b. Water-seal drainage is used to keep the system airtight (see Figure 43-29, p. 733)
G. When caring for persons with chest tubes, you need to (see Box 43-8, p. 734):
  1. Keep the drainage system below the level of the person's chest
  2. Measure the person's vital signs as directed by the nurse
    a. Report changes immediately
  3. Report signs and symptoms of hypoxia and respiratory distress immediately
  4. Report complaints of pain or difficulty breathing immediately
  5. Keep connecting tubing coiled on the bed; allow enough slack so the tubes are not dislodged when the person moves
  6. Make sure that the tubing is not kinked
  7. Observe chest drainage; report changes to the nurse immediately
  8. Record chest drainage according to agency policy
  9. Turn and position the person as directed
  10. Assist the person with coughing and deep breathing as directed; assist with incentive spirometry as directed
  11. Note bubbling activity in the drainage system; tell your supervisor immediately if the bubbling increases, decreases, or stops
  12. Tell your supervisor if any part of the system is loose or disconnected
  13. Make sure petrolatum gauze is at the bedside in case a tube comes out
  14. Call for help immediately if a chest tube comes out; cover the site with a sterile petrolatum gauze; stay with the person until a nurse arrives

Classroom Activities

1. Use Box 27-1, p. 633 in the textbook to review the respiratory system with students.
  a. Display the overhead transparency showing the respiratory system. Use this as the basis to review the structures and functions of the respiratory system.

2. Write on the chalkboard: "Major factors affecting oxygen use are:"

a. Call on students to identify the factors affecting oxygen use. Write the correct answers on the chalkboard.

b. Allow time for questions and discussion.

3. Call on students to describe the three processes involved in respiratory system function.

4. Write each of the following terms on a separate index card: Hypoxia, Tachypnea, Hypoxemia, Bradypnea, Apnea, Hypoventilation, Hyperventilation, Dyspnea, Cheyne-Stokes respirations, Orthopnea, Biot's respirations, and Kussmaul's respirations.

a. Call on students to pick an index card and define the term on the card he or she picked.

5. Write each of the following common tests used to determine causes of altered respiratory function in a different color on a flip chart. Allow space after each term to write in the definition.

a. Chest x-ray
b. Lung scan
c. Bronchoscopy
d. Thoracentesis
e. Pulmonary function tests
f. Arterial blood gases
g. Pulse oximetry

Call on students to define each test. Write the correct answers on the flip chart.

6. Call on students to describe the difference between saliva and sputum.

7. Write the following measures on the chalkboard:
a. Positioning
b. Coughing and deep breathing
c. Frequent position changes
d. Incentive spirometry

Call on students to discuss the importance of each measure in promoting oxygenation.

8. Ask students who is responsible for starting and maintaining oxygen therapy.
a. What is the role of the nursing assistant?

9. Have available the various devices used to administer oxygen (nasal cannulas, simple face mask, partial-rebreathing mask, non-rebreathing mask, and Venturi mask). Encourage students to handle the equipment and become familiar with how each item is used.

a. Stress the importance of knowing and following all safety rules when handling oxygen equipment.

b. Remind students that oxygen is treated as a drug.

10. Write on the chalkboard "Artificial airways are used when:"

a. _____

b. _____

c. _____

d. _____

Call on students to describe when artificial airways are used. Write the correct answers on the chalkboard.

11. Display a diagram showing the three parts of a tracheostomy tube (see Figure 43-23, p. 729) on an overhead transparency. Describe the function of each part.

12. Have available the various airways and tracheostomy tubes for students to manipulate.
a. Call on students to identify and define the following types of airways: (Oropharyngeal airway, Nasopharyngeal airway, Endotracheal tube, and Tracheostomy tube).

13. Display the principles and safety measures in Box 43-6, p. 731 in the textbook, on an overhead transparency.
a. Carefully review each of the safety measures with students.
b. Remind students that suctioning can seriously harm the person if not done correctly.

14. Arrange for a respiratory therapist to visit the class. He or she should:
a. Show slides of normal lungs and diseased lungs (cancer, tuberculosis, COPD)
b. Demonstrate the use of oxygen administration equipment.
c. Demonstrate how mechanical ventilation works.
d. Demonstrate how chest tubes work.

Allow time for questions and discussion.

15. Use the procedure checklists provided.

a. Demonstrate the procedures in this chapter.

b. Remind students that before performing the procedures in this chapter they must make sure that:

   (1) Their province or territory allows support workers to perform the procedure.

   (2) The procedure is in their job description.

   (3) They have the necessary education and training.

   (4) A nurse is available to answer questions and supervise them.

c. Have each student practice and return demonstrate the procedures in this chapter. When appropriate, have each student assume the role of the patient/resident when practicing and return demonstrating a procedure.

   (1) Ask students to share how it felt to be the patient/resident.

   (2) How will the experience help them provide better care.

   (3) Use a simulator or anatomical model when appropriate.

Homework Assignments

Ask students to answer the questions at the end of Chapter 43 in the textbook. Tell students the date and time that this assignment must be completed and turned in.

If the accompanying student workbook is being used, assign the Chapter 43 workbook exercises. Tell students the date and time that this assignment must be completed and turned in.

Name _____

Date _____

Oxygen Needs

The doctor orders tests to determine the cause of altered respiratory function. Match the following tests with the correct definitions.

a. Chest x-ray

b. Lung scan

c. Bronchoscopy

d. Thoracentesis

e. Pulmonary function tests

f. Arterial blood gasses

1. _____ Tests that measure the amount of air moving in and out of the lungs and how much air the lungs can hold.

2. _____ The pleura is punctured and air or fluid is aspirated from it. Also done to remove fluid for laboratory study or to inject anti-cancer drugs.

3. _____ A radiograph is taken of the chest to evaluate changes in the lungs.

4. _____ A scope is passed into the trachea and bronchi to inspect for bleeding or tumors. The doctor may also take tissue samples or remove mucous plugs and foreign objects.

5. _____ A radial or femoral artery is punctured to obtain arterial blood. Laboratory tests measure the amount of oxygen in the blood.

6. _____ The person inhales a radioactive gas and is injected with a radioisotope. The lungs are scanned to see what areas are not getting air.

7. What are the signs and symptoms of hypoxia?

a. _____

b. _____

c. _____

d. _____

e. _____

f. _____

g. _____

h. _____

i. _____

j. _____

k. _____

l. _____

m. _____

n. _____

o. _____

Chapter 43 Student Assignment

Name _____

Date _____

Oxygen Needs

8. List the important aspects of care for persons receiving mechanical ventilation.

a. _____

b. _____

c. _____

d. _____

e. _____

f. _____

g. _____

h. _____

i. _____

j. _____

k. _____

l. _____

m. _____

n. _____

o. _____

p. _____

q. _____

9. When caring for persons with chest tubes, you need to:

a. _____

b. _____

c. _____

d. _____

e. _____

f. _____

g. _____

h. _____

i. _____

j. _____

k. _____

l. _____

m. _____

n. _____

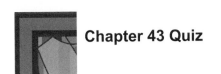

Chapter 43 Quiz

Name _____

Date _____

Oxygen Needs

True or False

Mark **T** *for true or* **F** *for false.*

1. _____ Altered function of any system affects the body's ability to meet its oxygen needs.

2. _____ Hypoxia is life-threatening.

3. _____ In adults, normal respirations occur between 25 and 30 times per minute.

4. _____ Orthopnea is a normal breathing pattern.

5. _____ Altered respiratory function may be acute or chronic.

6. _____ Pulse oximetry reduces the need for good observation.

7. _____ Sputum and saliva are the same. They are produced by the salivary glands in the mouth.

8. _____ Persons with breathing difficulties often prefer to sit up in bed and lean forward.

9. _____ Support workers are responsible for administering oxygen.

10. _____ Do not perform any procedure that you do not understand.

11. _____ The alarm on Mr. Adams' ventilator sounds. You should turn off the alarm and call your supervisor.

Multiple Choice

Circle the BEST answer.

12. The lack or absence of breathing is:
    a. Dyspnea.
    b. Apnea.
    c. Hypoxia.
    d. Orthopnea.

13. Which pulse oximetry measurement is within normal range?
    a. 82%
    b. 90%
    c. 92%
    d. 96%

14. Using a machine to move air in and out of the lungs is:
    a. Lung scan.
    b. Hyperventilation.
    c. Mechanical ventilation.
    d. Intubation.

15. Which measure does not promote oxygenation?
    a. Placing the client in the semi-Fowler's position
    b. Coughing and deep breathing exercises
    c. Having the person use an incentive spirometer
    d. Allowing the client to rest in the same position for 4 hours

16. Mr. Adams has a tracheostomy. Which measure will not help prevent aspiration?
    a. Ensuring dressings have no loose gauze or lint
    b. Keeping the stoma covered when outside.
    c. Taking a shower instead of a tub bath
    d. Covering the stoma when shaving

17. When performing oropharyngeal suctioning on an adult, a suctioning cycle is no longer than:
    a. 10 to 15 seconds.
    b 5 seconds.
    c. 15 to 20 seconds.
    d. 25 seconds.

18. Which statement about chest tubes is incorrect?
    a. The drainage system is airtight.
    b. Keep the drainage system at chest level.
    c. Keep connecting tubing coiled on the bed.
    d. Make sure the tubing is not kinked.

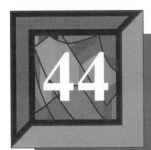

Assisting with the Physical Examination

Instructor's Preparation

I. Read Chapter 44 in the textbook. Carefully review chapter objectives, key terms, and review questions.

II. Read the outline in Chapter 44 of the instructor's guide. Carefully review the classroom activities, the student assignment, and the quiz.

III. If you are using the accompanying student workbook, review the activities for Chapter 44.

IV. Gather all necessary supplies and equipment for classroom activities and student assignments.
   A. Prepare appropriate flip charts
   B. Prepare overhead transparencies
   C. Gather coloured markers
   D. Gather the necessary equipment and supplies needed to demonstrate and have each student return demonstrate the procedures in this chapter
   E. Gather any other items that will be needed for classroom activities
   F. Assemble items in the order they will be used

V. Make sure that the necessary equipment is available and in good working order.

Objectives

- Define the key terms listed in this chapter
- Explain what to do before, after, and during a physical examination
- Identify the equipment used during a physical examination
- Describe how to prepare a person for an examination
- Describe four examination positions and how to drape the person for each position
- Explain the guidelines for assisting with a physical examination
- Learn the procedure described in this chapter

Key Terms

dorsal recumbent position
horizontal position
knee-chest position
laryngeal mirror
lithotomy position
nasal speculum
ophthalmoscope
otoscope
percussion hammer
reflex hammer
Sims' position
supine position
tuning fork
vaginal speculum

<hr>

Outline

Assisting with the Physical Examination

I. INTRODUCTION
  A. Physical examinations are done for many reasons
    1. Routinely to promote health
    2. Pre-employment
    3. To diagnose and treat disease
    4. Some long-term care facilities require new residents to have a physical exam on arrival
    5. Other facilities or agencies require residents to have yearly physicals
    6. In a facility, you may be asked to assist
    7. In the community, assisting with a physical is unlikely in your job description
II. YOUR RESPONSIBILITIES
  A. Depend on agency policies and procedures
  B. You may:
    1. Collect linens
    2. Collect equipment and supplies
    3. Prepare the room
    4. Transport the person
    5. Provide enough lighting
    6. Measure vital signs, height, and weight
    7. Position and drape the person
    8. Hand equipment and instruments to the examiner
    9. Stay with the client before or during the exam for support and to help prevent falls
    10. Label specimen containers
    11. Dispose of linens and discard used disposable supplies
    12. Clean reusable equipment
    13. Help the person dress and get comfortable after the examination
III. EQUIPMENT
  A. You need to know the following instruments (see Figure 44-1, p. 739):
    1. The ophthalmoscope is a lighted instrument used to examine the internal structures of the eye
    2. The otoscope is a lighted instrument used to examine the external ear and eardrum
    3. The percussion hammer (reflex hammer) is used to tap body parts to test reflexes
    4. The vaginal speculum is used to open the vagina so it and the cervix can be examined
    5. The nasal speculum is used to examine the inside of the nose
    6. The tuning fork is vibrated to test hearing

    7. The laryngeal mirror is used to examine the mouth, teeth, and throat
  B. Items may be on an examination tray
    1. If not, they are collected and arranged on a tray or table
IV. PREPARING THE CLIENT
  A. Factors that cause anxiety include:
    1. Concern about possible findings
    2. Discomfort
    3. Embarrassment
    4. Fear of exposure
    5. Not knowing the procedure
  B. The client is prepared physically and psychologically
    1. The doctor or RN explains the purpose of the examination and what to expect
      a. The procedure is explained
      b. The resident must give consent
    2. The resident may want a different examiner
    3. The resident may want a family member present
  C. Usually all clothes are removed; right to privacy is protected
    1. The person is covered with a drape
    2. Usually a hospital gown is worn
  D. Explain to the person that some exposure is necessary during the examination
    1. Only the body part being examined is exposed
    2. Screen the person and close the door
  E. Focus on children
    1. Young children are allowed to leave undergarments on; they are removed only as necessary
  F. The person urinates before the examination
    1. Obtain a urine specimen if needed (see Chapter 29)
  G. The person is protected from chilling and drafts
  H. The examiner may want height, weight, and vital signs measured
  I. Preparing the Person for an Examination ▶ p. 740
V. POSITIONING AND DRAPING
  A. Some examination positions are uncomfortable and embarrassing
  B. Before helping the person assume a position, explain the following:
    1. The need for the position
    2. How the position is assumed
    3. How the body is draped
    4. How long the person can expect to be in the position

C. Examination positions (see Figure 44-2, p. 741)
 1. The supine position (also called the dorsal recumbent or horizontal position)—the person is flat on his or her back with the legs together
  a. If the perineal area is to be examined, the knees are flexed and hips externally rotated; drape as for perineal care (see Figure 44-2A, p. 741)
 2. The lithotomy position—the person lies on her back and her hips are brought to the edge of the examination table (see Figure 44-2B, p. 741)
  a. The knees are flexed, hips are externally rotated, and feet are supported in stirrups
  b. Drape as for the dorsal recumbent position (see Chapter 27)
 3. The knee-chest position—the person kneels on the bed or examination table (see Figure 44-2C, p. 741)
  a. The person rests his or her body on the knees and chest, the head is turned to one side, the arms are above the head or flexed at the elbows
  b. The drape is applied in a diamond shape to cover the back, buttocks, and thighs
  c. This position is rarely used for older persons
   (1) The side-lying position is used
 4. The Sims' position—a side-lying position (see Figure 44-2D, p. 741)
  a. The upper leg is sharply flexed so that it is not on the lower leg; the lower arm is behind the person
  b. The drape is applied in a diamond shape

VI. ASSISTING WITH THE EXAMINATION
 A. Follow the rules in Box 44-1, p. 742 in the textbook
 B. Focus on children
  1. A parent is present for the examination of an infant or child
   a. The parent may hold the child
    (1) Being kept still may frighten an infant
    (2) A child may fear separation from a parent
    (3) Some fear being physically harmed
   b. Remember that the parent may be anxious too

  c. Toys are used to assess development
  d. Vaginal speculums are not used
 C. Focus on older persons
  1. Persons with dementia may resist the examiner's efforts
   a. The person is not restrained or forced to have the procedure
   b. The person may react better at another time
   c. Having a family member present may help
   d. The person's rights are always respected
 D. After the examination
  1. The person is taken back to the room
   a. In a clinic, the person dresses in the examination room
  2. Assist as needed
   a. Lubricant used during the examination is wiped or cleaned before the person dresses or returns to the room
   b. Used disposable items are put in a waste container
   c. Replace supplies so the tray is ready for the next examination
   d. Reusable items are cleaned according to agency policy and returned to the tray
   e. The examination table is covered with a clean drawsheet or paper
   f. All specimens are labeled and sent to the laboratory with a requisition slip
   g. The person's unit or examination room should be neat and orderly
   h. Follow agency policy for soiled linens

Classroom Activities

1. Ask students to discuss the responsibilities of support workers in assisting with the physical examination.
 a. Write the following on the chalkboard: "Your responsibilities may include:"
  (1) Call on students to list responsibilities.
  (2) Write correct responses on the chalkboard.

2. Make available the following instruments used in physical examinations: ophthalmoscope, otoscope, percussion hammer, vaginal speculum, nasal speculum, tuning fork, and laryngeal mirror.
 a. Call on students to identify each instrument and describe its use.
 b. Allow students to handle each instrument.

3. Divide students into groups of three. Provide each group with several sheets of notebook paper. Ask students to discuss and answer the following questions about the physical examination:
   a. What factors cause anxiety?
   b. How is the person's quality of life promoted?
   c. What are some special needs of children?

   Allow 15 minutes for discussion. Then call on one student from each group to report on one question. Other students should give input as appropriate.

4. Use the procedure checklist provided.
   a. Demonstrate the procedure in this chapter.
   b. Have each student practice and return demonstrate the procedure in this chapter. Have each student assume the role of the patient/resident when practicing and return demonstrating the procedure.

5. Display an overhead transparency showing the examination positions (Figure 44-2, p. 741).
   a. Describe each position carefully. Allow time for discussion.
   b. Ask each student to assume the positions commonly used for examinations.
   c. Have each student stay in a position for 15 minutes. Ask students to discuss how they felt physically and psychologically. How will their experience help them to provide better care?

6. Display the guidelines for assisting with the examination listed in Box 44-1, p. 742 in the textbook on an overhead transparency.
   a. Carefully review each rule with students. Encourage questions.

7. Divide students into two groups. Provide each group with a flip chart and colored markers.
   a. One group should write "Focus on children" at the top of a sheet. The other group should write "Focus on older persons" at the top of a sheet.
   b. Allow each group 10 minutes to list special needs of the persons in their group.
   c. Call on one student from each group to report to the class. Allow time for discussion after each report.

8. Call on students to list the responsibilities of nursing assistants after the physical examination.

9. Discuss opportunities for cross training.

Homework Assignments

Ask students to answer the questions at the end of Chapter 44 in the textbook. Tell students the date and time that this assignment must be completed and turned in.

If the accompanying student workbook is being used, assign the Chapter 44 workbook exercises. Tell students the date and time that this assignment must be completed and turned in.

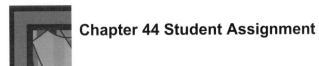

Name _____

Date _____

Assisting with the Physical Examination

1. List the rules for assisting with the physical examination.

a. _____

b. _____

c. _____

d. _____

e. _____

f. _____

g. _____

h. _____

i. _____

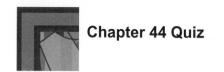

Name _____

Date _____

Assisting with the Physical Examination

True or False

Mark **T** *for true or* **F** *for false.*

1. _____ A physical examination causes anxiety for many people.

2. _____ Usually all clothes are removed for a complete physical examination.

3. _____ The person urinates after the examination.

4. _____ The examiner wants the person's height, weight, and vital signs measured. These are obtained before the examination.

5. _____ An ophthalmoscope is used to examine the inside of the nose.

6. _____ Parents are not allowed to be present during the examination of a child.

7. _____ Wash your hands before and after assisting with an examination.

Multiple Choice

Circle the BEST answer.

8. This instrument is vibrated to test hearing.
   a. Otoscope
   b. Ophthalmoscope
   c. Laryngeal mirror
   d. Tuning fork

9. You are preparing Mrs. Cliff for a physical examination. Which is incorrect?
   a. You need to be sensitive to her feelings.
   b. She urinates before the examination.
   c. Reassure her by telling her that there is no exposure during the examination.
   d. Screen her and close the door to the room.

10. The person is weighed before an examination. Which is correct?
    a. Pajamas and a robe are worn.
    b. Shoes are worn.
    c. The person urinates before being weighed.
    d. All of the above.

11. Mr. Lopez is confused. He resists your efforts to prepare him for a physical examination. Which is incorrect?
    a. The examination may need to be tried at another time.
    b. He is restrained if necessary.
    c. Having a family member present may help calm him.
    d. His rights are respected.

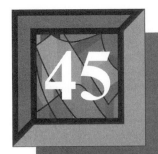

45

The Patient Having Surgery

Instructor's Preparation

I. Read Chapter 45 in the textbook. Carefully review chapter objectives, key terms, and review questions.

II. Read the outline in Chapter 45 of the instructor's guide. Carefully review the classroom activities, the student assignment, and the quiz.

III. If you are using the accompanying student workbook, review the activities for Chapter 45.

IV. Gather all necessary supplies and equipment for classroom activities and student assignments.

A. Prepare overhead transparencies

B. Prepare situation/index cards

C. Gather anatomical models

D. Gather simulators

E. Gather the necessary equipment and supplies needed to demonstrate and have each student return demonstrate the procedures in this chapter

F. Gather any other items that will be needed for classroom activities

G. Assemble items in the order they will be used

V. Make sure that the necessary equipment is available and in good working order.

Objectives

- Define the key terms listed in this chapter
- Describe the common fears and concerns of surgical patients
- Explain how people are physically and psychologically prepared for surgery
- Describe how to prepare a room for the postoperative patient
- List the signs and symptoms to report to the nurse postoperatively
- Explain how circulation is stimulated after surgery
- Describe how to meet hygiene, nutrition, fluid, and elimination needs after surgery
- Learn the procedures described in this chapter

Key Terms

anesthesia
elective surgery
embolus
emergency surgery
general anesthesia
local anesthesia
postoperative
preoperative
regional anesthesia
thrombus
urgent surgery

Outline

The Patient Having Surgery

I. INTRODUCTION
  A. Surgery is done for many reasons
    1. Removing a diseased organ or body part
    2. Removing a tumor
    3. Repairing injured tissue
    4. To diagnose disease
    5. To improve appearance
    6. To relieve symptoms
  B. Many surgeries require hospital stays; ambulatory (outpatient) surgeries are quite common
  C. Types of surgeries
    1. Elective surgery is done for the person's well-being
      a. Not life saving
      b. May not be necessary for the person's health (e.g. cosmetic)
      c. Surgery is scheduled in advance
    2. Urgent surgery is needed for the person's health
      a. Must be done soon to prevent further damage or disease
      b. Examples are cancer and coronary artery bypass surgery
    3. Emergency surgery is done immediately to save a person's life or limb
      a. The need is sudden and unexpected
      b. Examples of emergency situations are accidents, stabbings, and bullet wounds
  D. The person is prepared for what happens before, during, and after surgery
II. PSYCHOLOGICAL CARE
  A. Illness and injury cause many fears and concerns; Box 45-1, p. 746 in the textbook, lists common fears
    1. Surgery increases fears
  B. Feelings are affected by past experience
    1. Some have had surgery before, some have not
    2. Family and friends may share their experiences
    3. Most people know about tragic surgical events experienced by others
  C. Some people talk about their fears, others are quiet
  D. You must respect the person's fears and concerns
    1. The health team must show the person warmth, sensitivity, and caring

E. Patient information
  1. Before surgery
    a. The physician explains the need for surgery
      (1) The person is told about surgical procedures, risks, and possible complications
      (2) Risks from not having surgery are explained
    b. Information is given about who will do the surgery, when it is scheduled, and how long it will take
    c. Questions and misunderstandings are cleared up
    d. Instructions about care are given
    e. Information is given by the physician or the nurse
  2. After surgery
    a. The physician tells the patient and family about results
      (1) The physician decides what and when to tell them
      (2) The health care team may have information before the person is told
        (a) Do not tell of any diagnosis
        (b) Do not give incomplete or inaccurate information
        (c) Your supervisor tells you what and when the patient and family were told
F. Your role
  1. If you are involved in preoperative and postoperative care:
    a. Listen to the person voice fears or concerns
    b. Refer questions about the surgery or its results to the nurse
    c. Explain procedures you will perform and why they are being done
    d. Communicate effectively-- use verbal and nonverbal communication (see Chapter 12)
    e. Report verbal and nonverbal signs of patient fear or anxiety to the nurse
    f. Report a person's request to see clergy to the nurse
III. THE PREOPERATIVE PERIOD
  A. The preoperative period may be many days or just a few minutes
  B. Good preoperative preparation prevents complications after surgery
  C. Preoperative teaching
    1. Done by a nurse

2. Teaching includes:
   a. Preoperative activities
   b. Deep breathing, coughing, and leg exercises
   c. The recovery room (see Figure 45-1, p. 747)
   d. Vital signs
   e. Food and fluids
   f. Turning and repositioning
   g. Early ambulation
   h. Pain
   i Needed treatments and equipment
   j. Position restrictions

3. Focus on children
   a. The child and parents are prepared for surgery
   b. Often play is used to help the child understand
   c. A tour of the operating and recovery rooms is common
   d. The child and parents are introduced to staff

D. Special tests
1. Ordered to evaluate the person's circulatory, respiratory, and urinary systems
   a. A chest x-ray
   b. A complete blood count
   c. Urinalysis
   d. Electrocardiograms
2. Typing and crossmatching of blood may be done
3. Other tests depend on the person's condition and the surgery
   a. The person is prepared for tests as needed

E. Nutrition and fluids
1. A light meal is usually allowed
2. The person is NPO 6 to 8 hours before surgery
   a. This reduces the risk of vomiting and aspiration during anesthesia and after surgery
   b. An NPO sign is placed in the person's room
   c. The water pitcher and glasses are removed from the person's room

F. Elimination
1. Enemas may be required before surgery
   a. Common before abdominal and intestinal surgery; needed to clear the colon of feces
   b. Also given when straining or a bowel movement could cause postsurgical problems
2. Some surgeries require catheters
   a. The bladder must be empty for pelvic and abdominal surgeries (to prevent injury to the bladder)
   b. Catheters also allow accurate output measurements during and after surgery

G. Personal care
1. Personal care before surgery usually involves the following:
   a. A complete bed bath, shower, or tub bath is taken
     (1) Special soap or cleanser may be ordered
   b. Makeup and nail polish are removed
     (1) Done so the lips, skin, and nail beds can be observed for color and circulation
   c. Long hair is braided; all hairpins, clips, combs, and similar items are removed
     (1) Wigs and hair pieces are also removed
     (2) Some agencies require persons to wear surgical caps
   d. Oral hygiene is performed to promote comfort
     (1) Remember that the person is NPO
     (2) See Focus on Children box, p. 747 in the textbook
   e. Dentures are removed before pre-operative medications are given
     (1) Dentures are cleaned and kept moist in a denture cup
     (2) Dentures are kept in a safe place

H. Valuables
1. Removed for safekeeping
2. A note is made on the person's chart about the valuables removed and where they are kept
3. The patient may want to wear a wedding band or religious item
   a. Secure these in place with gauze or tape

I. Skin preparation
1. The skin cannot be sterilized
2. A skin prep can reduce the number of microbes
3. Hospital policy and the surgeon's preference determine the area to be prepared for a specific surgery
   a. The incision site and a large area around the site are prepped (see Figure

45-2, p. 749)

4. The skin preparation is done right before surgery

5. Disposable prep kits are used for shaving (see Figure 45-3, p. 750)

6. Be very careful not to cut, scratch, or nick the skin (see Figure 45-4, p. 750)

   a. Any break in the skin is a possible infection site

7. Standard Precautions are followed

8. The Surgical Skin Prep ▶ p. 750

J. The preoperative checklist (see Figure 45-5, p. 752)

1. Placed on the front of the person's chart

2. The RN makes sure the checklist is completed

3. Promptly report when you complete each task

4. Report any observations

K. Preoperative medications

1. Given 45 minutes to 1 hour before surgery

   a. One helps the person relax and feel drowsy

   b. One dries up respiratory secretions to prevent aspiration

2. Falls and accidents are prevented after drugs are given

   a. Bed rails are raised

   b. The person is not allowed out of bed

     (1) The person voids before drugs are given

   c. Smoking is not allowed

3. Follow agency policy for bed position

4. Move furniture out of the way to make room for the stretcher

5. Clean off the overbed table and bedside stand

6. Raise the bed to the highest position for transferring the patient from the bed to a stretcher

L. Transport to the operating room

1. The patient is transferred onto a stretcher and covered with a bath blanket

2. Falling is prevented

   a. Safety straps are secured and side rails raised

3. Identification checks are made

4. The person's chart is given to the operating room (OR) staff member

5. Focus on children

   a. Some agencies allow a parent to be with the child while anesthesia is given

IV. ANESTHESIA

A. The loss of feeling or sensation produced by a drug

1. General anesthesia produces unconsciousness and loss of feeling or sensation

   a. Given by IV or an inhaled gas

2. Regional anesthesia produces loss of sensation or feeling in a large area of the body

   a. The person does not lose consciousness

   b. A drug is injected into a body part

3. Local anesthesia produces loss of sensation in a small area

   a. A drug is injected at the specific site

V. THE POSTOPERATIVE PERIOD

A. The person is taken to the recovery room (RR) or postanesthesia room (PAR) or postanesthesia recovery unit (PACU)

1. The person recovers from the anesthetic

B. The person leaves the recovery room when:

1. Vital signs are stable

2. The person has good respiratory function

3. The person can respond and call for help when needed

C. Preparing the person's room

1. The room is prepared after the person is taken to the OR; preparations include:

   a. Making a surgical bed (see Chapter 24)

   b. Placing equipment and supplies in the room; see Preparing the Patient's Room, p. 753 in the textbook, for a list of items

   c. Raising the bed to its highest position

   d. Lowering bed rails

   e. Moving furniture out of the way for the stretcher

D. Return from the recovery room

1. The person is transported by the recovery room nurses

2. Assist in transferring the person from the stretcher to the bed as needed

3. Help position the person

4. Vital signs are taken and observations made

5. The nurse checks dressings, catheters, IV infusion, and other tube placements and functions

6. Bed rails are raised and the signal light is placed within reach

7. Necessary care and treatments are given

8. The family is allowed to see the person
E. Measurements and observations
   1. Often you will measure vital signs and observe the person
   2. Vital signs are usually measured:
     a. Every 15 minutes the first hour
     b. Every 30 minutes for 1 to 2 hours
     c. Every hour for 4 hours
     d. Then every 4 hours
   3. The nurse tells you how often to check the person
   4. Be alert for the signs and symptoms listed in Box 45-2, p. 754 in the textbook
   5. Report them to the nurse immediately
F. Positioning
   1. Proper positioning promotes comfort and prevents complications
   2. The type of surgery affects positioning
   3. Position restrictions may be ordered
   4. Position for ease and comfort in breathing
   5. Stress on the incision is prevented
   6. Position to prevent aspiration
   7. Repositioning every 1 to 2 hours helps prevent respiratory and circulatory complications
   8. Turn the person carefully
   9. Pillows and other devices may be used (see Chapters 21 and 22)
   10. The nurse tells you when to reposition the person and the positions allowed
   11. See Focus on Older Adults box, p. 754 in the textbook
G. Coughing and deep breathing
   1. Respiratory complications are prevented
     a. Pneumonia is an inflammation and infection in the lung
     b. Atelectasis is the collapse of a portion of the lung
       (1) Coughing, deep breathing, and incentive spirometry help prevent these complications (see Chapter 43)
   2. See Focus on Older Adults box, p. 754 in the textbook
H. Stimulating circulation
   1. Is especially important in the legs
     a. If blood flow is sluggish, clots (thrombi) may form (see Figure 45-6A, p. 755)
   2. A blood clot can break loose and travel

through the bloodstream and becomes an embolus (see Figure 45-6B, p. 755)
   3. An embolus that lodges in the lung (pulmonary embolus) can cause severe respiratory problems and death
   4. Focus on older persons
     a. Blood is pumped through the body with less force
     b. There is increased risk for thrombi and emboli
   5. Leg exercises
     a. Increase venous blood flow; help prevent thrombi
     b Your supervisor tells you when to do exercises
     c. Exercises are done with the person supine
     d. Done at least every 1 to 2 hours while the person is awake
     e. Exercises are done five times; have the person:
       (1) Make circles with the toes
       (2) Dorsiflex and plantar flex the feet
       (3) Flex and extend one knee and then the other (see Figure 45-7, p. 755)
       (4) Raise and lower one leg off of the bed and then the other (see Figure 45-8, p. 755)
   6. Elastic stockings—bandages
     a. Help prevent thrombi
     b. Often ordered for postoperative patients and for those with heart disease and circulatory disorders
     c. Both elastic stockings and bandages could harm the patient if applied improperly and that is why most hospitals only allow nurses to apply them
     d. If you are assigned this task make sure it is in your scope of practice and employer policy allows you to do it
     e. Make sure you are properly trained and have close supervision
     f. Applications are discussed in Chapter 28 in the textbook
     g. Applied to an extremity
     h. Have the same purpose as elastic stockings
     i. Also provide support and reduce swelling from musculoskeletal injuries
     j. Applied from the lower part of an extremity to the top part

k. The nurse gives you directions
l. When applying bandages:
   (1) Use the correct size
   (2) Position the extremity in good alignment
   (3) Face the person
   (4) Expose fingers or toes if possible
   (5) Apply with firm, even pressure
   (6) Check the color and temperature of the extremity every hour
   (7) Reapply a loose, wrinkled, moist, or soiled bandage
I. Early ambulation
   1. Prevents postoperative circulatory complications
   2. Prevents thrombi, pneumonia, atelectasis, constipation, and urinary tract infections
   3. The person dangles first
      a. Blood pressure and pulse are measured (see Chapter 21)
   4. Usually the person does not walk very far
      a. Distance increases as the person gains strength
   5. The nurse tells you when to ambulate
J. Wound healing
   1. The incision needs protection
   2. Healing is promoted and infection prevented
   3. Wound healing is discussed in Chapter 41 in the textbook
K. Nutrition and fluids
   1. The person has an IV infusion on return from the OR
      a. Continued IV therapy depends on the type of surgery and the person's condition
   2. The person's diet progresses from NPO, to clear liquids, to full liquids, to a light diet, to a regular diet
      a. The diet is ordered by the doctor
   3. Frequent oral hygiene is important when the person is NPO
   4. A patient with a nasogastric (NG) tube is NPO and receives IV therapy (see Chapter 26)
L. Elimination
   1. Normal bowel and urine elimination are affected by:
      a. Anesthesia
      b. The surgery
      c. Being NPO
      d. Pain medications
   2. The measures to promote elimination are practiced (see Chapters 16 and 17 in the textbook)
   3. Intake and output are measured postoperatively
      a. The person must urinate within 8 hours after surgery
      b. Report time and amount of the first voiding
      c. Some patients have catheters after surgery; see Chapter 29 in the textbook for care of the person with a catherer
   4. Suppositories and enemas may be ordered for constipation
   5. Rectal tubes may be ordered for flatulence
M. Comfort and rest
   1. Pain is common after surgery
      a. The degree of pain depends on the extent of surgery, the incision site, and the presence of tubes, casts, or other devices
   2. Pain medication is ordered by the physician
   3. The RN uses the nursing process to promote comfort and rest
   4. Many measures listed in Chapter 20 in the textbook are part of the care plan
N. Personal hygiene
   1. Important for physical and mental well-being
   2. Frequent oral hygiene, hair care, and a complete bed bath the day after surgery help refresh and renew the person physically and psychologically
   3. The gown is changed whenever it becomes wet or soiled (see Chapter 27)

Classroom Activities

1. Write on the chalkboard: "Surgery is done for many reasons:"
   a. Call on students to list the common reasons that surgery is done.
      (1) Write the correct answers on the chalkboard.

2. Write the following terms on the chalkboard:
   a. Elective surgery
   b. Urgent surgery
   c. Emergency surgery

Call on students to define and give an example of each term. Write the correct answers on the chalkboard after the appropriate term.

3. Display the common fears and concerns caused by illness and injury on an overhead transparency (see Box 45-1, p. 746 in the textbook). Use this as a basis for discussion.

4. Write each of the following items related to preoperative preparation on separate index cards: Preoperative teaching, Special tests, Nutrition and fluids, Elimination, Personal care, Valuables, and Skin preparation. Divide students into pairs or groups of three. Distribute one index card to each pair or group.
   a. Write on the chalkboard: "Good preoperative preparation prevents complications after surgery."
   b. Ask each pair or group to discuss how the item on their index card relates to good preoperative preparation. Allow 15 minutes for discussion. Then call on one student from each pair or group to report to the class.
      (1) Allow time for discussion.

5. Call on students to discuss the measures to use to prevent falls after the preoperative medications are given.

6. Tell the students that the patient's room is prepared after the person is taken to the OR. Write on the chalkboard: "Preparations Include:"
   a. Call on students to list the preparations. Write the correct answers on the chalkboard.

7. Write the following postoperative care measures on separate index cards: Measurements and Observations, Positioning, Coughing and Deep Breathing, Stimulating Circulation, Early Ambulation, Nutrition and Fluids, Elimination, Comfort and Rest, and Personal Hygiene.
   a. Divide students into pairs. Distribute one index card to each pair.
   b. Tell the students that each index card lists an important measure of postoperative care. Ask students to identify the importance of the measure on their index card and describe what the measure involves.

c. Allow students 15 minutes for discussion. Then call on one student from each pair to report to the class.
   (1) Allow time for questions and discussion after each presentation.

8. Use the procedure checklists provided.
   a. Demonstrate the procedures in this chapter.
   b. Have each student practice and return demonstrate the procedures in this chapter.
      (1) Use simulators and anatomical models as appropriate.

9. Demonstrate the leg exercises described in this chapter. Have each student practice and return demonstrate the leg exercises.
   a. Each student should take a turn as the patient/resident.

10. Ask students to share any personal experiences they may have had with surgery.
   a. How did members of the health team meet their physical and psychological needs?
   b. How will their experience help them provide better care?

Homework Assignments

Ask students to answer the questions at the end of Chapter 45 in the textbook. Tell students the date and time that this assignment must be completed and turned in.

If the accompanying student workbook is being used, assign the Chapter 45 workbook exercises. Tell students the date and time that this assignment must be completed and turned in.

Chapter 45 Student Assignment   Name _____

                                      Date _____

The Patient Having Surgery

1. List the common fears of surgical patients. Fear of:

   a. _____

   b. _____

   c. _____

   d. _____

   e. _____

   f. _____

   g. _____

   h. _____

   i. _____

   j. _____

   k. _____

   l. _____

   m. _____

   n. _____

2. Personal care before surgery usually involves the following:

   a. _____

   b. _____

   c. _____

   d. _____

   e. _____

3. You prepare the room for the person's return from the recovery room. Preparations include:

   a. _____

   b. _____

   c. _____

   d. _____

   e. _____

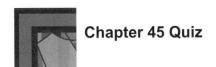

Chapter 45 Quiz

Name _____

Date _____

The Patient Having Surgery

True or False	Multiple Choice

Mark **T** *for true or* **F** *for false.*

1. _____ Elective surgery is done immediately to save the person's life.

2. _____ The person is prepared physically and psychologically for surgery

3. _____ The water pitcher and glass are removed from the room when the person is NPO.

4. _____ The skin is sterilized before surgery to prevent infection.

5. _____ Nursing assistants are responsible for obtaining the person's written consent for surgery.

6. _____ After preoperative medications are given, bed rails are raised and the person is not allowed out of bed.

7. _____ Regional anesthesia causes unconsciousness and loss of feeling or sensation.

8. _____ Coughing and deep breathing exercises help prevent pneumonia.

9. _____ Proper positioning helps prevent postoperative complications.

10. _____ The person must urinate within 4 hours after surgery.

11. _____ The changes of aging increase the older person's risk for respiratory complications.

12. _____ The person is usually on bedrest for 2 days after surgery.

Circle the **BEST** *answer.*

13. You assist in the psychological care of the surgical patient. Which is incorrect?
   a. Listen to the person who voices fears about surgery.
   b. Carefully explain the surgical procedure to the person.
   c. Perform procedures and tasks with skill and ease.
   d. Use verbal and nonverbal communication.

14. You prepare the room for the person's return from the recovery room by:
   a. Making a closed bed.
   b. Placing equipment and supplies in the room.
   c. Lowering the bed to the lowest position.
   d. Raising the bed rails.

15. Which statement about positioning the person after surgery is incorrect?
   a. Stress on the incision is prevented.
   b. Turn the person with smooth, gentle motions.
   c. Repositioning every 4 hours helps prevent respiratory complications.
   d. Pillows and other positioning devices are often used.

16. Elastic bandages are ordered for Mr. Randall. Elastic bandages:
   a. Are applied from the upper part of the extremity to the lower part of the extremity.
   b. Come in one size.
   c. Are applied to cover the fingers and toes.
   d. Are reapplied when loose or wrinkled.

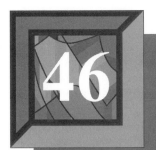

46

Caring for a Client Who Is Dying

Instructor's Preparation

I. Read Chapter 46 in the textbook. Carefully review chapter objectives, key terms, and review questions.

II. Read the outline in Chapter 46 of the instructor's guide. Carefully review the classroom activities, the student assignment, and the quiz.

III. If you are using the accompanying student workbook, review the activities for Chapter 46.

IV. Gather all necessary supplies and equipment for classroom activities and student assignments.
   A. Prepare the correct number of handouts
   B. Prepare appropriate flip charts
   C. Prepare overhead transparencies
   D. Prepare situation/index cards
   E. Gather coloured markers
   F. Gather the necessary equipment and supplies needed to demonstrate and have each student in turn demonstrate the procedures in this chapter
   G. Gather any other items that will be needed for classroom activities
   H. Assemble items in the order they will be used

V. Make sure that the necessary equipment is available and in good working order.

VI. Contact guest speakers to confirm the day, date, time, and location that they are expected.
   A. Ask the speakers if they require any special equipment or supplies; ensure these are available.

Objectives	Key Terms
• Define the key terms listed in this chapter	advance directive
• Explain how culture, religion, and age influence attitudes about death	anticipatory grief
• Describe the five stages of grief	grief
• Explain how to help meet a dying person's needs	living will
• Describe the needs of the family of a dying person	palliative care
• Describe palliative care	postmortem care
• Explain the importance of the advance directive	rigor mortis
• Identify the signs of approaching death and the signs of death	
• Describe how to assist in giving postmortem care	
• Learn the procedure described in this chapter	

Outline

Caring for a Client Who Is Dying

I. INTRODUCTION

  A. Dying people are often cared for in facilities or at home

    1. Many are in hospice programs

  B. Health team members see death often

  C. Your attitudes about death and dying affect the care you give

  D. Understanding the dying process helps you approach the dying person with care, kindness, and respect

II. LIFE-THREATENING ILLNESS

  A. An illness or injury for which there is no reasonable expectation of recovery

  B. Health-care professionals cannot predict the exact time of death

  C. Hope and the will to live influence living and dying

III. ATTITUDES ABOUT DEATH

  A. Experiences, culture, religion, and age influence attitudes about death

    1. Attitudes and beliefs often change as the person grows older

  B. Family is often involved in the person's care

    1. The family also comforts each other

  C. Many adults and children have never had contact with a dying person

    1. It is frightening, morbid, and a mystery

  D. Culture and religion

    1. American practices and attitudes are different from those of other cultures (see Respecting Diversity box, p. 761)

    2. Attitudes about death are closely related to culture and religion

      a. Reincarnation is the belief that the spirit or soul is reborn in another body or another form of life

    3. Many persons strengthen their religious beliefs when dying

    4. Religion provides comfort for the dying person and the family

    5. Many religions have rites and rituals that are practiced during the dying process and at time of death

  E. Beliefs about death

    1. Adults fear pain and suffering, dying alone, and invasion of privacy

      a. Also fear loneliness and separation from family and loved ones

      b. Worry about who will care for and support those left behind

      c. Adults may resent death; it interferes with plans, hopes, and dreams

    2. Focus on children

      a. Ideas about death change as people grow older

      b. Infants and toddlers have no concept of death

      c. Children between the ages of 3 and 5 years:

        (1) Are curious about death

        (2) Recognize death of family members, pets, other animals, or bugs

        (3) Think death is temporary

        (4) Often blame themselves

        (5) See death as punishment for being bad

        (6) Are often given answers that cause fear and confusion when they ask questions about death

      d. Children between the ages of 5 and 7 years:

        (1) Know death is final

        (2) Do not think they will die

        (3) Think death happens to others

        (4) Think death can be avoided

        (5) Associate death with punishment and body mutilation

        (6) Associate death with witches, ghosts, goblins, and monsters

        (7) Ideas come from fairy tales, movies, cartoons, video games, and television

    3. Focus on older persons

      a. Usually have fewer fears than younger adults

      b. Accept that death will occur

      c. Have had more experience with dying and death

      d. Some welcome death as freedom from pain, suffering, and disability

      e. Death means reunion with those who have died first

      f. Persons often fear dying alone

IV. THE STAGES OF GRIEF

  A. Dr. Elizabeth Kübler-Ross describes 5 stages:

    1. Denial

      a. Persons refuse to believe that they are dying

      b. The person responds, "No, not me"

      c. The person cannot deal with problems or decisions about the illness or injury

        (1) Some people are still in denial when they die

    2. Anger

      a. The person thinks "Why me?"

b. The person feels anger and rage

c. The person envies and resents those who have life and health

d. The person blames others

   (1) Anger is normal; do not take it personally

3. Bargaining

a. The person says, "Yes me, but…"

b. The person bargains with God for more time

c. Promises are made in exchange for more time

d. Bargaining is usually done privately and on a spiritual level

4. Depression

a. The person thinks "yes me" and is very sad

b. The person mourns over losses

c. The person may cry and say little

d. The person may talk about people and things that will be left behind

5. Acceptance

a. The person is calm and at peace

b. Unfinished business is completed

c. Reaching this stage does not mean death is near

B. Dying persons do not always go through all five stages

1. A person may never move beyond a certain stage

2. Some move back and forth between stages

3. Some are in one stage until death

C. Family also experience the five stages of grief, and often not at the same time as the person who is dying

D. Members of the health care team also experience the stages of grief

1. Caring for a dying person is a moving and emotional experience

E. Supporting a grieving family can by very difficult and you will grieve the loss of clients you have cared for

F. It is important that you examine your feelings about loss and grief

1. Do not turn away feelings, and develop your own support system (see Box 46-1, p. 762)

V. PALLIATIVE CARE

A. Focuses on the physical, emotional, social, and spiritual needs of dying persons and their families

B. Care does not focus on cures or life-saving procedures

C. Pain relief and comfort measures are stressed

D. The goal is to improve the dying person's quality of life

E. May be part of a hospital, or in a facility, or at home

F. Follow-up care and support groups for survivors are provided

G. Some cities and towns have community hospice organizations run by volunteers who work closely with home care programs

H. Hospices are homes that provide a comfortable, peaceful setting and provide palliative care

I. The most common facility setting is the palliative care unit within a hospital

1. Many long-term care facilities also have palliative care

J. Palliative care requires a team of many different professions along with the person and family (who are the key members of the team)

K. The person is an active participant in his or her own care

VI. CARING FOR A PERSON WHO IS DYING

A. Dying people continue to have psychological, social, and spiritual needs

B. The person has the right to die in peace and dignity (see Box 46-2, and Providing Compassionate Care box, p. 763)

C. They may want family and friends present

D. Some want to be alone

E. They often need to talk at night

F. Listening and touch are very important to the dying person

1. Listening

a. The dying person needs to talk, express feelings, and share worries and concerns

b. Do not worry about saying the wrong thing

c. Being there for the person is what counts

2. Touch

a. Touch conveys caring and concern when words cannot

b. Silence along with touch is a powerful and meaningful way to communicate

c. Respect the person's beliefs

G. Spiritual needs are important

1. The person may wish to see a priest, rabbi, minister, or other cleric

2. The person may want to take part in religious practices
  a. Provide privacy
  b. Courtesy is given to the clergy
3. The person is allowed to have religious objects nearby
  a. Handle these items like other valuables

VII. PHYSICAL NEEDS
A. There is general slowing of body processes, weakness, and changes in levels of consciousness
B. The person is encouraged to be as independent as possible
  1. As the person weakens more help is provided
C. Pain relief and comfort
  1. Some people have severe pain
  2. Health care professionals administer medications to relieve pain
  3. The care plan may call for other measures such as back massages and relaxation techniques
  4. Skin care, personal hygiene, and good alignment promote comfort
  5. Follow the care plan
D. Comfort and positioning
  1. Frequent position changes, good body alignment, and supportive devices promote comfort
  2. Turn the person slowly and gently
  3. Persons with breathing difficulties usually prefer the semi-Fowler's position
E. Vision, hearing, and speech
  1. Vision and eye care
    a. Blurs and gradually fails
     (1) Explain what you are doing
    b. The person naturally turns toward light
     (1) A dark room may be frightening
     (2) The room should be well lit
      (a) Avoid bright lights and glares
    c. Eyes may be half open
    d. Secretions collect in the corners of the eyes
     (1) Good eye care is essential
     (1) Follow the care plan
  2. Hearing
    a. One of the last functions lost
    b. Even if unconscious, the person may hear
     (1) Always assume the person can hear you
     (2) Speak in a normal voice

     (3) Provide reassurance and give explanations about care
     (4) Offer words of comfort
     (5) Avoid topics that could upset the person
  3. Speech
    a. Becomes difficult
     (1) May be hard to understand
    b. Sometimes the person cannot speak
     (1) You must anticipate the person's needs
     (2) "Yes or no" questions are asked
     (3) Question are kept at a minimum
    c. You must still talk to the person
F. Mouth, nose, and skin
  1. Oral hygiene is essential for comfort
    a. Routine care is given if the person can eat and drink
    b. Frequent oral hygiene is given as death approaches and when there is difficulty taking oral fluids
     (1) Also important if the person cannot swallow
    c. Offer ice chips or small sips of fluids for dry mouth
  2. Crusting and irritation of the nostrils can occur
    a. The nose is carefully cleaned
    b. Apply a lubricant as directed by the care plan
  3. Skin Care
    a. Circulation fails and body temperature rises as death approaches
    b. The skin is cool, pale, and mottled
    c. Perspiration increases
    d. Good skin care, bathing, and prevention of pressure ulcers are necessary
    e. Linens and gowns are changed as needed
    f. Only light bed coverings are needed
G. Elimination
  1. The dying person may have urinary and fecal incontinence
    a. Bed protectors or incontinence briefs are used
    b. Perineal care is given as necessary
  2. Some persons have constipation or urinary retention
    a. The care plan may call for the use of enemas and catheter care

VIII. THE FAMILY
A. They are going through a stressful time
B. Show your feelings to the family by being available, courteous, and considerate; use

touch
C. Family are allowed to spend a lot of time with their loved one
1. Normal visiting hours do not apply
D. Respect the family's right to privacy
1. You cannot neglect care just because the family is present
E. Let families help with care if they wish (most facilities will allow)
F. Family may be tired, sad, and tearful
1. They need support and understanding
2. Treat them with courtesy and respect
3. Visiting with a clergy may be comforting
a. Communicate the request to your supervisor immediately

IX. LEGAL ISSUES
A. Much attention is given to the right to die
1. Many people do not want machines or other measures to keep them alive
2. Consent is needed for any treatment
a. All provinces and territories have legislation about the need for consent (see Chapter 10)
3. Most clients make their own decisions but if unable because of confusion or dementia, a substitute decision-maker will decide on care
B. Advance Directive (living will)—legal document that states the person's wishes about future health care, treatmen,t and personal care
1. Used when the person can no longer make or express wishes
2. Allows people to control their future health care
3. Without an advance directive decisions must be made by family members and this can cause conflict
4. Every province and territory has legislation about advance directives
5. Serve two purposes: appoint a proxy to make medical decisions, and give written instructions about medical care/treatment/personal care
6. People often use advance directives to forbid certain types of treatment and care when there is no hope of recovery (e.g., tube feedings)
7. Known by different names and have different powers depending on province or territory
8. It is important to know the legislation in your province or territory, as there are differences

C. "Do not resuscitate" orders
1. This means that no attempt will be made to resuscitate the person
a. The person is allowed to die in peace and with dignity
2. Orders are written after consulting with the person or family
3. Some advance directives address resuscitation

X. SIGNS OF DEATH
A. Signs may occur rapidly or slowly
1. Movement, muscle tone, and sensation are lost
2. Peristalsis and other gastrointestinal functions slow down
3. Circulation fails and body temperature rises
a. The person feels cool or cold, looks pale, and perspires heavily
b. The pulse is fast, weak, and irregular
c. The blood pressure starts to fall
4. The respiratory system fails (causes the "death rattle")
a. Cheyne Stokes respirations are common
5. Pain decreases as the person loses consciousness
a. Some people are conscious until death occurs
B. The signs of death include no pulse, respirations, or blood pressure
1. The pupils are fixed and dilated
C. A doctor determines that death has occurred and pronounces the person dead
a. In some parts of the country, RN's are able to pronounce death in the home
D. Focus on home care
1. Know your employer's policies and call your supervisor

XI. CARE OF THE BODY AFTER DEATH
A. Called postmortem care
B. You may be asked to assist
C. Care begins as soon as the death is pronounced
D. Standard Precautions are followed
E. Done to maintain the body's appearance; discoloration and skin damage are prevented
F. Includes gathering valuables and personal items for the family
G. The right to privacy and to be treated with dignity and respect apply after death
H. Rigor mortis develops within 2 to 3 hours after death
1. Stiffness or rigidity of skeletal muscles

2. Postmortem care involves positioning the body in normal alignment before rigor mortis sets in

I. The body should appear in a comfortable and natural position for viewing by the family

J. Movement of the body can cause remaining air in the lungs, stomach, and intestines to be expelled

   1. The body produces sounds, do not be alarmed

K. Assisting with Postmortem Care ▶ p. 767

Classroom Activities

1. Using the round table discussion format, ask students to share any personal feelings and experiences related to death.
   a. Discuss the role of culture and religion.
   b. How will the students' personal experience and feelings affect the care they provide?

2. Write on the chalkboard:
   a. Beliefs about death are affected by the person's age
   (1) Adults
   (2) Children
   (3) Older persons

   Ask students what beliefs adults, children, and older persons have about death. Write the correct answers on the chalkboard. Allow time for questions and discussion.

3. Display the five stages of dying described by Dr. Helen Kübler-Ross on an overhead transparency. Use this as a basis to discuss the five stages with students.
   a. Allow time for questions and discussion.

4. Write each of the following terms on a separate index card: Vision; Hearing; Speech; Mouth, nose, and skin; Elimination; Comfort and positioning; and The person's room.
   a. Divide students into seven groups. Provide each group with several sheets of notebook paper.
   b. Ask one person from each group to choose an index card. Then ask each group to write down the following information about the term on their index card.
   (1) What measures are needed to meet the dying persons needs related to the term on each index card.
   c. Allow 15 minutes for this exercise. Then call on one student from each group to report to the

class. Allow time after each presentation for questions and discussion.

5. Call on students to discuss how the needs of the family are met.

6. Invite a pastor who works in a hospital or nursing center to talk to the class about the role of the pastor in meeting the needs of the dying person and his or her family.
   a. Also discuss the role of the pastor in helping members of the health care team deal with the death of persons they care for.
   (1) Allow time for questions and discussion.

7. Arrange for a representative from hospice to visit the class. He or she should provide materials that explain the hospice philosophy and describe the services they provide.
   a. Allow time for questions and discussion.

8. Write the following on the chalkboard: "The Dying Persons' Bill of Rights"
   a. Call on students to list the rights. Write the correct answers on the chalkboard.

9. Ask students, "What are the signs of death?" Write the correct answers on the chalkboard.

10. Invite the coroner or a representative from the coroner's office to discuss when a death is a coroner's case.
    a. Ask students to write key points in a notebook for future reference.
    b. Allow time for questions.

11. Use the procedure checklist.
    a. Demonstrate the procedure in this chapter.
    b. Have each student practice and return demonstrate the procedure in this chapter.

Homework Assignments

Ask students to answer the questions at the end of Chapter 46 in the textbook. Tell students the date and time that this assignment must be completed and turned in.

If the accompanying student workbook is being used, assign the Chapter 46 workbook exercises. Tell students the date and time that this assignment must be completed and turned in.

Chapter 46 Student Assignment

Name _____

Date _____

Caring for a Client Who Is Dying

Write your answers in the blanks provided.

1. You will help to meet the dying person's

   _____,

   _____,

   _____, and

   _____ needs.

2. Ideas about death change as people grow older. What do persons in the following age groups understand and feel about death?

   a. Infants and toddlers—

   _____

   _____

   _____

   _____

   b. Children between 3 and 5 years of age—

   _____

   _____

   _____

   _____

   c. Children between 5 and 7 years of age—

   _____

   _____

   _____

   _____

   d. Adults—

   _____

   _____

   _____

   _____

   e. Older persons—

   _____

   _____

   _____

   _____

3. _____ and

   _____ are

   two very important aspects of communication when dealing with the dying person.

Name _____

Date _____

Caring for a Client Who Is Dying

4. Define these terms:

   a. Patient Self-determination Act —

   _____

   _____

   _____

   _____

   b. Advance directives—

   _____

   _____

   _____

   _____

   c. Living will—

   _____

   _____

   _____

   _____

   d. Durable power of attorney for health care—

   _____

   _____

   _____

   _____

   e. "Do no resuscitate" order—

   _____

   _____

   _____

   _____

Chapter 46 Quiz

Name _____

Date _____

Caring for a Client Who Is Dying

| True or False | Multiple Choice |

*Mark **T** for true or **F** for false.*

1. _____ Attitudes about death are closely related to culture and religion.

2. _____ Children between the ages of 3 and 5 years of age know death is final.

3. _____ Older persons usually have fewer fears about death than younger adults.

4. _____ Dying people continue to have psychological, social, and spiritual needs.

5. _____ A darkened room provides comfort to the dying person.

6. _____ Hearing is one of the last functions to be lost.

7. _____ Normal visiting hours apply if the person is dying.

8. _____ Hospice care focuses on cures and life-saving procedures.

9. _____ A "do not resuscitate" order means that the person is allowed to die in peace and with dignity.

10. _____ Postmortem care begins as soon as a doctor pronounces the person dead.

11. _____ The right to privacy and the right to be treated with dignity and respect apply after death.

*Circle the **BEST** answer.*

12. Mrs. Jansen is dying. She is very sad. She cries a lot and says little. She is in the stage of:
    a. Denial.
    b. Depression.
    c. Anger.
    d. Acceptance.

13. Mrs. Jansen asks to see a priest at two o'clock in the morning. You should:
    a. Ask her why she wants to see the priest.
    b. Report her request to the nurse immediately.
    c. Tell her to go back to sleep.
    d. Tell her you will ask the nurse to call the priest in the morning.

14. Care of the dying person includes all of the following except:
    a. Providing frequent oral hygiene.
    b. Providing good skin care.
    c. Positioning the person in good body alignment.
    d. Active and passive range-of-motion exercises.

15. The stiffness or rigidity of skeletal muscles that occurs after death is called:
    a. Rigor mortis.
    b. Postmortem.
    c. Peristalsis.
    d. DNR.

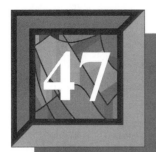

Basic Emergency Care

Instructor's Preparation

I. Read Chapter 47 in the textbook. Carefully review chapter objectives, key terms, and review questions.

II. Read the outline in Chapter 47 of the instructor's guide. Carefully review the classroom activities, the student assignment, and the quiz.

III. If you are using the accompanying student workbook, review the activities for Chapter 47.

IV. Gather all necessary supplies and equipment for classroom activities and student assignments.
   A. Prepare the correct number of handouts
   B. Prepare appropriate flip charts
   C. Prepare overhead transparencies
   D. Prepare situation/index cards
   E. Gather coloured markers
   F. Gather anatomical models
   G. Gather simulators/CPR mannequins
   H. Gather the necessary equipment and supplies needed to demonstrate and have each student return demonstrate the procedures in this chapter
   I. Gather any other items that will be needed for classroom activities
   J. Assemble items in the order they will be used

V. Make sure that the necessary equipment is available and in good working order.

VI. Contact guest speakers to confirm the day, date, time, and location that they are expected.
   A. Ask the speakers if they require any special equipment or supplies; ensure these are available.

Objectives

- Define the key terms listed in this chapter
- Describe the signs, symptoms, and emergency care for cardiac arrest and obstructed airway
- Describe the signs, symptoms, and emergency care for hemorrhage
- Describe the signs, symptoms, and emergency care for shock
- Describe different types of seizures and how to care for a person during a seizure
- Describe the causes, types, and emergency care for burns
- Identify the common causes of and emergency care for fainting
- Describe the signs of and emergency care for stroke
- Learn the procedures described in this chapter

Outline

Basic Emergency Care

I. INTRODUCTION
  A. Knowing what to do in an emergency can mean the difference between life and death
II. GENERAL RULES OF EMERGENCY CARE
  A. First aid is the emergency care given to an ill or injured person before medical help arrives
    1. The goals are to prevent death and prevent injuries from becoming worse
  B. When an emergency occurs, activate the local Emergency Medical Services (EMS) system
    1. Involves emergency personnel trained and educated to give emergency care
      a. They know how to treat, stabilize, and transport persons with life-threatening conditions
    2. In many areas the EMS system is activated by dialing 911
      a. Calling the local fire department, police department, or telephone operator also activates the system
  C. Each emergency is different
    1. Guidelines in Box 47-1, p. 773 in the textbook, apply to any emergency
  D. In facilities, a nurse decides when to activate the EMS system
    1. The nurse tells you what to do to help
    2. Some allow nursing assistants to do cardiopulmonary resuscitation (CPR), others do not
      a. Know your center's policy
    3. Some residents are not resuscitated
      a. The nurse and the care plan tell you which residents have Do Not Resuscitate (DNR) orders (see Chapter 46)
  E. In community settings, you decide when to activate the EMS system
    1. Home care agencies have guidelines about when to activate EMS systems and when to call your supervisor
    2. Some home care agencies do not allow support workers to start CPR, so know your employer's policies
III. BASIC LIFE SUPPORT (BLS)
  A. Cardiac arrest is when the person's heart and breathing stop suddenly and without warning
    1. Can occur anywhere at any time
    2. The person suffers permanent brain damage unless breathing and circulation are restored
  B. Respiratory arrest is when breathing stops, but the heart still pumps blood for several minutes
    1. Causes of respiratory arrest include
      a. Drowning
      b. Stroke
      c. Foreign body airway obstruction (FBAO)—choking on an object (see Page 784)
      d. Drug overdose
      e. Electric shock (including lightning)
      f. Smoke inhalation
      g. Suffocation
      h. Heart attack
      i. Coma
      j. Injuries from motor vehicle accidents or other trauma
    2. If breathing is not restored, cardiac arrest occurs
    3. If the person still has a pulse, rescue breathing can prevent cardiac arrest
  C. Chain of Survival
    1. The Heart and Stroke Foundation of Canada's basic life support courses teach this
      a. The actions in the chain are taken for heart attack, cardiac arrest, stroke, and FBAO
      b. Any delay reduces the person's chance of surviving
    2. Early recognition
      a. You must realize the person is having a medical emergency
      b. You must know the warning signs (see Chapter 31, and p. 784 in the textbook)
    3. Early access to the emergency response system
      a. Means activating the EMS system to get help as quickly as possible
      b. Phone the emergency number before you do anything else

c. 911 is the emergency number in most Canadian cities and towns

d. Confirm the EMS number in your community

e. Facilities have codes that are called for life-threatening emergencies

4. Early CPR—see below

5. Early defibrillation—see p. 789 in the textbook

6. Early advanced care—given by EMS staff, physicians, and nurses

   a. May include medications and other life-saving measures

D. Cardiopulmonary resuscitation (CPR)

   1. There are three major signs of cardiac arrest:
      a. No pulse
      b. No breathing
      c. No response

   2. CPR must be started as soon as cardiac arrest occurs
      a. Provides oxygen to vital organs until more advanced care can be given

   3. CPR has three basic parts:
      a. Airway
      b. Breathing
      c. Circulation

   4. The person must be supine on a hard, flat surface
      a. Arms are positioned at the sides
      b. If turning is necessary, logroll the person; the person may have other injuries

   5. Airway
      a. The respiratory passages must be open to restore breathing
      b. The head-tilt/chin-lift maneuver is used to open the airway (see Figure 47-1 and Figure 47-2, p. 774)
         (1) Place one hand on the person's forehead
         (2) Apply pressure on the forehead with the palm to tilt the head back
         (3) Place the fingers of the other hand under the bony part of the chin
         (4) Lift the chin forward as the head is tilted backward with the other hand
      c. When the airway is open, check for vomitus, loose dentures, or other foreign bodies

         (1) Remove dentures; protect from loss or damage
         (2) Wipe vomitus away with the index and middle fingers
            (a) Wear gloves or cover your fingers with a cloth

6. Breathing
   a. The person must get oxygen
      (1) Otherwise permanent brain and organ damage occurs
   b. Rescue breathing is done for the person
   c. Before you start, determine breathlessness (see Figure 47-3, p. 775)
      (1) Should take no more than 10 seconds to:
         (a) Maintain an open airway
         (b) Place your ear over the person's mouth and nose
         (c) Observe the person's chest
         (d) Look—to see if the chest rises and falls
         (e) Listen—for the escape of air
         (f) Feel—for the flow of air on your cheek
   d. Mouth-to-mouth resuscitation
      (1) Most common method of rescue breathing (see Figure 47-4, p. 775)
      (2) Airway is kept open
      (3) Pinch the person's nostrils shut with the thumb and index finger of the hand on the forehead
      (4) Take a deep breath; place your mouth tightly over the person's mouth
      (5) Slowly blow air into the person's mouth
      (6) The person's chest should rise as the lungs fill with air
      (7) You should hear air escape as the person exhales
      (8) After giving a ventilation, remove your mouth from the person's mouth
         (a) Take in a quick, deep breath
   e. Mouth-to-nose technique
      (1) Used when:
         (a) You cannot ventilate the victim's mouth
         (b) You cannot open the mouth
         (c) You cannot make a tight seal for mouth-to-mouth resuscitation

(d) The mouth is severely injured

(2) The mouth is closed

(3) The head-tilt/chin-lift method is used to open the airway

(4) Pressure is placed on the chin to close the mouth

(5) Place your mouth over the person's nose and blow air into the nose (see Figure 47-6, p.776)

   (a) After ventilation, remove your mouth from the person's nose

f. Mouth-to-stoma ventilation (stoma in the neck), see Figure 47-7, p.776)

(1) Seal your mouth around the stoma and blow air into the stoma

(2) Before giving mouth-to-mouth or mouth-to-nose ventilation, check for a neck stoma

g. Barrier devices prevent contact with the person's mouth, blood, body fluids, secretions, and excretions

(1) Mouth-to-barrier device is another method of rescue breathing (see Figure 47-5, p. 776)

(2) The barrier device is placed over the person's mouth and nose

(3) Make sure the seal is tight

(4) Breathe into the barrier device

h. When CPR is started:

(1) Give two breaths first; exhale after each breath

(2) Then give breaths at the rate of one every 5 seconds

(3) During CPR, give two breaths after every 15 chest compressions

7. Circulation

a. Blood flow to the brain and other organs must be maintained

b. The heart stops beating in cardiac arrest

(1) Blood must be pumped in some other way

c. Artificial circulation is accomplished by chest compressions

(1) Before starting chest compressions, determine pulselessness

   (a) Use the carotid artery on the side near you, for adults

   (b) Use brachial pulse for infants

   (c) Place the tips of your index

and middle fingers on the person's trachea; slide your fingertips down off the trachea to the groove of the neck (see Figure 47-9, p. 777)

   (d) To find brachial pulse in infants place your thumb on the outside of the infant's arm, just above the elbow; place your middle and index fingers on the inside of the arm between the elbow and the shoulder (see Figure 47-10, p. 777); press gently to feel the pulse

d. The heart lies between the sternum and the spinal column (see Figure 47-11, p. 778)

(1) Pressure applied to the sternum compresses the heart

e. For effective chest compressions, the person is supine on a hard, flat surface

f. Proper hand position is important (see Fig. 47-11, p. 778 in the textbook)

(1) Use two or three fingers to find the lower part of the person's rib cage on the side near you; use the hand closest to the person's feet

(2) Move your fingers up along the rib cage to the notch at the centre of the chest; the notch is where the ribs and breastbone meet; place your middle finger in the notch; place your index finger beside your middle finger

(3) Place the heel of your other hand on the lower half of the sternum next to your index finger

(4) Remove your index and middle fingers from the notch

(5) Place that hand on the hand already on the sternum

(6) Extend or interlace your fingers; keep your fingers off the chest (see Figure 47-11, p.778)

g. Proper body position:

(1) Your elbows are straight

(2) Your shoulders are directly over the person's chest

(3) Exert firm downward pressure

   (a) Depress the sternum 4-5 cm (1/2 to 2 inches) in the adult

(4) Release the pressure without re-

moving your hands from the chest

(5) Give compressions in regular rhythm at a rate of 100 compressions per minute

8. Performing CPR

a. CPR is done for cardiac arrest

b. Determine if cardiac arrest or fainting has occurred

c. CPR is done when there is unresponsiveness, breathlessness, and pulselessness

d. BLS for the adult involves the following sequence:

(1) Determine unresponsiveness (tap, shake, shout)

(2) Activate the EMS system immediately if the person is unresponsive

(3) Determine breathlessness (look, listen, feel)

(4) Open the airway; give two breaths if the person is not breathing

(5) Determine pulselessness

(6) Start chest compressions if the person has no pulse

e. You can do CPR alone or with another person

f. Never practice CPR on another person

(1) Mannequins are used

g. Adult CPR—One Rescuer ▶ p. 780

h. Adult CPR—Two Rescuer ▶ p. 781

E. Basic life support for infants and children

1. Cardiac arrest due to heart disease is rare in children

a. Sudden infant death syndrome (SIDS), respiratory diseases, airway obstruction, drowning, infection, and nervous system diseases are the most common causes in children under 1 year of age

b. Injuries are the most common cause in children older than 1 year

2. Sequence of BLS for infants and children (1 to 8 years old)

a. Do not move or shake the child to determine unresponsiveness; tap or shout (head, neck, and spinal cord injuries are possible)

b. Shout for help or send a second rescuer to activate the EMS system

c. If alone, provide BLS for 1 minute before activating the EMS system

d. If there are no injuries and the person is small, carry the person to the telephone

e. Move any person from a dangerous location; also move if you cannot perform CPR where the person is lying

f. If you must move the person, make sure the head does not roll, twist, or tilt

g. Use the head-tilt/chin-lift maneuver for infants and children (see Figure 47-15, p. 782)

(1) Do not hyperextend the head

(2) Tilt the head to a normal, neutral position

h. If a neck injury is suspected, use the jaw-thrust maneuver (see Figure 47-2, p.774)

(1) Place two or three fingers under each side of the lower jaw at the angle of the jaw

(2) Use your other finger to lift the jaw upward and outward

(3) Rest your elbows on the surface on which the child is lying

i. Keep the airway open throughout CPR

j. Only use one hand for chest compressions on a child (see Figure 47-17, p. 784); use only two or three fingers on an infant (see Figure 47-16, p. 784)

(1) Keep the other hand on the forehead to maintain the head tilt

(2) For children, use both hands for the head-tilt/chin-lift maneuver when giving breaths

k. Compress the chest at a rate of 100 per minute

l. Give 5 chest compressions followed by 1 slow rescue breath

m. Repeat 20 sets of 5 compressions followed by 1 rescue breath; twenty sets will take slightly longer than 1 minute to complete

F. Foreign body obstruction (FBAO) in adults and children

1. Can lead to cardiac arrest

a. The body does not get oxygen

2. Foreign bodies can cause airway obstruction

a. Large, poorly chewed pieces of meat

b. Dentures

c. Laughing and talking while eating

d. Weakness, poorly fitting dentures,

dysphagia and chronic illness are common causes in older adults
   e. Infants and young children are at risk because they are likely to put small objects in their mouths
   f. Many foods such as hot dogs and popcorn can easily cause FBAO in children (see Chapter 16)
3. Can occur in unconscious persons
   a. Common causes are aspirating vomitus and the tongue falling back into the airway
     (1) Can occur during cardiac arrest
4. Partial obstruction
   a. The person moves some air in and out of the lungs
   b. The person is conscious
   c. Forceful coughing often removes the object
5. Complete airway obstruction
   a. The person clutches at the throat (see Figure 47-18, p. 785)
   b. The person cannot breathe, speak, or cough
   c. The person is pale and cyanotic
   d. Air does not move in and out of the lungs
   e. If conscious, the person is very apprehensive
   f. The obstruction must be removed before cardiac arrest occurs
   g. Is an emergency; the EMS system must be activated
6. The Heimlich maneuver
   a. Used to relieve an obstructed airway caused by a foreign body
   b. Involves abdominal thrusts (see Figure 47-19, p. 786)
   c. Performed with the person standing, sitting, or lying down
     (1) The finger sweep is used with the Heimlich maneuver when an adult becomes unconscious
   d. Not effective in extremely obese persons and in pregnant women
     (1) Chest thrusts are used (see Box 47-2, p. 785)
7. FBAO—The Responsive Adult or Child ▶ p. 786
8. FBAO in Infants
   a. Responsive infants with airway obstruction require back blows and chest thrusts
   b. If the infant becomes unresponsive,

follow same procedure as for adults
   c. Infections and allergic reactions can also cause obstruction
   d. Unless you witness or strongly suspect that the infant has FBAO do not try to clear this obstruction but activate EMS at once
   e. FBAO—The Responsive Infant ▶ p. 786
9. Finding an unconscious adult
   a. You did not see the person lose consciousness; you do not know the cause
     (1) You cannot assume the cause is choking
     (2) You need to establish unresponsiveness and attempt rescue breathing
     (3) Abdominal thrusts are done if you cannot ventilate the person
       (a) The finger sweep maneuver is used
10. The Unresponsive Adult, Child, or Infant ▶ p. 788
G. Recovery position
  1. A side-lying position (see Figure 47-22, p. 788)
  2. Used when the person is breathing and has a pulse
   a. Logroll the person into the recovery position
     (1) Keep the head, neck, and spine straight
   b. Keep the person in good alignment
   c. An arm supports the head
  3. Keeps the airway open and prevents aspiration
  4. Do not use if the person might have neck injuries or other trauma
H. Self-administered Heimlich maneuver
  1. You can perform the Heimlich maneuver to relieve an obstructed airway on yourself; to do so:
   a. Make a fist with one hand
   b. Place thumb side of the fist above your navel and below the lower end of the sternum
   c. Grasp your fist with your other hand
   d. Press inward and upward quickly
   e. Press the upper abdomen against a hard surface if thrust did not relieve the obstruction
   f. Use as many thrusts as needed
IV. AUTOMATED EXTERNAL DEFIBRILLATORS (AEDs)

A. Early defibrillation is the fourth link in the heart and Stroke Foundation of Canada's Chain of Survival

B. Ventricular Fibrillation (VF) causes cardiac arrest

C. Heart does not beat at a regular beat but shakes and quivers and no blood is pumped to the heart, brain, and other organs

D. VF must be stopped and a regular heart rhythm restored

E. A defibrillator delivers a shock to the heart, which stops VF, and a regular rhythm starts

F. AEDs are computerized devices found in hospitals, long-term care facilities, other health care agencies, and many businesses and institutions

G. Most basic life support courses now teach health care providers and members of the general public how to use them

V. HEMORRHAGE

A. If a blood vessel is cut or torn, bleeding occurs

   1. The larger the blood vessel, the greater the bleeding

B. Hemorrhage is the excessive loss of blood in a short period of time

   1. If not stopped, death results

C. Can be internal or external

   1. Internal hemorrhage

     a. Cannot be seen

     b. Bleeding occurs inside the body into tissues and body cavities

     c. Signs include pain, shock, vomiting blood, coughing up blood, and loss of consciousness

     d. You must activate the EMS system; then:

       (1) Keep the person warm, flat, and quiet

       (2) Do not give fluids

     e. Follow Standard Precautions

   2. External bleeding

     a. Usually seen; may be hidden by clothing

     b. Bleeding from an artery is bright red and occurs in spurts

     c. There is a steady blood flow from a vein

     d. To control external hemorrhage, follow the guidelines listed in Box 47-1, p. 773 in the textbook

       (1) Activate the EMS system

       (2) Practice Standard Precautions

         (a) Wear gloves if possible

       (3) Place a sterile dressing directly over the wound (see Figure 47-23, p. 789)

         (a) Use any clean material, if sterile material is not available

       (4) Apply pressure with your hand directly over the bleeding site

         (a) Do not release pressure until bleeding is controlled

       (5) If direct pressure does not control bleeding, apply pressure over the artery above the bleeding site (see Figure 47-24, p. 790)

         (a) Use your first three fingers to apply pressure on the artery

         (b) Bind the wound when the bleeding stops; tape or tie the dressing in place

         (c) You can use a scarf, belt, or piece of clothing

         (d) If the dressing is around a limb, check for good circulation

VI. SHOCK

A. Results when there is not enough blood supply to organs and tissues

B. Causes include blood loss, myocardial infarction (MI), burns, and severe infection

C. Signs and symptoms include:

   1. Low or falling blood pressure

   2. Rapid and weak pulse

   3. Rapid respirations

   4. Cold, moist, and pale skin

   5. Thirst

   6. Restlessness

   7. Confusion and loss of consciousness

D. To prevent and treat shock, follow the guidelines listed in Box 47-1, p. 773 in the textbook

   1. Keep the person lying down

   2. Maintain an open airway

   3. Control hemorrhage

   4. Keep the person warm

   5. Reassure the person

E. Anaphylactic shock

   1. Anaphylaxis is a life-threatening sensitivity to an antigen

     a. In severe cases, anaphylactic shock occurs in seconds

   2. Signs and symptoms include:

     a. Sweating

b. Shortness of breath

c. Low blood pressure

d. Irregular pulse

e. Respiratory congestion

f. Swelling of the larynx

g. Hoarseness

h. Dyspnea

3. Is an emergency; the EMS system must be activated

   a. The person needs special drugs to reverse the allergic reaction

   b. Keep the person lying down

   c. Keep the airway open

   d. CPR is necessary if cardiac arrest occurs

VII. SEIZURES

  A. Violent and sudden involuntary contractions of muscles

  B. Causes include head injuries, high fever, brain tumors, poisoning, seizure disorders, central nervous system infection, and lack of blood flow to the brain

  C. Major types:

    1. Partial seizures

     a. Only part of the brain is involved

     b. The person does not lose consciousness

    2. Generalized seizures

     a. The whole brain is involved

     b. The generalized tonic (grand mal seizure) clonic seizure has two phases:

      (1) The tonic phase

       (a) The person loses consciousness; falls if standing or sitting

       (b) The body is rigid; all muscles contract at once

      (2) The clonic phase

       (a) Muscle groups contract and relax; causes jerking and twitching movements of the body

       (b) Urinary and fecal incontinence may occur

      (3) After the seizure, the person usually falls into a deep sleep

       (a) May have confusion and headache on awakening

    3. Generalized absence (petit mal) seizure

     a. Usually lasts for a few seconds

     b. There is loss of consciousness; twitching of eyelids and staring

     c. No first aid is necessary

    4. The following measurer are performed for a generalized tonic-clonic seizure:

     a. Follow the guidelines listed in Box 47-1, p. 773 in the textbook (includes activating the EMS system)

     b. Do not leave the person alone

     c. If the person is not in bed, lower the person to the floor to protect them from falling

     d. Place a folded blanket, towel, cushion under the person's head (see Figure 47-25, p. 791)

     e. Turn the person onto their side (left side is best); ensure the head is turned to the side

     f. Loosen jewelry and clothing (ties, scarves etc.) around the neck

     g. Move furniture, equipment, or any object the person could strike during uncontrolled body movements

     h. Do not restrain body movements during the seizure

     i. Do not put your fingers between the person's teeth

     j. Do not insert any object into the person's mouth as this could cause choking

VIII. BURNS

  A. Can severely disable a person

  B. Most burn injuries occur in the home

  C. Common causes are:

    1. Dry heat—fire, stoves

    2. Moist heat—hot liquids, steam

    3. Chemicals—oven cleaner, drain cleaner

    4. Electricity—faulty electrical equipment, live wires, or lightning (see Figure 47-27, p. 792)

    5. Radiation—sunlight

  D. Types of burns—some are minor and others severe

    1. Burns are more severe and require emergency help when:

     a. They are located on the head, face, neck, hands, feet, or genitals

     b. They are spread over a large area of the body

     c. The burned person is under 2 or over 50 years of age or has a pre-existing medical condition (such as diabetes or

hypertension)
2. First-degree burns are the least severe
   a. Only top layer of skin is affected
   b. Skin is red or discolored, and mild swelling and a moderate amount of pain are present
   c. May not require medical attention
3. Second-degree burns involve the dermis and part of the epidermis
   a. Skin is red or mottled and blistering
   b. Burns are very painful because nerve endings are exposed
   c. Severe sunburn and burns caused by hot liquids are examples
   d. They are serious and require medical attention
4. Third-degree burns are very deep, affecting the dermis and the entire epidermis
   a. Most severe and require emergency medical attention
   b. Fat, muscle, and bone may be injured or destroyed
   c. Skin may look black, white, or charred
   d. Often covers a large surface area (see Figure 47-26, p. 792)
   e. Person may have excruciating pain if nerves are exposed, or no pain at all

E. Treatment
1. For minor first-degree burns that are limited to a small area
   a. Immediately cool the injury to reduce pain, swelling, and blistering and tissue damage
   b. Immerse in cool water and cover with a clean, wet, cool cloth
   c. Once pain is reduced, gently pat dry and cover with dry, lint-free, clean cloth
   d. Do not apply oil, butter, salve, or ointments
   e. Report the burn to your supervisor
   f. Seek medical attention if necessary
2. Emergency care of second and third-degree burns includes the following
   a. Follow the guidelines listed in Box 47-1, p. 773 in the textbook (includes activating EMS and following Standard Precautions)
   b. For chemical burns—brush off any loose powder, flush the area with large amounts of cool water for 15 to 20 minutes; remove contaminated clothing
   c. For electrical burns—do not touch the person if still in contact with electrical source
      (1) Turn off power or remove electrical source using an object that does not conduct electricity (i.e., wood)
      (2) Do not apply water as may increase risk of shock
   d. For heat source—stop the burning process, protect yourself, and extinguish the flames
   e. Remove hot clothing that is not sticking to the skin, jewelry, and tight clothing before injury swells
   f. Provide CPR as needed
   g. Cool the burned skin with cool water.
      (1) Do not use cold water on large, third-degree burns, cover with a clean, moist compress and reapply up to 20 minutes
   h. Loosely cover the burn wounds with a clean, dry covering and secure
   i. Do not use oil, butter, or any ointment on burns
   j. Do not break blisters
   k. Keep the person warm
   l. Watch for shock and stay with the person until help arrives

IX. POISONING
   A. Many household products can cause poisoning (see Chapter 16)
   B. Children and people with confusion or dementia are at risk
   C. In the community, make sure the phone number of the local poison control centre is posted near the telephone
   D. Signs of poisoning include empty pill bottle or hazardous products lying about; the person suddenly collapses, vomits, or has difficulty breathing
   E. If you suspect poisoning
      1. Follow the guidelines listed in Box 47-1, p. 773 in the textbook
      2. Gather any evidence that could help determine what has been ingested

X. FAINTING
   A. Sudden loss of consciousness from inadequate blood supply to the brain
   B. Hunger, fatigue, fear, and pain are common causes; also standing in one position too long and being in a warm, crowded room

C. Dizziness, perspiration, and blackness before the eyes are warning signals
   1. The person looks pale
   2. Pulse is weak
   3. Respirations are shallow if consciousness is lost
D. Emergency care includes:
   1. Have the person sit or lie down before fainting
   2. If sitting, the person bends forward and places the head between the knees
   3. If the person is lying down, elevate the legs
   4. Loosen tight clothing
   5. Keep the person lying down if fainting has occurred
   6. Do not let the person get up until all-symptoms have subsided for about 5 minutes
   7. Help the person to a sitting position after recovery
XI. STROKE
A. Is described in Chapter 31 in the textbook
B. The brain is suddenly deprived of its blood supply
   1. Usually only part of the brain is affected
C. May be caused by a thrombus, embolus, or cerebral hemorrhage
D. Signs vary; they depend on the size and location of brain injury
   1. Loss of consciousness or semiconsciousness, rapid pulse, labored respirations, elevated blood pressure, vomiting, hemiplegia, and aphasia are signs
   2. Seizures may occur
E. Emergency care includes (follow guidelines in Box 47-1, p.773):
   1. Place the person in the recovery position in the unaffected side (see Figure 47-22, p. 788)
   2. Elevate the head without flexing the neck
   3. Loosen tight clothing
   4. Keep the person quiet and warm
   5. Reassure the person
   6. Provide CPR and emergency care if necessary
XII. COMPASSIONATE CARE
A. Must be protected during emergencies
   1. The person is treated with dignity and respect
B. The right to privacy and confidentiality is protected
   1. Do not expose the person unnecessarily
   2. Onlookers are threats to privacy and confidentiality
C. The right to personal choice is protected
   1. The person has the right to choose which hospital to be taken to
D. Personal possessions are protected
E. The person needs to feel safe and secure
   1. Physical and psychological safety are important
   2. Reassurance, explanations about care, and a calm approach are important

Classroom Activities

1. Arrange for an EMT or paramedic to talk to the class about how the EMS system is activated and functions in your community.
   a. Ask students to write key points in a notebook for future reference.
   b. Allow time for questions and discussion.

2. Display the guidelines in Box 47-1, p. 773 in the textbook, on an overhead transparency.
   a. Carefully review each rule with students.
   b. Allow time for questions and discussion.

3. Write the following terms on the chalkboard:
   a. Cardiac arrest
   b. Respiratory arrest

   Call on students to define each term. Write the correct answers on the chalkboard.

4. Provide students with information about how to become certified in basic life support in your community. You can help students enroll in classes.

5. Write the following on a flip chart:
   a. The three major signs of cardiac arrest:

   (1) _____

   (2) _____

   (3) _____

   b. The three basic parts of CPR:

   (1) _____

   (2) _____

   (3) _____

Call on students to provide the answers. Write the correct answers on the flip chart. Use this as a basis to discuss the process of CPR.

6. Divide students into two groups. Provide each group with a flip chart and colored markers.
   a. Ask one group to list the sequence of CPR for the adult.
   b. Ask one group to list the sequence of CPR for infants and children.

   Allow 10 minutes for this exercise. Then call on one student from each group to report to the class. Discuss why the sequence is different for different age groups.

7. Write "Obstructed Airway" on the chalkboard.
   a. Call on students to list the causes.
   b. Call on students to describe the differences between a partial airway obstruction and a complete airway obstruction.

8. Write the word "Hemorrhage" on the chalkboard. Call on students to define the term. Write the correct answer on the chalk.

9. Divide students into two groups. Provide each group with a flip chart and colored markers.
   a. Ask one group to describe internal hemorrhage. They should also describe what must be done for a person with internal hemorrhage.
   b. Ask one group to describe external hemorrhage. They should also describe what must be done for the person with external hemorrhage.

   Allow 10 minutes for this exercise. Then call on one student from each group to report to the class. Allow time after each presentation for questions and discussion.

10. Write each of the following terms on a separate index card: Shock, Anaphylactic shock, Seizures, Burns, Fainting, and Stroke.
    a. Divide students into six groups. Provide each group with several sheets of notebook paper.
    b. Ask one person from each group to choose an index card. Then ask each group to write down the following information about the term on their index card:
    (1) Definition
    (2) Causes
    (3) Signs and symptoms
    (4) Types (if applicable)
    (5) Emergency measures to perform

Allow 20 minutes for this exercise. Then call on one student from each group to report to the class. Allow time after each presentation for questions and discussion.

11. Using a round table discussion format, ask students to describe how quality of life is protected in emergency situations.
    a. Discuss the person's rights and how they are protected.

12. Use the procedure checklists provided. Demonstrate each procedure in this chapter.
    a. Have each student practice and return demonstrate each procedure in this chapter. Use a simulator and CPR mannequins when appropriate.

Homework Assignments

Ask students to answer the questions at the end of Chapter 47 in the textbook. Tell students the date and time that this assignment must be completed and turned in.

If the accompanying student workbook is being used, assign the Chapter 47 workbook exercises. Tell students the date and time that this assignment must be completed and turned in.

Chapter 47 Student Assignment

Name _____

Date _____

Basic Emergency Care

Write your answers in the spaces provided.

1. You must activate the emergency medical services (EMS) system. What information should you give the operator?

   a. _____

   b. _____

   c. _____

   d. _____

   e. _____

   f. _____

2. Use the _____
   _____
   on the side near you to check for pulselessness.

3. List the three basic parts of CPR.

   a. _____

   b. _____

   c. _____

4. The _____
   _____ is used to relieve an obstructed airway caused by a foreign body.

5. What measures can you take to control external hemorrhage?

   a. _____

   b. _____

   c. _____

   d. _____

   e. _____

6. Do the following to prevent and treat shock:

   a. _____

   b. _____

   c. _____

   d. _____

   e. _____

   f. _____

   g. _____

7. Emergency care for fainting includes:

   a. _____

   b. _____

   c. _____

   d. _____

   e. _____

   f. _____

   g. _____

400

Chapter 47 Quiz

Name _____

Date _____

Basic Emergency Care

True or False

*Mark **T** for true or **F** for false.*

1. _____ Respiratory arrest is when breathing stops and the heart stops.

2. _____ Basic life support procedures support breathing and circulation.

3. _____ For effective chest compressions, the person must be supine and on a soft, comfortable surface.

4. _____ Cardiopulmonary resuscitation is done for cardiac arrest and fainting.

5. _____ Do not move or shake a child to determine responsiveness.

6. _____ The airway must be open to restore breathing.

7. _____ Choking can lead to cardiac arrest.

8. _____ With complete airway obstruction, the conscious person clutches at the throat.

9. _____ Internal bleeding is easily controlled by applying direct pressure to the bleeding site.

10. _____ High blood pressure and a slow, weak pulse are signs of shock.

11. _____ Anaphylaxis is a life-threatening sensitivity to an antigen.

12. _____ A person is having a seizure. You must restrain the person's body movements to promote safety.

13. _____ Full-thickness burns are very painful.

14. _____ The right to privacy and confidentiality are protected during an emergency.

Multiple Choice

Circle the BEST answer.

15. The emergency care given to an ill or injured person before medical help arrives is called:
    a. Emergency medical system.
    b. First aid.
    c. Basic life support.
    d. Cardiopulmonary resuscitation.

16. When providing emergency care, which is incorrect?
    a. Know your limits. Do not do more than you are able.
    b. Call for help.
    c. Move the person to a more comfortable place.
    d. Keep the person warm.

17. The most common method of rescue breathing is:
    a. Mouth-to-mouth resuscitation
    b. Mouth-to-nose resuscitation
    c. Mouth-to-stoma resuscitation
    d. Mouth-to-barrier device resuscitation

18. Before starting chest compressions:
    a. Check for breathlessness.
    b. Check for a blood pressure.
    c. Check for pulselessness.
    d. All of the above.

19. When doing chest compressions, which is incorrect?
    a. Your elbows are straight.
    b. Your shoulders are directly over the person's chest.
    c. Exert firm downward pressure.
    d. Depress the sternum $2^1/2$ to 3 inches.

20. Adult CPR is being given by two people. Breaths are given:
    a. After every 10 compressions.
    b. After every compression.
    c. After every 15 compressions.
    d. After every 5 compressions.

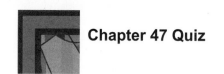

Name _____

Date _____

Basic Emergency Care

21. You find a person unconscious, which is *incorrect?*
    a. You can assume that the person is choking.
    b. You need to establish unresponsiveness.
    c. If the person is unresponsive, attempt rescue breathing.
    d. Abdominal thrusts are done if you cannot ventilate the person.

22. Do the following to prevent and treat shock *except:*
    a. Keep the person lying down.
    b. Control hemorrhage.
    c. Keep the person cool.
    d. Reassure the person.

23. Emergency care of burns includes all of the following *except:*
    a. Remove the person from the fire or burn source.
    b. Leave the burns open to the air.
    c. Remove hot clothing that is not sticking to the skin.
    d. Provide basic life support as needed.

24. Emergency care for the person having a stroke includes all of the following *except:*
    a. Elevate the head without flexing the neck.
    b. Loosen tight clothing.
    c. Turn the person away from the affected side.
    d. Keep the person quiet and warm.

Medical Terminology

Instructor's Preparation

I. Read Chapter 48 in the textbook. Carefully review chapter objectives, key terms, and review questions.

II. Read the outline in Chapter 48 of the instructor's guide. Carefully review the classroom activities, the student assignment, and the quiz.

III. If you are using the accompanying student workbook, review the activities for Chapter 48.

IV. Gather all necessary supplies and equipment for classroom activities and student assignments.
   A. Prepare appropriate flip charts
   B. Prepare flash cards
   C. Gather coloured markers
   D. Gather any other items that will be needed for classroom activities
   E. Assemble items in the order they will be used.

V. Make sure that the necessary equipment is available and in good working order.

Objectives

- Define the key terms listed in this chapter
- Identify three word elements used in medical terms
- Learn the meanings of common Greek and Latin prefixes, roots, and suffixes
- Combine word elements into medical terms
- Learn the meanings of common medical terms
- Identify the four abdominal regions
- Define the directional terms that describe the positions of the body in relation to other body parts
- Identify and define the abbreviations used in health care

Key Terms

abbreviation
anterior
combining vowel
distal
dorsal
lateral
medial
posterior
prefix
proximal
root
suffix
ventral
word element

Outline

Medical Terminology

I. INTRODUCTION
   A. Knowing medial terminology is important in your work
      1. Learning medical terms can be fun and educational
II. WORD ELEMENTS
   A. Medical terms are made up of parts or word elements
      1. Important word elements are prefixes, roots, and suffixes
   B. Prefixes are word elements placed at the beginning of a word
      1. Prefixes are always combined with other word elements
      2. They are never used alone
      3. See p. 799 in the textbook for a list of prefixes used in medical terminology
   C. Roots contain the basic meaning of the word
      1. A root is combined with another root, with prefixes, and with suffixes in various combinations to form a medical term
      2. A vowel may be added; the vowel is called a combining vowel and is usually an "o"
         a. A combining vowel makes pronunciation easier
      3. See pp. 799-800 in the textbook for a list of the most common roots and their combining vowels
   D. Suffixes are placed at the end of a root to change the meaning of the word
      1. Suffixes are not used alone
      2. When translating medical terms, begin with the suffix
      3. You need to learn the suffixes listed on p. 800 in the textbook
   E. Combining word elements
      1. Medical terms are formed by combining word elements
      2. A root can be combined with prefixes, roots, or suffixes
      3. The more complex combinations of prefixes, roots, and suffixes are:
         a. Two prefixes, a root, and a suffix
         b. A prefix, two roots, and a suffix
         c. Two roots, and a suffix
      4. Prefixes always come before roots and suffixes always come after roots
      5. Practice forming medical terms by combining the word elements listed in this chapter

III. ABDOMINAL REGIONS
   A. The abdomen is divided into the following regions
      1. Right upper quadrant (RUQ)
      2. Left upper quadrant (LUQ)
      3. Right lower quadrant (RLQ)
      4. Left lower quadrant (LLQ)
IV. DIRECTIONAL TERMS
   A. Certain terms describe the position of one body part in relation to another
      1. They give the direction of the body part when the person is standing and facing forward
         a. Anterior (ventral)—located at or toward the front of the body or body part
         b. Distal—the part farthest from the center or from the point of attachment
         c. Lateral—relating to or located at the side of the body or body part
         d. Medial—relating to or located at or near the midline of the body or body part
         e. Posterior (dorsal)—located at or toward the back of the body or body part
         f. Proximal—the part nearest to the center or point of origin
V. ABBREVIATIONS
   A. Shortened forms of words or phrases
      1. They save time and space
      2. Each agency has a list of accepted abbreviations
      3. Common abbreviations are listed on the inside back cover of the textbook

Classroom Activities

1. Write the following word elements on the chalkboard: Prefix, Root, and Suffix.
   a. Call on students to define each word element. Write the correct answers on the chalkboard.
   b. Explain how these word elements are combined to form medical terms.

2. Have each student practice forming medical terms by combining various word elements.

3. Write the four abdominal regions on the chalkboard. Ask students to stand up and point to each of the abdominal regions on their own bodies.

4. Write the following terms on a flip chart using different colored markers:
   a. Anterior
   b. Distal
   c. Lateral
   d. Medial
   e. Posterior
   f. Proximal

   Call on students to come forward and write the definition after each term. Clarify any wrong answers.

5. Make flash cards with medical terms.
   a. Divide students into pairs. Distribute a set of flash cards to each pair. Ask students to use the flash cards to help them memorize medical terms.
      (1) Ask students to exchange their set of flash cards with another pair every 5 minutes. Allow 20 minutes for this exercise.
   b. Encourage students to use flash cards at home to help them memorize medical terms.

6. Make flash cards with common abbreviations and have students work in pairs to identify common abbreviations.
   a. Encourage students to use flash cards at home to help them memorize abbreviations.

Homework Assignments

Ask students to answer the questions at the end of Chapter 48 in the textbook. Tell students the date and time that this assignment must be completed and turned in.

If the accompanying student workbook is being used, assign the Chapter 48 workbook exercises. Tell students the date and time that this assignment must be completed and turned in.

Name _____

Date _____

Medical Terminology

Write your answers in the spaces provided.

1. Word elements used in medical terminology are:

   a. _____

   b. _____

   c. _____

2. The four regions of the abdomen are:

   a. _____

   b. _____

   c. _____

   d. _____

3. Define the following directional terms.

   a. Distal _____

   _____

   _____

   b. Proximal _____

   _____

   _____

   c. Anterior (ventral) _____

   _____

   _____

   d. Medial _____

   _____

   _____

   e. Posterior (dorsal) _____

   _____

   _____

   f. Lateral _____

   _____

   _____

4. What is the meaning of each of the following prefixes?

   a. bi _____

   _____

   _____

   b. dys _____

   _____

   _____

   c. hypo

   _____

   _____

   _____

   d. mal _____

   _____

   _____

   e. post _____

   _____

   _____

Medical Terminology

5. What is the meaning of each of the following roots?

   a. cephal(o) _____

   _____

   _____

   b. derma _____

   _____

   _____

   c. lith(o) _____

   _____

   _____

   d. ocul(o) _____

   _____

   _____

   e. phleb(o) _____

   _____

   _____

6. What is the meaning of each of the following suffixes?

   a. ectomy _____

   _____

   _____

   b. graphy _____

   _____

   _____

   c. osis _____

   _____

   _____

   d. plegia _____

   _____

   _____

   e. uria _____

   _____

   _____

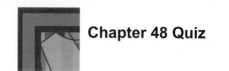

Name _____

Date _____

Medical Terminology

True or False	Multiple Choice

Mark **T** *for true or* **F** *for false.*

   1. _____ Knowing medical terminology is important in your work.

   2. _____ A prefix is a word element placed at the end of a word.

   3. _____ A prefix is often used alone.

   4. _____ The root contains the basic meaning of the word.

   5. _____ Suffixes are not used alone.

   6. _____ When translating medical terms, begin with the root.

Circle the BEST answer.

   7. Shortened forms of words or phrases are:
     a. Suffixes.
     b. Word elements.
     c. Abbreviations.
     d. Medical terms.

   8. The prefix "ab" means:
     a. Toward.
     b. Against.
     c. Double.
     d. Away from.

   9. Gastritis is:
     a. Inflammation of the stomach.
     b. A reddened tongue.
     c. A rapid pulse.
     d. An abdominal incision.

  10. What is the word that means inflammation of a joint?
     a. Apnea
     b. Hemiplegia
     c. Arthritis
     d. Thoracotomy

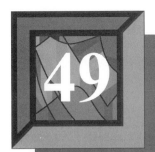

49

Your Job Search

Instructor's Preparation

   I. Read Chapter 49 in the textbook. Carefully review chapter objectives, key terms, and review questions.

  II. Read the outline in Chapter 49 of the instructor's guide. Carefully review the classroom activities, the student assignment, and the quiz.

 III. If you are using the accompanying student workbook, review the activities for Chapter 49.

 IV. Gather all necessary supplies and equipment for classroom activities and student assignments.

     A. Prepare the correct number of handouts

     B. Prepare appropriate flip charts

     C. Prepare overhead transparencies

     D. Prepare situation/index cards

     E. Gather correct slides

     F. Gather any other items that will be needed for classroom activities

     G. Assemble items in the order they will be used

   V. Make sure that the necessary equipment is available and in good working order.

 VI. Contact guest speakers to confirm the day, date, time, and location that they are expected.

     A. Ask the speakers if they require any special equipment or supplies; ensure these are available

Objectives

- Learn the key terms listed in this chapter
- List three tools you need to organize yourself for your job search
- Explain the difference between a chronological résumé and a functional résumé
- List three sources of advertised positions
- Identify methods for finding out about unadvertised positions
- List five details that are important in a letter of application
- Explain why you should take time completing application forms
- List what interviewers are trying to determine during an interview
- Explain why the interview is a key element in the job search
- Explain why it is important to practise and plan before an interview
- Describe three ways to make a good impression at an interview
- Explain why it is important to write a thank-you note following an interview

Key Terms

chronological résumé
cover letter
functional résumé
letter of application
reference
résumé
solicited letter of application
unsolicited letter of application

Outline

Your Job Search

I. INTRODUCTION
   A. Finding a job takes discipline, focus and hard work but it can be an exciting opportunity to learn about yourself and meet other people
II. GETTING ORGANIZED
   A. You will need the following tools to help you get organized:
      1. A computer and printer
      2. A telephone with an answering machine
      3. Office supplies—paper, envelopes, etc.
      4. Resources—books on résumé writing, telephone directories, etc.
      5. Box 49-1, p. 807 in the textbook, contains a list of useful resources
III. SETTING PRIORITIES AND GOALS
   A. Before writing your résumé you must decide what type of support work you want to do, whether you want to work in the community or a facility, and whether you want full or part-time work
   B. If you are undecided, then apply for positions in more than one setting
IV. PREPARING YOUR RESUME
   A. Introduction
      1. A résumé should be a concise one to two-page summary of your experience, education, work-related skills, and personal qualities
      2. Employers use résumés to decide who will be interviewed for the job
      3. When you prepare your résumé, keep in mind that employers pay attention to spelling and grammar; they also use the résumé to determine your fit in their setting
   B. Elements of a résumé
      1. Experience
      2. Education
      3. As options you can include:
         a. Objective of your career goals
         b. Profile of your particular skills and experience
         c. Interests related to the job
   C. Getting started on your résumé
      1. Start by making a list of your experiences, skills, and qualities
      2. Make list of the skills and qualities an employer would want to see in a support worker
      3. Compare the lists and expand on the

areas of your expertise that an employer might be interested in
   D. Organizing your résumé
      1. Chronological résumé
         a. Highlights employment history, starting with your most current employment, and working backward (see Figure 49-1, p. 808)
         b. Best for candidates who have a steady history of employment, with at least two years experience, and few gaps in employment
      2. Functional résumé
         a. Highlights skills or functions and briefly lists positions held (see Figure 49-2, p. 809)
         b. Best for those who have little work experience, long periods of not working, or frequent job changes
   E. Writing your résumé—as you write your résumé ask these questions:
      1. Is the information relevant?
      2. Have I been completely honest?
      3. Have I expressed myself clearly?
      4. Is my résumé consistent?
      5. Is my résumé correct?
   F. Formatting and printing
      1. Choose a simple, professional-looking format
      2. Do not use more than one font
      3. Keep graphics to a minimum
      4. Do not crowd too much type onto the page
      5. Print on good-quality white or ivory paper; staple pages together if more than two
V. FINDING AND FOLLOWING LEADS
   A. Advertised positions
      1. Employment advertisements
      2. Internet
      3. College career services
   B. Unadvertised positions can be found by:
      1. Contacting people you know
      2. Checking with your district home care program
      3. Looking in the yellow pages
      4. Checking your local library
      5. Attending job fairs
      6. Checking with your Canada Employment Centre
   C. Selecting References
      1. Choose people who can speak to a potential employer about your skills, abilities, and personal qualities

2. Use previous employers or teachers, rather than friends or family
3. Make sure that you ask the person for a reference, their contact information is correct, you keep your references informed if you are asked for an interview, and you let them know if you get the job

VI. PREPARING A LETTER OF APPLICATION (ALSO CALLED A COVER LETTER)
A. Solicited letter of application responding to an advertisement (see Figure 49-3, p. 812)
B. Unsolicited letter of application inquiring about potential job openings (see Figure 49-4, p. 813)
  1. Determining the employer's needs
    a. If responding to an advertisement, describe how you match your skills with the employer's needs
    b. If writing an unsolicited, letter find out as much as you can about the employer, their goals, and philosophies, and highlight your skills to enhance their agency or facility
  2. Organizing a letter or application
    a. The letter in Figure 49-4, p. 813 in the textbook, shows the different parts of a standard letter that you must include:
     (1) Front matter—return address, date, name and title, address of prospective employer, and greeting
     (2) Body—refer to page 814 for content; see Figure 49-3 and Figure 49-4, p. 812-813 in the textbook, for some examples
     (3) Closing—refer to page 814 for content; see Figure 49-3 and Figure 49-4, p. 812-813 in the textbook, for some examples
  3. Writing your letter
    a. You will need to write several drafts and revise your letter, but make sure you answer the following questions:
     (1) Have I emphasized relevant skills and qualities?
     (2) Have I emphasized accomplishments and skills?
     (3) Have I used an appropriate tone?
     (4) Is my letter concise?
     (5) Does my letter sound and look professional?
  4. Delivering your letter
    a. Hand deliver your letter of application and résumé whenever possible
    b. You can courier your application and follow-up with a phone call to check if everything arrived
    c. Many employers may ask for a fax or e-mail submission; it is always wise to also deliver a hard copy, if possible, as often technology can shut down transmission and your application may not arrive

VII. COMPLETING A JOB APPLICATION FORM
A. For some positions, you may be asked to complete an application form
B. The employer may use this information to make sure your have acceptable reading and writing skills
C. Make sure you answer all questions honestly and without any grammar or spelling errors, and don't leave any areas blank
D. These forms often require detailed information about your previous experience, reasons for leaving a job, etc.; always be honest in your answers
E. Always ask someone to proofread your application; a mistake we miss might be easily spotted by someone else
F. If submitting your application online, be just as careful, and have someone else read it before sending it

VIII. THE JOB INTERVIEW
A. The employer's chance to get to know and evaluate you
B. Lets you find out more about the agency or facility
C. Box 49-2, p. 816 in the textbook, lists common interview questions
  1. Prepare your answers
  2. Prepare a typed list of your skills to give to the interviewer
D. Your appearance is important
E. You must be on time
  1. A dry run may be helpful
F. When you arrive, tell the receptionist your name and why you are there
  1. Give the interviewer's name
  2. Wait in a professional manner
  3. Remember to smile
G. Greet the interviewer in a polite, courteous manner
  1. A firm handshake is best
  2. Address the interviewer as Mr., Mrs., Ms., Miss, or Doctor
  3. Use good posture

4. Maintain good eye contact
5. Avoid distracting habits
6. Keep your mind on the interview
H. Answer questions honestly
I. Speak clearly and with confidence
J. Avoid short "yes" or "no" responses
K. Give the interviewer your skills list
L. Explain that you are willing to learn
M. At the end of the interview, you will have the chance to ask questions
   1. The interviewer's answers will help you decide whether the job is right for you
N. Review the job description with the interviewer
   1. Ask questions at this time
   2. Advise the interviewer of any functions you cannot perform for training, legal, ethical, or religious reasons
O. The interviewer signals when the interview is over
   1. Ask the interviewer when you can check on your application
   2. Thank the interviewer before leaving
P. A written thank you note is advised
   1. It must be neat and legible
IX. THE EMPLOYMENT OFFER
A. You may be offered the job at the end of the interview, within a few days, or in a few weeks
B. If you are not offered the job, review the interview and ask yourself the questions in Box 49-3, p.819 in the textbook
C. Before accepting an offer of employment find out as much as you can about the terms of your employment
D. Clarify your wages, hours of work, requirements, and expectations
   1. If hired by an agency, most have procedure manuals to answer your questions
   2. If a contract position, find out the length and terms of the contract
   3. If hired by a client or their family, clarify the terms of employment and read Revenue Canada's booklet *Employee or Self-employed* (available at your local Canada Customs and Revenue Agency Office)

Classroom Activities

1. Obtain job application forms from the agencies to which students will be applying for jobs.
   a. Have each student practice completing a job application. Allow 15 minutes. Answer any questions. Collect the completed applications. Check them for completeness. Discuss the importance of accuracy, neatness, and completeness.
   b. Applications can be returned at the end of class or at the beginning of the next class.

2. Ask students to divide into small groups of three or four. Ask each group to discuss what qualities they would look for if they were responsible for hiring support workers for an agency. Allow 15 minutes for discussion. Have each group answer the following questions and report back to the class:
   a. What qualities and characteristics are most important to you? Why?
   b. What would you look for during the interview process?

3. Divide students into pairs. Provide each with the Classified Ads section of a local newspaper.
   a. Ask students to find ads for support workers job openings. Ask them to identity what information about the job the ad gives them.
      (1) What questions about the job do they have?
      (2) What makes one ad more appealing than the others?
   b. Allow 10 to 15 minutes for discussion, and then have one student from each pair report to the class. Allow time for discussion.

4. Have students compile a list of questions they would ask an interviewer before accepting a job. Allow 15 minutes. Randomly call on students to read one of their questions. Initiate discussion from the class. Encourage students to discuss what they are looking for in a job.

Homework Assignments

Ask students to answer the questions at the end of Chapter 49 in the textbook. Tell students the date and time that this assignment must be completed and turned in.

If the accompanying workbook is being used, assign the Chapter 49 workbook exercises. Tell students the date and time that this assignment must be completed and turned in.

Chapter 49 Student Assignment

Name _____

Date _____

Your Job Search

Write your answers in the spaces provided.

1. When writing your résumé what questions should you ask yourself?

   a. _____

   b. _____

   c. _____

   d. _____

   e. _____

2. List resources you can use to find job openings.

   a. _____

   b. _____

   c. _____

   d. _____

3. List 10 things that will help you make a good impression at an interview.

   a. _____

   b. _____

   c. _____

   d. _____

   e. _____

   f. _____

   g. _____

   h. _____

   i. _____

   j. _____

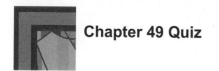

Chapter 49 Quiz

Name _____

Date _____

Your Job Search

True or False

Mark **T** *for true or* **F** *for false.*

1. _____ Lying on a job application is illegal.

2. _____ Tardiness and absences are among the most common reasons for losing a job.

3. _____ You feel that you are being harassed at work. You should ignore it to avoid causing trouble.

4. _____ How you dress is not important for a job interview.

5. _____ Every employee is responsible for job safety.

Multiple Choice

Circle the BEST answer.

6. To function at your best, you must by physically and mentally healthy. Which is incorrect?
   a. Adequate sleep and rest are needed.
   b. Never report to work under the influence of alcohol.
   c. Eat foods high in fats and salt.
   d. Good vision is needed.

7. Professional appearance involves all of the following except:
   a. Uniforms are clean, pressed, and mended.
   b. Hairstyles are simple and attractive.
   c. Wear your name badge or photo ID.
   d. Wear a lot of jewelry and bright nail polish.

8. You are ill and cannot come to work. Which is correct?
   a. Call a co-worker to report your illness.
   b. Do not call anyone. You are sick and need your rest.
   c. Call your supervisor.
   d. Call the administrator.

9. When formatting your résumé which should you NOT do.
   a. Choose a simple font
   b. Use only one font
   c. Do not crowd too much onto one page
   d. Use graphic devices and use bold to emphasize important points.

10. References should not include :
    a. past employers
    b. family
    c. previous teachers
    d. previous supervisor

414

FINAL EXAMINATION — VERSION 1

True or False

Mark **T** *for true. Mark* **F** *for false.*

1. _____ The goal of health promotion is to reduce the risk of illness.

2. _____ You can never refuse to perform a delegated task.

3. _____ You feel that you are being harassed at work. You should ignore it to avoid causing trouble.

4. _____ Everyone who works at an agency has the right to read the patient's or resident's records.

5. _____ Listen and use silence when dealing with an angry person.

6. _____ During systole, the heart chambers fill with blood.

7. _____ The pancreas is called the master gland.

8. _____ The rate of growth and development is even and at a set pace.

9. _____ All persons age at the same rate.

10. _____ Long-term care facilities are designed to meet the special needs of older and disabled persons.

11. _____ Pillows are used to position infants.

12. _____ Restraints are used only after trying all other alternatives.

13. _____ Household cleaners are kept in locked storage areas out of the reach of children.

14. _____ Transmission-based Precautions are used in the care of all persons.

15. _____ The muscles in the lower back are used to lift heavy objects from the floor.

16. _____ Push, slide, or pull heavy objects rather than lift them.

17. _____ You are going to transfer Mrs. Jones from the bed to a chair. Move her from the direction of the weak side of her body.

18. _____ The call system is always kept within the person's reach.

19. _____ Soiled linen is placed on the floor in the person's room until you finish making the bed.

20. _____ Plastic bags or dry cleaning bags can be used in the home to protect the mattress.

21. _____ You are giving oral care to an unconscious person. The person's mouth is held open with your fingers.

22. _____ The towel bar can be used for support when the person gets in or out of the tub.

23. _____ Cut hair to remove matted or tangled hair.

24. _____ Support workers cut and trim toenails.

25. _____ The healthy adult excretes about 1500 ml of urine per day.

26. _____ Catheterization increases the risk of urinary tract infection.

27. _____ Ignoring the need to defecate can lead to constipation.

28. _____ Good oral hygiene and denture care improve the ability to taste.

29. _____ Support workers regulate IV solution flow rates.

30. _____ The brachial artery is used most often for taking a pulse.

31. _____ The blood pressure cuff is applied over clothing.

32. _____ The person with a contracture is permanently deformed and disabled.

33. _____ Illness and injury decrease the need for rest and sleep.

34. _____ Pain is personal. It differs for each person.

35. _____ Admission to a health care facility often causes anxiety and fear.

36. _____ You help orient the person to the new environment.

37. _____ Parents are not allowed to be present during the examination of a child.

38. _____ The skin is sterilized before surgery to prevent infection.

39. _____ Coughing and deep breathing exercises help prevent pneumonia.

40. _____ Infants and children are at risk for pressure ulcers.

41. _____ Tape is used to secure a dressing. Tape should encircle the entire body part.

42. _____ Hot compresses and packs are left in place for 30 to 35 minutes.

43. _____ Infants and children are at great risk for rapid changes in body temperature.

44. _____ Altered respiratory function may be acute or chronic.

45. _____ The alarm on Mr. Adams' ventilator sounds. You should turn off the alarm and call the nurse.

46. _____ Self-care is a major goal of rehabilitation.

47. _____ A person may be unaware of gradual hearing loss.

48. _____ Glaucoma is always sudden in onset.

49. _____ Chemotherapy affects only cancer cells.

50. _____ Cigarette smoking is the most common cause of emphysema.

51. _____ Anxiety is seen in all mental health disorders.

52. _____ Depression is uncommon in older persons.

53. _____ Dementia is a normal part of aging.

54. _____ Confused and demented persons do not have the right to personal choice.

55. _____ Epilepsy cannot be controlled. It always interferes with learning.

56. _____ Attitudes and sex needs stay the same as a person ages.

57. _____ You have finished bottle-feeding a baby. The formula remaining in the bottle is stored in the refrigerator.

58. _____ Cardiopulmonary resuscitation is done for cardiac arrest and fainting.

59. _____ With complete airway obstruction, the conscious person clutches at the throat.

60. _____ A person is having a seizure. You must restrain the person's body movements to promote safety.

61. _____ Dying people continue to have psychological, social, and spiritual needs.

62. _____ Hospice care focuses on cures and life-saving procedures.

63. _____ A prefix is a word element placed at the end of a word.

Multiple Choice

Circle the BEST answer.

64. The Charter of Rights and Freedoms guarantees our right to:
    a. mobility
    b. vote
    c. life, liberty and security
    d. all of the above

65. These statements are about pressure sores. Which is *false?*
    a. a reddened area is the first sign of a pressure sore
    b. bony areas are the common site for pressure sores
    c. shearing and friction can cause pressure sores
    d. abdominal folds are the most common site of pressure sores

66. There are many advantages of home care. Which is *not?*
    a. lower costs
    b. greater comfort
    c. slower rate of recovery
    d. lower risk of infection

67. A person's photograph is taken without permission. This is called:
    a. Malpractice.
    b. Negligence.
    c. Invasion of privacy.
    d. Assault.

68. Stress is (choose the best answer):
    a. the way one copes with and adjusts to everyday living
    b. a response or change in the body caused by some factor
    c. a mental or emotional response
    d. a thought or idea

69. Wrinkling of the skin is caused by
    a. an increase in subcutaneous fat
    b. loss of elasticity in the skin
    c. a decrease in subcutaneous fat
    d. an increase in elasticity in the skin

70. A child is deprived of food and clothing. This is:
    a. Physical neglect.
    b. Physical abuse.
    c. Emotional neglect.
    d. Sexual abuse.

71. Looking at things from another's point of view is called:
    a. Courtesy.
    b. Empathy.
    c. Work ethics.
    d. Politeness.

72. A co-worker tells you that a doctor and nurse are dating. This is:
    a. Gossip.
    b. Eavesdropping.
    c. Confidential information.
    d. Sexual harassment.

73. Universal precautions
    a. are just for nurses
    b. involves treating all persons as it they were in-fected
    c. means wearing gloves whenever you can
    d. means you must wear long gowns when making beds and giving a bed bath

74. Measures in the nursing care plan are carried out. What step of the nursing process is this?
    a. Nursing diagnosis
    b. Planning
    c. Implementation
    d. Evaluation

75. You answer a person's phone in the hospital. How should you answer?
    a. "Good morning. Mrs. Kemp's room."
    b. "Good morning. Third floor."
    c. "Hello."
    d. "Good morning. Mrs. Kemp's room. Joan Bates, support worker, speaking."

76. The following statements relate to basic needs. Which is *incorrect*?
    a. People normally meet their own needs.
    b. Higher level needs must be met before lower level needs.
    c. Need for self-actualization is rarely totally met.
    d. The need for self-esteem is affected by illness.

77. As a patient, Sally Jones has the right to:
    a. Considerate and respectful care.
    b. Information about her diagnoses, treatment, and prognoses.
    c. Refuse treatment.
    d. All of the above.

78. The largest part of the brain and the center of thought and intelligence is the:
    a. Cerebellum.
    b. Midbrain.
    c. Brain stem.
    d. Cerebrum.

79. Where does digestion begin?
    a. In the stomach
    b. In the esophagus
    c. In the mouth
    d. In the duodenum

80. The outer layer of the skin is called the:
    a. Dermis.
    b. Epidermis.
    c. Integument.
    d. Myelin.

81. Which is not a developmental task of adolescence?
    a. Accepting change in appearance
    b. Becoming independent from parents and adults
    c. Developing leisure time activities
    d. Developing morals, values, and attitudes needed to function in society

82. Changes in psychological and social functioning are called:
    a. Growth.
    b. Development.
    c. A reflex.
    d. A stage.

83. Residents of long-term care facilities have the right to:
    a. Make telephone calls in private.
    b. Participate in planning their care.
    c. Receive mail unopened.
    d. All of the above.

84. Retirement usually results in:
    a. Lowered income.
    b. Physical changes from aging.
    c. Companionship and usefulness.
    d. Financial security.

85. When cleaning up a spill of body fluid
    a. always wear gloves
    b. use paper towels to absorb fluid
    c. dispose of the towels in waterproof bags
    d. all of the above

86. You are dealing with an agitated person. Which is *incorrect*?
    a. Stand as close to the person as possible.
    b. Position yourself close to the door.
    c. Do not touch the person.
    d. Talk to the person in a calm manner.

87. Errors in care are reported:
    a. At the end of your shift.
    b. Only if the person was injured.
    c. To the person's family when they visit.
    d. Immediately to your supervisor.

88. Why is age a factor in safety?
    a. Young children have not learned what is safe and what is dangerous.
    b. Infants are helpless.
    c. Physical changes from aging can affect balance and movements.
    d. All of the above.

89. A microbe that is harmful and causes infection is:
    a. A reservoir.
    b. A pathogen.
    c. A nonpathogen.
    d. Normal flora.

90. Mrs. Adams is in isolation. Which is *incorrect?*
    a. Say hello from the doorway often.
    b. Treat her with respect, kindness, and dignity.
    c. Provide hobby materials if possible.
    d. Spend as little time in her room as possible.

91. Standard precautions:
    a. Are used for all persons.
    b. Prevent the spread of pathogens through the air.
    c. Require gowns, masks, gloves, and protective eyewear.
    d. nvolve medical and surgical asepsis.

92. When logrolling a person, you must:
    a. Make sure the bed is in the Fowler's position.
    b. Lower the bed to the lowest position.
    c. Lower both bed rails.
    d. Turn the person as a unit in alignment with one motion.

93. The person's unit:
    a. Is arranged for staff convenience.
    b. Should always have dim lighting.
    c. Should be as personal and homelike as possible.
    d. Is kept clean by the person.

94. The overbed table is not used:
    a. For eating.
    b. As a working surface.
    c. To store the urinal.
    d. To store shaving articles.

95. Which is correct when handling linens?
    a. Shake linens in the air to remove wrinkles.
    b. Place dirty linen on the floor.
    c. Collect linens in the order of use.
    d. Return unused linen to the linen closet.

96. You are giving Mr. Wilson a back massage. Which is *incorrect?*
    a. Warm the lotion before applying it.
    b. The massage should last about 1 minute.
    c. Use firm strokes.
    d. Always keep your hands in contact with his skin.

97. The infestation of the body with lice is:
    a. Pediculosis corporis.
    b. Dandruff.
    c. Pediculosis pubis.
    d. Pediculosis capitis.

98. You assist Mr. Gomez with shaving. Which is *incorrect?*
    a. Soften the skin before shaving.
    b. Hold the skin taut as necessary.
    c. Shave away from the direction of hair growth.
    d. Report nicks or cuts to the nurse immediately.

99. Frequent urination at night is:
    a. Polyuria.
    b. Nocturia.
    c. Dysuria.
    d. Urgency.

100. The goal of bladder training is to:
    a. Remove the catheter.
    b. Allow the person to walk to the bathroom.
    c. Gain voluntary control of urination.
    d. All of the above.

101. A person has an ileostomy. Which is *incorrect?*
    a. The stool is formed.
    b. Good skin care is essential.
    c. The entire large intestine has been removed.
    d. The pouch must fit well.

102. Which is *false?*
    a. Enema solutions should be 40.5° C (105° F).
    b. The left Sims' position is used for an enema.
    c. The enema bag is held 12 inches above the anus.
    d. The enema solution is administered rapidly.

103. Dietary guidelines for Canadians include all of the following *except:*
    a. Eat a variety of food.
    b. Maintain a healthy weight.
    c. Choose a diet low in fat.
    d. Choose a high-sodium diet.

104. Mrs. Sanchez has an order for NPO. This means that:
    a. Fluids are restricted.
    b. Records are kept of oral intake.
    c. She cannot eat or drink anything.
    d. She is encouraged to drink a variety of fluids.

105. Which food groups contain the most fat?
    a. Breads, cereal, rice, and pasta
    b. Fruits
    c. Milk, yogurt, and cheese
    d. Meat, poultry, fish, dry beans, eggs, and nuts

106. Which statement about feeding a person is *false*?
    a. Ask if he or she wants to pray before eating.
    b. A fork is used to feed the person.
    c. The person is asked the order in which to serve foods.
    d. Engage the person in a pleasant conversation.

107. When charting what should you *not* do?
    a. Record in a logical manner
    b. Use a pencil
    c. Chart a procedure after it is completed
    d. Make an error and correct while charting

108. Normal respirations are:
    a. Between 10 and 20 per minute.
    b. Quiet and effortless.
    c. Regular, with both sides of the chest rising and falling equally.
    d. All of the above.

109. Bed cradles are used to:
    a. Keep the weight of top linens off the feet.
    b. Keep the hips abducted.
    c. Prevent plantar flexion.
    d. Prevent the mattress from sagging.

110. Which statement about range-of-motion (ROM) exercises is *incorrect*?
    a. ROM exercises can cause injury if not done correctly.
    b. The nurse tells you which joints to exercise.
    c. The joint is moved past the point of pain.
    d. The joint is moved slowly, smoothly, and gently.

111. Which statement about ambulation is *false?*
    a. A transfer belt is used if the person is weak or unsteady.
    b. The person is allowed to shuffle or slide when walking after bedrest.
    c. Walking aids may be needed permanently or temporarily.
    d. Crutches, canes, walkers, and braces are common walking aids.

112. Pain that is felt in a part of the body that is no longer there is:
    a. Acute pain.
    b. Phantom pain.
    c. Radiating pain.
    d. Chronic pain.

113. Mr. Smith has difficulty sleeping, and he awakens several times during the night. He has difficulty answering your questions and seems moody. His pulse is irregular and his eyes are red and puffy. He is showing signs of:
    a. Insomnia.
    b. Sleep deprivation.
    c. Enuresis.
    d. Distraction.

114. You are admitting Mrs. Dillan. While you are taking her vital signs, she complains of severe abdominal pain. You should:
    a. Call the doctor.
    b. Finish the admissions process. Then report Mrs. Dillan's complaint of pain to the nurse.
    c. Call the nurse immediately.
    d. Tell Mrs. Dillan not to worry because her doctor will see her soon.

115. You are preparing Mrs. Cliff for a physical examination. Which is *incorrect?*
    a. You need to be sensitive to her feelings.
    b. She urinates before the examination.
    c. Reassure her by telling her that there is no exposure during the examination.
    d. Screen her and close the door to the room.

116. Which statement about positioning the person after surgery is *incorrect?*
    a. Stress on the incision is prevented.
    b. Turn the person with smooth, gentle motions.
    c. Repositioning every 4 hours helps prevent respiratory complications.
    d. Pillows and other positioning devices are often used.

117. You can assist in Mr. Long's psychological preparation by explaining:
    a. The reason for the surgery.
    b. The procedures you are doing.
    c. The risks and possible complications of surgery.
    d. What to expect during the preoperative and postoperative periods.

118. A laceration is:
    a. A closed wound caused by a blow to the body.
    b. A partial-thickness wound caused by the scraping away of skin.
    c. An open wound with torn tissue and jagged edges.
    d. The collection of blood under the skin and tissue.

119. Which drainage is green, yellow, or brown?
    a. Serous drainage
    b. Sanguineous drainage
    c. Serosanguineous drainage
    d. Purulent drainage

120. A wound appears red and swollen. The area around it is warm to the touch. These are signs of:
    a. The inflammatory phase of wound healing.
    b. The proliferative phase of wound healing.
    c. Healing by primary intention.
    d. Healing by secondary intention.

121. Heat applications are used for all of the following *except* to:
    a. Relieve pain.
    b. Control bleeding.
    c. Relax muscles.
    c. Decrease joint stiffness.

122. These statements are about moist heat applications. Which is *false?*
    a. Water is in contact with the skin.
    b. The effects of moist heat are less than those of a dry heat application.
    c. Moist heat penetrates deeper than dry heat.
    d. The temperature of a moist heat application is lower than a dry heat application.

123. The lack or absence of breathing is:
    a. Dyspnea.
    b. Apnea.
    c. Hypoxia.
    d. Orthopnea.

124. The worst way to manage stress is to:
    a. deny it
    b. adapt to it
    c. modify it
    d. avoid it

125. You prevent pressure ulcers by:
    a. Providing good skin care.
    b. Turning and repositioning the person as directed.
    c. Performing range-of-motion exercises as directed.
    d. All of the above.

126. You are caring for Mr. Clark. You are feeling frustrated by his slow progress. You should:
    a. Tell him that you are frustrated.
    b. Be firm. Tell him that he must work harder.
    c. Discuss your feelings with the nurse.
    d. Ask a co-worker to care for Mr. Clark.

127. Which statement is *false?*
    a. Sympathy and pity help the person adjust to the disability.
    b. You should know how to apply self-care devices.
    c. You should know how to use equipment used in the person's care.
    d An attitude of hopefulness must be conveyed to the person.

128. Cataract is an eye disorder in which:
    a. The optic nerve is damaged.
    b. Pressure within the eye is increased.
    c. The lens becomes cloudy.
    d. Severe eye pain is common.

129. Mrs. Linn has had a stroke. Which is incorrect?
    a. Rehabilitation starts about 1 week after the stroke.
    b. Give emotional support and encouragement.
    c. Give good skin care.
    d. Encourage coughing and deep breathing.

130. Which statement about multiple sclerosis is *correct?*
    a. The onset is sudden.
    b. Symptoms usually start after age 60.
    c. Men are affected more than women.
    d. Blurred vision and double vision occur first.

131. Vomiting is dangerous because of the possibility of:
    a. Aspiration.
    b. Cardiac arrest.
    c. Fluid retention.
    d. Stroke.

132. These statements are about HIV and AIDS. Which is *false?*
    a. Standard precautions are practiced and the Bloodborne Pathogen Standard is followed.
    b. There may be signs and symptoms of central nervous system damage.
    c. The person is at risk for infection.
    d. The person always shows some signs and symptoms.

133. The set of attitudes, values, behaviors, and traits of a particular person is:
    a. Phobia.
    b. Personality.
    c. Affect.
    d. Id.

134. The most common type of dementia is:
    a. Multi-infarct dementia.
    b. Alzheimer's disease.
    c. Stroke.
    d. Syphilis.

135. Sundowning means that:
    a. The person becomes sleepy when the sun sets.
    b. Behaviors become worse in the late afternoon and evening hours.
    c. Behavior improves at night.
    d. The person is in the third stage of the disease.

136. Spastic means:
    a. The person is mentally retarded.
    b. Continuous writhing motions of the trunk, arms, and legs.
    c. Uncontrolled contractions of the skeletal muscles.
    d. Paralysis of both arms and legs.

137. MSDS stands for:
    a. metals and solvents data sheet
    b. material safety data sheet
    c. medical survey data sheet
    d. none of the above

138. Sexual activity:
    a. Always involves intercourse.
    b Is not allowed in nursing centers.
    c. Involves handholding, touching, and embracing.
    d. Is unhealthy for older persons.

139. Mr. Cole is masturbating in the dining room. You should do all the following *except:*
    a. Cover him and take him quietly to his room.
    b. Scold him for his bad behavior.
    c. Provide privacy and protect his rights.
    d. Report the behavior to the nurse.

140. A pinkish brown vaginal drainage that lasts for about 10 days after birth is called:
    a. Lochia serosa.
    b. Cesarean.
    c. Lochia rubra.
    d. Lochia alba.

141. Zach's cord has not yet healed. His diaper should be:
    a. Loose over the cord.
    b. Snug over the cord.
    c. Below the cord.
    d. Disposable.

142. When providing emergency care, which is *incorrect?*
    a. Know your limits. Do not do more than you are able.
    b. Call for help.
    c. Move the person to a more comfortable place.
    d. Keep the person warm.

143. Which of these steps would *not* be helpful in caring for a confused patient?
    a. call the person by name each time you have contact with him/her
    b. keep clocks and calendars in the person's room
    c. maintain a daily routine of activities
    d. prior to beginning care, describe your plan for the entire shift

144. Care of the dying person includes all of the following *except:*
    a. Providing frequent oral hygiene.
    b. Providing good skin care.
    c. Positioning the person in good body alignment.
    d. Active and passive range-of-motion exercises.

145. Shortened forms of words or phrases are:
    a. Suffixes.
    b. Word elements.
    c. Abbreviations.
    d. Medical terms.

FINAL EXAMINATION — VERSION 2

True or False

---

*Mark **T** for true. Mark **F** for false.*

1. _____ Rehabilitation helps persons return to their highest level of physical and psychological functioning.

2. _____ Support workers supervise other support workers.

3. _____ Lying on a job application is illegal.

4. _____ When answering the phone in a patient's home, simply answer with "hello".

5. _____ Patients have the right to refuse treatment.

6. _____ The ball-and-socket joint allows movement in all directions.

7. _____ Male sex cells are called sperm.

8. _____ Development relates to physical changes that are measured and occur in a steady and orderly manner.

9. _____ Incontinence is normal for clients over 80 years of age.

10. _____ Bed rails are safe for patients trying to get out of bed without help.

11. _____ If you feel threatened in a person's home, you should leave and call your supervisor.

12. _____ The person is called by name to accurately identify the person before giving care.

13. _____ To properly wash your hands, hold your hands and forearms higher than your elbows throughout the procedure.

14. _____ Using a lift sheet to move a person up in bed reduces shearing and friction.

15. _____ Base of support is the area on which an object rests.

16. _____ Persons with spinal cord injuries are logrolled.

17. _____ Mr. Jones hoards food in the drawer of his bedside stand. You must wait until he leaves the room and remove the food.

18. _____ When removing dirty linens, roll the linens toward you.

19. _____ Wash your hands before handling clean linens and after handling dirty linens.

20. _____ Hot water is used for cleaning dentures.

21. _____ Pressure ulcers usually occur over bony areas.

22. _____ You never trim or shave a beard or moustache without the person's consent.

23. _____ Clothing is removed from the person's strong side first.

24. _____ Catheters treat the cause of urinary incontinence.

25. _____ Adhesive tape is used to secure condom catheters.

26. _____ The person is positioned in the right side-lying position for a cleansing enema.

27. _____ When preparing meats, roasting, broiling, and baking are better than frying.

28. _____ Support workers are responsible for IV therapy.

29. _____ Axillary temperatures are more reliable than oral temperatures.

30. _____ Respirations are counted right after taking a pulse. The person should be unaware that you are counting respirations.

31. _____ If a person starts to fall, ease him or her to the floor.

32. _____ Acute pain is felt suddenly and generally lasts less than 6 months.

33. _____ Changes in a person's usual environment can affect the amount and quality of sleep.

34. _____ The person will feel safer and more secure if you explain what you are doing and why.

35. _____ A robe and slippers are worn when the person is weighed and measured.

36. _____ Usually all clothes are removed for a complete physical examination.

37. _____ Support workers are responsible for obtaining the person's written consent for surgery.

38. _____ Proper positioning helps prevent postoperative complications.

39. _____ Wound care involves preventing infection and preventing further injury.

40. _____ Incorrect application of binders can cause severe discomfort, skin irritation, and circulatory and respiratory problems.

41. _____ Dirty linen can be placed on the floor to avoid contact with clean linen.

42. _____ Moist cold applications penetrate deeper than dry ones.

43. _____ Altered function of any system affects the body's ability to meet its oxygen needs.

44. _____ Persons with breathing difficulties often prefer to sit up in bed and lean forward.

45. _____ Rehabilitation focuses on the person's disabilities.

46. _____ Hearing loss may cause speech problems.

47. _____ Surgery is the only treatment for cataracts.

48. _____ A malignant tumor grows slowly and does not invade healthy tissue.

49. _____ Traction is removed when making the person's bed.

50. _____ Unmet needs at any age affect personality development.

51. _____ Panic is the highest level of anxiety.

52. _____ Acute confusion is usually permanent.

53. _____ Persons with Alzheimer's disease choose to be agitated and rude.

54. _____ Developmental disabilities are always severe. Persons need constant support.

55. _____   Sexuality is not important for older persons.

56. _____   Do not leave a baby unattended on a table, bed, sofa, high chair, or other high surface.

57. _____   A vaginal discharge during the post-partum period is a sign of infection.

58. _____   Basic life support procedures support breathing and circulation.

59. _____   Choking can lead to cardiac arrest.

60. _____   Internal bleeding is easily controlled by applying direct pressure to the bleeding site.

61. _____   Attitudes about death are closely related to culture and religion.

62. _____   The right to privacy and the right to be treated with dignity and respect apply after death.

63. _____   The root contains the basic meaning of the word.

Multiple Choice

Circle the BEST answer.

64. A health care agency or program for persons who are dying is:
    a. Case management.
    b. Hospice.
    c. Managed care.
    d. A preferred provider organization.

65. The goal of the health team is to:
    a. Provide quality care.
    b. Make money.
    c. Provide case management.
    d. Assign tasks and responsibilities.

66. If a fire occurs which of these steps should be done first?
    a. use a fire extinguisher to put out the fire
    b. close all doors and windows
    c. sound the nearest fire alarm
    d. move persons who are in danger to a safe place

67. A person is tied in a chair to prevent the person from wandering. This is called:
    a. Slander.
    b. False imprisonment.
    c. Assault.
    d. Verbal abuse.

68. The best behaviour of a support worker when feeding a resident is:
    a. telling a resident the value of each type of food.
    b. appearing patient and calm.
    c. feeding one kind of food before starting another.
    d. talking about her family without knowing if they visit.

69. The stiffness or rigidity of skeletal muscles that occurs after death is called:
    a. Rigor mortis.
    b. Postmortem.
    c. Peristalsis.
    d. DNR.

70. The intentional attempt or threat to touch a person's body without the person's consent is:
    a. Assault.
    b. Battery.
    c. Defamation.
    d. False imprisonment.

71. You are ill and cannot come to work. Which is correct?
    a. Call a co-worker to report your illness.
    b. Do not call anyone. You are sick and need your rest.
    c. Call your supervisor.
    d. Call the administrator.

72. You are on your meal break. Which is *false?*
    a. You can make personal phone calls.
    b. Family members can meet you.
    c. You can take a few extra minutes if necessary.
    d. The RN needs to know that you are off the unit.

73. Which is *incorrect* when recording on a patient's or resident's chart?
    a. Communicate clearly and concisely.
    b. Use a pencil in case you make a mistake.
    c. Record in a logical manner.
    d. Record only what you observed and did yourself.

74. Which is a symptom?
    a. Redness
    b. Vomiting
    c. Pain
    d. Pulse rate of 78

75. These statements are about recording. Which is *false?*
    a. Use the person's exact words when possible.
    b. Record only what you observed and did yourself.
    c. Do not skip lines.
    d. To save time, chart a procedure before it is completed.

76. The values and beliefs of a group passed from one generation to the next is:
    a. Self-actualization.
    b. Religion.
    c. Culture.
    d. Holism.

77. Which is *false?*
    a. A person's culture influences health and illness practices.
    b. Culture and religion influence food practices.
    c. A person's religious and cultural practices are not allowed in the health care agency.
    d. A person may not follow all of the beliefs and practices of his or her religion or culture.

78. The basic unit of body structure is:
    a. An organ.
    b. A cell.
    c. Tissue.
    d. Mitosis.

79. The substance in red blood cells that carries oxygen and gives blood its color is:
    a. Protoplasm.
    b. Plasma.
    c. Hemoglobin.
    d. Leukocytes.

80. Besides hearing, the ear is involved with:
    a. Regulating body movements.
    b. Balance.

c. Smoothness of body movements.
d. Controlling involuntary muscles.

81. Newborns have certain reflexes. Which reflex is necessary for feeding? (It guides the baby's mouth to the nipple.)
    a. Sucking reflex
    b. Rooting reflex
    c. Startle reflex
    d. Grasping reflex

82. Reproductive organs begin to function and secondary sex characteristics appear during:
    a. Late childhood.
    b. Preadolescence.
    c. Puberty.
    d. Early adulthood.

83. A resident refuses a bath. You must:
    a. Call the resident's family.
    b. Get help and give the bath.
    c. Report the refusal to the nurse.
    d. Change the resident's care plan.

84. Death of a partner results in the loss of a:
    a. Friend.
    b. Lover.
    c. Companion.
    d. All of the above.

85. Who decides how to style a resident's hair?
    a. The resident
    b. The nurse
    c. The support worker
    d. The family

86. Paralysis on one side of the body is called:
    a. Hemiplegia.
    b. Paraplegia.
    c. Coma.
    d. Quadriplegia.

87. A restraint attached to the person's body and a stationary object is a(an):
    a. Chemical restraint.
    b. Passive physical restraint.
    c. Active physical restraint.
    d. Full bed rail.

88. You are caring for an infant and young children. Which measure is unsafe?
    a. Checking children in cribs often
    b. Keeping one hand on a child in a crib if you need to look away

c. Propping a baby bottle on a rolled towel or blanket

d. Keeping plastic bags away from children

89. An infection acquired after admission to a health care agency is a:
    a. Communicable disease.
    b. Nosocomial infection.
    c. Nonpathogen.
    d. Hepatitis infection.

90. Masks prevent the spread of microbes from:
    a. The gastrointestinal tract.
    b. The skin.
    c. The respiratory tract.
    d. All of the above.

91. When cleaning equipment, do all of the following *except:*
    a. Rinse the item in cold water before cleaning.
    b. Wash the item with soap and hot water.
    c. Use a brush if necessary.
    d. Clean from the dirtiest area to the cleanest.

92. The back-lying position is the:
    a. Sims' position.
    b. Semi-Fowler's position.
    c. Dorsal recumbent position.
    d. Prone position.

93. To provide full visual privacy for persons, you must:
    a. Provide care with the room door open.
    b. Pull the curtain around the bed only if the person has a roommate.
    c. Pull the curtain around the bed only if the person asks you to.
    d. Always pull the curtain completely around the person's bed when care is given.

94. Which does *not* prevent or reduce odors?
    a. Placing fresh flowers in the room
    b. Emptying bedpans promptly
    c. Using room deodorizers
    d. Practicing good personal hygiene

95. The type of bed used for a person arriving on a stretcher is:
    a. A closed bed.
    b. A surgical bed.
    c. An open bed.
    d. An occupied bed.

96. Good oral hygiene:
    a. Prevents mouth odor and infection.
    b. Is only done once a day.
    c. Is not important for unconscious persons.
    d. Allows buildup of tartar and plaque.

97. Hair loss is:
    a. Hirsutism.
    b. Pediculosis.
    c. Alopecia.
    d. Decubitus.

98. Which of the following statements about foot care is *incorrect?*
    a. Feet are easily infected and injured.
    b. Assistive personnel use scissors to cut toenails.
    c. Dirty feet and socks harbor microbes.
    d. Cleaning toenails is easier after soaking.

99. Mrs. Andrews has an indwelling catheter. Which is *incorrect?*
    a. Attach the drainage bag to the bed rail.
    b. She should not lie on the tubing.
    c. Keep the drainage bag below the bladder.
    d. Provide perineal care daily and after bowel movements.

100. You are instructed to strain Mr. Powers' urine. You know that straining urine is done to find:
    a. Hematuria.
    b. Stones.
    c. Nocturia.
    d. Urgency.

101. Mrs. Harvey complains of abdominal discomfort. Watery stool has been leaking from her rectum. This is probably:
    a. Diarrhea.
    b. Anal incontinence.
    c. A fecal impaction.
    d. Constipation.

102. You note a black, tarry stool. This is called:
    a. Melena.
    b. Feces.
    c. Hemostool.
    d. Occult blood.

103. The breathing of fluid or an object into the lungs is:
    a. Gavage.
    b. Aspiration.
    c. Dysphagia.
    d. Regurgitation.

104. Which vegetable is not allowed on a 1000 mg sodium diet?
    a. Steamed carrots
    b. Steamed broccoli
    c. Sauerkraut
    d. Lettuce

105. Fats, oils, and sweets:
    a. Should be used in moderate amounts.
    b. Are low in calories.
    c. Should be used sparingly.
    d. Have great nutritional value.

106. A person is bleeding from an IV site. You should:
    a. Remove the IV catheter or needle.
    b. Apply direct pressure.
    c. Call for the RN immediately.
    d. Apply a dressing to the site.

107. A person with a persistent blood pressure measurement above 140/90 has:
    a. Tachycardia.
    b. Hypertension.
    c. Hypotension.
    d. Anxiety.

108. When taking a blood pressure, you should do all of the following *except:*
    a. Take the blood pressure in the arm with an IV infusion.
    b. Apply the cuff to a bare upper arm.
    c. Turn off the television and radio.
    d. Locate the brachial artery.

109. Muscle atrophy is:
    a. The abnormal shortening of a muscle.
    b. Bending backward.
    c. A decrease in the size or a wasting away of the muscle tissue.
    d. Excessive straightening of a body part.

110. Mr. Brown has an ankle brace. You notice a reddened area on the ankle bone when you remove the brace. You should:
    a. Put a bandage on the reddened area.
    b. Massage the reddened area.
    c. Report your observation to the nurse.
    d. Do all of the above.

111. Passive range-of-motion exercises are performed by:
    a. The person.
    b. A health team member.
    c. The person with the assistance of another.
    d. The person with the use of a trapeze.

112. Which of the following is *not* a measure used to promote sleep?
    a. Drinking alcoholic beverages at bedtime
    b. Following bedtime rituals
    c. Eating a bedtime snack
    d. Reducing noise

113. These statements are about sleep. Which is *false?*
    a. Tissue healing and repair occur during sleep.
    b. Voluntary muscle activity increases during sleep.
    c. Sleep refreshes and renews the person.
    d. Ill and injured persons need more sleep than healthy persons do.

114. A person with dementia is being admitted to a long-term care facility. Which statement is correct?
    a. Family members are asked to leave to help the person adjust.
    b. The admission process is completed as quickly as possible.
    c. The person's confusion may increase in new surroundings.
    d. All of the above.

115. Mr. Lopez is confused. He resists your efforts to prepare him for a physical examination. Which is *incorrect?*
    a. The examination may need to be tried at another time.
    b. He is restrained if necessary.
    c. Having a family member present may help calm him.
    d. His rights are respected.

116. You prepare the room for the person's return from the recovery room by:
    a. Making a closed bed.
    b. Placing equipment and supplies in the room.
    c. Lowering the bed to the lowest position.
    d. Raising the bed rails.

117. Mr. Long's preoperative medication was given. He:
    a. Must remain in bed.
    b. Is allowed to smoke with supervision.
    c. Can use the commode to void.
    d. Is allowed only sips of water.

118. An open wound on the lower legs and feet caused by poor return blood flow from veins is called:
    a. A stasis ulcer.
    b. An arterial ulcer.
    c. A pressure ulcer.
    d. A thrombus.

119. You are changing a nonsterile dressing. Before you begin:
    a. Review the procedure with the nurse.
    b. Allow pain medications time to take effect.
    c. Collect all needed equipment and supplies.
    d. Do all of the above.

120. The skin and underlying tissues are pierced. This is:
    a. A penetrating wound.
    b. An incision.
    c. A contusion.
    d. An abrasion.

121. Hypothermia is a:
    a. Very low body temperature.
    b. Bluish discoloration of the skin.
    c. Very high body temperature.
    d. Moist cold application.

122. These statements are about sitz baths. Which is *false?*
    a. The pelvic area is immersed in warm or hot water for 20 minutes.
    b. The sitz bath lasts 25 to 30 minutes.
    c. They clean the perineum, relieve pain, increase circulation, and stimulate voiding.
    d. Weakness or fainting can occur.

123. Which measure does not promote oxygenation?
    a. Positioning the person in the semi-Fowler's position
    b. Coughing and deep breathing exercises
    c. Having the person use an incentive spirometer
    d. Allowing the person to rest in the same position for 4 hours

124. Hypoxia is:
    a. A deficiency of oxygen in the blood.
    b. The amount of hemoglobin that contains oxygen.
    c. A deficiency of oxygen in the cells.
    d. The lack of carbon dioxide.

125. Rehabilitation begins when the person:
    a. Leaves the hospital.
    b. Enters a subacute rehabilitation program.
    c. Seeks health care.
    d. Goes home with home health care.

126. Mr. Juarez does not feel that he is making progress. He is angry. You should:
    a. Tell him that being angry will only make things worse.
    b. Try to understand his feelings. Offer support.
    c. Offer sympathy.
    d. Call his doctor.

127. Mr. Olson's rehabilitation begins with preventing:
    a. Angry feelings.
    b. Contractures and pressure ulcers.
    c. Illness and injury.
    d. Loss of self-esteem.

128. To communicate with the speech-impaired person, you should:
    a. Listen and give the person your full attention.
    b. Ask the person to repeat or rephrase, if necessary.
    c. Watch the person's lips move.
    d. Do all of the above.

129. Which is *incorrect* when caring for a person with a hip fracture.
    a. Give good skin care.
    b. Prevent external rotation of the hip.
    c. Perform range-of-motion exercises as directed.
    d. Keep the operated leg adducted at all times.

130. The HIV virus is spread by:
    a. Sneezing.
    b. Insects.
    c. Unprotected oral sex.
    d. Holding hands.

131. A person has angina pectoris. Which is true?
    a. Damage to the heart muscle occurs.
    b. The pain is described as crushing, stabbing, or squeezing.
    c. The pain is relieved with rest and nitroglycerin.
    d. All of the above.

132. A person has cystitis. This is:
    a. A kidney infection.
    b. Kidney stones.
    c. A urinary tract infection.
    d. An inflammation of the bladder.

133. Mr. Jansen is 75 years old. His daughter notices that he is agitated, has poor grooming, complains of not sleeping and feeling tired all the time. These are signs and symptoms of:
    a. Aging.
    b. A phobia.
    c. Abusive personality.
    d. Depression.

134. Agitated and restless behavior may be the result of:
    a. Pain or discomfort.
    b. Too much stimuli.
    c. Lack of sleep.
    d. All of the above.

135. Joe Dunn has dementia. Dementia describes:
    a. A false belief.
    b. An illness caused by changes in the brain.
    c. Seeing, hearing, or feeling something that is not real.
    d. Alzheimer's disease.

136. A congenital defect of the spinal column is:
    a. A convulsion.
    b. Spina bifida.
    c. Hydrocephalus.
    d. Paralysis.

137. The person with epilepsy has:
    a. Seizures.
    b. Diplegia.
    c. Athetoid.
    d. Spastic movements.

138. You promote sexuality by:
    a. Helping a patient apply make up.
    b. Draping and screening the person appropriately.
    c. Allowing privacy for masturbation.
    d. All of the above.

139. Mr. Dawson is being sexually aggressive. The behavior may be:
    a. An attempt to prove he is still attractive and able to perform sexually.
    b. Due to confusion and disorientation.
    c. Done on purpose.
    d. All of the above.

140. Which action is correct when bottle-feeding the baby?
    a. Hold the baby close to you and relax.
    b. Prop the bottle and lay the baby down.
    c. Leave the baby alone with the bottle.
    d. Burp the baby every 10 minutes.

141. Zach is a 2-month-old infant. Which is *false?*
    a. Zach's crib should be within hearing distance of caregivers.
    b. Zach should have a pillow for sleep.
    c. Zach should be positioned on his back for sleep.
    d. Crib rails should be up at all times.

142. Emergency care of burns includes all of the following *except:*
    a. Removing the person from the fire or burn source.
    b. Leaving the burns open to the air.
    c. Removing hot clothing that is not sticking to the skin.
    d. Providing basic life support as needed.

143. How many breaths are given at the beginning of CPR?
    a. 1
    b. 2
    c. 3
    d. 4

144. The person's written statement about the use of life-sustaining measures is called:
    a. A durable power of attorney.
    b. A "do not resuscitate" order.
    c. A living will.
    d. Hospice care.

145. The prefix "ab" means:
    a. Toward.
    b. Against.
    c. Double.
    d. Away from.

Chapter 1

1. c
2. e
3. s
4. r
5. a
6. f
7. n
8. j
9. o
10. b
11. h
12. m
13. d
14. g
15. l
16. q
17. i
18. t
19. p
20. k

Chapter 2

1. a. Personal care
   b. Assistance with activities of daily living
   c. Assistance with home management
2. Strategies that improve or maintain health and independence
3. Strategies that prevent the occurrence of disease or injury
4. *(Any six of the following answers in any order.)*
   a. Income
   b. Social status
   c. Social support networks

d. Education
e. Employment
f. Working conditions
g. Environment
h. Personal health practices
i. Coping skills

Chapter 3

1. *(Any 5 of the following.)*
   a. Hospital
   b. Acute care
   c. Community day programs
   d. Long-term care facilities
   e. Assisted living facilities
   f. Retirement residences
   g. Community nursing agencies
2. *(In any order.)*
   Acute care
   a. Intended to diagnose an immediate health issue
   b. Intended to treat an immediate health issue
   c. Appears suddenly
   d. Lasts a short time
   e. Symptoms can be severe
   Chronic care
   a. On going condition
   b. Slow or gradual onset
   c. Grows worse over time
   d. Sometimes can be controlled
   e. Complications can sometimes be prevented
3. *(Any two for each setting.)*
   Community day programs
   a. Working closely with a team or supervisor
   b. Working in a structured environment
   c. Must be very organized
   d. Meeting multiple needs

For Clients

a.Terms of employment

b. Establishing work limits

Facility

a. Structured environment

b. Meeting multiple needs and demands

c. Doing many tasks in a short periods of time

d. respecting your scope of practice

e. Working shifts

(Students may identify specific issues for hospitals or facilities.)

Chapter 4

1. c
2. d
3. a
4. e
5. b
6. *(Any 8 of the following answers in any order.)*
   a. Nature of illness or condition
   b. Person's age
   c. Person's level of physical fitness
   d. Amount and degree of pain and discomfort the person experience
   e. The prognosis
   f. Person's emotional, social, intellectual, and spiritual health
   g. Person's personality and ability to cope with difficulties
   h. Person's culture
   i. Presence of emotional, social, and financial support

Chapter 5

1. A function, procedure, or activity that you assist with or perform for the client
2. A process by which an RN authorizes another health care provider to perform certain tasks; transfer or function
3. A meeting attended by the health care team and family members to discuss a client's care
4. A list of the tasks you are to do for each client
5. A team of health care providers and specialists who work together for the benefit of the client

(Answers for 6 to 14 may be in any order.)

6. The task is beyond the legal limits of your role.
7. The task is not in your job description.
8. You are not prepared to perform the task safely.
9. The task could harm the person.
10. The person's condition has changed.
11. You do not know how to use supplies or equipment.
12. Directions are unethical, illegal, or against policy.
13. Directions are unclear or incomplete.
14. The nurse is not available for supervision.

Chapter 6

1. Showing acceptance and regard for another person
2. The connection between two or more people
3. A person who assumes responsibilities for an ill or disabled person in the home
4. being open to and trying to understand the experiences and feelings of others
5. Caring about another person's misfortune and suffering
6. *(Any 3 of the following.)*
   a. Oxygen
   b. Water
   c. Food
   d. Elimination
   e. Rest
   f. Shelter
7. *(Any 3 of the following.)*
   a. Protection from harm
   b. Protection from danger
   c. Protection from fear
   d. Protection from pain
8. *(Any 3 of the following.)*
   a. Romantic love
   b. Physical desire
   c. Need to belong to a group
   d. Need to belong to a family
   e. Need to have personal belongings
   f. Need to have contact with other people
9. *(Any 2 of the following.)*
   a. Offering encouragement
   b. Praise the person's successes
   c. Recognize efforts
   d. Provide the person with honest, constructive feedback

Chapter 7

1. a
2. f
3. g
4. d
5. c
6. e
7. b
8. S
9. S
10. O
11. S
12. O

13. O
14. O
15. S
16. S
17. O

Chapter 8

1. Consult your supervisor when:
   (Any 5 of the following.)
   a. There is an emergency
   b. You observe a change in the client's condition or normal functioning
   c. The client becomes ill
   d. The client is in distress
   e. You believe the client's safety is at risk
   f. A problem arises involving medications
   g. The client complains about their condition or care
   h. The client asks you a question about diagnosis, condition or treatment plans
   i. The client or family member asks you to do something that contradicts the care plan
   j. You have a conflict with a client or family member
   k. A question or problem arises with which you need help

2. SMART:
   a. **S**pecific
   b. **M**easurable
   c. **A**chievable
   d. **R**ealistic
   e. **T**imely

3. *(Any 3 of the following.)*
   a. Is the situation or issue affecting you, a co worker, your supervisor, or one of your clients?
   b. Should you be concerned about the situation?
   c. Can you influence or contribute to a positive outcome?
   d. Does the issue require immediate attention?

Chapter 9

1. a. Autonomy
   b. Justice
   c. Beneficence
   d. Nonmalefience
2. *(Any 5 of the following.)*
   a. Provide high quality personal care and support services
   b. Provide compassionate care to all clients
   c. Value the dignity and value of all clients

   d. Respect their client's choice about how they receive or participate in care
   e. Respect their client's right to privacy and confidentiality
   f. Do not misuse their position of trust
   g. Are reliable
   h. Promote and maintain their client's safety
3. *(Any 4 of the following.)*
   a. Being concerned for all clients
   b. Do not betray their trust
   c. Respect their privacy
   d. Perform you services competently and skillfully
   e. Keep information confidential
   f. Do not snoop in the person's home
   g. Do not gossip with your friends or co workers
   h. Never speak about a client where others may overhear you
   i. Do not pry into the person's private life

Chapter 10

1. a. The right to be treated with dignity and respect
   b. The right to privacy and confidentiality
   c. The right to give or withhold informed consent
   d. The right to autonomy
2. a. Adult Care Regulations
   b. Community Care Facility Act
3. *(Any 4 of the following.)*
   a. Knock on the person's door
   b. Ask others to leave the room before giving care
   c. Close the door and use curtains or screens
   d. Drape properly during personal care
   e. Keep the person covered when moving through the facility
   f. Close the bathroom door when the person is using the bathroom
   g. Do not open or read the person's mail
   h. Do not touch or examine the person's belongings without permission
   i. Allow the person to visit or telephone in private
   j. Do not pry into the persons' private life
   k. Keep information confidential
   l. Do not discuss a client with your family, friends, or the client's family
4. e
5. a
6. h
7. b
8. c
9. d
10. f
11. g

Chapter 11

1. Could be any combination from single parent families, stepparents, same sex couples, families with children or without children; could include any other family members such as grandparents, aunts, uncles, etc.
2. Always respect your client's cultural beliefs
3. *(Any 3 of the following.)*
   a. Language
   b. Values
   c. Beliefs
   d. Habits
   e. Way of life
   f. Rules of behaviour
   g. Traditions
4. groups of people who share similar features
5. the characteristics of a group of people
6. the area immediately around one's body
7. an verly simple or exaggerated impression of a person or a group of people
8. an attitude that judges a person based on his or her membership in a group
9. children, grandparents, grandchildren, aunts, uncles and cousins
10. behaviour that treats people unfairly based on their group membership

Chapter 12

1. a. Asking closed question
   b. Open ended question
   c. Active listening
   d. Using silence
2. c, a, d, e, b,
3. *(Any of the following.)*
   a. To exchange information
   b. To get to know another person
   c. To provide support or comfort to another
   (Students may identify many other functions.)
4. Exchange information
5. a. volume
   b. tone
   c. speed
   d. pitch
6. a. sender
   b. message
   c. receiver
   d. feedback

Chapter 13

1. a. Nucleus
   b. Cell membrane
   c. Cytoplasm

2. a. Epithelial tissue—covers internal and external body surfaces. Tissue that lines the nose, mouth, respiratory tract, stomach, and intestines is epithelial tissue. So are the skin, hair, nails, and glands.
   b. Connective tissue—anchors, connects, and supports other body tissues. Connective tissue is found in every part of the body.
   c. Muscle tissue—allows the body to move by stretching and contracting.
   d. Nerve tissue—receives and carries impulses to the brain and back to body parts.
3. organs; one or more functions
4. a. The integumentary system—the skin is the body's natural covering. The protective covering of the body.
   b. The musculoskeletal system—provides the framework for the body and allows the body to move. It protects and gives the body shape.
   c. The nervous system—controls, directs, and coordinates body functions.
   d. The circulatory system—made up of the blood, heart, and blood vessels. The blood carries food, oxygen, and other substances to cells and removes waste. It aids in the regulation of body temperature.
   e. The respiratory system—brings oxygen into the lungs and eliminates carbon dioxide.
   f. The digestive system—breaks down food, physically and chemically, so it can be absorbed for use by the cells.
   g. The urinary system—removes waste products from the blood and maintains water balance within the body.
   h. The reproductive system—male and female reproductive systems are different. The difference allows for the process of reproduction. It produces male and female sex cells.
   i. The endocrine system—made up of glands that secrete hormones into the blood stream. Hormones regulate the activities of other organs and glands in the body.
   j. The immune system—protects the body from disease and infection.

Chapter 14

(Answers can be in any order.)
1. Growth and development occur from fertilization until death.
2. The process proceeds from simple to complex.
3. Growth and development occur in a certain direction.
4. Growth and development occur in a sequence, order, and pattern.

5. The rate of growth and development is uneven, not at a set pace.
6. Each stage has its own characteristics and developmental tasks.

Chapter 15

1. *(Any 3 for each setting.)*
Integumentary system
a. Less elastic
b. Losses strength
c. Brown spots
d. Fewer nerve endings and blood vessels
e. Fatty tissue layer is lost
f. Skin thins and sags
g. Dry skin
h. Itching
i. Nails thicken
Nervous system
a. Vision, hearing, taste, smell and touch decrease
b. Reduce sensitivity to pain
c. Reduce blood flow to brain
d. Cell shrinkage
e. Shorter memory, forgetfulness
f. Slower ability to respond
g. Changers in sleep pattern
h. dizziness
Respiratory system
a. Respiratory muscles weakens
b. Lung tissue becomes less elastic
c. Difficulty breathing
d. Decreased strength for coughing
(Any others listed on page 164 of textbook.)
2. a. Respect your client's clothing and grooming preferences
b. Accept the client's sexual relationships
c. Allow privacy
3. a. Young old 60-74
b. Middle old 75-84
c. Old-old over 85
4. Sex is the physical activities involving the reproductive organs. The activities are done for pleasure or to produce children. Sexuality involves the personality and the body. A person's attitudes and feelings are involved. It affects how a person behaves, thinks, dresses, and responds to others.

Chapter 16

(Answers within each number can be in any order.)
1. a. Low blood pressure when standing or sitting
b. Drowsiness
c. Fainting
d. Dizziness
e. Poor muscle coordination

f. Unsteadiness
g. Frequent urination
h. Confusion and disorientation
i. Visual impairment
(Any 5 of the following.)
2. a. Smoking in bed
b. Spilling hot liquids
c. Children playing with matches
d. Charcoal grills
e. Fireplaces
f. Stoves
3. a. Choking on an object
b. Drowning
c. Inhaling gas or smoke
d. Strangulation
e. Electrical shock
4. a. "No Smoking" signs are placed on the person's door and near the bed.
b. Patients, residents, and visitors are reminded not to smoke in the person's room.
c. Smoking materials are removed from the room.
d. Electrical equipment is turned off before it is unplugged.
e. Wool blankets and synthetic fibers that cause static electricity are removed from the person's room.
f. Electrical equipment is removed from the person's room.
g. Candles and incense are not used in the person's room.
h. Materials that ignite easily are removed from the person's room.

Chapter 17

1. *(Any 6 of the following.)*
a. Bowel problems
b. Bladder problems
c. Cognitive decline
d. Cuts and bruises
e. Dehydration
f. Emotional harm
g. Fractures
h. Infections
i. Joint problems
j. Nerve injuries
k. Pressure ulcers
l. Strangulation
2. a. Never used to discipline a person
b. Never used to punish or penalize a person
c. Never used for staff convenience
3. *(Any 10 of the following.)*
a. Use the restraint noted in the care plan
b. Follow employer policies and procedures
c. Use restraint only after being instructed about

its proper use

d. Use the correct size

e. Use only restraints that have manufacturer instructions and warning label

f. Read the warning labels

g. Follow the manufacturer's instructions

h. Do not use sheets, towels or other items to restrain

i. Use intact restraints

j. Do not use to position client on toilet

k. Do not use to position on furniture that does not allow for correct application

l. Position client in good alignment

m. Pad bony areas

n. Secure the restraint

o. Crisscross vest restraints in front

p. Tie according to employer policy

q. Secure straps out of client's reach

r. Secure to movable part of the bed frame at waist level

s. Never secure to bed rails

t. Keep bed rails up

u. Use a belt restraint with chairs or wheelchairs

v. Do not use back cushions

w. Use bed rails only if on care plan

x. Check circulation every 15 minutes if mitt, wrist or ankle restraint used

y. Check the client every 15 minutes if restrained

z. If client in supine position monitored constantly

aa. Do not use restraint near a fire, flame or smoking materials

4. b
5. e
6. f
7. c
8. g
9. a
10. d

Chapter 18

(Answers can be listed in any order.)

1. a. Fever
   b. Increased pulse and respiratory rates
   c. Pain or tenderness
   d. Fatigue and loss of energy
   e. Loss of appetite
   f. Nausea
   g. Vomiting
   h. Diarrhea
   i. Rash
   j. Sores on mucous membranes
   k. Redness or swelling
   l. Discharge or drainage

2. a. Exposure incident—any eye, mouth, other mucous membrane, nonintact skin, or parenteral contact with blood or other potentially infectious materials.
   b. Parenteral—piercing the mucous membrane or skin barrier.
   c. Source individual—any person whose blood or other potentially infectious material may be a source of an occupational exposure to employees.

Chapter 19

1. Physical abuse
2. Verbal abuse
3. Involuntary seclusion
4. Financial abuse
5. Mental abuse
6. Sexual abuse
7. Emotional neglect
8. Physical abuse
9. Sexual abuse
10. Rape
11. Molestation
12. Incest
13. Child pornography
14. Child prostitution
15. *(Any 5 of the following.)*
    a. Using restraints inappropriately
    b. Handling the client roughly
    c. Isolating the client in his/her room
    d. Not checking of the client for long periods of time
    e. Leaving the client in soiled linen or clothes
    f. Providing care against the client's wishes
    g. Failing to provide privacy
    h. Failing to keep information confidential
    (Students may identify many other examples and should be given credit for these.)

16. *(Any 4 of the following.)*
    a. Fear of the abuser
    b. Do not know where or how to get help
    c. Afraid they will be forced to move to a LTC facility
    d. May not be able to report because of physical or mental condition
    e. If the abuser is one of their children, they may be ashamed that their child could do this

Chapter 20

1. a. Admission—official entry of a person into an agency or nursing unit
   b. Discharge—official departure of a person from an agency or nursing unit

c. Transfer—moving a person from one room, nursing unit, or agency to another

2. a. Completing an admission checklist
   b. Weighing and measuring the person
   c. Obtaining a urine specimen if one is ordered
   d. Orienting the person to the room, nursing unit, and agency

(Answers can be in any order.)

3. a. Empty and clean bedpans, urinals, commodes, and kidney basins promptly
   b. Change soiled linens and clothing promptly
   c. Dispose of soiled linen and clothing
   d. Clean persons who are wet or soiled
   e. Dispose of incontinent products promptly
   f. Dispose of ostomy products promptly
   g. Keep soiled laundry containers closed
   h. Provide the person with good personal hygiene
   i. Use room deodorizers when necessary and if allowed

(Answers can be in any order.)

4. a. Comfort
   b. Sleep
   c. Elimination
   d. Nutrition
   e. Personal hygiene
   f. Activity
   g. Communication

(Answers can be in any order.)

5. a. Aching
   b. Burning
   c. Cramping
   d. Crushing
   e. Dull
   f. Gnawing
   g. Knifelike
   h. Piercing
   i. Pressure
   j. Sharp
   k. Sore
   l. Squeezing
   m. Stabbing
   n. Throbbing
   o. Viselike

(Answers can be in any order.)

6. a. Changes in speech
   b. Crying
   c. Gasping
   d. Grimacing
   e. Groaning
   f. Grunting
   g. Holding the affected part
   h. Irritability
   i. Maintaining one position
   j. Moaning
   k. Quietness
   l. Restlessness
   m. Rubbing
   n. Screaming

Chapter 21

1. i
2. g
3. d
4. j
5. c
6. b
7. h
8. a
9. f
10. e
11. Wide
12. Close
13. Face; twisting
14. Push; slide; pull
15. Hips; knees

Chapter 22

1. a. Flexion
   b. External rotation
   c. Supination
   d. Adduction
   e. Extension
   f. Pronation
   g. Dorsiflexion
   h. Internal rotation
   i. Hyperextension
   j. Abduction
   k. Rotation

2. a. Exercise only the joints that the nurse tells you to exercise.
   b. Expose only the body part being exercised.
   c. Use good body mechanics.
   d. Support the extremity being exercised.
   e. Move the joint slowly, smoothly, and gently.
   f. Do not force a joint beyond its present range-of-motion or to the point of pain
   g. Perform ROM to the neck only if allowed by agency policy.

Chapter 23

1. *(Any 6 of the following.)*
   a. Set priorities
   b. Set a routine
   c. Use your time well
   d. Finish tasks and put items away
   e. Set time limits for each task

f. Focus on the task

g. Put the client's needs first

2. *(Any 7 of the following.)*

   a. Read all labels carefully

   b. Never mix cleaning products

   c. Wear utility gloves

   d. Never use products in unlabelled containers

   e. Store products in their original containers

   f. Keep cleaning products away from food

   g. Keep cleaning products out of reach of children and adults with dementia

   h. Use products only for their intended purpose

   i. Keep aerosol cans away from heat source

   j. Ask the client before using a strong cleaner on a surface

   k. Rinse strong, abrasive cleaners immediately after use

   l. Do not scrub vigorously

3. *(Any 4 of the following.)*

   a. Wipe surfaces with cloth and hot, soapy water

   b. Rinse and dry

   c. Scrub with disinfectant and rinse with boiling water; if the surfaces were in contact with raw poultry, meat, fish or eggs, dry with paper towels

   d. Use baking soda to remove stubborn counter stains

   e. Wipe table with cloth and hot, soapy water

4. *(Any 4 of the following.)*

   a. Remove lint from the filter

   b. Do not overload the dryer

   c. Use cooler temperatures according to garment label

   d. Do not put woolens in the dryer, lay flat to dry on a towel

   e. Use a sheet of fabric softener (with permission of the client)

   f. Remove garments when dryer stops to prevent wrinkles

   g. Remove lint from the filter

Chapter 24

1. a. Mattress pad

   b. Bottom sheet

   c. Plastic drawsheet

   d. Cotton drawsheet

   e. Top sheet

   f. Blanket

   g. Bedspread

   h. Pillow cases

   i. Bath towels

   j. Hand towel

   k. Wash cloth

   l. Hospital gown

   m. Bath blanket

2. Dirty; away from

Chapter 25

1. i

2. a

3. d

4. b

5. e

6. c

7. j

8. g

9. f

10. h

(Answers can be in any order.)

11. a. Used to eating with family so had no interest in preparing meal for themselves

   b. Can't drive to grocery store

   c. Can't carry groceries

   d. No one to help buy groceries

   e. No one to help prepare meals

   f. Low income

   g. Poor appetite

   h. Poor vision makes food preparation difficult

   i. Oral problems

   j. medication side-effects

12. a. 180

   b. 90

   c. 60

   d. 240

   e. 150

   f. 120

   g. 300

Chapter 26

1. a. Through the nose to the stomach

   b. Through the nose to the small intestine

   c. Through an opening (stoma) into the stomach

2. *(Answers can be in any order.)*

   a. Cancer

   b. Trauma

   c. Coma

   d. Paralysis

   e. Dysphagia

   f. Dementia

   g. Surgery

   h. Ostomy

3. a. Frequent oral hygiene

   b. Lubricant to the lips

   c. Mouth rinses

   d. Nose and nostrils cleaned every 4-6 hours

e. Secure the tube with tape tie the tube to the client's gown to relieve pressure
4. *(Any 4 of the following.)*
   a. Cannot take fluids by mouth
   b. Replace minerals and vitamins lost because of illness or injury
   c. Provide sugar for energy
   d. Administer medications and blood
   e. Provide hyperalimentation

Chapter 27

(Answers can be in any order.)
1. a. Dry, cracked, swollen, or blistered lips
   b. Redness, swelling, irritation, sores, or white patches in the mouth or on the tongue
   c. Bleeding, swelling, or excessive redness of gums
   d. Any loose teeth

(Answers can be in any order.)
2. a. The color of the skin, lips, nail beds, and sclera
   b. The location and description of rashes
   c. Dry skin
   d. Bruises or open skin areas
   e. Pale or reddened areas
   f. Drainage or bleeding from wounds or body openings
   g. Skin temperature
   h. Complaints of pain or discomfort

Chapter 28

(Answers can be in any order.)
1. a. Culture
   b. Personal choice
   c. Skin and scalp condition
   d. Health history
   e. Self-care abilities

(Answers can be in any order.)
2. a. Follow Standard Precautions and the Bloodborne Pathogen Standard
   b. Protect the bed linens
   c. Soften the skin before shaving
   d. Encourage the person to do as much as possible
   e. Hold the skin taut as necessary
   f. Shave in the direction of hair growth
   g. Shave upward, starting at the ankle when shaving legs
   h. Rinse the body part thoroughly
   i. Apply direct pressure to any nicks or cuts
   j. Report nicks and cuts to the nurse immediately

(Answers can be in any order.)
3. a. Provide for privacy; do not expose the person
   b. Encourage the person to do as much as possible

c. Allow the person to choose what to wear
d. Remove clothing from the strong side first
e. Put clothing on the weak side first
f. Support the arm or leg when removing or putting on a garment

Chapter 29

1. e
2. b
3. g
4. a
5. f
6. c
7. d
8. a. Urge incontinence—the involuntary loss of urine after feeling a strong need to void
   b. Stress incontinence—the loss of small amounts of urine with exercise and certain movements
   c. Mixed incontinence—a combination of stress and urge incontinence
   d. Overflow incontinence—the loss of urine when the bladder is too full
   e. Functional incontinence—the involuntary, unpredictable loss of urine
   f. Unconscious or reflex incontinence—the loss of urine at predictable intervals

Chapter 30

1. d
2. j
3. f
4. a
5. c
6. h
7. e
8. g
9. b
10. i
11. a. Tap water enema
    b. Soapsuds enema
    c. Saline enema
    d. Oil-retention enema
    e. Commercial enema

Chapter 31

(Answers can be in any order.)
1. a. A family history of cancer
   b. Exposure to radiation
   c. Exposure to certain chemicals
   d. Smoking
   e. Alcohol

f. High-fat, high-calorie diet

g. Food additives

h. Viruses

i. Hormones

2. Osteoarthritis

(Answers can be in any order.)

3 a. Lack of estrogen after menopause

b. Lack of dietary calcium

c. Smoking

d. High alcohol intake

e. Lack of exercise

f. Bedrest and immobility

(Answers can be in any order.)

4. a. To reduce and immobilize fractures

b. For muscle spasms

c. To correct or prevent deformities

d. For other musculoskeletal injuries

(Answers can be in any order.)

5. a. Stab or bullet wounds

b. Motor vehicle accidents

c. Workplace accidents

d. Falls

e. Sports injuries

(Answers can be in any order.)

6. a. Chronic bronchitis

b. Emphysema

c. Asthma

(Answers can be in any order.)

7. a. Sudden weakness or numbness of the face, arm, or leg on one side of the body

b. Sudden dimness or loss of vision, particularly in one eye

c. Loss of speech, or trouble talking or understanding speech

d. Sudden, severe headaches with no known cause

e. Unexplained dizziness, unsteadiness, or sudden falls (especially with any of the other signs)

(Answers can be in any order.)

8. a. Sex (male gender)

b. Age (more common in older persons)

c. Obesity

d. Cigarette smoking

e. Lack of exercise

f. A diet high in fat and cholesterol

g. Hypertension

h. Family history of CAD

i. Uncontrolled diabetes

9. The heart cannot pump blood normally

(Answers can be in any order.)

10. a. Unprotected anal, vaginal, or oral sex with an infected person

b. Needle sharing among IV drug users

c. HIV-infected mothers before or during childbirth

d. HIV-infected mothers through breast-feeding

Chapter 32

1. The person seeks health care

2. Remaining abilities

3. Physical, psychological, social, economic

4. a. The person

b. The doctor

c. The nursing team

d. Other health team members

e. The family

5. a. Hospitals

b. Subacute care centers

c. Home care agencies

d. Day care centers

e. Rehabilitation centers

f. Long-term care facilities

Chapter 33

1. *(Any 4 of the following.)*

a. Depressed mood

b. Irritability

c. Reduced interest in almost all activities

d. Significant weight gain or weight loss

e. Insomnia or too much sleep

f. Too much or too little motor activity

g. Fatigue or loss of energy

h. Feeling of worthlessness or quilt

i. Reduced ability to concentrate or think

j. Difficulties making decisions

k. Recurrent thoughts of death

2. a. A mental state in which perception of reality is impaired

b. False beliefs

c. Seeing, hearing, and feeling things that are not real

d. No appetite and has a great fear of weight gain and obesity

e. Characteristic that marks a person as different or flawed

3. *(Any 4 of the following.)*

a. Experience many losses

b. Loss of physical health

c. Loss of cognitive abilities

d. Depression

e. Loneliness

f. Facing death because of serious illness

Chapter 34

(Answers can be in any order.)
1. a. Drugs
   b. Alcohol
   c. Delirium
   d. Depression
   e. Tumors
   f. Heart, lung, and blood vessel problems
   g. Head injuries
   h. Infection
   i. Vision and hearing problems

(Answers can be in any order.)
2. a. Gradual loss of short-term memory
   b. Problems finding or speaking the right words
   c. Not recognizing objects
   d. Forgetting how to use simple everyday things
   e. Forgetting to turn off the stove, close windows, or lock doors
   f. Mood and personality changes
   g. Agitation
   h. Poor judgement

(Answers can be in any order.)
3. a. Family members can no longer meet the person's needs
   b. The person no longer knows the caregiver
   c. Family members have health problems
   d. Money problems occur
   e. The person has behaviors that are dangerous to self or others

Chapter 35

1. *(Any 3 of the following.)*
   a. Genetic problems
   b. Conditions present at birth
   c. Brain injury
   d. Disease
   e. Hearing loss
   f. Brain tumors
   g. Problems involving the structures used for speech
2. a. Interpreting the message
   b. Sending the message
   c. Sending and interpreting the message
3. *(Any 4 of the following.)*
   a. Frustration
   b. Depression
   c. Anger
   d. Low self esteem
   e. Shame
   f. Guilt
   g. Stress
4. *(Any 5 of the following.)*
   a. Minimize distractions

b. Adjust the lighting
c. Give the client your full attention
d. Ask the client questions to which you know the answer
e. Determine the subject being discussed
f. Follow the client's lead
g. Speak slowly, clearly and in a normal tone of voice
h. Give the client time to respond
i. Use simple words and short sentences
j. Be patient
k. Use positive statements
l. Use appropriate questioning and paraphrasing techniques
m. Provide cues as needed
n. Try other communication methods

Chapter 36

1. Hearing, balance
(Answers can be in any order.)
2. a. Speaking too loudly
   b. Leaning forward to hear
   c. Turning and cupping the better ear toward the speaker
   d. Asking questions or responding inappropriately
   e. Asking for words to be repeated
3. The optic nerve
4. Respect, dignity, pity

Chapter 37

(Answers can be in any order.)
1. a. Has jaundice
   b. Looks sick
   c. Has redness or drainage around the cord stump or circumcision
   d. Has a high temperature
   e. Is limp and slow to respond
   f. Cries all the time and does not stop crying
   g. Is flushed, pale, or perspiring
   h. Has noisy, rapid, difficult, or slow respirations
   i. Is coughing or sneezing
   j. Has reddened or irritated eyes
   k. Turns his or her head to the side or puts a hand to one ear
   l. Screams for a long time
   m. Has skipped feedings
   n. Has vomited most of the feeding or vomits between feedings
   o. Has hard, formed stools or watery stools
   p. Has a rash
(Answers can be in any order.)

2. a. Fever of 100.4° F or greater
   b. Abdominal or perineal pain
   c. Foul-smelling vaginal discharge
   d. Bleeding from an episiotomy or cesarean section incision
   e. Redness, swelling, or drainage from an episiotomy or c-section incision
   f. Saturating a sanitary napkin within 1 hour of application
   g. Red lochia after lochia has changed color
   h. Burning on urination
   i. Leg pain, tenderness, or swelling
   j. Sadness or feelings of depression
   k. Breast pain, tenderness, or swelling

(Answers can be in any order.)

3. a. The baby must be delivered to save the baby's or mother's life
   b. The baby is too large to pass through the birth canal
   c. The mother has a vaginal infection that could be transmitted to the baby
   d. A normal vaginal delivery will be difficult for the baby or mother

Chapter 38

(Answers can be in any order.)

1. a. Mental retardation
   b. Down syndrome
   c. Cerebral palsy
   d. Autism
   e. Epilepsy
   f. Spina bifida

(Answers can be in any order.)

2. a. Childhood diseases
   b. Head injuries
   c. Near drowning
   d. Mercury poisoning
   e. Lead poisoning
   f. Poor nutrition
   g. Child abuse

3. Every citizen in Canada

Chapter 39

1. a. Right medication
   b. Right person
   c. Right dose
   d. Right route
   e. Right time

2. *(Any 5 of the following.)*
   a. Capsules
   b. Lozenges
   c. Tablets

   d. Ointments
   e. Suppositories
   f. Transdermal disks or patches
   g. Elixirs
   h. Suspensions
   i. Syrups
   j. Drops
   k. Liquids for injection
   l. Aerosols

3. a. Pharmacy name
   b. File number or prescription number
   c. Drug name and dose
   d. Refills
   e. Physician's name
   f. Date filled

4. a. Client's name
   b. Name of medication
   c. Dose of medication and administration instructions

Chapter 40

1. a. 95.8° F
   b. 98.4° F
   c. 100.2° F
   d. 101° F
   e. 102.6° F
   f. 35.5° C
   g. 36.5° C

2. a. 80-180
   b. 80-160
   c. 80-130
   d. 80-120
   e. 70-110
   f. 60-100

3. a. 35
   b. 30
   c. 25
   d. 23
   e. 21
   f. 20
   g. 19
   h. 18
   i. 16-18

4. a. 152
   b. 86

Chapter 41

(Answers can be in any order.)

1. a. Are confined to a bed or chair
   b. Are unable to move
   c. Have loss of bowel or bladder control
   d. Have poor nutrition

e. Have altered mental awareness

f. Have problems sensing pain or pressure

g. Have circulatory problems

h. Are older, obese or very thin

2. a. Stage 1—the skin is red. Color does not return to normal when pressure is relieved.

b. Stage 2—the skin cracks, blisters, or peels. There may be a shallow crater.

c. Stage 3—the skin is gone and the underlying tissue is exposed. There may be drainage.

d. Stage 4—muscle and bone are exposed and damaged. Drainage is likely.

3. a. Primary intention—the wound edges are brought together. This closes the wound.

b. Secondary intention—wounds are cleaned and dead tissue removed. Edges are not brought together and the wound gaps.

c. Tertiary intention—involves leaving a wound open and closing it later.

4. a. Hemorrhage—the excessive loss of blood in a short period of time

b. Infection—contaminated wound appears inflamed and has drainage

c. Dehiscence—the separation of the wound layers

d. Evisceration—the separation of the wound along with protrusion of abdominal organs

Chapter 42

(Answers can be in any order.)

1. a. Complaints of pain, numbness, or burning

b. Excessive redness

c. Blisters

d. Pale, white, or gray skin

e. Cyanosis

f. Shivering

2. a. 106° F to 115° F; 41.1° C to 46.1° C

b. 98° F to 106° F.; 36.6° C to 41.1° C

c. 93° F to 98° F; 33.8° C to 36.6° C

d. 80° F to 93° F; 26.6° C to 33.8° C

e. 65° F to 80° F; 18.3° C to 26.6° C

f. 50° F to 65° F; 10.0° C to 18.3° C

Chapter 43

1. e

2. d

3. a

4. c

5. f

6. b

(Answers can be in any order.)

7. a. Restlessness

b. Dizziness

c. Disorientation

d. Confusion

e. Behavior/personality changes

f. Difficulty concentrating

g. Apprehension

h. Anxiety

i. Fatigue

j. Agitation

k. Increased pulse rate

l. Increased rate and depth of respiration

m. Sitting position/leaning forward

n. Cyanosis

o. Dyspnea

(Answers can be in any order.)

8. a. Keep the signal light within reach.

b. Make sure there is enough slack on hoses and connecting tubes.

c. Answer signal lights promptly.

d. Always explain who you are and what you are going to do.

e. Orient the person to day, date, and time.

f. Tell the nurse if the person shows signs of respiratory distress.

g. Do not change any settings on the ventilator or reset alarms.

h. Provide a means of communication.

i. Use established hand or eye signals for "yes" and "no."

j. Ask questions that have simple answers.

k. Watch what you say within the person's hearing distance.

l. Watch your nonverbal communication.

m. Take time to comfort and reassure the person.

n. Meet the person's basic needs for hygiene, elimination, and activity.

o. Apply a moist cloth or lubricant to the lips as directed by the nurse.

p. Use touch.

q. Tell the person when you are leaving and when you will return.

(Answers can be in any order.)

9. a. Keep the drainage system below the level of the person's chest.

b. Measure the person's vital signs as directed by the nurse; report changes to the nurse immediately.

c. Report signs and symptoms of hypoxia and respiratory distress to the nurse immediately.

d. Report complaints of pain or difficulty breathing to the nurse immediately.

e. Keep connecting tubing coiled on the bed; allow enough slack so the tubes are not dislodged when the person moves.

f. Make sure that the tubing is not kinked.

g. Observe chest drainage; report changes to the nurse immediately.

h. Record chest drainage according to agency policy..

i. Turn and position the person as directed by the nurse

j. Assist the person with coughing and deep breathing as directed by the nurse; assist with incentive spirometry as directed.

k. Note bubbling activity in the drainage system; tell the nurse immediately if the bubbling increases, decreases, or stops.

l. Tell the nurse if any part of the system is loose or disconnected.

m. Make sure petrolatum gauze is at the bedside in case a tube comes out.

n. Call for help immediately if a chest tube comes out; cover the site with a sterile petrolatum gauze; stay with the person until a nurse arrives.

j. Tubes, needles, and other equipment

k. Complications

l. Prolonged recovery

m. More surgery or treatments

n. Separation from family and friends

(Answers can be in any order.)

2. a. A complete bed bath, shower, or a tub bath.

b. Makeup and nail polish are removed.

c. Long hair is braided. All hair pins, clips, combs, and other items are removed. A surgical cap may be worn.

d. Oral hygiene is performed.

e. Dentures are removed before preoperative medications are given.

(Answers can be in any order.)

3. a. Making a surgical bed

b. Placing equipment and supplies in the room

c. Raising the bed to its highest level

d. Lowering bed rails

e. Moving furniture out of the way for the stretcher

Chapter 44

(Answers can be in any order.)

1. a. Wash your hands before and after the examination.

b. Provide for privacy. Expose only the body part being examined.

c. Assist the person in assuming positions as directed by the examiner.

d. Place instruments and equipment in a handy location for the examiner.

e. Stay in the room when a female is examined (unless you are a male).

f. Protect the person from falling.

g. Anticipate the examiner's need for equipment.

h. Place paper or paper towels on the floor if the person is asked to stand.

i. Practice medical asepsis and Standard Precautions. Follow the Bloodborne Pathogen Standard

Chapter 45

(Answers can be in any order.)

1. a. Cancer

b. Disfigurement and scarring

c. Disability

d. Pain during surgery

e. Dying during surgery

f. Affects of anesthesia

g. Going to sleep or not waking up after surgery

h. Exposure

i. Pain or discomfort after surgery

Chapter 46

1. Physical, psychological, social, spiritual

2. a. Infants and toddlers—have no concept of death.

b. Children (3 to 5)—start to be curious about death. Recognize the death of family members and pets. See death as punishment.

c. Children (5 to 7)—know death is final. Do not think that they will die. Death happens to other people.

d. Adults—fear pain and suffering, dying alone, and invasion of privacy. Fear loneliness and separation from loved ones. Often resent death.

e. Older persons—usually have fewer fears. They accept that death will occur. Some welcome death as a freedom from pain and suffering. Often fear dying alone.

3. Listening, touch

4. a. Patient Self-determination Act—gives persons the right to accept or refuse medical treatment. Also the right to make advance directives.

b. Advance directives—a written document stating a person's wishes about health care when that person can no longer make his or her own decisions.

c. Living will—a person's written statement about the use of life-sustaining measures.

d. Durable power of attorney for health care—the power to make decisions about health care is given to another person.

e. "Do not resuscitate" order—an order written by the doctor. It means that no attempt will be made to resuscitate the person. The person is allowed to die with dignity.

Chapter 47

(Answers can be in any order.)
1. a. Your location—street, address, city
   b. Telephone number that you are calling from
   c. What happened (e.g., heart attack, accident)
   d. How many people need help
   e. Condition of victims, obvious injuries, and any life-threatening situations
   f. What aid is being given
2. Carotid artery
3. a. Airway
   b. Breathing
   c. Circulation
4. Heimlich maneuver

(Answers can be in any order.)
5. a. Activate the EMS system
   b. Practice Standard Precautions and follow the Bloodborne Pathogen Standard
   c. Place a sterile dressing directly over the wound
   d. Apply pressure with your hand directly over the bleeding site
   e. If direct pressure does not control bleeding, apply pressure over the artery above the bleeding site

(Answers can be in any order.)
6. a. Keep the person lying down
   b. Maintain an open airway
   c. Control hemorrhage
   d. Keep the person warm
   e. Reassure the person
   f. Activate the EMS system
   g. Follow Standard Precautions and the Bloodborne Pathogen Standard

(Answers can be in any order.)
7. a. Have the person sit or lie down before fainting occurs
   b. If sitting, the person bends forward and places the head between the knees
   c. If the person is lying down, elevate the legs
   d. Loosen tight clothing
   e. Keep the person lying down if fainting has occurred
   f. Do not let the person get up until symptoms have subsided for about 5 minutes
   g. Help the person to a sitting position after recovery

Chapter 48

1. a. Prefix
   b. Root
   c. Suffix
2. a. Right upper quadrant (RUQ)
   b. Left upper quadrant (LUQ)
   c. Right lower quadrant (RLQ)
   d. Left lower quadrant (LLQ)
3. a. Distal—the part farthest from the center or point of attachment
   b. Proximal—the part nearest to the center or point of origin
   c. Anterior (ventral)—located at or toward the front of the body
   d. Medial—relating to or located at or near the midline
   e. Posterior (dorsal)—located at or toward the back of the body
   f. Lateral—relating to or located at the side of the body
4. a. Bi—double, two, twice
   b. Dys—bad, difficult, abnormal
   c. Hypo—under, decreased, less than normal
   d. Mal—bad, illness, disease
   e. Post—after, behind
5. a. Cephal(o)—head
   b. Derma—skin
   c. Lith(o)—stone
   d. Ocul(o)—eye
   e. Phleb(o)—vein
6. a. Ectomy—excision, removal of
   b. Graphy—making a record
   c. Osis—condition
   d. Plegia—paralysis
   e. Uria —condition of the urine

Chapter 49

1. a. Is the information relevant
   b. Have I been completely honest
   c. Have I expressed myself clearly
   d. Is my resume consistent
   e. Is my resume correct
2. *(Any 4 of the following.)*
   a. Employment advertisements
   b. The internet
   c. College career services
   d. Contact people you know
   e. Check with your district home care program

f. Look in the yellow pages for agencies
g. Attend job fairs
h. Check with your Canada Employment Centre.

3. *(Any 10 of the folowing in any order; students may also have very valid tips.)*
   a. Neat and clean hair
   b. Fresh breath a nd clean teeth
   c. Not too much make up
   d. Minimum amount of jewelry
   e. Cover tattoos
   f. Remove excess body ornaments
   g. Do not use perfume
   h. Clean and trimmed nails
   i. Wear business clothes
   j. Shoes in good repair
   k. Arrive 5-10 minutes early
   l. Do not chew gum
   m. Do not talk on the phone while waiting
   n. Use a firm handshake
   o. Listen carefully
   p. Take your time answering questions

QUIZ ANSWERS

Chapter 1

1. T
2. T
3. F
4. F
5. b
6. d
7. a
8. d
9. a

Chapter 2

1. T
2. F
3. T
4. T
5. d
6. c
7. b
8. a

Chapter 3

1. T
2. F
3. F
4. T
5. T
6. T
7. c
8. a
9. d
10. d

Chapter 4

1. F
2. F
3. T
4. T
5. T
6. F
7. T
8. c
9. d
10. d
11. a

Chapter 5

1. F
2. F
3. T
4. T
5. d
6. d
7. b
8. *(Any 3 of the following.)*
   a. Right task
   b. Right circumstances
   c. Right person
   d. Right directions and communication
   e. Right supervision

Chapter 6

1. F
2. T
3. F

4. T
5. T
6. T
7. T
8. F
9. F
10. F
11. a
12. b
13. d
14. e
15. d

Chapter 7

1. F
2. T
3. F
4. F
5. F
6. c
7. d
8. c
9. b

Chapter 8

1. T
2. T
3. T
4. T
5. F
6. F
7. T
8. e
9. b

10. c
11. a

Chapter 9

1. F
2. T
3. F
4. a
5. a
6. b
7. d

Chapter 10

1. T
2. T
3. F
4. T
5. T
6. F
7. F
8. d
9. c
10. c
11. d

Chapter 11

1. F
2. T
3. T
4. F
5. T
6. T
7. T
8. c
9. a
10. c
11. e
12. b

Chapter 12

1. F
2. F
3. T
4. F
5. T
6. T
7. T
8. a
9. c
10. d
11. b

12. c

Chapter 13

1. F
2. T
3. T
4. F
5. T
6. F
7. F
8. T
9. F
10. T
11. T
12. F
13. F
14. F
15. b
16. a
17. b
18. d
19. c
20. d
21. c
22. a
23. b
24. c
25. b

Chapter 14

1. F
2. T
3. T
4. T
5. F
6. b
7. b
8. d
9. c
10. c

Chapter 15

1. T
2. F
3. F
4. T
5. T
6. T
7. F
8. F
9. T
10. T

11. T
12. d
13. c
14. b
15. d
16. c
17. d
18. a

Chapter 16

1. F
2. T
3. T
4. F
5. T
6. F
7. F
8. F
9. F
10. F
11. T
12. b
13. d
14. a

Chapter 17

1. F
2. T
3. T
4. T
5. T
6. F
7. F
8. T
9. c
10. b
11. e

Chapter 18

1. F
2. F
3. T
4. F
5. F
6. T
7. F
8. T
9. F
10. b
11. b
12. c
13. a

14. a
15. c
16. d

Chapter 19

1. T
2. F
3. T
4. F
5. F
6. F
7. T
8. T
9. b
10. d
11. c
12. d

Chapter 20

1. T
2. F
3. T
4. T
5. T
6. F
7. T
8. T
9. T
10. T
11. F
12. T
13. T
14. F
15. T
16. T
17. F
18. T
19. T
20. F
21. b
22. c
23. c
24. b
25. c
26. a
27. b
28. d
29. a
30. c
31. a
32. b
33. a
34. a

35. c

Chapter 21

1. F
2. F
3. T
4. F
5. T
6. c
7. c
8. d
9. b
10. a

Chapter 22

1. T
2. F
3. F
4. T
5. F
6. c
7. b
8. a
9. c
10. d
11. d
12. c

Chapter 23

1. F
2. T
3. T
4. F
5. F
6. F
7. T
8. c
9. b
10. d
11. d

Chapter 24

1. F
2. T
3. F
4. F
5. T
6. F
7. T
8. F
9. F

10. T
11. d
12. c
13. c
14. b
15. d

Chapter 25

1. T
2. F
3. T
4. T
5. F
6. T
7. F
8. T
9. T
10. F
11. c
12. d
13. a
14. c
15. b
16. c

Chapter 26

1. F
2. F
3. F
4. T
5. T
6. F
7. F
8. T
9. F
10. T
11. a
12. a
13. a
14. d

Chapter 27

1. F
2. T
3. T
4. F
5. T
6. F
7. T
8. F

9. F
10. a
11. c
12. b
13. c

Chapter 28

1. F
2. T
3. F
4. T
5. T
6. F
7. F
8. a
9. c
10. c
11. b
12. a

Chapter 29

1. T
2. F
3. F
4. T
5. F
6. T
7. T
8. F
9. T
10. T
11. F
12. b
13. d
14. b
15. a

Chapter 30

1. T
2. F
3. F
4. F
5. T
6. F
7. F
8. T
9. T
10. b
11. c
12. a
13. d

14. a

Chapter 31

1. F
2. T
3. F
4. F
5. T
6. T
7. F
8. T
9. T
10. F
11. T
12. T
13. T
14. F
15. T
16. b
17. a
18. d
19. a
20. d
21. c
22. a
23. b
24. b
25. a
26. d
27. c

Chapter 32

1. F
2. T
3. T
4. F
5. T
6. c
7. d
8. d
9. b
10. a
11. c

Chapter 33

1. T
2. F
3. F
4. T
5. T
6. F

7. c
8. b
9. b
10. c
11. d
12. d
13. b

Chapter 34

1. F
2. T
3. F
4. F
5. F
6. T
7. T
8. F
9. T
10. F
11. T
12. T
13. b
14. c
15. d
16. d
17. a
18. c

Chapter 35

1. T
2. F
3. T
4. T
5. T
6. T
7. T
8. F
9. a
10. a
11. d

Chapter 36

1. F
2. T
3. T
4. F
5. F
6. T
7. F
8. F
9. a
10. c

11. c
12. d
13. c
14. b

Chapter 37

1. F
2. T
3. F
4. T
5. T
6. F
7. T
8. F
9. F
10. T
11. T
12. T
13. F
14. T
15. F
16. T
17. T
18. F
19. T
20. F
21. b
22. c
23. a
24. b
25. a

Chapter 38

1. T
2. F
3. F
4. T
5. T
6. F
7. T
8. F
9. b
10. c
11. c
12. d

Chapter 39

1. F
2. F
3. F
4. T

5. F
6. T
7. T
8. b
9. d
10. d

Chapter 40

1. F
2. F
3. T
4 F
5. T
6. F
7. T
8. T
9. F
10. T
11. T
12. F
13. T
14. b
15. b
16. a

Chapter 41

1. T
2. T
3. T
4. T
5. F
6. T
7. F
8. F
9. T
10. a
11. c
12. a
13. d
14. d
15. d

Chapter 42

1. T
2. T
3. F
4. T
5. T
6. T

7. F
8. T
9. b
10. a
11. d

Chapter 43

1. T
2. T
3. F
4. F
5. T
6. F
7. F
8. T
9. F
10. T
11. F
12. b
13. d
14. c
15. d
16. c
17. a
18. b

Chapter 44

1. T
2. T
3. F
4. T
5. F
6. F
7. T
8. d
9. c
10. c
11. b

Chapter 45

1. F
2. T
3. T
4. F
5. F
6. T
7. F
8. T
9. T
10. F
11. T

12. F
13. b
14. b
15. c
16. d

Chapter 46

1. T
2. F
3. T
4. T
5. F
6. F
7. F
8. F
9. T
10. T
11. T
12. b
13. b
14. d
15. a

Chapter 47

1. F
2. T
3. F
4. F
5. T
6. T
7. T
8. T
9. F
10. F
11. T
12. F
13. F
14. T
15. b
16. c
17. a
18. c
19. d
20. d
21. a
22. c
23. b
24. c

Chapter 48

1. T
2. F
3. F
4. T
5. T
6. F
7. c
8. d
9. a
10. c

Chapter 49

1. T
2. T
3. F
4. F
5. T
6. c
7. d
8. c
9. d
10. b

ANSWERS TO FINAL EXAMINATIONS

Answers to Final Examinations—Version 1

1. T	26. T	50. T	74. c	98. c	122. b
2. F	27. T	51. T	75. d	99 b	123. b
3. F	28. T	52. F	76. b	100. c	124. a
4. F	29. F	53. F	77. d	101. a	125. d
5. T	30. F	54. F	78. d	102. d	126. c
6. F	31. F	55. F	79. c	103. d	127. a
7. F	32. T	56. F	80. b	104. c	128. c
8. F	33. F	57. F	81. c	105. d	129. a
9. F	34. T	58. F	82. b	106. b	130. d
10. T	35. T	59. T	83. d	107. b	131. a
11. F	36. T	60. F	84. a	108. d	132. d
12. T	37. F	61. T	85. d	109. a	133. b
13. T	38. F	62. F	86. a	110. c	134. b
14. F	39. T	63. F	87. d	111. b	135. b
15. F	40. T	64. d	88. d	112. b	136. c
16. T	41. F	65. d	89. b	113. b	137. b
17. F	42. F	66. c	90. d	114. c	138. c
18. T	43. T	67. c	91. a	115. c	139. b
19. F	44. T	68. b	92. d	116. c	140. a
20. F	45. F	69. c	93. c	117. b	141. c
21. F	46. T	70. a	94. c	118. c	142. c
22. F	47. T	71. b	95. c	119. d	143. d
23. F	48. F	72. a	96. b	120. a	144. d
24. F	49. F	73. c	97. a	121. b	145. c
25. T					

Answers to Final Examinations—Version 2

1. T	26. F	50. T	74. c	98. b	122. b
2. F	27. T	51. T	75. d	99. a	123. d
3. T	28. F	52. F	76. c	100. b	124. c
4. T	29. F	53. F	77. c	101. c	125. c
5. T	30. T	54. F	78. b	102. a	126. b
6. T	31. T	55. F	79. c	103. b	127. b
7. T	32. T	56. T	80. b	104. c	128. d
8. F	33. T	57. F	81. b	105. c	129. d
9. F	34. T	58. T	82. c	106. c	130. c
10. F	35. F	59. T	83. c	107. b	131. c
11. T	36. T	60. F	84. d	108. a	132. d
12. F	37. F	61. T	85. a	109. c	133. d
13. F	38. T	62. T	86. a	110. c	134. d
14. T	39. T	63. T	87. c	111. b	135. b
15. T	40. T	64. b	88. c	112. a	136. b
16. T	41. F	65. a	89. b	113. b	137. a
17. F	42. T	66. d	90. c	114. c	138. d
18. F	43. T	67. b	91. d	115. b	139. d
19. T	44. T	68. b	92. c	116. b	140. a
20. F	45. F	69. a	93. d	117. a	141. b
21. T	46. T	70. a	94. a	118. a	142. b
22. T	47. T	71. c	95. b	119. d	143. b
23. T	48. F	72. c	96. a	120. a	144. c
24. F	49. F	73. b	97. c	121. a	145. d
25. F					

ANSWERS TO WORKBOOK

Chapter 1

1. F; The risk of acquiring a serious illness increases with age.
2. T
3. T
4. F; Discretion means having good judgment about when information should be kept private and when it should be shared.
5. F; Keep personal matters out of the workplace.
6. T
7. T
8. T
9. a. RN
   b. Physician
   c. Respiratory therapist
   d. Dietician
   e. Physical therapist
   f. Occupational therapist
   g. Speech-language pathologist
   h. Spiritual advisor
   i. Social worker
10. a. Eating
    b. Bathing
    c. Grooming
    d. Dressing
11. a. Personal care
    b. Support for nurses and other professionals
    c. Family support
    d. Social support
    e. Housekeeping/home management
12. patient/resident/client
13. a. Dignity
    b. Independence

c. Preferences
d. Privacy
e. Safety
14. *(Any five of the following.)*
    • A positive attitude
    • A sense of responsibility
    • A professional appearance
    • Discretion about client information
    • Discretion about personal matters
    • Acceptable speech and language
15. *(Any five of the following.)*
    • Follow dress code policies
    • Wear a clean, well-fitting, modest uniform
    • Wear clean stockings and socks
    • Wear comfortable, well-polished shoes
    • Wear underclothing that cannot be seen through the uniform
    • Keep hair away from face and off the collar
    • Use make-up sparingly
    • Do not wear perfume, cologne, or aftershave
    • Keep fingernails clean, short, and neatly shaped
    • Do not wear jewellery
    • Cover tatoos
16. a. Priorities of support work
    b. Client's viewpoint
    c. Scope of practice
    d. Supervisor's viewpoint
17. a. The training program
    b. Employer's policies
    c. Supervisor
18. Choose from the following:
    • Older adults
    • People with disabilities
    • People with medical problems
    • People having surgery
    • People with mental health problems

455

- People needing rehabilitation
- Children
- Mothers and newborns
- People requiring special care

19. c

Chapter 2

1. a. Public administration
   b. Comprehensiveness
   c. Universality
   d. Portability
   e. Accessibility
2. Choose from the following:
   - Nursing care
   - Physiotherapy
   - Occupational therapy
   - Speech therapy
   - Nutrition counseling
   - Social work
   - Respiratory therapy
3. Strategies that improve or maintain health and independence.
4. Strategies that prevent the occurrence of disease or injury.
5. a. Older adults
   b. Families with children
   c. People with mental, physical, or developmental disabilities
   d. People with short-term medical conditions
   e. People with long-term medical conditions
   f. People in the recovery, rehabilitative, or life-ending stages of disease
6. a. Immunization programs
   b. Prenatal and parenting classes
   c. Information campaigns (e.g., to reduce drinking during pregnancy, unsafe sex, and tobacco use)
   d. Efforts to improve housing, decrease poverty, monitor safe drinking water, and protect the environment
7. By providing nonmedical care and services that can help prevent major health problems.
8. F; The federal government is responsible for delivering health care services to Aboriginal people.
9. F; The Canadian health care system has seen a shift in focus from hospital care to home care.
10. T
11. T
12. T
13. F. Income and social status are key factors that determine a person's health.
14. F; In the Canada Health Act, the principle of portability ensures that people keep their health coverage even if they are unemployed or change jobs.

15. T
16. 1930
17. 1947
18. 1972
19. 1961
20. P
21. P
22. S
23. P
24. S
25. P

Chapter 3

1. c
2. e
3. a
4. d
5. f
6. g
7. h
8. b
9. An on-going illness, slow or gradual in onset, that usually worsens over time and cannot be cured. Examples of chronic illnesses: Diabetes, multiple sclerosis, Alzheimer's disease
10. An illness that appears suddenly and usually lasts a short time, usually less than three months. Examples of acute illnesses: pneumonia, influenza
11. Working on your own, taking direction from different professionals, maintaining professional boundaries, providing for client safety, providing for personal safety
12. a. Rehabilitation
    b. Counselling for people with mental illness
    c. Recreational activities
13. People who cannot care for themselves at home but do not need acute medical care or high-level nursing care.
14. To maintain the residents' health and independence to the greatest extent possible, and to meet residents' physical, emotional, social, intellectual, and spiritual needs.
15. F; Residents must pay the full cost.
16. T
17. T
18. F; Support workers in community day programs work closely with a team and supervisor.
19. T
20. T
21. F; Convalescent care is another term for subacute care.

Chapter 4

1. c
2. a
3. b
4. e
5. d
6. g
7. c
8. f
9. a
10. d
11. e
12. h
13. b
14. F; A social support system is an informal group of people who help each other.
15. T
16. T
17. F; A disability is the loss of physical or mental function; an illness is the loss of physical or mental health.
18. T
19. F; Discrimination is treating people unfairly because of their group membership.
20. F; To promote independence, clients should always be encouraged to make decisions for themselves if they are able.
21. T
22. Well-being in all dimensions of one's life
23. a. Physical health
    b. Emotional health
    c. Social health
    d. Intellectual health
    e. Spiritual health
24. *(In any order.)*
    - Following a nutritious diet
    - Exercising regularly
    - Living in a smoke-free environment
    - Drinking alcohol moderately or not at all
    - Having a good night's sleep
    - Following safety practices
    - Seeking medical attention when needed
25. *(Students can come up with their own examples. The text says the following.)*
    - Encourage residents to participate in games and outings
    - Encourage residents to read
    - Help residents do crossword puzzles or crafts
    - Talk with residents about community and world events
26. *(Any five of the following.)*
    - The nature of the illness or condition
    - The person's age
    - Level of physical fitness
    - Amount of pain and discomfort
    - The prognosis
    - The person's emotional, social, intellectual, and spiritual health
    - The person's personality and ability to cope with difficulties
    - The person's culture
    - The presence or absence of emotional, social, and financial support
27. a. Fear and anxiety
    b. Sadness and grief
    c. Depression
    d. Denial
    e. Anger
28. *(Any six of the following.)*
    - Change in routine
    - Change in work life
    - Change in family life
    - Change in sexual function
    - Loss of independence
    - Loss of dignity
    - Change in self-image

Chapter 5

1. e
2. a
3. f
4. b
5. d
6. c
7. g
8. b
9. c
10. e
11. a
12. d
13. e
14. b
15. c
16. d
17. a
18. T
19. F; Some provinces allow RPNs to supervisor support workers in long-term care facilities.
20. F; Talking about work problems with clients could destroy the client's trust in the facility or agency.
21. T
22. F; You must have sound reasons for refusing to do a task.
23. T
24. F
25. a
26. c
27. a

28. d

29. a. Opportunities for collaboration
    b. Opportunities for communication
    c. A wide array of abilities, skills, and perspectives
    d. Better decision making and problem solving
    e. A positive, trusting atmosphere

30. a. Physicians
    b. Nurses
    c. Social workers
    d. Support workers
    e. Therapists
    f. The resident and the resident's family

31. a. Teach the task
    b. Assess performance
    c. Monitor over time to ensure the person remains able to perform the task correctly and safely

32. *(Any six of the following.)*
    - The client's condition
    - Support worker's ability to perform the task
    - Risks involved in performing the task
    - Frequency required of task
    - Level of supervision available
    - Availability of a nurse should the client's condition change or problems arise
    - Time available for the support worker to perform the task
    - Legislated restrictions on the kinds of acts and procedures support workers are allowed to perform
    - The support worker's job description

33. *(In any order.)*
    - The client
    - The client's family
    - A case manager
    - A family physician
    - Nurse(s)
    - Support worker(s) and their supervisors
    - Social worker
    - Therapist(s)

Chapter 6

1. g
2. e
3. d
4. f
5. h
6. a
7. c
8. b
9. a
10. c
11. e

12. a
13. b
14. c
15. a
16. c
17. a
18. a
19. d
20. a

21. a. Personality
    b. Family background
    c. Environment
    d. Life circumstances

22. a. Explain why a procedure needs to be done
    b. Explain who will do the procedure
    c. Explain how the procedure will be performed
    d. Describe what sensations or feelings to expect

23. *(Student can think up various situations; the text's examples include the following.)*
    - A married couple with or without children
    - An unmarried couple living together, with or without children
    - A widowed grandparent raising grandchildren
    - Divorced parent living with a partner
    - Two women or two men living together in a same-sex relationship
    - Older parents, adult children, and grandchildren living together

24. *(Student can think up various situations; the text's examples include the following.)*
    - Accepting the client's values, feelings, lifestyle, and decisions
    - Being courteous and polite
    - Recognizing the client's need for privacy and independence
    - Encouraging clients to express preferences, make personal choices, and do as much as they can for themselves

25. A professional helping relationship is established to benefit the client, whereas a friendship is a personal social relationship that benefits both people involved.

26. a. Self-actualization
    b. Self-esteem
    c. Love and belonging
    d. Safety
    e. Physical

Chapter 7

1. e
2. f
3. b
4. a

5. d
6. c
7. b
8. b
9. d
10. a
11. b
12. Sight, smell, touch, hearing
13. Subjective
14. Objective
15. a. S
   b. S
   c. O
   d. O
   e. O
   f. S
   g. S
   h. O
   i. O
   j. O
16. a. S
   b. O
   c. S
   d. O
   e. O
   f. S
17. a. 1100
   b. 0800
   c. 1600
   d. 0730
   e. 1845
   f. 1200
   g. 0300
   h. 0450
   i. 1730
   j. 2245
   k. 2355
   l. 2115
18. title
19. a. Ability to respond
   b. Movement
   c. Pain or discomfort
   d. Skin
   e. Eyes, Ears, Nose, and Mouth
   f. Respirations
   g. Bowels and bladder function
   h. Appetite
   i. Activities of daily living
20. a. Is the person easy or difficult to arouse?
   b. Can the person state his or her name, the time, and the location?
   c. Can the person identify others correctly?
   d. Can the person answer questions correctly?
   e. Does the person speak clearly?
   f. Can the person follow instructions correctly?
   g. Is the person calm, restless, or excited?
   h. Is the person quiet or able to coverse?
21. a. Can the person squeeze your fingers with each hand?
   b. Can the person move his or her arms and legs?
   c. Are the person's movements shaky or jerky?
   d. Does thee person complain of stiff or painful joints?
22. *(Any eight of the following.)*
- Aching
- Burning
- Cramping
- Dull
- Gnawing
- Knifelike
- Piercing
- Pressure
- Sharp
- Sore
- Squeezing
- Stabbing
- Throbbing
- Vice-like
23. a. Do both sides of the person's chest rise and fall with respirations?
   b. Is breathing noisy?
   c. Does the person complain of difficulty breathing?
   d. What is the amount and colour of the sputum?
   e. What is the frequency of the person's cough? Is it dry or productive?
24. a. Is the skin pale or flushed?
   b. Is the skin cool, warm, or hot?
   c. Is the skin moist or dry?
   d. What colour are the lips and nails?
   e. Is the skin intact? If not, where are the broken areas?
   f. Are sores or reddened areas present?
   g. Are bruises present? Where?
   h. Does the person complain of itching?
25. *(In any order.)*
- Is the abdomen firm or soft?
- Does the person complain of gas?
- Amount, colour, and consistency of stool?
- Frequency of bowel movements?
- Can the person control bowel movement?
- Pain or difficulty urinating?
- Amount of urine?
- Does urine have a foul smell?
- Can the person control the passage of urine?
- Frequency of urination?
26. a. Can the person perform personal care without help (e.g., bathing, brushing teeth, combing

hair, shaving)?

   b. Can the person use the toilet, commode, bedpan, or urinal?

   c. Can the person feed himself or herself?

   d. Can the person walk?

   e. What amount and kind of assistance are needed?

27. a. prompt/thorough/accurate
   b. name/room and bed numbers/the time you made your observation or gave care
   c. what you observed and did yourself
   d. often as the client's condition requires
   e. any changes in the client's condition
   f. information about care given, the client's response, observations, the client's activities, special treatments, and medications

28. a. 0200
   b. 1030
   c. 0500
   d. 0930
   e. 6:00 a.m.
   f. 11.45 a.m.
   g. 6:00 p.m.
   h. 10:00 p.m.

29. F; Always use ink.
30. T
31. T
32. F; Use only employer-approved abbreviations.
33. T
34. F; Never use an eraser; make a single line through the error, write "error" over it, and sign your initials.
35. T
36. F; Do not skip lines; draw a line through the blank space of a partially completed line or to the end of a page.
37. T
38. F; Record only what you observed and did yourself.
39. F; Chart care and treatments after they are completed.
40. F; Only record observations; do not record your interpretations, judgments, assumptions, or opinions.
41. T
42. T
43. F; Use the client's exact words.
44. T
45. F; Do not omit information.
46. T

Chapter 8

1. f
2. d
3. a
4. g
5. c
6. b
7. h
8. e
9. F; Stressors that last for a short period of time usually create only mild stress.
10. T
11. T
12. F; Children may show the same signs of stress as do adults.
13. T
14. F; You should plan ahead but remain flexible and responsive to changes.
15. F; Report all conflicts with clients, even if they are resolved.
16. T
17. F; Older adults can cope with stress as well as other adults.
18. F; Some stress motivates us to perform well.
19. *(Any four of the following.)*
- Develop self-awareness
- Think positively
- Assert yourself
- Ask for help and support
- Practise calming exercises

20. a. Identify priorities to focus on what is important
   b. Set goals
   c. Make daily plans
   d. Make weekly plans

21. a. Identify and solve problems before they become major issues
   b. Explain the situation to your supervisor and ask for advice
   c. Arrange a private meeting with the person with whom you have a conflict
   d. Explain the problem to the person, focusing on facts, not on the person
   e. Listen to the other person's response without interrupting
   f. Identify ways to resolve the conflict, offering your own ideas and asking for the other person's ideas
   g. Implement the solutions, and review the situation as needed

22. *In the following order.*
- Identify the problem and determine whether it requires your attention.
- Analyze the problem. Decide if it is one you can solve on your own. Always ask your super-

visor for help if you are uncertain.
- Devise a plan. Think of as many solutions as you can, and decide which is the most practical and helpful. Keep safety in mind. Implement the plan. Involve your supervisor if necessary.

23. *(Students can think up their own examples.)*
24. *(Any five of the following.)*
- Rapid pulse
- Rapid respirations
- Increased blood pressure
- Rapid speech, higher-pitched voice
- A "lump" in the throat
- "Butterflies" in the stomach
- Dry mouth
- Sweaty palms
- Sore muscles in neck, arms, and back
- Perspiration
- Nausea
- Diarrhea
- Urinary frequency
- Urinary urgency
- Difficulty sleeping
- Change in appetite
- Change in weight

25. *(Any three of the following.)*
- Anxiety
- Depression
- Anger
- Worry
- Fear
- Burnout
- Irritability
- Loss of self-esteem
- Fatigue
- Dissatisfaction
- Forgetfulness
- Poor concentration
- Difficulty focusing or following directions
- Emotional outbursts
- Smoking
- Drinking
- Talking about the stressor

26. *(Any five of the following.)*
- There is an emergency
- There is a change in the client's condition or normal functioning
- The client becomes ill
- The client is in distress
- The client's safety may be at risk
- A problem arises involving medications
- The client complains about his or her condition or care
- The client asks you a question about his or her diagnosis, condition, or treatment plans

- The client or family asks you to do something that contradicts the care plan
- You have a conflict with a client or family member
- A question or problem arises with which you need help

27. a. Specific
    b. Measurable
    c. Achievable
    d. Realistic
    e. Timely

28. a. Explain the situation to your supervisor and ask for advice
    b. Ask the person if you can meet privately
    c. Agree on a time and place to talk
    d. Meet in a private setting where others cannot see or hear you
    e. Explain the problem by listing facts and specific behaviours; focus on the problem and not on the person
    f. Listen to the person's response without interrupting
    g. Identify ways to resolve the problem; offer your ideas and ask for the other person's ideas
    h. Schedule a date and time to review the situation later
    i. Thank the person for meeting with you
    j. Implement the solutions
    k. Review the situation as needed

Chapter 9

1. e
2. c
3. d
4. b
5. f
6. a
7. F; Support work is an unregulated profession and therefore has no formal code of ethics.
8. T
9. T
10. F; You should never talk about a client with anyone who is not a member of the care team.
11. F; You should not become personally involved with clients or their families.
12. F; Only discuss the client with members of the care team who need to know.
13. T
14. The moral principles or values that guide us when deciding what is right and what is wrong, what is good and what is bad.
15. *(Students can make up their own. The text suggests the following, in any order.)*

- Support workers provide high-quality personal care and support services
- They provide compassionate care to all clients
- They value the dignity of all clients
- They respect their clients' choices about how they receive or participate in their care
- They respect their clients' rights to privacy and confidentiality
- They do not misuse their position of trust
- They are reliable
- They promote and maintain their clients' safety

16. a. Autonomy
    b. Justice
    c. Beneficence
    d. Nonmaleficence
17. Consider the four principles of health care ethics. Collect as much information about the situation as possible. Consider all possible options. Ask yourself: Does the option respect the client's wishes and preferences? Does it treat the client justly and fairly? Does it provide the client with a short-term or long-term benefit? And, could it cause harm or increase the risk of harm?
18. If the client is at risk for injury, you must involve the supervisor.
19. a

Chapter 10

1. e
2. g
3. c
4. J
5. b
6. d
7. h
8. I
9. f
10. a
11. F; Human rights legislation protect against harassment.
12. T
13. T
14. T
15. F; Support workers are never responsible for obtaining written consent.
16. T
17. T
18. F; Opening a client's mail is never appropriate; doing so would be an invasion of privacy.
19. T
20. T
21. a
22. b

23. b
24. a
25. d
26. c
27. a. Freedom of conscience and religion
    b. Freedom of thought, belief, opinion, and expression
    c. Freedom of peaceful assembly and association
    d. The right to vote
    e. The right to enter, remain in, and leave Canada
    f. The right to life, liberty, and security of the person
    g. The right to equality before and under the law, without discrimination based on race, ethnic origin, colour, religion, sex, age, or disability
28. Choose from the following:
    - To be treated with dignity and respect
    - To life in a safe and clean environment
    - To be properly sheltered, clothed, groomed, and cared for
    - To keep and display personal possessions, pictures, and furnishings in their rooms
    - To have family present 24 hours a day if the person is dying
    - To be free from abuse
    - To discuss problems or suggest changes to any aspect of the services provided to them
    - To privacy privacy and confidentiality
    - To give or withhold informed consent
    - Autonomy (the right to make decisions)
29. *(Students can make up their own examples. The text's examples include the following.)*
    - Be courteous
    - Respect the person's belonging and property
    - Address an adult by title and last name, unless the person tells you to do otherwise
    - Allow clients to do things for themselves
    - Assist with personal care and grooming whenever necessary
    - Be patient
    - Listen attentively
    - Make eye contact and use touch, if culturally appropriate
    - Never scold, laugh at, or embarrass the person
30. accurate / complete information
31. a. The reason for the treatment or service
    a. What will be done
    b. How it will be done
    c. Who will be doing it
    d. The expected outcomes
    e. Potential risks and side effects of the treatment
    f. Other treatment options
    g. The likely consequences of not having the treatment

32. negligent
33. privacy
34. *(Students can make up their own examples. The text's examples include the following.)*
    - Knock on the client's door and wait for a reply before entering
    - Ask others to leave the room before giving care
    - Close the door, drapes, and shades and use curtains or screens when providing care
    - Drape the client during personal care procedures, and only expose the body part involved in the treatment or procedure
    - Keep clients covered when moving them throughout the facility
    - Close the bathroom door when a client is using it
    - Do not open or read clients' mail
    - Do not touch clients' belongings without permission
    - Allow clients to visit with others and use the telephone in private
    - Do not pry into clients' private lives
    - Keep all personal and health information confidential
35. a. Not performing a task or procedure correctly.
    b. Performing a task or procedure for which you are not qualified
    c. Making a mistake.
36. Recording every procedure
37. Choose from the following:
    •Human rights legislation
    •Occupational health and safety legislation
    •Employment standards legislation
    •Labour relations legislation
    •Workers' compensation legislation
    •Long-term care facilities legislation
    •Community services legislation
38. Employers and employees both have responsibilities to ensure job safety.
39. a. exposed
    b. others
    c. in private
    d. send/receive
    e. care/treatment/condition

Chapter 11

1. d
2. f
3. g
4. e
5. a
6. c
7. b

8. F; Some cultures are uncomfortable with casual touch from strangers and tend to avoid touching.
9. F; In Western cultures, personal space is usually about 90 cm (3 feet).
10. T
11. T
12. T
13. F; Some folk remedies may interfere with medical treatments.
14. F Prejudice frequently leads to discrimination
15. T
16. T
17. T
18. a. Communication
    b. Family and social organization
    c. Religion and worship
    d. Health care practices and reactions to illness
19. a. Touch
    b. Personal space
    c. Eye contact
    d. Facial expressions
20. a. Pain
    b. Surprise
    c. Embarrassment
    d. Happiness
21. Parents, grandparents, children, aunts, uncles, cousins
22. An older person can feel greatly stressed and disappointed when their children reject their culture.
23. *(Any seven of the following.)*
    - Daily living habits
    - Behaiours
    - Relationships with others
    - Diet
    - Healing
    - Days of worship
    - Birth and birth control
    - Medicine
    - Death
24. a. How your culture influences you
    b. How cultural influences clients' behaviours and attitudes
    c. Each client is unique, and individuals may not follow every belief and practice of their culture and religion.
25. smile
26. *(Any four of the following.)*
    - Convey comfort by the tone of your voice and with your body language
    - Do not speak loudly or shout
    - Speak slowly and distinctly
    - Keep messages short and simple
    - Be alert for words the client seems to understand

- Use gestures and pictures
- Repeat the message in different ways
- Avoid using medical terms, abbreviations, and slang
- Be certain the client understands what is going to happen and consents before you begin a procedure
- Learn a few useful phrases in the client's language

Chapter 12

1. c
2. k
3. a
4. I
5. e
6. g
7. b
8. J
9. h
10. d
11. f
12. T
13. F; Touch is a powerful form of nonverbal communication.
14. F; When paraphrasing, use fewer words than the person used to send the message.
15. T
16. F; Older adults, like everyone else, are aware of messages sent through body language.
17. T
18. T
19. T
20. F; Positioning yourself at eye level shows caring and respect.
21. F Pet names are patronizing and thus create a barrier to communication.
22. F Assertive communication is expressing oneself positively and directly, without offending others. Aggressive communication is usually not respectful and is threatening.
23. *(Any eight of the following.)*
    - Choose words carefully
    - Use simple, everyday language
    - Speak clearly, slowly, and distinctly
    - Control the volume and tone of voice
    - Be brief and consise
    - Present information in a logical manner
    - Ask one question at a time
    - Determine understanding
    - Do not pretend to understand
24. *(Any five of the following.)*
    - Posture

- Appearance
- Facial expressions
- Body movements
- Eye contact
- Gestures
25. a. A sender sends a message
    b. A receiver receives the message
    c. The receiver interprets the message
    d. The receiver provides feedback
26. *(Any four of the following.)*
    - Facing the person
    - Making eye contact
    - Leaning toward the person
    - Responding to the person
    - Avoiding communication barriers
27. a. Start a conversation
    b. Find out about a client's needs and preferences
28. a. Hearing problems
    b. Vision problems
    c. Nervous system disorders
    d. Cultural differences
    e. Loud noises
    f. Lack of privacy
    g. Distractions
29. a. Interrupting
    b. Answering your own questions
    c. Giving advice
    d. Minimizing problems
    e. Using patronizing language
    f. Failing to listen
30. a. Rapid movements
    b. Pacing
    c. Clenched fists
    d. Reddened face or neck
31. a. Explain why the procedure is done
    b. Explain who will do it
    c. Explain how it will be done
    d. Describe what sensations or feelings they can expect
32. a. Tell the person the steps in the task
    b. Show the person how to do each step
    c. Have the person try each step
    d. Review the person's success with each step
33. *(Any five of the following.)*
    - Put the client at ease
    - Start wit small, easy steps
    - Observe and listen
    - Use positive statements
    - Let the client set the pace
    - Provide support and offer encouragement
    - Allow time for practice
34. communicating
35. nonverbal
36. body

37. support worker
38. barrier
39. a. Acknowledge that the person feels frustrated or frightened.
    b. Treat the person with respect and dignity.
    c. Answer the person's questions clearly and thoroughly.
    d. Tell the person what you are going to do and when
    e. Do not keep the person waiting for long periods.
    f. Stay calm and professional.
    g. Do not argue.
    h. Listen and use silence.
    i. Protect yourself from violent behaviours.
    j. Leave and call your supervisor if you think you are in danger.
    k. Report the person's behaviour to your supervisor.

Chapter 13

1. a
2. J
3. b
4. c
5. I
6. f
7. h
8. d
9. g
10. e
11. M
12. S
13. S
14. M
15. M
16. S
17. d
18. b
19. e
20. c
21. J
22. g
23. I
24. a
25. L
26. h
27. f
28. k
29. c
30. e
31. b
32. f

33. d
34. a
35. a. Cell membrane
    b. Nucleus
    c. Cytoplasm
36. mitosis
37. a. Epithelial tissue—covers internal and external body surfaces
    b. Connective tissue—anchors, connects, and supports other body tissues
    c. Muscle tissue—allows the body to move by stretching and contracting
    d. Nerve tissue—relays information to and from the brain and throughout the body
38. a. bear the weight of the body
    b. allow skill and ease in movement
    c. protect the organs
    d. allow various degrees of movement and flexibility
39. a. allows movement in all directions
    b. allows movement in one direction
    c. allows turning from side to side.
40. bones/conscious control
41. The nervous system controls, directs, and coordinates body functions.
42. spinal cord
43. a. sight
    b. hearing
    c. taste
    d. smell
    e. touch
44. amplify/inner ear/malleus, incus, stapes
45. a. Blood
    b. Heart
    c. Vessels
46. The function of the lungs is to allow respiration—breathing.
47. The digestive system breaks down food physically and chemically so it can be absorbed for use by the cells.
48. stool
49. kidney
50. a. Release ova
    b. Secrete the hormones estrogen and progesterone
51. pituitary gland
52. a. Causes growth of muscles, bones, and other organs.
    b. Enables thyroid gland function.
    c. Stimulates the adrenal gland.
    d. Prevents the kidneys from excreting excessive amounts of water.
    e. Causes the uterine muscles to contract during childbirth.

53. metabolism
54. calcium
55. a. Regulate metabolism of carbohydrates
    b. Regulate the amount of salt and water that are absorbed and lost by the kidneys
56. a. Attack and destroy abnormal or unwanted substances
    b. Cause the body to produce antibodies
    c. Digest and destroy microorganisms and other unwanted substances
    d. Produce antibodies
    e. Cause the production of antibodies that circulate in the plasma
    f. Destroy invading cells or attract other cells that destroy invading cells
57. a. Hinge joint; elbow
    b. Pivot joint; located at the base of the skull
    c. Ball and socket; hips
58. a. Cerebrum
    b. Cerebellum
    c. Brainstem
59. a. Right atrium; Receives blood from body tissues.
    b. Right ventricle; Pumps blood to the lungs for oxygen.
    c. Left atrium; Receives oxygenated blood from the lungs.
    d. Left ventricle; Pumps oxygenated blood to all parts of the body.
    e. Superior vena cava; Carries blood from the head and arms to the right atrium.
    f. Aorta; A large artery that receives blood directly from the left ventricle and then branches into other arteries that carry the blood to all parts of the body.
60. This will have to be done.
61. a. Pharynx
    b. Trachea
    c. Right main bronchus
    d. Left main bronchus
    e. Diaphragm
    f. Pleura
    g. Alveolus
62. a. Salivary glands
    b. Pharynx (throat)
    c. Esophagus
    d. Stomach
    e. Small intestine
    f. Large intestine
    g. Rectum
    h. Anus
    i. Liver
    j. Pancreas
    k. Gall bladder

64. a. Kidneys
    b. Ureters
    c. Urinary bladder
    d. Urethra
65. To be consistent with other questions, maybe just have students identify and not describe function a. Urethra; The outlet for both urine and sperm.
    b. Testis; Male sex gland that produces sperm and secretes testosterone.
    c. Epididymis; Coiled tube that sperm travel through after leaving the testes.
    d. Vas deferens; Tube leading from the epididymus to the seminal vesicle.
    e. Seminal vesicle; Stores sperm and produces semen.
    f. Urinary bladder; Stores urine.
    g. Prostate gland; Secretes fluid into the semen.
    h. Penis; Releases semen.
    i. Rectum; Stores feces.
66. a. Mons pubis
    b. Clitoris
    c. Labia minora
    d. Urethra
    e. Labia majora
    f. Vagina
    g. Anus

Crossword Puzzle

Across
2. Vein
4. Peristalsis
7. Hemoglobin
9. Artery
10. Tissue
12. Cell
13. Immunity

Down
1. Metabolism
3. Menstruation
5. Capillary
6. Digestion
7. Hormone
8. Organ
11. System

Chapter 14

1. 3 years
2. 5 years
3. 7 years
4. 2 months
5. 1 year
6. 3 years

7. 3 months
8. 3 years
9. 8 months
10. 6 months
11. 5 months
12. a. Growth and development occur from the moment of fertilization until death.
    b. The process proceeds from the simple to the complex.
    c. Growth and development occur from the head to the foot and from the centre of the body outward.
    d. Growth and development occur in a sequence, order, and pattern; each stage lays the foundation for the next stage.
    e. Growth and development do not occur at a set pace; some children develop rapidly, and others, slowly.
    f. Each stage of growth and development has its own characteristics and developmental tasks.
13. growth
14. development
15. newborn
16. opposite
17. 8 years
18. Puberty
19. middle age
20. Middle adulthood
21. Preschool
22. 7 years
23. 2 years
24. 10-14 years
25. Birth-4 weeks
26. Young adulthood
27. 8 months
28. 10-14 years
29. 2 1/2 years
30. Adolescence
31. 3 years
32. 8 years
33. Middle adulthood
34. 5 years
35. Middle adulthood
36. Young adulthood
37. 6 years
38. c
39. b
40. a
41. d
42. b
43. d
44. f
45. h
46. b

47. f
48. a
49. I
50. e
51. d
52. c
53. b
54. g
55. e
56. d
57. a
58. c
59. b
60. h
61. f
62. a

Chapter 15

1. a
2. a
3. b
4. b
5. c
6. c
7. b
8. a
9. c
10. a
11. a
12. b
13. b, c
14. a
15. b, c
16. b
17. c
18. d
19. a
20. e
21. f
22. g
23. c
24. c
25. F; The person chooses what to wear; respect the client's clothing routines.
26. T
27. F; Do not judge the person.
28. T
29. T
30. F; Older people have the right to develop new relationships.
31. T
32. F; Respect the client's grooming routines.
33. d

34. c
35. 60/74
36. 75/84
37. old-old
38. a. Separation from children.
    b. Lack of companionship.
39. Sometimes the roles reverse—the child cares for the parent.
40. a. Getting involved in the new activities in the community
    b. Being involved with grandchildren and family
    c. Home care clients can participate in a "friendly visitor" program, and long-term care residents can participate in social activities offered in the facility
41. Women usually live longer than men.
42. a. Physical/mental health problems
    b. The will to live/suicide
43. a. Move away or die
    b. to talk to/speak the same language as others in the community
44. a. Skin breakdowns, tears, and pressure ulcers may result.
    b. Fewer nerve endings affects the ability to sense heat, cold, and pain.
    c. The person may have decreased mobility, thus increasing the risk of falls.
    d. Bones may break easily—sometimes even turning in bed can cause fractures.
    e. Older people may not feel pain when ill or injured and not tend to the illness or injury, or they may not feel heat and burn themselves.
    f. Risk of falls increase. Reduced blood flow to the brain may cause dizziness and fainting. Energy levels, memory, and reflexes are also affected.
45. a. Protect the person from drafts.
    b. Offer socks, sweaters, blankets.
    c. Ask to raise the thermostat setting.
46. a. Activity—Encourage the person to be as active as possible.
    b. Diet—The diet should be rich in protein, calcium, and vitamins.
47. heat/cold
48. a. Musculoskeletal
    b. Integumentary
    c. Nervous
    d. Respiratory
49. eating/digestive
50. decreased kidney function/not drinking enough fluids
51. the bladder muscles/the size of the bladder
52. difficulty urinating/frequent urination
53. adequate fluids

54. To reduce the need to urinate during the night.
55. a. Not covering the client's chest with heavy bed linens
    b. Placing the client in semi-Fowler's position
    c. Encouraging the client to be as active as possible
56. a. holding hands
    b. touching
    c. caressing
    d. embracing
57. c
58. c
59. d
60. b

Chapter 16

1. d
2. a
3. c
4. c
5. a
6. b
7. b
8. c
9. b
10. d
11. a
12. b
13. a
14. b
15. d
16. c
17. g
18. a
19. e
20. g
21. b
22. d
23. c
24. e
25. f
26. a. Do not use baby walkers.
    b. Secure the child using the waist and crotch straps, and lock the tray after securing the child. Keep the highchair away from stoves, tables, and counters.
    c. Keep crib rails up and locked. Check children in cribs often. Make sure there are no toys or soft, fluffy items in the crib; the crib is placed far away from blinds, shades, or drapes; and the mattress fits snugly and is firm.
    d. Never leave live extension cord lying out. Put safety plugs in all unused electrical outlets. Do

not let electrical cords hang down from tables or counters where children could pull on them.

   e. Do not let children wear necklaces, strings, cords, or other items around their necks. Remove or tie up cords or drawstrings on clothing. Tie cords up or use a cord shortener on blinds. Do not hang items with strings, cords, or elastic around cribs or playplens.

   f. Keep all poisonous substances in a high, locked area away from children. Do not store harmful substances in food containers or juice bottles. Keep childproof caps on harmful substances. Put away cleaners immediately after use. Never call medications "candy."

27. a. Always supervise children who are in or near water.

   b. Keep bathroom doors closed to prevent drowning in toilets or bathtubs.

   c. Keep diaper pails locked, and keep sinks, tubs, basins, and buckets empty when not in use.

28. a. Stiff joints and weak muscles—movements are slower and less steady

   b. Poor balance

   c. Less sensitive to heat, smell, taste, and touch

   d. Poor vision and hearing

   e. Memory problems

29. People who are confused, disoriented, drowsy, hearing-impaired, or distracted may answer to any name.

30. Bed rails are used when they are called for in the care plan.

31. *(Any ten answers listed in Box 16-3, p. 173 in the textbook, in any order.)*

32. *(Any ten answers listed in Box 16-5, p. 176 in the textbook, in any order.)*

33. *(Any ten answers listed in Box 16-4, p. 175 in the textbook, in any order.)*

34. *(Any ten answers listed in Box 16-6, p. 177 in the textbook, in any order.)*

35. a. Having written safety policies

   b. Training and educating employees about these safety policies

   c. Creating a health and safety committee to identify workplace hazards and investigate accidents.

   d. Responding to reports of workplace hazards

   e. Warning employees about safety hazards and correcting these hazards whenever possible

   f. Reporting all accidents promptly to the government department responsible for OH&S

   g. Making sure that all necessary equipment is available and in good working order

36. a. Following all safety policies and procedures

   b. Using all recommended protective equipment

and clothing

   c. Reporting all safety hazards and concerns to the supervisor or the health and safety committee

   d. Completing an incident report after an accident

37. *(Any six answers listed in Box 16-8, p. 179 in the textbook, in any order.)*

38. identify recurring problems/revise safety policies as needed.

39. In the material safety data sheet (MSDS).

40. a. The health risks and safety hazards presented by the product.

   b. How to safely handle the product.

   c. How to safety use the product.

   d. How to safely store the product.

   e. How to safely dispose of the product.

   f. First aid measures required in case of an accident or emergency

41. a. Product information

   b. Supplier information

   c. Hazard symbol

   d. Risk phrases that describe the health hazard

   e. Precautionary statements that describe safety measures to take when using the product

   f. First aid measures in case of accident or emergency

   g. Reference to the MSDS

42. roll/cover/smother

43. *(Any six answers listed in Box 16-12, p. 191 in the textbook, in any order.)*

44. Carry the keys in your strong hand and extend one key. If necessary, use this key to slash at the attacker's face.

45. a. Kick

   b. Push your thumbs into the attacker's eyes

   c. Scratch

46. a

47. c

48. d

49. a

50. a

51. a

52. b

53. d

54. b

55. F; An electric plug that is not grounded could cause an electric shock.

56. T

57. T

58. T

59. F; Always position infants on their backs.

60. F; Sound the alarm before attempting to put out a fire.

61. F; Different extinguishers are used for different types of fire.

62. T
63. F; Leave all labeling on containers.
64. F; Check the MSDS before cleaning attempting these tasks.
65. a. The cord is frayed.
    b. It is not grounded with a third prong.

Chapter 17

1. h
2. b
3. e
4. f
5. d
6. c
7. a
8. g
9. F; The least restrictive device is used.
10. T
11. T
12. F; Restraints must not be used to position a person on the toilet.
13. F; Vest restraints are crisscrossed in the front.
14. b
15. a
16. c
17. a
18. c
19. b
20. protect clients from harming themselves or others
21. a. A client tries to pull out an IV and feeding tube. Without these tubes, the client could die.
    b. A client with severe mental illness tries to strangle a staff member.
    c. A child tries to rip out her stitches, thus risking serious infection.
22. Medications used to control behaviour or movement.
23. last resort and less restrictive measures have failed.
24. *(Any twelve in any order.)*
    - Use diversions to calm and distract the client (e.g, TV, music)
    - Encourage the client to follow routines and habits
    - Provide attention and companionship
    - Reduce noise levels and provide a calm, quiet setting
    - Explain procedures and care measures
    - Closely supervise the client
    - Allow the client to wander in a safe area
    - Orient confused clients to people, time, and place
    - Place the call bell within reach

- Meet food, fluid, and elimination needs promptly
- If ordered, help the client use padded hip protectors, pillows, wedge cushions, posture and positioning aids
- Follow safety precautions to prevent falls; if ordered, use floor cushions and roll guards
- Promote uninterrupted sleep

25. false imprisonment charges
26. informed consent/cannot
27. a. every 15 minutes
    b. food/fluid/comfort/elimination
28. combative or agitated clients can hurt themselves and the worker; several workers can apply restraints quickly and safely.
29. Confusion may increase because the person is agitated or doesn't understand what is happening.
30. as short a time as possible
31. Treat the person with kindness, caring, respect, and dignity. Visit the person often, offer repeated explanations and reassurance. Be a good listener.
32. good body alignment/padded/pressure/injury
33. discomfort/agitation/restricted breathing/restricted circulation
34. strangulation
35. a. Remove the restraint
    b. Reposition the client
    c. Meet elimination needs
    d. Give skin care
    e. Perform range of motion exercises or ambulate the client, according to the care plan
    f. Offer food and fluids
36. a. The type of restraint applied
    b. The reason for the restraint
    c. Safety measures taken, as listed in the care plan (e.g., bed rails padded and raised)
    d. The time restraint was applied
    e. The time restraint was removed
    f. The care given when the restraint was removed
    g. Skin colour and condition
    h. The pulse felt in the restrained part
    i. Complaints of a tight restraint, difficulty breathing, and pain, numbness, or tingling in the restrained part

Chapter 18

1. microbes
2. people, animals, food, water, soil, inanimate objects
3. warm/dark/water/nourishment
4. Hold your hands down so that the dirty water washes down the sink and not onto your clean skin.

5. Hand-operated faucets are contaminated, so you would contaminate your hands if you touched them after washing.

6. a. Redness in the area
   b. Swelling of the area
   c. Complaints of pain or tenderness
   d. Fever
   e. Chills
   f. Increased pulse
   g. Increased respiratory rate
   h. Fatigue and loss of energy
   i. Loss of appetite
   j. Discharge from the infected area that may have a foul odour

7. It can exit through the discharge from the wound.

8. Pathogens enter through a portal of entry in the new host—body openings and breaks in the skin or mucous membranes.

9. Caregivers must wash their hands before and after caring for Mr. Fox.

10. The gown should be removed immediately because it is contaminated when wet.

11. after admission to a health care facility

12. a. Respiratory tract
    b. Urinary tract
    c. Gastrointestinal tract
    d. Skin

13. (Any three of the following answers in any order.)
    a. Immediately before and after giving care
    b. Whenever the hands are visibly soiled
    c. After contact with her own or another's blood, body fluids, secretions, or excretions
    d. After touching objects that are contaminated (e.g., soiled linen, garbage bags)
    e. Before and after preparing and handling food
    f. Before feeding the client
    g. Before putting on and after removing gloves
    h. After personal body functions (e.g., going to the bathroom, sneezing)

14. warm or hot water makes organic material thick, sticky, and hard to remove.

15. a. Wear PPEs when cleaning items that may be contaminated with blood, body fluids, secretions, or excretions.
    b. Wash the item with soap and hot water
    c. Scrub the item thoroughly.
    d. Rinse the item in warm water.
    e. Dry the item.

16. reusable items/irritate hands

17. white vinegar/water/vinegar solution

18. boiling water

19. a. Blood
    b. All body fluids, secretions, and excretions (except sweat)

    c. Nonintact skin (skin with open breaks)
    d. Mucous membranes

20. procedures or tasks likely to cause splashes or sprays of blood, body fluids, secretions, or excretions.

21. contaminated

22. Place used disposable sharp items in a puncture-resistant container.

23. The front of the mask.

24. a. Children may be afraid if they cannot see your face.
    b. Clients with confusion or dementia may be afraid if they cannot see your face.

25. (Any seven of the following answers in any order.)
    • Washing hands properly and at appropriate times
    • Assisting clients with hand washing as necessary
    • Cleaning, disinfecting, sterilizing equipment, as appropriate
    • Maintaining personal hygiene
    • Keeping vaccinations up to date
    • Keeping tables, countertops, wheelchair trays, and other surfaces clean and dry
    • Washing contaminated areas with soap and water.
    • Providing for the client's skin care and oral hygiene, according to the care plan
    • Covering nose and mouth when coughing and sneezing. Washing hands afterward.
    • Ensuring clients have their own care equipment, and not sharing items among clients
    • Not taking equipment and supplies from one client's room and using for another client
    • Holding equipment and linens away from the uniform
    • Covering bedpans and commodes with a lid when transporting
    • Avoiding sitting on a client's bed
    • Not using items that have touched the floor
    • Disinfecting tubs, showers, shower chairs, bedpans, urinals, and commodes after each use.

26. tasks and procedures/material that may be highly contaminated

27. gloves (always) and a gown if you will have substantial contact with the person or if the person is incontinent or has diarrhea, an ileostomy, colostomy, or wound drainage.

28. cuts or open areas on your skin, fever, vomiting, diarrhea, sore throat, or a cough

29. (Any five of the following answers in any order.)
    • Wear PPE as required.
    • Collect all needed equipment before entering the room.

- Prevent contamination of equipment and supplies. If anything drops on the floor, do not use it.
- Use mops wetted with a disinfectant solution to clean floors.
- Prevent drafts.
- Use paper towels to handle contaminated items.
- Remove items from the room in sturdy, leakproof plastic bags.
- Double bag items if the outer part of the bag is contaminated.
- Follow employer policy for removing and transporting disposable and reusable items.
- Do not touch your hair, nose, mouth, eyes, or other body parts when providing care.
- Do not touch any clean area if your hands are contaminated.
- Place clean items that you bring in to the room on paper towels.
- Do not shake linen.
- Use paper towels to turn faucets on and off.

30. a. According to employer policy
    b. In a container that is tightly capped
    c. In a container that is puncture-resistant
    d. In a container that is leakproof
31. a. Do not sort or rinse linen in client care areas.
    b. Hold soiled linens away from your uniform.
    c. Remove soiled linens by folding them with the dirties areas in the centre
    d. Linen contaminated with blood, body fluids, secretions, or excretions must be placed in a sturdy, leakproof laundry bag labelled with the biohazard symbol. Wear gloves.
    e. Bag soiled linen in the room where it was used.
32. c
33. b
34. d
35. c
36. c
37. d
38. d
39. a
40. c
41. b
42. c
43. c
44. b
45. d
46. b
47. c
48. a
49. b
50. c
51. a

52. c
53. a
54. c
55. F; Some microbes do not need or get oxygen from the reservoir.
56. F; Microbes thrive in a warm, dark environment
57. T
58. F; The person only needs to wear a clean gown or pyjamas and an isolation gown.
59. T
60. T
61. F
62. F; If a sterile item is below your waist, it is considered contaminated.
63. thumbs, knuckles, sides of hands, little fingers, and under the nails.
64. The outside of the gown and its waist strings
65. The interior 1-inch margin around the sterile field is considered contaminated.

Chapter 19

1. e
2. d
3. b
4. a
5. c
6. e
7. a
8. c
9. d
10. b
11. T
12. F; Similar numbers of women and men report being abused by their partners.
13. T
14. F Slapping is physical abuse.
15. F Financial abuse is the most common for older adults
16. T
17. F; Failing to provide privacy is violating the person's rights and is a form of abuse.
18. T
19. T
20. F; Provide for privacy and safety and then tell your supervisor about the situation.
21. T
22. F Sexual harassment is a form of sexual abuse.
23. F The event that triggers abuse often has nothing to do with the victim.
24. F; People who were abused as children are more likely to abuse their own children.
25. T; However, report the abuse or suspicions of abuse to your supervisor.

26. c
27. a
28. a. Tension-building phase
    b. Abusive phase
    c. Honeymoon phase
29. a. Has problems with alcohol or drugs
    b. Has a mental illness or severe personality flaws
    c. Has been abused as a child
    d. Is going through a period of high stress
30. a. Family crisis
    b. Single-parenting
    c. Isolation
    d. Caring for children with special needs.
31. a. They may fear the abuser.
    b. They may not know where or how to get help.
    c. They may fear being forced to move into a facility if the abuser is the primary caregiver.
    d. They may have physical or mental disabilities that prevent them from reporting.
32. *(The student can think up their own examples; the following are from the text.)*
    • Using restraints inappropriately
    • Handling the client roughly
    • Isolating the client
    • Stealing from the client
    • Not reviewing the care plan regularly
    • Not responding to a call for help
    • Not checking of the client for long periods of time
    • Leaving the client in soiled linen or clothes
    • Violating a client's rights
33. *(Any five of the following answers in any order.)*
    • Swearing, name calling, and using racial or cultural slurs
    • Threats
    • Denial of meal breaks, drinking water, bathroom use, or hand washing facilities
    • Hitting, pushing, kicking, spitting, biting, pinching, or other physical attacks
    • Inappropriate touching
    • Sexual assault or harassment
34. a. Stay calm, and stand up so as not to be dominated by the client, but far enough away so that the person cannot reach you.
    b. Position yourself close a door, and note the location of call bells, alarms, and other security devices.
    c. Keep your hands free, but do not touch the client.
    d. Listen to the client. Restate what the person says in your own words. Do not raise your voice, argue, scold, or interrupt.
    e. Tell the person you will get your supervisor to speak to him or her. In a facility, make sure the

person is safe, then quickly leave the room. Tell a nurse or security officer about the situation. If you cannot leave the room, sound the call bell, alarm, or other security device.
    f. In a client's home, leave the house immediately if you think you are in danger. Go to a safe place, and call your supervisor. If you cannot leave the house and feel threatened, call the police.
35. *(Any three within each context, in any order.)*
    Physical abuse
    • Physical injuries (e.g., burns, bumps, cuts, bruises, etc.)
    • New injuries appear while older ones are still healing
    • Frequent injuries
    • Injuries in the shape of an object (e.g., a welt in the shape of a hand)
    • Unexplained missing or loose teeth
    Sexual abuse
    • Irritation, injury of the thighs, perineum, or breasts
    • Intense fear of bathing or perineal care
    • Torn, stained, or bloody underwear
    • Vaginal discharge, genital odour, and painful urination
    • Difficulty walking or sitting
    • Avoidance of touching
    Emotional abuse
    • A change in behaviour
    • Person seems fearful or withdraw
    • Person's behaviour changes when the caregiver (i.e., the potential abuser) leaves and enters the room
    • The person is not permitted to socialize or has withdrawn from family and friends
    • Caregiver insists on being present or within hearing distance of all conversations
    • Caregiver's behaviour is erratic
    • Caregiver does not show affection toward the person
    • Caregiver often complains about the person
    Financial abuse
    • The caregiver refuses to spend money on caring for the person
    • The person has many unpaid bills
    • There is a lack of adequate food, clothing, personal care items, etc.
    • The caregiver seems more concerned about the cost rather than the quality of the person's care
    • The potential abuser does not have a job and is secretive about his or her income
    • The person must ask for permission to write cheques or spend money

Neglect
- Living conditions are unsafe, unclean, or inadequate
- Personal hygiene is poor (e.g., ingrown nails, untreated sores, matted hair)
- Signs of poor nutrition and fluid intake (e.g., weight loss, sunken eyes, dry skin)
- Pressure sores
- Medications not purchased
- The person is left unsupervised or unattended for long periods of time

36. a. Listen attentively. Recognize the person's feelings.
    b. Reassure the person that you believe him or her. Do not deny or ignore the problem.
    c. Assure the person that you will do what you can to help.
    d. Notify your supervisor at once. You are also legally responsible for reporting child abuse directly to child protection authorities.
    e. Provide emotional support for the person no matter what he or she decides to do. A competent adult may make the informed decision to live with the abuse.
37. a. Physical abuse
    b. Sexual abuse
    c. Neglect
    d. Sexual abuse
    e. Neglect
    f. Emotional abuse>
38. Negligence—U
39. Invasion of privacy—I
40. Assault—I
41. Negligence—U
42. Invasion of privacy—I
43. False imprisonment—I
44. Negligence—U
45. Slander—I
46. Assault—I
47. Battery—I
48. Invasion of privacy—I
49. Slander—I
50. False imprisonment—I

Chapter 20

1. a
2. e
3. d
4. d
5. b
6. d
7. c
8. e

9. T
10. F; Support workers must have the person's permission before throwing away personal items.
11. T
12. T
13. c
14. c
15. d
16. c
17. a
18. the person has pain
19. acute pain
20. a. Past experience with pain lets the person know what to expect, and this can either help or hinder pain management. Not having experience and not knowing what to expect may make the person fearful.
    b. Anxiety can make the pain feel worse.
    c. Not enough rest and sleep can make pain feel worse.
    d. The more attention the person gives to the pain, the worse it feels.
    e. Pain means different things to different people, and they react accordingly. For example, Some see pain as a sign of weakness and therefore try to deny or ignore it.
    f. Pain is easier to deal with when family and friends offer comfort and support.
    g. Culture influences how people respond to pain. For example, in some cultures people show no reaction to pain, and in others, they have strong verbal and nonverbal reactions.
    h. Young children may not know words to express that they are in pain. Changes in behaviour may be the only indicator of pain. Older adults may have decreased pain sensations. Older adults with dementia may not be able to communicate that they are in pain. Changes in behaviour may indicate pain.
21. a. Ask where the pain is. Ask the client to point to the area of the pain.
    b. Ask when the pain started and how long it has lasted.
    c. Ask the client to rate the pain on a scale of 1 to 10.
    d. Ask the client to describe the pain. Write down the person's exact words.
    e. Ask what the client what he or she was doing before the pain started and when the pain started.
    f. Ask if you may check vital signs. Pulse, respirations, and blood pressure often increase with pain.
    g. Ask the client if he or she has other symptoms

that often occur with pain (e.g., dizziness, nausea, weakness)

22. a. Pain may be accepted as the will of God.
   b. Pain may be stoically accepted until very severe.
   c. Pain may be ignored, and pain relief measures may have to be offered more than once before they are accepted.
23. Older adults have decreased pain sensations, so they may not feel pain until it becomes severe. Because pain alerts a person to illness or injury, not being able to feel pain may result in undetected disease or injury.
24. a. Increased pulse, respirations, and blood pressure
   b. Nausea
   c. Pale skin
   d. Sweating
   e. Vomiting
25. *(Any four of the following.)*
   • Keep hospital beds in the lowest position.
   • Follow the care plan for bed rail use.
   • Check on the person every 10 to 15 minutes.
   • Provide assistance when the person is up.
   • Provide heat or cold applications as directed in the care plan.
   • Provide a calm, quiet, darkened environment.
26. 30 minutes
27. a. Direct the person's attention away from the pain (e.g., conversation, music, tv, games)
   b. Means absence of mental or physical stress. The nurse or therapist teaches the person how to breathe deeply and slowly and to contract and relax muscle groups. Make sure the person is in a comfortable position and the room is quiet.
   c. Involves creating an image in the mind and focusing on it. Soft music, a blanket for warmth, and a darkened room may help.
28. The person may tell you about the pain, or the person's body language and behaviour may indicate pain.
29. crying, fussing, change in behaviour
30. Plan care activities so that the person has time to rest without interruptions. Do not rush clients or push them beyond their limits when providing care. Allow rest periods as needed.
31. a. 12-14 hours
   b. 11-12 hours
   c. 8-9 hours
   d. 7-8 hours
   e. 5-7 hours
32. milk, cheese, beef
33. a. Discomfort, pain, nausea, and coughing can hinder sleep. Often clients are awakened for treatment or medication.
   b. Foods and drink with caffeine prevent sleep; certain protein in milk, cheese, and beef promote sleep.
   c. Exercising just before bed may delay sleep.
   d. Most people sleep better in their own beds and in familiar surroundings. A change in the environment, noise, and light and disrupt sleep.
   e. Some medications promote sleep and drowsiness, and others interfere with sleep. Alcohol may make the person drowsy, but then cause the person to wake up and have difficulties falling back to sleep.
   f. Any type of change causes stress and may disrupt sleep.
   g. Fear, worry, anxiety, and depression disrupt sleep.
34. a. Make sure bed linens are clean, dry, and wrinkle-free.
   b. Provide for warmth (blankets, socks).
   c. Reduce noise.
   d. Darken the room.
35. a. Caffeinated drinks (colas, coffee, etc)
   b. Alcohol
36. a. Encourage residents to choose their furnishings.
   b. Encourage residents to display personal items in their rooms.
   c. Help family members arrange the room and hang pictures.
   d. Provide a warm welcome.
37. a. Birth to 1 year.
   b. 65 years and over.
38. a. Higher toilets are easier for people in wheelchairs to use.
   b. They are easier for people with joint problems.
39. refreshments/the staff and roommate/pictures
40. The person's physician, nurse, or social worker
41. a. How the person tolerated the transfer.
   b. Whether a nurse will bring the person's chart and medications.
42. Tell a nurse immediately.
43. c
44. a
45. d
46. b
47. b
48. b
49. a
50. a
51. b
52. b
53. b

54. a
55. a
56. b
57. b
58. d
59. b

Chapter 21

1. Friction
2. Posture
3. Shearing
4. Gait belt
5. Logrolling
6. Supine
7. Lateral
8. Fowler's
9. Sims'
10. Alignment
11. Drawsheet
12. Dangle
13. Prone
14. Wheelchair
15. *(In any order.)*
    - Assess the situation before you begin lifting.
    - Face your work area.
    - Bend and your knees. and hips and squat when lifting or setting down objects below your waist.
    - Tighten your stomach muscles and tuck in your pelvis as you lift.
    - Hold objects close to your body when lifting, moving, or carrying them.
    - Avoid unnecessary bending and reaching.
    - Turn your whole body as one unit when changing the direction of your movement.
    - Push, slide, or pull heavy objects whenever you can, rather than lifting them.
16. Stand with your feet and legs apart for a wide base of support.
17. injury
18. shearing
19. To prevent the head from hitting the headboard when being moved up.
20. *(Any six of the following.)*
    - Check with your supervisor and the care plan about limits or restrictions in moving or positioning for the client.
    - Decide how to move the client and how much help you need before attempting the move.
    - Ask for help before starting the move
    - Communicate directions with your helper by counting 1-2-3, and then moving together.
    - Move the client in small increments.

- Cover and screen the client for privacy.
- Make sure tubes or drainage containers connected to the client are not pulled, tangled, or pinched during the move.
- Position the client in good alignment after the move.
- Make sure linens are wrinkle-free after moving.
21. To limit how much the support worker has to bend and reach.
22. To provide more support for clients with fragile bones and joints.
23. Communicate directions when lifting; count 1-2-3 and then lift together.
24. pain/skin damage/lifted more evenly
25. So that the person is close to you and you do not have to reach and stretch as much when turning.
26. a. Clients with arthritic spines or knees
    b. Clients recovering from hip fractures
    c. Clients with spinal cord injuries
    d. Clients recovering from spinal cord surgery
27. a. Pulse and respirations (if instructed to do so)
    b. Pale or bluish skin colour
    c. Complaints of dizziness, light-headedness, or difficulty breathing
    d. How well the activity was tolerated
    e. The length of time the person dangled
    f. The amount of help needed
    g. Other observations or complaints
28. unsteady/disabled
29. Depends on the client's physical abilities, condition, and size.
30. To promote the client's comfort.
31. They are used when a client cannot help with a transfer.
32. a. You are trained to use the lift.
    b. The lift works
    c. The client's weight does not exceed the lift's weight limit.
33. *(Any nine of the following.)*
    - Check with your supervisor and the care plan for the best position for the client
    - Follow the scheduled times for repositioning the client.
    - Use good body mechanics.
    - Ask for help before beginning the process.
    - Explain the procedure to the client.
    - Be gentle when moving the client.
    - Provide for privacy.
    - Leave the client in good body alignment—use pillows as directed in the care plan for comfort and support.
    - Make sure linens are wrinkle-free.
    - In facilities, place the call bell within the client's reach.

34. a. Promotes comfort and well-being
    b. Makes breathing easier
    c. Improves circulation
    d. Helps prevent many complications (e.g., pressure ulcers and contractures)
35. T
36. F; Hold objects close to your body.
37. F; Bend at your knees and hips and squat when lifting objects from the floor.
38. F Having help also protects the worker from injury.
39. T
40. F; You should be primarily concerned that you transfer the person safely.
41. F; Clients are repositioned at least every 2 hours.
42. a
43. c
44. a
45. Fowler's position
46. Supine position
47. prone/ankles
48. prone/the edge of the mattress
49. the lateral position
50. Sims' position
51. Shoulders, upper arms, hips, and thighs

Chapter 22

1. f
2. g
3. c
4. I
5. a
6. b
7. d
8. e
9. h
10. g
11. J
12. o
13. c
14. n
15. a
16. m
17. h
18. L
19. p
20. I
21. b
22. e
23. f
24. k
25. d
26. a. Some ADL are allowed (e.g., self-feeding, oral hygiene, bathing, shaving, and hair care)
    b. Everything is done for the client. No ADL allowed.
    c. The client can use the bedside commode for elimination needs.
    d. The client can use the bathroom for elimination needs.
27. a. Reduces physical activity
    b. Reduces pain
    c. Encourages rest
    d. Helps the person regain strength
    e. Promotes healing
28. A footboard prevents plantar flexion and footdrop.
29. Trochanter roll
30. A hip abduction wedge keeps the hips abducted (turning away from the midline of the body). It is placed between the client's legs.
31. exercise
32. a. Clients do the exercises by themselves.
    b. Someone moves the client's joints through the range-of-motion exercises.
    c. The client does the exercises with some help from another person.
33. A gait belt (transfer belt)
34. If you try to stop the fall, you could injure the person or fall yourself. Easing the person to the floor lets you control the direction of the fall and protect the person's head.
35. On the strong side
36. a. Move the cane forward 15 to 25 cm
    b. Move the weak leg (which is opposite the cane) forward so that it is even with the cane.
    c. Move the strong leg forward and ahead of the cane and the weak leg.
37. A walker gives more support than a cane, so some people feel safer with a walker than with a cane.
38. 15 to 20 cm
39. d
40. c
41. a
42. b
43. b
44. c
45. d
46. F; Exercise only the joints you are instructed to.
47. T
48. F; Do not force a joint to the point of pain
49. F; The person should wear nonskid street shoes.
50. T
51. F; Attachments on the walker can carry needed items, making the person less dependent on others.
52. a. flexion, extension, hyperextension
    b. abduction, adduction
    c. external rotation, internal rotation

53. a. Supination
    b. Pronation

Crossword Puzzle
Across
4. atrophy
5. pronation
6. contracture
7. rotation
9. extension
10. range of motion
12. supination
13. dorsiflexion
14. syncope
Down
1. footdrop
2. adduction
3. hyperextension
8. abduction
11. flexion

Chapter 23

1. e
2. b
3. d
4. a
5. f
6. c
7. F; Work from cleanest to dirtiest
8. T
9. F; Wear utility gloves
10. F; Because some cleaners scratch surfaces, use special cleaners for the bathroom.
11. T
12. T
13. F; Use only dishwashing detergents in the dishwasher.
14. T
15. F; Items should be soaked for 30 minutes, but only use bleach with the client's permission.
16. T
17. F; Never mix bleach and ammonia—doing so creates a toxic gas.
18. *(Any six of the following.)*
    • Set priorities
    • Set a routine
    • Use your time well—start with tasks that have a waiting period or run automatically, and then go on to other tasks.
    • Finish tasks, and put items away
    • Set time limits for each task
    • Focus on the task
    • Put the client's needs first

19. a. Rinse in cold water.
    b. Soak in a solution of 1 L warm water, 2 mL liquid (hand) dishwashing detergent, and 15 mL ammonia for 30 minutes.
    c. Rinse in cool water.
    d. Soak in a solution of 1 L warm water and 15 mL vinegar for 1 hour
    e. Machine wash with chlorine bleach (with permission) and detergent. Dry as usual.
20. To clean items without damaging them.
21. *(In any order.)*
    • Do not pour dirty or contaminated liquids down the kitchen sink.
    • Use one cloth for counters, another for wiping floors, and another for dishes.
    • Use paper towels to dry your hands.
    • Change cloths daily as needed. Wash in bleach and hot water.
    • Use paper towels when possible.
    • Clean the microwave after every use.
    • Do not put soiled diapers into the kitchen garbage.
22. *(Any five of the following.)*
    • Rinse and dry bar soaps after use.
    • Flush the toilet with the seat down to prevent splashing.
    • Rinse the sink after used for washing, shaving, or oral hygiene.
    • Remove and dispose of hair from the sink, tub, or shower.
    • Hang damp towels and bath mats up to dry.
    • Wash bath mats, the wastebasket, and the laundry hamper every week.
    • Wipe out the bathtub or shower immediately after use.
    • Open shower doors.
    • Do not put dirty or contaminated liquids in the sink. Flush them down the toilet.
23. *(Any six of the following.)*
    • Read all labels carefully.
    • Never mix cleaning products.
    • Wear utility gloves.
    • Never use products in unlabelled containers.
    • Store products in their original containers.
    • Keep cleaning products away from food.
    • Keep cleaning products out of reach of children and adults with dementia.
    • Use products only for their intended purpose.
    • Keep aerosol cans away from heat sources.
    • Ask the client before using a strong cleaner on a surface.
    • Rinse strong, abrasive cleaners immediately after use.
    • Do not scrub vigorously.

24. *(Any six of the following.)*
    - Clear away clutter.
    - Work from higher to lower.
    - Work from far to near.
    - Work from dry to wet.
    - Work from cleanest to dirtiest.
    - Change cloths and water frequently.
    - Use a damp cloth for dusting.
    - Rinse and dry washed surfaces.
    - Avoid soiling a clean area.

Chapter 24

1. a. Top linens are pulled up, and the bedspread is neatly pulled over the pillow.
   b. Top linens are folded back so the client can easily get into bed.
   c. A bed made with the client in it.
   d. Top linens are folded for transferring the client to or from a stretcher.
2. To protect the mattress and bottom linens from dampness and soiling.
3. Plastic retains heat and may make the client uncomfortable; Also, plastic drawsheets are hard to keep tight and wrinkle-free.
4. Shaking bed linens spreads microbes.
5. warmth/privacy
6. a. Make sure the client must is in good body alignment
   b. Know about restrictions or limits in the client's movement or positioning.
   c. Make sure the client knows each step of the procedure before it is done.
7. Making one side of the bed before going to the other saves the worker time and energy.
8. a. Bumper pads must fit snugly against the slats.
   b. They must be secured in place with at least six ties.
   c. The ties must be away from the baby—avoid long ties.
   d. Bumper pads must be removed when the baby can stand in the crib.
9. a. Flat
   b. Fowler's position
   c. Semi-Fowler's position
   d. Trendelenburg's position
   e. Reverse Trendelenburg's position
10. - Bedspread: 7
    - Plastic drawsheet: 3
    - Bath towel: 9
    - Bottom sheet: 2
    - Bath blanket: 13
    - Cotton drawsheet: 4
    - Hospital gown: 12
    - Washcloth: 11
    - Mattress pad: 1
    - Top sheet: 5
    - Pillowcases: 8
    - Blanket: 6
    - Hand towel: 10
11. F; A closed bed is made when the person is up for most of the day.
12. T
13. F; Contact your supervisor.
14. T
15. F; Fanfold the linens to the side of the bed farthest from the door.
16. b
17. b
18. a
19. a. Old cotton drawsheet
    b. Old plastic drawsheet
    c. Old bottom sheet and mattress pad
    d. Clean bottom sheet and mattress pad
    e. Clean cotton drawsheet
    f. Clean plastic drawsheet
20. C, A, B, D

Chapter 25

1. a. 180 cc
   b. 240 cc
   c. 1000 cc
   d. 480 cc
   e. 120 cc
   f. 150 cc
   g. 360 cc
   h. 120 cc
2. a 4
   b. 9
   c. 4
3. 10 months
4. a. Eat a variety of foods
   b. Emphasize cereals, breads, other grain products, vegetables, and fruit
   c. Choose lower-fat dairy products, leaner meats, and foods prepared with little or not fat.
   d. Participate in regular physical activity and healthy eating.
   e. Limit salt, alcohol, and caffeine.
5. 50-100 g
6. India
7. a. Help the person move to a sitting position in bed.
   b. Help the person to the dining room.
8. a. Assist with elimination and hand washing
   b. Change clothing and provide clean linen if necessary

c. Be sure dentures, eyeglasses, and hearing aids are in place.
    d. Assist with menu choices.
    e. Make the setting attractive.
 9. a. May cause difficulty swallowing.
    b. Affects appetite and enjoyment of food.
    c. Makes digestion of fried and fatty foods difficult, and may cause indigestion.
    d. Can affect chewing.
    e. Results in slower emptying of the stomach and colon, causing flatulence and constipation.
10. Cooked fruits and vegetables
11. a. So the person does not feel rushed
    b. To show caring and respect
    c. Spoons are less likely to cause injury than are forks
    d. This portion is easy to chew and swallow
    e. Fluids help with chewing and swallowing
    f. To show caring and respect
    g. To show that you have time to spend with the person; also, facing the client allows you to observe for choking and for problems with chewing and swallowing
    h. To encourage independence
12. a. clear-liquid
    b. high-fibre
    c. high-calorie
    d. fat-controlled/low-cholesterol
    e. High-protein
13. water/heart
14. fruits and vegetables
15. a certain blood sugar level
16. The food is puréed.
17. a. low fluid intake
    b. vomiting
    c. diarrhea
    d. bleeding
    e. excess sweating
    f. increased urine production
18. 1500 mL
19. 2000 to 2500 mL
20. To keep the mucous membranes of the mouth moist.
21. *(In any order.)*
    • Grain products 5-12 servings/day
    • Vegetables and fruit 5-10 servings/day
    • Milk products 2-4 servings/day
    • Meat & alternatives 2-3 servings/day
22. a. Grain
    b. Meat and alternatives
    c. Vegetables and fruit
    d. Vegetables and fruit
    e. Meat and alternatives
    f. Milk products

g. Other foods
    h. Grain products
    i. Vegetables and fruit
    j. Milk products
23. a. decrease/fewer calories are needed
    b. increase/to aid in digestion, kidney function, chewing and swallowing
    c. Increase/for tissue growth and repair
    d. Increase/to prevent constipation
    e. Decrease/these are hard to digest
    f. Increase/to aid in chewing and swallowing <In next edition, this question should be revised to avoid implying that all older adults should eat pureed foods, etc)
24. b
25. b
26. d
27. b
28. d
29. F; Tissues swell if too much sodium is retained.
30. F;
31. T
32. F; Foods high in sodium are omitted.
33. T
34. F; Snacks are also necessary
35. T
36. T
37. T
38. e
39. a
40. c
41. b
42. d
43. c
44. g
45. e
46. J
47. I
48. a
49. b
50. d
51. f
52. h
53. b
54. d
55. e
56. a
57. c
58. f
59. *Label the plate as per page, 379 (number each segment so it looks like the face of a clock).*
    a. At 6:00 and 7:00
    b. Between 12:00 and 1:00

Chapter 26

1. T
2. F; Formula is given at room temperature.
3. T
4. F; The client needs frequent oral hygiene to relieve dry mouth and dry lips.
5. F Central venous sites are the subclavian vein and the internal jugular vein.
6. a
7. c
8. a
9. d
10. a. Through the nose into the stomach (nasogastric tube)
    b. Through the nose into the small intestine (nasointestinal tube)
    c. Into the stomach through a surgically created opening (gastrostomy tube)
    d. Into the intestines through a surgically created opening (jejunostomy tube)
    e. Into the stomach through a surgically created opening and an endoscop is through the mouth and into the stomach (percutaneous endoscopic gastrostomy [PEG] tube)
11. a Cancers of the head, neck, and esophagus
    b. coma
    c. dysphagia caused by paralysis
    d. trauma or surgery to the face, head, mouth or neck
    e. dementia
12. a coughing
    b. sneezing
    c. vomiting
    d. suctioning
    e. poor positioning
13. a Insert feeding tubes
    b. Test the position of the tube
    c. Give the first dose of a tube feeding
14. 4/400/20
15. electronic feeding pump
16. semi-Fowler's/1 to 2 hours/regurgitation
17. a. To relieve dry mouth
    b. To relieve dry lips
    c. To relieve dryness of the nasal passages
    d. To relieve dryness
18. This position prevents the stomach from emptying.
19. a. Nausea
    b. Discomfort during the tube feeding
    c. Vomiting
    d. Diarrhea
    e. Distended abdomen
    f. Coughing

g. Complaints of indigestion or heart burn
h. Redness, swelling, drainage, odour, or pain at the ostomy site
i. Elevated temperature
j. Signs and symptoms of respiratory distress
k. Increased pulse rate
l. Complaints of flatulence

20. a. Receive fluids
    b. Receive minerals and vitamins
    c. Receive sugar for energy
    d. Receive medications and blood
    e. Receive hyperalimentation (a solution highly concentrated with nutrients)
21. a. Back of the hand, forearm, or crease of the elbow
    b. On the head
    c. In the subclavian vein or the internal jugular vein
    d. The cephalic or basilic veins in the arm
22. a. Practice Standard Precautions
    b. Do not move the needle or catheter
    c. Follow the safety measures for restraints if the nurse restrains the extremity to prevent movement the needle or catheter from moving
    d. Protect the IV bag, tubing, and needle or catheter when ambulating the client
    e. Assist the client with turning and repositioning.
    f. Move the bag to the side of the bed on which the person is lying, allowing enough slack in the tubing
    g. Notify your supervisor immediately if bleeding occurs from the insertion site.
    h. Notify your supervisor immediately if you notice signs or symptoms of complications
23. a. Bleeding
    b. Puffiness or swelling
    c. Pale or reddened skin
    d. Complaints of pain at or above the IV site
    e. Hot or cold skin near the site
    f. Fever
    g. Itching
    h. Drop in blood pressure
    i. Tachycardia
    j. Irregular pulse
    k. Cyanosis (bluish skin colour)
    l. Changes in mental function
    m. Loss of consciousness
    n. Difficulty breathing
    o. Shortness of breath
    p. Decreasing or no urine output
    q. Chest pain
    r. Nausea
    s. Confusion

Chapter 27

1. b
2. b, d
3. d
4. a, b, d, c
5. b, c
6. d
7. a. Upon awakening
   b. After each meal
   c. At bedtime
   d. Before meals (if the client wishes)
8. a. Illness and disease
   b. Some medications and diseases
   c. Some medications and diseases
   d. Oxygen, smoking, decreased fluid intake, anxiety
9. 3
10. *(In any order.)*
    • Dry, cracked, swollen, or blistered lips
    • Redness, swelling, irritation, sores, or white patches in the mouth or on the tongue
    • Bleeding, swelling, or redness of the gums
    • Loose teeth
    • Rough, sharp, or chipped areas on dentures
    • Complaints of pain or discomfort
11. To make the surface soft so that if that dentures are dropped, they will not break.
12. warp
13. To prevent them from drying out and warping.
14. a. To remove plaque and tartar from the teeth
    b. To remove food particles from between the teeth
15. on one side with the head turned well to the side/aspiration
16. a. To clean the skin and mucous membranes of the genital and anal areas
    b. To remove microbes, dead skin, perspiration, and excess oils
    c. To refresh and relax the client
    d. To stimulate circulation and exercise body parts
17. care plan
18. a. They do not understand what is happening or why
    b. They may fear harm or danger
19. a. Not rushing the person
    b. Using a calm, pleasant voice
    c. Diverting the person's attention
    d. Calming the person and trying again later
20. a. To prevent making the water soapy and to reduce the risk of slips and falls in the tub or shower
    b. To remove all soap residue and prevent irritation
    c. Pat, rather than rub, to gently dry the skin and

avoid damaging it
    d. To remove microbes and prevent skin irritation
21. a. Reduce drafts by closing doors and windows
    b. Use a bath blanket to cover the person before and after the bath
22. under the breasts, under the arms, in the groin area, and sometimes between the toes
23. The powder can cake and crust, causing skin irritation.
24. infants, young children, and older adults/fragile skin
25. a. Dry the bathroom or shower room floor
    b. Check hand rails, grab bars, hydraulic lifts, and other safety aids. They must be in working order.
    c. In tubs or showers without a nonskid surface, place a bath mat inside.
    d. Place needed items within the person's reach
    e. Place the call bell with the person's reach.
    f. Have the person use safety bars when getting in and out of the tub or shower. The person must not use towel bars for support.
    g. Do not use bath oils because they make the surfaces slippery.
    h. Keep bar soap in the dish to prevent the person from slipping on it.
    i. Do not leave weak or unsteady people unattended.
    j. Stay within hearing distance if the person can be left alone.
26. *(Any eight of the following.)*
    • The colour of the skin, lips, nail beds, and sclera
    • The location and description of rashes
    • Dry skin
    • Bruises or open skin areas
    • Pale or reddened areas, particularly over bony parts
    • Drainage or bleeding from wounds or body openings
    • Swelling of the feet and legs
    • Corns or calluses on the feet
    • Skin temperature
    • Complaints of pain or discomfort
27. a. Face
    b. hands
    c. Underarms
    d. Back
    e. Buttocks
    f. Perineal area
28. the spread of microbes and infection
29. a. The client is unconscious
    b. The client is paralyzed
    c. The client is in a cast or traction
    d. The client is weak from illness or surgery

30. This temperature will keep the person warm but will not burn or scald the person.
31. a. Placing a bath towel over the chest area.
    b. Lifting the towel slightly.
    c. Reaching under the towel to wash the breasts and chest.
32. a. Certain heart diseases
    b. Back injuries
    c. Back surgeries
    d. Skin diseases
    e. Some lung disorders
33. urethral area/anal area
34. *(Any three of the following.)*
    a. Odours
    b. Redness, swelling, discharge, or irritation
    c. Complaints of pain, burning, or other discomfort
    d. Signs of urinary or fecal incontinence
35. d
36. d
37. a
38. b
39. b
40. a
41. c
42. a
43. d
44. T
45. F; Follow the care plan and the client's preferences
46. T
47. F; They are used to keep the skin soft and prevent drying
48. T
49. See Figure 27-1, p. 402 in the textbook
50. See Figure 27-9, page 415 in the textbook
51. See Figure 27-24, page 427 in the textbook

Chapter 28

1. tangles
2. a. Use a wide-tooth comb
   b. Wet the hair or use petroleum jelly to make combing easier
   c. Begin at the neckline and comb upward, lifting and fluffing hair outward. Continue until you reach the forehead.
3. a. Support the back of the client's head with one hand and shampoo with the other. If the person must lean forward, have the person place a folded washcloth over the eyes, and support the forehead with one hand as you shampoo with the other.
   b. Make sure wheelchair is securely locked in

place. If the person is leaning back over the sink, place a folded towel over the sink edge to protect the neck. Give the person a folded washcloth to hold over the eyes. Use assistive devices or a shampoo rinse tray.
   c. Lock the stretcher wheels and use the safety straps. Follow the care plan for side rail use. Place a folded towel over the edge of the sink. Help the person tilt his or her head over the edge of the sink. Place a folded washcloth over the person's eyes.
   d. Place a shampoo tray under the client's head to protect linens and mattress. Place a folded washcloth over the person's eyes.
4. Ask your supervisor for permission.
5. people with limited range of motion in their necks and upper backs
6. Razor blades can cause nicks and cuts. Follow Standard Precautions to prevent contact with blood.
7. oil gland secretion increases during puberty, and so they tend to have oily hair
8. plastic garbage bags
9. Apply a warm washcloth or face towel to the face for a few minutes
10. a. Apply direct pressure to the nick or cut.
    b. Report the nick or cut to your supervisor at once.
11. Do not treat corns, bunions, or blisters.
12. a. Harbour microbes
    b. Provide a warm, moist environment for the growth of microbes.
    c. Cause blisters or ingrown nails
    d. Prolongs healing. Foot infections and injuries can therefore become very serious for someone with poor circulation.
    e. Cause poor circulation
    f. Can cause nicks, cuts, and other injuries
13. Gangrene/amputation
14. Right after soaking them or bathing
15. *(Any four of the following.)*
    a. Very dry skin
    b. Food odours
    c. Cracks or breaks in the skin, especially between the toes
    d. Ingrown nails
    e. Loose nails
    f. Reddened, irritated, or calloused areas on the feet, heels, or ankles
    g. Drainage or bleeding
    h. Change in colour or texture of nails, especially black, thick, or brittle nails
    i. Corns, bunions, or blisters
16. 5 (Remove pullover), 3 (Remove garments that

open in front), 1 (Cover the person), 4 (Undo buttons), 6 (Remove pants), 2 (Remove garments that open in back)
17. c
18. b
19. b
20. b
21. b
22. c
23. b
24. g
25. f
26. J
27. e
28. I
29. a
30. d
31. h
32. F; How one's hair look affects emotional well-being.
33. T
34. F; Begin at the end of the hair and gently comb through. Working up to the scalp, add small sections of hair.
35. T
36. F; Older people need to shampoo less frequently because of decreased oil gland secretion.
37. T
38. F; The skin should be held taut.
39. F; Fingernails should only be trimmed with nail clippers, never with scissors.

Chapter 29

1. 1500 mL per day
2. a. at bedtime
   b. after getting up in the morning
   c. before meals
3. a. Increase urine production
   b. Decreases urine production
   c. Cause red-coloured urine
   d. Cause bright yellow urine
   e. Cause a change in urine odour
4. a. By clients in casts
   b. By clients in traction
   c. By clients with limited back motion
   d. By clients with fragile bones or painful joints
   e. After a hip fracture
5. To hook to the bed rail or other place within the client's reach
6. Running water, flushing the toilet, or playing music can mask the sound.
7. call bell/toilet tissue
8. a. Offer the person something to read

   b. Allow the person enough time
9. perineal/wash his or her hands
10. To protect against contacting urine or feces.
11. flow back into the bladder/infection
12. Adhesive tape does not expand, so blood flow to the penis could be restricted and thus injure the penis.
13. In a spiral part way around the penis
14. *(Any ten of the following.)*
    • Record the person's voidings
    • Answer all calls for assistance promptly
    • Promote normal urinary and bowel elimination
    • Encourage urination at scheduled intervals
    • Follower the person's bladder training program
    • Encourage the person to wear clothing that is easy to remove
    • Encourage the person to do pelvic muscle exercises, as directed by the care plan
    • Help prevent urinary tract infections by providing adequate fluids, encouraging the person to wear cotton undergarments, and providing perineal care as needed.
    • Decrease fluid intake before bedtime
    • Provide good skin care
    • Provide dry garments and linens
    • Observe for signs of skin breakdown
    • Use incontinence produces as directed by the care plan
15. a. urinary tract infections, nervous system disorders, bladder cancer, diabetes
    b. weakened pelvic floor, enlarged prostate, some medications, immobility, restraints, unanswered calls for help, confusion, difficulty removing clothing, certain surgeries
16. Skin irritation, breakdown, and infection
17. Voluntary control of urination
18. a. The person attempts to urinate within 15 or 20 minutes at scheduled times.
    b. If the person has a catheter, it is clamped to prevent urine from draining out of the bladder. Usually the catheter is clamped for 1 hour at first, and then is clamped for 3 to 4 hours at a time. When the catheter is removed, voiding is encouraged every 3 to 4 hours or as directed by the care plan.
19. voiding/into the stream of urine
20. The urine is chilled on ice or refrigerated during the collection period to prevent the growth of microbes.
21. To see if there are stones in the urine.
22. dysuria
    a. urinary tract infection
    b. trauma
    c. urinary tract obstruction

23. hematuria
    a. kidney disease
    b. urinary tract infection
    c. trauma
24. nocturia
    a. excessive fluid intake
    b. kidney disease
    c. prostate disease
25. oliguria
    a. inadequate fluid intake
    b. shock
    c. burns
    d. kidney disease
    e. heart failure
26. polyuria
    a. drugs
    b. excessive fluid intake
    c. diabetes
    d. hormone imbalance
27. An artificial opening between the ureter and the abdomen.
28. a
29. c
30. b
31. a
32. b
33. b
34. a
35. c
36. F; You should pratise medical asepsis and Standard Precautions.
37. T
38. F; A fracture pan would be the most comfortable.
29. T
40. F; A clean container is adequate.
41. F; Label it with the person's full name, address, or room and bed number, date, and time.
42. T
43. F; Place the specimen container in a plastic bag for transportation to the laboratory.
44. See Figure 29-11, pg. 479 in the textbook (note the position of the arrow).
    a. Increases or decreases in the amount of urine (after emptying drainage bag)
    b. Complaints of pain, burning, need to urinate, or irritation.
    c. Colour, clarity, and odour of urine
    d. Presence of particles
45. a. Catheter
    b. Drainage tubing
    c. Safety pin, to secure the drainage tubing on the bed
    d. Drainage bag
    e. Clamp

46. To prevent the tubing from looping below the drainage bag. If the tubing fell below the drainage bag, the urine would not be able to flow into the drainage bag.
47. The catheter is taped to the man's abdomen to prevent movement of the catheter and friction at the insertion site.

Crossword Puzzle
Across
4 Glysocsuria
6 Polyuria
7 Catheter
9 frequency
10 hematuria
11 dysuria
13 micturition
14 acetone
Down
1 Oliguria
2 Nocturia
3 Catheterization
5 Voiding
8 Urgency
12 Urination

Chapter 30

1. feces
2. enema
3. ileostomy
4. defecation
5. peristalsis
6. ostomy
7. suppository
8. flatus
9. stool
10. diarrhea
11. chyme
12. stoma
13. a. bleeding in the stomach
    b. Bleeding in the lower colon or rectum; also, beets
    c. A diet high in green vegetables
14. a. Abnormalities in colour
    b. Abnormalities in amount
    c. Abnormalities in consistency
    d. Abnormalities in odour
    e. Abnormalities in shape
    f. Abnormalities in size
    g. Abnormalities in frequency
    h. Complaints of pain
15. Feces become hard and dry when fluid intake is poor.

16. Bacterial action causes the stools' odour.
17. *(Any three of the following.)*
    - Abdominal discomfort and swelling
    - Cramping
    - A feeling of fullness or pain in the rectum
    - Nausea or vomiting
    - Fever
    - Increased need or decreased ability to urinate
    - Liquid feces seeping from the anus
18. a. A low-fibre diet
    b. Ignoring the urge to defecate
    c. Decreased fluid intake
    d. Inactivity
    e. Medications
    f. Aging
    g. Certain diseases
19. *(Any six of the following.)*
    - Assist the client to the toilet or commode, or provide the bedpan, as soon as requested.
    - Wheel the client into the bathroom on the commode if possible, to provide privacy.
    - Provide for privacy (Ask visitors to leave the room, close doors, pull privacy curtains, and close window curtains, blinds, or shades)
    - Make sure the bedpan is warm.
    - Position the client in a normal sitting or squatting position.
    - Cover the client for warmth and privacy when using a bedpan.
    - Allow enough time for defecation. Do not rush the client.
    - Place the call bell and toilet tissue within reach.
    - Stay with the client if he or she is weak or unsteady.
    - Leave the room if the client can be alone, but stay within hearing distance.
    - Provide perineal care.
    - Dispose of stood promptly.
    - Assist the client with hand washing after elimination.
    - Follow the care plan if the client has fecal incontinence.
    - Follow Standard Precautions.
20. a. Skin irritation
    b. Skin breakdown
    c. Pressure ulcers
21. Promptly respond to all requests for help using the bathroom, bedpan, or commode.
22. dehydration
23. a. Abdominal cramping or pain.
    b. Shortness of breath
    c. Swollen abdomen, or "bloating"
24. a. To gain control of bowel movements
    b. To develop a regular pattern of elimination,

thus preventing fecal impaction, constipation, and fecal incontinence
25. meal/breakfast
26. defecation
27. a. To remove feces
    b. To relieve constipation or fecal impaction
    c. To clean the bowel of feces before certain surgeries or X-ray procedures
    d. To relieve flatulence and intestinal distension
28. Add 5 to 10 mL of table salt to 500 to 1000 mL of tap water.
29. By irritating and distending the rectum.
30. You have given enough when the return solution is clear and free of feces.
31. Usually about 40.5 degrees C for adults.
32. saline
33. Remind the person not to flush the toilet.
34. If you release pressure, the solution would be drawn from the rectum back into the bottle.
35. The pouch collects feces and flatus.
36. feces is present/balloons or bulges with flatus
37. 3-7 days, and whenever it leaks
38. a. Provide good hygiene
    b. Empty the pouch
    c. Encourage the client to avoid gas-forming foods
    d. Put deodorants into the pouch, according to the care plan
39. before breakfast
40. The feces in the small intestine contain digestive juices that are very irritating to the skin.
41. Specimens are taken immediately to the laboratory when the test requires a warm stool sample.
42. Blood in stools that cannot be detected by simply looking.
43. d
44. b
45. b
46. a
47. b
48. d
49. a
50. a
51. a
52. b
53. d
54. c
55. c
56. c
57. a. 30 cm
    b. 45 cm
58. 7.5 to 10 cm
59. Sims' position

Chapter 31

1. *(Any six of the following.)*
   - A cough that goes on for more than two weeks
   - Blood in the stool
   - Any change in bowel habits
   - Indigestion that continues more than a few days
   - Unexplained aches and pains that go on for more than two weeks
   - Difficulty urinating or blood in the urine
   - Unexplained bleeding of any sort
   - Any lump or mass
   - A sore that does not heal
   - A new growth on the skin
   - Patches of skin that bleed, itch, or are red
   - Any change in moles or birthmarks

2. Radiation therapy can cause skin breakdown, so the physician may order special skin care procedures.

3. a. Discomfort
   b. Nausea and vomiting
   c. Fatigue
   d. Anorexia (loss of appetite)
   e. Diarrhea
   f. Skin breakdown

4. range of motion in the hips and knees

5. Because pain occurs with weight-bearing and joint motion.

6. a. Physicians may order aspirin for pain
   b. heat or cold applications may be ordered
   c. Obese people may be advised to lose weight
   d. A low-fat, low-calorie diet may be ordered
   e. A cane or walker may be used for support

7. juvenile rheumatoid arthritis

8. a. Maintain joint motion
   b. Control pain
   c. Prevent deformities

9. the person turns in bed or gets up from a chair

10. *(Any five of the following.)*
    - Limb looks bent or out of position
    - Pain
    - Swelling
    - Limited movement of limb or loss of function
    - Bruising and colour changes in the skin at the fracture site
    - Bleeding (internal or external)

11. a. a pressure ulcer could have developed, or there could be poor circulation or nerve damage
    b. reduced blood flow to the part
    c. reduced blood flow to the part
    d. reduced blood flow to the part
    e. infection
    f. pressure on a nerve
    g. pressure on a nerve
    h. cool skin means poor circulation; hot skin means inflammation
    i. infection
    j. infection

12. *(Any four of the following.)*
    - Do not cover the cast with blankets, plastic, or other material
    - Turn the client as directed by the care plan.
    - Do not place a wet cast on a hard surface
    - Support a wet cast with your palms when turning and positioning the client
    - Protect the client from rough cast edges
    - Keep a plaster cast dry
    - Do not allow the client to insert anything into the cast
    - Elevate a casted arm or leg on pillows
    - Have enough help when turning and repositioning the client
    - Position the client as directed by your supervisor and the care plan

13. a. Healing is slower for older people
    b. Older people are at risk for life-threatening postoperative complications (e.g., pneumonia)

14. *(Any six of the following.)*
    - Meet basic needs if the client is confined to bed, and prevent complications of bed rest
    - Transfer, turn, and reposition the person as directed
    - Keep the operated leg abducted at all times
    - Prevent external rotation of the hip
    - Provide range-of-motion exercises as directed
    - Provide a straight-backed chair with armrests
    - Place the chair on the unaffected side
    - Do not let the person stand on the affected leg unless allowed by the physician
    - Support and elevate the leg as directed when the person is in a chair
    - Apply elastic stockings as directed
    - Remind the person to not cross the legs while seated

15. a. body image
    b. daily activities
    c. work

16. *(Any seven of the following.)*
    - •Hemiplegia
    - Weakness on one side of the body
    - Loss of face control
    - Changing emotions
    - Difficulty swallowing
    - Dimmed vision or loss of vision
    - Loss of ability to speak or understand others
    - Changes in sight, touch, movement, and thought
    - Impaired memory
    - Urinary frequency, urgency, or incontinence

17. a. Assist with activities of daily living
    b. Encourage the client to do as much as possible
    c. Meet basic needs if the client is confined to bed; prevent complications of bed rest
    d. Assist with bladder or bowel training programs
    e. Assist with range-of-motion exercises
    f. Provide emotional support and encouragement
    g. Report any changes in the person's mood or behaviour
18. These help improve or maintain strength, posture, balance, and mobility.
19. a. activities of daily living
    b. promoting normal elimination
    c. speech
    d. movement
20. a. Conditions during birth
    b. Being shaken
    c. Childhood diseases
    d. Accidents
21. smoking
22. upright and slightly forward
23. Repeated attacks can damage the respiratory system.
24. a. Provide adequate fluids
    b. Position the person in Fowler's or semi-Fowler's position
    c. Assist with oxygen therapy, as needed
25. Airborne droplets
26. a. Standard Precautions
    b. Airborne Precautions
27. a. Flushed down the toilet
    b. Placed in a biohazard bag and disposed of following facility policy
28. a. Blood pressure tends to rise with age, beginning at about age 35
    c. Hypertension is more common among Canadians of South Asian, Aboriginal, and African descent
    d. If a parent has hypertension, the adult child has a greater change of also developing it; if both parents have hypertension, the risk increases even more
    e. The risk increases if the weight is stored around the abdomen
    f. Repeated exposure to stress may raise blood pressure levels
    g. May contribute to hypertension
    h. Excessive alcohol consumptionincreases blood pressure
29. a. the heart may enlarge
    b. blood vessels in the brain may burst and cause a stroke
    c. Blood vessels in eyes may be damaged
    d. Blood vessels in kidneys (and other organs)

may be damaged
30. a. Lack of exercise
    b. Excessive weight
    c. Smoking
    d. Excessive alcohol
    e. Stress
31. *(Any four of the following.)*
    • Pain on the left side that may travel (radiate) to the jaw, neck, shoulders, back, and/or arms
    • Shortness of breath
    • Nausea
    • Sweating
    • Dizziness or lightheadedness
    • Fatigue
    • Palpitations
32. a. Avoiding physical exertion
    b. Resting when the pain begins
    c. Avoiding stress
    d. Avoiding other triggers (extreme cold or heat, heavy meals, alcohol, smoking)
    e. Taking nitroglycerin
    f. Bypass surgery
33. *(Any seven of the following.)*
    • Sudden, severe chest pain, usually on the left side
    • Pain described as crushing, stabbing, or squeezing
    • Pain that radiates to the neck and jaw, and down the arm or to the sides
    • Pain that is more severe and lasts longer than angina
    • Pain that is not relieved by rest and nitroglycerin
    • Indigestion
    • Shortness of breath
    • Nausea or vomiting
    • Dizziness
    • Perspiration
    • Cyanosis
    • Cold and clammy skin
    • Low blood pressure
    • Weak and irregular pulse
34. a. Confusion and behaviour changes
    b. Low urine output
    c. Weight gain, swelling in feet and ankles, enlarged neck veins
35. *(Any five of the following.)*
    • Meet basic needs if the client is confined to bed; prevent complications of bed rest
    • Measure intake and output
    • Measure daily weight
    • Restrict fluids as ordered by the physician
    • Assist with transfers or ambulation
    • Assist with self-care activities

- Maintain good positioning and body alignment according to the care plan
- Apply elastic stockings to reduce leg swelling
36. Older adults usually have fragile skin. Combined with tissue swelling and poor circulation associated with CHF, this makes them at high risk for skin breakdown.
37. Provide good skin care and regular position changes
38. 2000-3000 mL
39. a. Measure and record urine output every hour
    b. Measure and record intake and output
    c. Restrict fluid intake
    d. Weigh the person daily using the same scale
    e. Provide frequent oral hygiene
    f. Meet basic needs if the client is confined to bed; prevent complications of bed rest
    g. Prevent infections
40. Up to one year. However, some people do not recover and develop chronic renal failure.
41. slowly destroyed
42. wastes and excess water from the blood
43. a. Limit fluids
    b. Measure blood pressure in the supine, sitting, and standing positions
    c. Measure weight daily with the same scale
    d. Use bath oils, lotions, and creams on the skin to prevent itching
    e. Provide frequent oral hygiene
    f. Encourage rest
    g. Meet basic needs if the client is confined to bed, and prevent complications of bed rest
44. a. Type 1 diabetes. Occurs most often in children and young adults.
    b. Type 2 diabetes. Usually develops in adulthood.
    c. Gestational diabetes. Develops during pregnancy.
45. Blindness, kidney disease, nerve damage, sexual dysfunction, circulatory disorders, stroke, heart attack, slow wound healing
46. Because a small injury on the foot may not heal (due to poor circulation and slow wound healing). This could lead to infection and gangrene. Amputation may be necessary.
47. *(Any eight of the following.)*
    - Nausea, vomiting, and abdomen pain
    - Dark urine
    - Jaundice
    - Light-coloured stools
    - Muscle pain
    - Drowsiness
    - Irritability
    - Itching

- Diarrhea
- General aching in the joints, accompanied by redness and swelling
48. gloves when assisting with perineal care, when cleaning incontinent clients, and when handling bedpans and rectal thermometers/Standard Precautions
49. a. Unprotected intercourse with an HIV-infected person
    b. Needle-sharing among IV drug users
    c. HIV-infected mothers to their babies at birth or during breastfeeding
    d. When infected body fluids come into direct contact with broken skin (not including saliva, tears, urine, sweat)
    e. Needlestick injuries
50. a. Swollen glands in the armpits, groin, neck; Red, brown, pin, or purplish blotches on the skin or inside the mouth, nose, or eyelids
    b. White spots or unusual blemishes on the tongue, in the mouth, or in the throat
    c. Memory loss, confusion, dementia
    d. Rapid weight loss, diarrhea that lasts for more than a week
51. AIDS reduces the person's ability to fight infections.
52. genital area, rectum, ears, mouth, nipples, throat, tongue, eyes, and nose
53. STDs
54. a. Hunger
    b. Vision changes
    c. Headach
    d. Rapid pulse
    e. Low blood pressure
    f. Confusion
    g. Convulsions
    h. Loss of consciousness
55. cancer
56. Emphysema
57. Multiple sclerosis
58. Stroke
59. Parkinson's disease
60. b
61. a
62. b
63. a
64. b
65. a
66. b
67. b
68. a
69. b
70. a
71. b

72. F; Stiffness often occurs after the person has not moved for a period
73. F; RA destroys connective tissue throughout the body, including connective tissue of the heart, lungs, eyes, kidneys, and skin.
74. T
75. F; Arthroplasty relieves pain and restores joint mobility, but does not cure arthritis.
76. T
77. F; Move the person slowly and gently to prevent fractures.
78. F; Protect from falls because the person is at risk for fractures.
79. T
80. T
81. F; Stroke occurs when brain cells are suddenly deprived of oxygen and nutrients.
82. F; Not all people with Parkinson's will have impaired mental function (but they still need to be treated with dignity and respect).
83. F; MS is a chronic and progressive disease.
84. T
85. F TB is caused by airborne droplets.
86. F; Anyone who has close, frequent contact with a person with TB is at risk.
87. F; Angina occurs when coronary arteries narrow or are blocked, causing the heart muscle to get insufficient oxygen. Chest pain occurs.
88. F; Inactivity (rest) usually relieves chest pain; activity triggers angina.
89. T
90. T
91. T
92. F Eventually all body systems are affected by chronic renal failure.
93. T
94. F; People infected with HIV can transmit the virus.
95. c
96. b
97. c
98. b
99. b
100. b
101. d
102. a
103. a
104. See Figure 31-8, p. 535 in the textbook (left diagram—shaded from the neck down)
105. See Figure 31-8, p. 535 in the textbook (right diagram—shaded from the waist down)

Chapter 32

1. c
2. a
3. b
4. a. To restore function to former levels
   b. To improve functional abilities
   c. To learn new skills
   d. To prevent further disability and illness
5. to be like the missing body part in function and/or appearance
6. splints, foot supports, and knee and back braces
7. a. Hospitals
   b. Specialized facilities
   c. Long-term care facilities
   d. Community care (e.g., home care and adult day programs)
8. *(Any eight of the following.)*
   • Acquired brain injury
   • Alcoholism
   • Amputation
   • Brain tumour
   • Burns
   • Cerebral palsy
   • Chronic obstructive pulmonary disease
   • Mental illness
   • Heart attack
   • Parkinson's disease
   • Spinal cord injury
   • Spinal cord tumour
   • Stroke
   • Substance abuse
9. To prevent further disability and illness
10. An electric toothbrush may make brushing the teeth easier for a person who has limited arm movement.
11. a. Allow the client to practice skills in private. Provide privacy for care procedures and elimination. Keep information about clients confidential
    b. Allow for personal choice whenever possible. Ask clients about their preferences.
    c. Focus on the positive. Remind clients of their progress, and stress their abilities and strengths. Be a good listener, and provide emotional support and encouragement. Be patient, and offer praise when even a little progress is made.
    d. Never force clients to do more than they are able. Allow time to rest. Follow the care plan for safety measures for each client. Keep the client in good alignment. Use safe transfer methods. Perform range-of-motion exercises as directed. Turn and position the client as directed. Report signs and symptoms of complications (e.g., pressure ulcers, contractures,

elimination problems, and depression). In facilities, make sure the call bell and overbed table are on the client's unaffected side.

e. Encourage the client to perform activities of daily living as independently as possible. Allow time for the client to complete the tasks. Be familiar with the client's self-help devices, and encourage their use whenever necessary. Practise the methods developed by the rehabilitation team when assisting the client. Practise the task the client must perform.

12. To identity any safety risks or health hazards and make the necessary changes to make the home more appropriate for the client.

13. F; A disability affects the whole person—the person's physical, emotional, social, intellectual, and spiritual dimensions

14. T

15. F; Because of the changes associated with aging, rehabilitation often takes longer for older adults than for other people.

16. T

17. F; Changes in the rehabilitation plan are made as needed.

Chapter 33

1. *(Any four of the following.)*
   - Biological factors
   - Childhood trauma or conflict
   - Social and cultural factors (e.g., poverty, discrimination, social isolation)
   - Stressful life events (e.g., death of loved one, divorce)
   - Poor physical health or disability

2. a. Psychoanalysis
   b. Behaviour therapy
   c. Group therapy
   d. Family therapy

3. a. Psychosis
   b. Delusions
   c. Hallucinations
   d. Paranoia

4. *(Any four of the following.)*
   - Feeling sad, "blue," or hopeless
   - Irritability
   - Reduced interest in almost all activities
   - Significant weight gain or loss, without dieting
   - Insomnia or too much sleep
   - Too much or too little motor activity
   - Fatigue or loss of energy
   - Feelings of worthlessness or guilt
   - Reduced ability to concentrate or think
   - Difficulties making decisions

   - Recurrent thoughts of death
5. a persistent thought or desire
6. the uncontrollable urge to perform an act
7. People sometimes act on obsessive ideas in order to deal with the recurring thought. (e.g., People obsessed with the idea that germs are on their hands will often wash their hands repeatedly.)
8. delusion of grandeur (unless, of course, the person is the prime minister!)
9. depression and mania
10. depression
11. bulimia/vomiting
12. The person takes diruretics to try to lose weight.
13. Schizrenia
14. anxiety
15. bipolar disorder
16. antisocial personality
17. d
18. c
19. c
20. c
21. a
22. d

Chapter 34

1. b
2. d
3. c
4. b
5. a, b
6. a
7. b
8. a
9. b
10. b
11. c
12. a
13. a
14. c
15. b
16. b
17. c
18. a
19. c
20. a
21. d
22. c
23. f
24. b
25. g
26. g
27. a
28. d

29. g
30. b
31. c
32. f
33. a
34. d
35. g
36. c
37. e
38. a. Memory loss that affects daily activities
    b. Confusion
    c. Problems finding the right words or following conversations
    d. Poor judgment
    e. Problems with common tasks
    f. Changes in mood, behaviour, or personality
    g. Loss of interest in activities or hobbies
39. older adults/physical
40. 65
41. AD impairs cognitive function and behaviour, thus the person does not recognize safety hazards. AD also causes movement and gait problems, increasing the risk of falls. <Change Alzheimer's disease to dementia>
42. a. Forgetfulness
    b. Problems finding words, finishing thoughts, following directions, and remembering names
    c. Poor judgment
    d. Occasional confusion
    e. Lack of spontaneity—less outgoing or interested in things
    f. Blames others for mistakes, forgetfulness, and other problems
    g. Irritable or defensive
    h. Problems performing everyday tasks
43. a. People with dementia often walk away, not knowing where they are going or how to get back. They may wander into traffic, become lost, or be at risk for heat or cold exposure.
    b. Sundowning is when signs, symptoms, and behaviours of dementia increase during hours of darkness. After the sun goes down, confusion, restlessness, anxiety, and agitation increase.
    c. Seeing, hearing, or feeling something that is not real.
    d. False beliefs. Delusions can cause intense fear or other emotions in the person.
    e. Extreme responses. The person acts as if there is extreme danger, a disaster, or tragedy.
    f. The person may fidget, pace, hit, or yell.
    g. The person may hit, pinch, grab, bite, or swear. They may result from agitation and restlessness.
    h. People in later stages of dementia may have poor communication skills and be very confused. They may scream to communicate.
    i. Sexual behaviours involve the wrong person, the wrong place, and the wrong time. Sometimes, people with dementia cannot control behaviour. They may undress or masturbate in public.
    j. People with dementia sometimes repeat themselves over and over. For example, they may ask the same question repeatedly, or fold the same napkin repeatedly.
44. By overstimulating the client (e.g., overwhelming the client with instructions or choices, or rushing the client).
45. a. Providing a calm, quiet setting
    b. Playing soft music
    c. Having the client wear his or her hearing aids and eyeglasses
    d. Having a family member or favourite caregiver comfort and calm the client
    e. Using touch to calm the client
46. Encourage the client's sexual partner to show affection; if the client masturbates in public, lead the client to his or her room and provide for privacy and safety. Notify your supervisor if the client repeatedly touches his or her genitals because this may be a sign of infection or pain.
47. a. The person may be tired or hungry
    b. The person may be frightened by poor light or shadows.
    c. The person may be afraid of the dark.
48. The person may become agitated or aggressive. Or the person may scream.
49. a. They cannot meet the person's needs
    b. Family members have their own health problems
    c. The person's behaviours present a danger to self or others
    d. The person no longer knows the family or caregiver
50. a. speak clearly and slowly
    b. you are going to do and why
    c. directions and answers to questions
    d. large numbers in the person's room and in other areas
    e. familiar objects and pictures within view
    f. clear and simple / to respond
    g. a calm, relaxed
    h. holidays, birthdays, and special events
51. a. Open curtains, shades, and drapes during the day
    b. Close them at night.
    c. Encourage the person to wear regular clothes during the day, not sleepwear

52. Follow a schedule for meals, bathing, exercise, TV, and other activities./This promotes a sense of order and what to expect.
53. Adult children who care for their own children and their parents are called the sandwich generation.
54. The person would not likely look for locks in these places. Therefore, these prevent the person from wandering away.
55. The person often cannot understand or follow reason.
56. F; Orient the person to date and time often.
57. T
58. F; Do not rearrange furniture or belongings; this may increase confusion
59. F; Delirium is a temporary, acute state of confusion
60. T
61. T
62. F; People with dementia cannot control their behaviours or what is happening to them.
63. F; Alzheimer's disease progresses at a different rate for different people.

Chapter 35

1. *(Any five of the following.)*
   - Genetic problems or conditions present at birth
   - Brain injury, which may be caused by accident, infection, drug abuse, stroke, and so on
   - Disease
   - Hearing loss
   - Brain tumours
   - Problems involving the structures used for speech
2. a. Receptive aphasia. Difficulty understanding language
   b. Expressive aphasia. Difficulty speaking or writing
   c. Expressive-receptive aphasia. Difficulty speaking and understanding language
3. inability to move the muscles used to speak/cannot control lip, jaw, or tongue movements and therefore cannot make the desired sounds and words
4. Difficulty speaking clearly because of weakness or paralysis in the muscles used to speak/usually have slurred, slow and soft speech and often have problems forming words, spacing their words, and breathing while speaking
5. *(Any four of the following.)*
   - Frustration
   - Depression
   - Anger
   - Low self-esteem
   - Shame
   - Guilt
6. *(Any four of the following.)*
   - Address questions and comments to the client, not to others who are present
   - Do not force a client to talk in front of others
   - Never show impatience, frustration, or worry when a client is having problems speaking or understanding
   - Encourage communication
   - Limit the number of choices to help the client express preferences
   - Be encouraging and supportive
   - Keep private information confidential
   - Learn to be comfortable with silence
   - Take extra time to explain procedures; do not explain all the steps at once.
   - Speak slowly and clearly
   - Be alert to signs the client has not understood you
7. *(Any six of the following.)*
   - Minimize distractions
   - Adjust the lighting; make sure the person can see your face clearly and that you can see the person's
   - Give the client your full attention; sit close by and face the person
   - Ask the client questions to which you know the answer; this helps you become familiar with the client's speech
   - Determine the subject being discussed; look for nonverbal clues
   - Follow the client's lead; change your communication method as needed
   - Speak slowly, clearly, and in a normal tone of voice
   - Give the client time to respond; do not answer your own questions
   - Use simple words and short sentences; focus mainly on action words and words for people, places, and things.
   - Be patient; repeat yourself as needed
   - Use positive statements
   - Use appropriate questioning and paraphrasing techniques; ask questions that require only a short answer or shake of the head, and summarize in your own words what the person has said
   - Provide cues as needed; encourage the use of gestures and pointing
   - Try other communication methods; follow the care plan and use writing and communication boards as needed
8. F; Most people with dementia have aphasia.
9. T

10. F; They are aware of their mistakes because they can understand what they are saying.
11. T
12. F; Speech disorders affect family relationships.
13. F; Routine tasks like shopping and cooking may be impossible for some people with speech and language disorders.
14. F; You still need to focus on communicating with these clients. Many require extra time and attention.
15. F; Allow the client time to answer questions and finish words.
16. T
17. F; Aphasia is often permanent.
18. a

Chapter 36

1. c
2. b
3. d
4. a
5. tired/lie down (You seem tired. Do you want to lie down?)
6. a. Because they cannot follow conversations. They may be afraid of embarrassing themselves by giving a wrong response.
   b. Because they cannot hear if someone else has something to say.
   c. Because they are under continual stress trying to compensate for their hearing loss.
7. a. Alert the person to your presence
   b. Adjust the lighting so the person can see your face for lip reading
   c. Reduce background noise
   d. Focus your attention on the client; stand or sit on the side of the unaffected ear, and do not do other tasks while speaking to the client
   e. Speak in a normal tone of voice; do not shout, and do not cover your mouth when talking
   f. Check communication aids; make sure the person is wearing hearing aids and eyeglasses, if used
   g. Adjust your language; state the topic of conversation clearly, and use simple words and short sentences; say things in a different way if the person does not understand you
   h. Use other communication methods (e.g., use body language or write key words on paper)
   i. Watch for signs of fatigue; avoid tiring the person
8. a. Check if the hearing aid is on.
   b. Check the battery position.
   c. Insert a new battery if needed.

d. Clean the ear mould if necessary.
9. a. Wash glass lenses with warm water and dry with a soft tissue. Use special cleaning solutions, tissues, and cloths to clean and dry plastic lenses.
   b. Store glasses in their case.
10. a. Wash the eye with mild soap and warm water. Rinse well.
   b. Line a container with a soft cloth or piece of gauze.
   c. Fill the container with water or a saline solution.
   d. Place the eye in the container. Close the container.
   e. Label the container with the client's name and room number
   f. Place the container in the drawer in the bedside stand or in another safe place as directed by the client.
   g. Wash the eye socket with warm water or saline. Use a washcloth or gauze square. Use a gauze square to remove excess moisture.
   h. Wash the eyelid with mild soap and warm water. Clean from the inner to the outer part of the eye. Dry the eyelid.
11. blind
12. *(Any six of the following.)*
   • Adjust the lighting to avoid glare; stand or sit in good light.
   • Alert the client to your presence; identify yourself when you enter the room, and tell the person when you are leaving the room.
   • Focus your attention on the client; do not turn or walk away while talking, and not do other tasks.
   • Speak in a normal tone; speak slowly and clearly, and do not cover your mouth when talking.
   • Assist with walking. Walk slightly ahead of the person at a normal pace. Offer your arm, and tell the person which are you are offering. Tell the person when you are approaching curbs or steps. Tell when you will step up or down. Inform the person of doors, turn, furniture, and other obstructions. Give specific directions (e.g., "on your left").
   • Assist with eating. Read menus to the person. Use the face of a clock to describe the location of the food on a plate. Or, guide the person's hand to each item on the tray. Cut meat, open containers, butter bread, and perform other activities as needed.
   • Provide a safe setting. Keep walkways clear and free of clutter. Keep doors opened or

closed, never partially opened. Do not re-arrange the furniture without the person's permission. Always replace items where you found them. Orient the person to a new setting. Describe the layout. Keep the call bell within reach.

13. Glaucoma
14. Ménière's disease
15. Cataract
16. c
17. b
18. b
19. d
20. d

Chapter 37

1. a
2. b
3. b
4. b
5. c
6. d
7. d
8. c
9. Doing so helps the baby feel loved and secure.
10. Keep one hand on the baby at all times. Gather all supplies before beginning the diaper change.
11. *(Any thirteen of the following.)*
    - Jaundice
    - Redness or drainage around the cord stump or circumcision
    - High temperature
    - Limpness and slowness to respond
    - Screaming or crying for a long time
    - Flushed or pale skin
    - Heavy perspiration
    - Rash
    - Noisy, rapid, difficult, or slow respirations
    - Coughing or sneezing
    - Reddened or irritated eyes
    - Turning head to one side or putting a hand to one ear (signs of an ear infection)
    - Not eating
    - Vomiting most of the feeding or between feedings
    - Hard, formed stools
    - Frequent watery, green, mucousy, or foul-smelling stools
    - Signs of dehydration (i.e., few than 6 wet diapers a day, dark yellow urine, decreased saliva and tears, dry lips, dry and wrinkled skin, sunken eyes and top of head)
    - Stiff neck

12. a. Wash your hands and remind the mother to wash hers.
    b. Help the mother to a comfortable position.
    c. Change the baby's diaper if necessary. Bring the baby to the mother.
    d. Offer to bring the mother a glass of water or juice.
    e. Offer the mother a blanket to cover the baby and herself.
    f. Help the mother burp the baby.
    g. Change the baby's diaper after the feeding if necessary.
    h. Lay the baby in the crib if the baby is asleep.
    i. Record what time the baby nursed and how long on each side. Report any problems or concerns.
13. a. Ready-to-feed formula. This is poured directly from the can into the baby bottle.
    b. Powdered formula. Add water according to the directions on the container.
    c. Concentrated formula. Add water according to the directions on the container.
14. *(Any nine of the following.)*
    - Place the bottle in a bowl of warm water until the formula feels warm to your wrist.
    - Tilt the bottle to check the flow of formula dropping out of the nipple.
    - Assume a comfortable position for feeding.
    - Hold the baby close to you.
    - Tilt the bottle so that the neck of the bottle and the nipple are always filled.
    - Do not prop the bottle and lay the baby down for the feeding.
    - Burp the baby when he or she has taken about half the formula. Also burp the baby at the end of the feeding.
    - Do not expect the baby to always finish all the formula. The feeding is over when the baby stops sucking and turns away from the bottle.
    - Discard remaining formula.
    - Wash the bottle, cap, and nipple after the feeding.
15. The baby is fed when he or she shows signs of hunger.
16. Washed thoroughly in hot, soapy water or in a dishwasher.
17. a. Hold the baby over your shoulder and gently pat or rub the baby's back.
    b. Support the baby in a sitting position on your lap. If under 3 months, support the baby's head and neck by cupping your hand under the baby's chin. Gently pat or rub the baby's back.
18. Tell your supervisor immediately/Because diarrhea can quickly upset the baby's water balance

and harm the baby.
19. Wash with mild soap and warm water.
20. Fold a cloth diaper in front for boys/Fold the diaper in the back for girls
21. a. Keeping the cord dry.
    b. Washing your hands before and after contact with the umbilical area.
    c. Keeping the cord clean. Gently wipe around the base of the cord with a cotton ball moistened with warm water.
    d. Keeping the top of the diaper below the cord.
    e. Reporting any signs of infection (e.g., redness, odour, drainage from the cord)
    f. Giving sponge baths until the cord falls off.
22. To allow for good hygiene and to possibly prevent certain cancers.
23. You cannot leave the baby to gather supplies after starting the bath. Therefore, all supplies must be gathered before beginning the procedure.
24. a. Never leave the baby alone on a table or in the bathtub.
    b. Hold the baby securely throughout the bath.
    c. Room temperature should be 24 to 27 degrees C. Turn up the thermostat and close windows and doors for 20 minutes before the bath.
    d. Water temperature must be between 37.8 and 40.6 degrees C. Measure bath temperature with a thermometer or test with the inside of your wrist.
25. At the beginning of the bath.
26. So that the babies do not scratch themselves or others
27. So that the baby does not squirm or fuss.
28. a. Fever of 38 degrees C or higher
    b. Chills, poor appetite, fatigue, nausea, or vomiting
    c. Lochia that soaks a sanitary pad within 1 hour of application
    d. Foul-smelling lochia
    e. Large number of clots in the lochia
    f. Painful, burning, or difficult urination
    g. Severe abdominal or perineal pain
    h. Bleeding, redness, swelling, or drainage from a cesarean-section incision
    i. Leg pain, tenderness, or swelling
    j. Breast pain, tenderness, or swelling
    k. Feelings of depression
29. cesarean section
30. T
31. F; Never warm bottles in a microwave because the formula could heat unevenly and burn the baby's mouth.
32. T
33. F; Diapers are also changed when they are wet.
34. F; Discard disposable diapers in the garbage, never in the toilet.
35. T
36. T
37. T

Chapter 38

1. a. Intellectual disabilities
   b. Down syndrome
   c. Cerebral palsy
   d. Autism
   e. Epilepsy
   f. Spina bifida
   g. Fetal alcohol syndrome
2. *(Any six of the following.)*
   • Abnormal genes inherited from one or both parents
   • Missing or extra chromosomes
   • Alcohol or drug use by the mother when pregnant
   • Poor nutrition
   • Exposure of the pregnant mother to certain environmental hazards (e.g., x-rays)
   • Illnesses of the mother during pregnancy (e.g., German measles)
   • Uncontrolled medical conditions in the pregnant mother (e.g., diabetes)
   • Premature birth
   • Low birth weight
   • Lack of oxygen to the baby during birth
   • Childhood disease (e.g., chickenpox)
   • Infections (e.g., meningitis)
   • Acquired brain injury (e.g., caused by accidents, disease, or abuse)
   • Severe malnutrition or neglect
3. intellectually disabled
4. Shaking the baby
5. a. live in families and be integrated into regular schools whenever possible.
   b. others who do not have disabilities
   c. to the fullest extent possible
   d. community/make choices and decision about their care and how they live
   e. love and be loved
   f. sexual abuse/sexuality issues
6. *(Any seven of the following.)*
   • Small head
   • Oval-shaped eyes that slant upward
   • Flat face
   • Short, wide neck
   • Large tongue
   • Wide-flat nose
   • Small ears

- Short stature
- Short, wide hands with stubby fingers
- Weak muscle tone
7. a. heart defects
   b. vision and hearing problems
   c. ear infections, respiratory infections, and thyroid gland problems
8. a. speech therapy
   b. language therapy
   c. physical therapy
   d. occupational therapy
9. a. are premature
   b. have a low birth weight
   c. do not cry in the first 5 minutes after birth
   d. need mechanical ventilation
   e. have bleeding in the brain
   f. have heart, kidney, or spinal cord abnormalities
   g. have blood problems
   h. have seizures
10. a. near drownings
    b. choking
    c. suffocation
    d. stroke
11. a. Movement is stiff and jerky. One or both sides of the body may be involved.
    b. Movement is involuntary and involves constant, slow weaving or writhing motions in the trunk, arms, hands, legs, and feet.
    c. weak muscle tone and difficulty coordinating movement
12. eating, writing, dressing, walking, moving
13. a. Intellectual disability
    b. Learning disability
    c. Hearing impairments
    d. Speech impairments
    e. Vision impairments
    f. Bowel and bladder control problems
    g. Seizures
    h. Attention deficit hyperactivity disorder
    i. Breathing problems
14. a. Communication
    b. Social skills
    c. Behaviour
15. a. Poor speaking skills
    b. Repeating words or phrases
    c. Not starting or maintaining conversation
    d. Repeating body movements
    e. Spending time alone
    f. Showing little reaction to pain
    g. Over-reacting to noise and touch
    h. Disliking cuddling
    i. Having frequent tantrums for no apparent reason
    j. Forming strong attachment to a singe item,

idea, activity, or person
    k. Needing routines
    l. Not fearing danger
    m. Not responding to others
    n. Being very active or very quiet
    o. Displaying aggressive or violent behaviour
16. a. Behaviour modification
    b. Speech and language therapy
    c. Music, auditory, recreation, and sensory therapies
    d. Occupational therapy
    e. Medication therapy
    f. Diet therapy
17. a. Foot weakness and bowel and bladder problems
    b. rarely causes impairments
    c. Leg paralysis and lack of sensation; bowel and bladder control impairments
18. a. The head will enlarge, which increases pressure on the brain
    b. intellectual disabilities
    c. Neurological damage
19. b
20. c
21. a
22. d
23. T
24. F; People with developmental disabilities have reproductive organs and sexual urges.
25. F; The degree of impairment differs with each individual.
26. T
27. T
28. F; Posture, balance, and movement are affected by spastic cerebral palsy
29. T
30. F; There is no cure for autism, but therapies can help the person control behaviours.
31. T
32. T
33. b
34. c

Chapter 39

1. d
2. f
3. h
4. a
5. i
6. e
7. j
8. c
9. b

10. g
11. F; An elixir is medication dissolved in a liquid containing alcohol or water and flavourings
12. F; The nurse or pharmacist teaches the person about side effects.
13. F; It is never the support worker's responsibility to fill pill boxes.
14. F; Apply water-soluble lubricant to suppositories. Do not use petroleum jelly because it is not water-soluble.
15. T
16. T
17. T; However, you may be assigned to sign the MAR on behalf of homecare clients who cannot do so for themselves.
18. T
19. F; Support workers may not purchase OTC medications for clients.
20. T
21. *(Any five of the following.)*
    • Reminding the client to take a medication
    • Bringing medication containers to the client
    • Bringing pre-poured medications, pre-filled syringes, or pill boxes to the client
    • Reading the prescription label to the client
    • Loosening or removing container lids or opening blister packs
    • Checking the dosage against the medication label
    • Providing water or other fluids as needed
    • Supervising the client as he or she pours the medication into hand, measuring spoon, or cup
    • Steadying the client's hand while he or she pours medications or administers eye drops, nasal sprays, and so on
22. an unwanted response that occurs along with the wanted response to the medication
23. a. The client's name
    b. The name, dose, and administration instructions for each medication
    c. A place to sign or initial after administering the medication
24. a. Oral. Taken by mouth and swallowed.
    b. Sublingual. Placed under the tongue and dissolved or absorbed into the body
    c. Topical. Applied to the skin or mucous membranes.
    d. Inhalant. Breathed in through the mouth or nose.
    e. Parenteral. Injected by needle into the muscle, a vein, or under the skin.
25. a. In a special place just for the person's medications.
    b. In a dry, cool place

c. Out of reach of adults with dementia and children
d. In the original labelled container, with the lid tightly closed
e. According to any special storage instructions
26. a. The right medication
    b. The right person.
    c. The right dose
    d. The right route
    e. The right time
27. a. Ointments, e.g., eye cream
    b. syrups, e.g., cough syrup
    c. Drops, e.g., nose drops
28. a. Ask the person to put the medication under the tongue
    b. Ask the person to close mouth and let the medication dissolve
    c. Remind the person not to chew or swallow the medication
    d. Do not give food or fluids while the medication is dissolving
29. a. Pharmacy name
    b. Date filled
    c. Expiration date
    d. Physician's name
    e. Times prescription can be refilled
    f. Drug name and dose
    g. Patient's name
    h. File number

Chapter 40

1. P
2. P
3. BP
4. BP
5. BP
6. BP
7. P
8. P
9. a
10. b
11. c
12. b
13. c
14. b
15. b
16. d
17. b
18. c
19. *(Any nine of the following.)*
    • During physical exams
    • When a person is admitted to a facility
    • Several times ad ay for hospital patients and

patients in subacute care units
- Before and after surgery
- Before and after complex procedures or diagnostic tests
- After certain care measures, such as ambulation
- After a fall or other injury
- When medications are taken that affect the respiratory or circulatory system
- Whenever the client complains of pain, dizziness, light-headedness, shortness of breath, rapid heart rate, or not feeling well
- As often as required by the client's condition
- As stated in the care plan (usually daily or weekly)

20. a. Is unconscious
    b. Has had surgery or an injury to the face, neck, nose, or mouth
    c. Has a nasogastric tube
    d. Is delirious, restless, confused, or disoriented
    e. Is paralyzed on one side of the body
    f. Has a sore mouth
    g. Has a convulsive disorder
    h. Is receiving oxygen therapy
21. a. Sides of the head
    b. Sides of the neck
    c. Inside of the elbows
    d. Wrists
    e. Top of inner thighs
    f. Knees
    g. Ankles
    h. Chest
22. a. Birth to 1 year
    b. 6 to 12 years
    c. 2 to 6 years
    d. 12 years and older
23. ear
24. 5 to 10 minutes
25. To prevent the spread of microbes
26. Do not let anything touch the tubing, and ask the client to be silent.
27. a. Elevated body temperature (caused by fever or exposure to hot environments)
    b. Exercise
    c. Pain
    d. Position change (pulse rate increases when a person sits or stands after lying down)
    e. Caffeine
    f. Emotions (excitement, fear, anger, anxiety)
    g. Medications (some increase pulse rate; others decrease it)
28. rhythm and force
29. You could mistake the pulse in your thumb for the client's pulse.
30. So that the client does not know that you are

counting respirations. Therefore, the client will not change breathing pattern.
31. a. Blood pressure increases with age, up to adulthood
    b. Women usually have lower blood pressures than men.
    c. The lower the blood volume, the lower the blood pressure (e.g., severe bleeding lowers blood pressure).
    d. Increases blood pressure.
    e. Usually increases blood pressure. However, severe pain causes shock, which significantly lowers the blood pressure.
    f. Increases blood pressure.
    g. Blood pressure is higher in overweight people.
    h. Blood pressure tends to be higher among people of South Asian, Aboriginal, and African descent.
    i. A high sodium diet increases the amount of water in the body. The extra fluid volume therefore increases blood pressure.
    j. Some medications raise blood pressure; others lower it.
    k. Blood pressure is lower when a person is lying down. It is higher when a person is standing. Sudden changes in position can cause changes in blood pressure. Standing suddenly may cause a sharp drop in blood pressure.
    l. Increases blood pressure.
    m. Increases blood pressure.
32. Measure the person's height while he or she is lying in bed.
33. A full bladder affects the weight.
34. top of the head/heels
35. *(Any twelve of the following.)*
    - Do not take blood pressure on an arm with an IV infusion, cast, or dialysis access site; an injured arm; or on the side where the client has had breast surgery.
    - Let the client rest for 10 to 20 minutes before measuring blood pressure.
    - Measure blood pressure with the client sitting or lying down (unless ordered otherwise by the physician).
    - Use the correct sized blood pressure cuff.
    - Apply the cuff to the bare upper arm.
    - Make sure the cuff is snug.
    - Place the diaphragm of the stethoscope firmly over the artery. The entire diaphragm must be in contact with the skin.
    - Make sure the room is quiet.
    - Have the manometer clearly visible.
    - Measure the systolic and diastolic pressures. The first sound is the systolic pressure. The

point where the sound disappears is the diastolic pressure.
- Take the blood pressure again if you are not
  sure of an accurate measurement. Wait 30 to
  60 seconds before repeating the measurement.
- Notify your supervisor at once if you cannot
  hear the blood pressure.
- Know the normal blood pressure ranges for
  the client. Immediately report any blood pressure measurement outside of the client's
  normal range.

36. a. 30-60 respirations/minute
    b. 20-30 respirations/minute
    c. 25-32 respirations/minute
    d. 12-20 respirations/minute
37. T
38. T
39. F; The hand-held unit is kept in a battery charger
    when not in use.
40. F; Subtract the radial pulse from the apical pulse
41. a. Earpieces
    b. Binaurals
    c. Rubber or plastic tubing
    d. Bell
    e. Chestpiece
    f. Diaphragm
42.

43.

44.

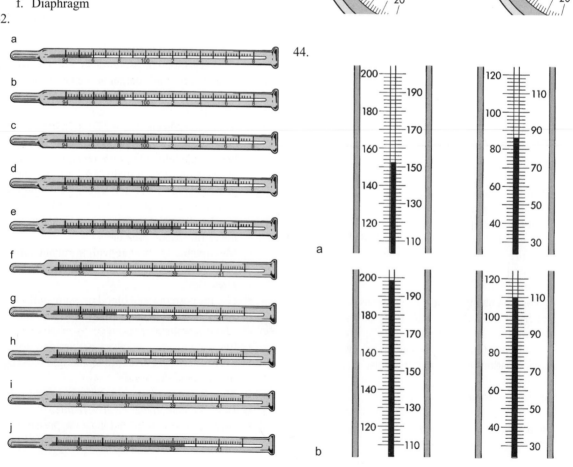

45. a. 101.4 degrees F
    b. 99.6 degrees F
    c. 97.2 degrees F

Crossword
Across
  2 Apical radial pulse
  5 Blood pressure
  6 Hypotension
  8 Stethoscope
  9 Bradycardia
  10 Respirations
  12 Hypertension
  13 Tachycardia
Down
  1 Diastole
  3 Pulse
  4 Sphygmomanometer
  7 Vital signs
  11 Systole

Chapter 41

1. f
2. a
3. h
4. k
5. c
6. b
7. g
8. e
9. d
10. I
11. J
12. c
13. a
14. b
15. d
16. c
17. b
18. c
19. a
20. d
21. a
22. b
23. c
24. b
25. c
26. c
27. a
28. b
29. a
30. poor blood return through the veins
31. A break or rip in the skin.
32. The hands, arms, and lower legs are common sites

for skin tears.
33. *(Any five of the following.)*
    • Keeping the skin moisturized.
    • Offering fluids.
    • Dressing and undressing the client carefully.
    • Dressing the client in soft clothing with long sleeves and long pants.
    • Keeping your fingernails short and smoothly filed.
    • Keeping the client's fingernails short and smoothly filed.
    • Not wearing rings with raised or large stones.
    • Following safety guidelines when lifting and transferring clients.
    • Preventing friction and shearing during lifting, moving, transferring, and repositioning (e.g., using a lift sheet).
    • Using pillows to support arms and legs.
    • Being patient and calm when the client resists care.
    • Padding bed rails and wheelchair arms, footrests, and leg supports.
    • Providing good lighting to help prevent the client from bumping into furniture or walls.
34. a. Pressure
    b. Friction
    c. Shearing
35. circulatory ulcers
36. shearing/blood vessels/tissues
37. a. Use proper lifting, positioning, and transferring procedures
    b. Do not raise the head of the bed more than 30 degress.
    c. Apply a thin layer of cornstarch to the bottom sheets.
38. *(Any five of the following.)*
    • Are confined to a bed or chair
    • Require moderate to complete help in moving
    • Have loss of bowel or bladder control
    • Have poor nutrition
    • Have altered mental awareness
    • Have problems sensing pain or pressure
    • Have circulatory problems
    • Are older
    • Are obese or very thin
39. is in contact with skin/friction
40. To reduce pressure on the heels by raising them off the bed.
41. the plastic does not touch the skin.
42. Soap can dry and irritate the skin.
43. moisture from urine, stool, perspiration, and wound drainage
44. a. To prevent skin from being in contact with skin
    b. To reduce moisture and friction
45. a. pale skin

b. A warm, reddened area
46. a. Lower legs
    b. Feet
47. a. High blood pressure
    b. Diabetes
    c. Aging
    d. Smoking
48. Dehiscence/evisceration
49. a. Is the wound red and swollen?
    b. Is the area around the wound warm to touch?
    c. Are sutures, staples, or clips intact or broken?
    d. Are wound edges closed or separated? Did the wound break open?
50. When large amounts of drainage are expected, a drain is applied to enable the drainage to leave the wound.
51. *(Any five of the following.)*
    • They protect wounds from injury and microbes.
    • They absorb drainage.
    • They remove dead tissue.
    • They promote comfort.
    • They cover unsightly wounds.
    • They provide a moist environment for wound healing.
    • When bleeding is a problem, pressure dressings help control bleeding.
52. a. Apply tape to the top, middle, and bottom of the dressing.
    b. Extend the tape several centimeters beyond each side of the dressing.
53. Paper and plastic tapes.
54. Wound odours, appearance, and drainage may be unpleasant and cause nonverbal reactions. Control nonverbal reactions so that you do not make the client ashamed, worried, or upset.
55. a. To remove tape, hold the skin down and gently pull the tape toward the wound. Remove adhesive from the skin.
    b. To remove dressings, lift the dressing very gently, and keep the soiled side of the dressing out of the person's sight.
56. a. Support wounds
    b. Hold dressings in place
    c. Reduce or prevent swelling by promoting circulation
    d. Promote comfort
    e. Prevent injury
57. a. After abdominal surgeries—to provide abdominal support and hold dressings in place.
    b. After breast surgeries—to support the breast after surgery.
    c. After rectal and perineal surgeries—to secure dressings in place.
58. a. Allow pain medications to take effect before giving care.
    b. Odours from wound drainage can take away appetite. Therefore, remove soiled dressings promptly from the room. Use room deodorizers as directed. Keep drainage containers of the client's sight. Tell your supervisor if the client has a taste for certain foods or beverages.
    c. Practice Standard Precautions. Carefully observe the wound. Immediately report any signs or symptoms of infection.
59. b
60. b
61. b
62. b
63. b
64. b
65. a
66. c
67. a
68. F; Never rub or massage reddened areas.
69. F; People in chairs should be reminded to shift their weight every 15 minutes.
70. F; Never rub vigorously. Always gently pat the skin.
71. T
72. F; Tape must never encircle a body part.
73. T
74. F; Never force the person to look at the wound.
75. F; Wear gloves when changing a dressing.
76. See Figure 41-1, A, p. 678 in the textbook
77. See Figure 41-1, B, p. 678 in the textbook
78. See Figure 41-1, C, p. 678 in the textbook
79. See Figure 41-1, D, p. 678 in the textbook
80. See Figure 41-1, E, p. 678 in the textbook
81. a. 1/The skin is red.
    b. 4/Muscle and bone are exposed and damaged.
    c. 3/The skin is gone, and the underling tissues are exposed. The exposed tissue is damaged.
    d. 2/The skin cracks, blisters, or peels. There may be a shallow crater.

Crossword
Across
5. decubitus ulcer
7. purulent
8. serous
9. shock
13. sanguineous
14. trauma
16. evisceration
Down
1. laceration
2. abrasion
3. stasis ulcer

4. hemorrhage
5. dehiscence
6. wound
10. contusion
12. incision
13. skin tear
15. hematoma

Chapter 42

1. Heat makes blood vessels dilate (open wider).
2. a. More blood flows through the vessels. Therefore, tissues have more oxygen and nutrients for healing.
   b. Excess fluid and wastes are removed from the area faster. Pain and swelling are reduced, and muscles relax.
3. a. Relieve pain
   b. Relax muscles
   c. Promote healing
   d. Reduce tissue swelling
   e. Decrease joint stiffness
4. Blood vessels constrict, and therefore blood flow decreases.
5. a. Infants
   b. Young children
   c. Older adults
   d. Fair-skinned people
   e. People who have decreased sensations (e.g., people with diabetes, spinal cord injuries, stroke)
   f. People with dementia or confusion
   g. People with metal implants
6. Moist
7. No longer than 20 minutes.
8. Sitz bath
9. a. Ice bag
   b. Ice collar
   c. Ice glove
10. Check every 5 minutes
11. a. Complaints of discomfort, pain, numbness, or burning
    b. Excessive redness
    c. Blisters
    d. Pale, white, or grey skin
    e. Cyanosis
    f. Shivering
12. (Any thirteen of the following.)
    • Apply only when ordered by a professional, allowed by your employer, and assigned to do so.
    • Know how to use the equipment
    • Measure the temperature of moist applications before applying.
    • Follow employer policies for safe temperature ranges.
    • Do not apply hot applications about 41.1 degrees C.
    • Ask your supervisor what the temperature of the application should be.
    • Know the precise site of the application.
    • Cover dry heat or cold applications before applying them. Use a flannel or terry cloth cover, towel, or pillowcase.
    • Do not leave clients at risk unattended. Observe them carefully.
    • Observe the skin for signs of complications. If any signs are observed, immediately remove the application and report to your supervisor.
    • Observe for changes in the client's behaviour, which may indicate pain.
    • Remind the client not to change the temperature of the application.
    • Prevent chills. Cover the client with a blanket or robe. Control room drafts.
    • Ask you supervisor how long to leave the application in place. Carefully watch the time. Applications are left on for no more than 20 minutes.
    • Provide for privacy.
    • If safe to leave, place the call bell within the client's reach or remain within hearing distance.
    • Practise Standard Precautions.
13. a
14. a
15. b
16. b
17. a
18. c
19. b
20. d
21. c
22. a
23. b

Chapter 43

1. a. Air moves into and out of the lungs
   b. O_2 and CO_2 are exchanged at the alveoli
   c. The blood transports O_2 to the cells and removes CO_2 from them.
2. a. Structures of the respiratory system must be intact and functioning. The airway must be open, and the alveoli must exchange O_2 and CO_2.
   b. Blood must flow to and from the heart. Narrowed vessels affect blood flow.
   c. The blood must have enough red blood cells because the hemoglobin in the red blood cells

picks up oxygen in the lungs and carries it to the cells.

d. Nervous system diseases and injuries can affect respiratory muscles. Some make breathing difficult or impossible.

e. Respiratory muscles weaken and lung tissue becomes less elastic with age. Also, strength needed for coughing decreases with age. Coughing removes secretions from the upper airway. If the person cannot cough, pneumonia can result. Older adults are at risk for respiratory complications after surgery.

f. Oxygen needs increase with exercise. For people with heart and respiratory diseases, even slight activity increases oxygen needs.

g. Oxygen needs increase when fever is present.

h. Pain increases the need for oxygen.

i. Some drugs depress the respiratory centre in the brain (e.g., narcotics).

j. Smoking causes lung cancer and chronic obstructive pulmonary disease.

k. Allergies may cause wheezing, congestion, and swelling of the upper airways. People with allergies are at risk for chronic bronchitis and asthma.

l. Some air pollutants (e.g., dust, fumes, toxins, sawdust) damage the lungs.

m. Good nutrition is needed to produce red blood cells (iron and vitamins are needed).

n. Alcohol depresses the brain. Excessive amounts of alcohol reduce cough reflex and increase the risk of aspiration. Obstructed airway and pneumonia are risks from aspiration.

3. deficiency of oxygen in the cells. The following are signs and symptoms of hypoxia:
   a. Restlessness
   b. Dizziness
   c. Disorientation
   d. Confusion
   e. Behaviour and personality changes
   f. Difficulty concentrating and following directions
   g. Apprehension
   h. Anxiety
   i. Fatigue
   j. Agitation
   k. Increased pulse rate
   l. Increased rate and depth of respirations
   m. Sitting position, often leaning forward
   n. Cyanosis
   o. Dyspnea

4. Remove the nail polish if the finger site is used.

5. a. The date and time
   b. What the client was dong at the time of the measurement
   c. Oxygen flow rate and the device used
   d. Reason for the measurement (routine or change in the client's condition)
   e. Other observations

6. To prevent the spread of infection—sputum is a body fluid.

7. pneumonia/atelectasis

8. Exhale slowly through pursed lips. Exhale until the ribs move as far down as possible.

9. a. Oxygen is delivered directly into each person's unit. Each unit is connected to a centrally located oxygen supply.
   b. Oxygen is stored in a metal tank. The tank may be placed at the bedside for clients who are confined to bed, or the tank may be transported on a wheeled cart or in a shoulder bag.
   c. Oxygen concentrators remove oxygen from the air and store it. If the concentrator is not portable, the client must stay close to the machine.

10. a. An oxygen mask that covers the nose and mouth. It has small holes in the sides. Room air enters the mask during inhalation, and CO_2 escapes during exhalation.
    b. A bag is added to the simple face mask. The bag is for exhaled air. When breathing in, the client inhales oxygen, some exhaled air, and some room air.
    c. Prevents exhaled air and room air from entering the bag. Exhaled air leaves through holes in the mask, so only oxygen from the bag is inhaled.
    d. Allows precise amounts of oxygen to be given.

11. Nothing. Bubbling means the humidifier is producing water vapour.

12. a. Secure connecting tubing (i.e., nasal cannula) in place. Tape or pin it to the client's garment according to employer policy.
    b. Make sure there are no kinks in the tubing
    c. Make sure the client does not lie on any part of the tubing.

13. *(Any eight of the following.)*
    • Place "No Smoking" signs in the room and on the room door.
    • Remove smoking materials form the room.
    • Remove materials from the room that ignite easily.
    • Keep oxygen source and tubing away from heat sources and open flames.
    • Turn off electrical items before unplugging them.
    • Use electrical equipment that is in good repair.
    • Use only electrical equipment with three-prong plugs.

- Do not use materials that cause static electricity (wool and synthetic fabrics).
- Know the location of fire extinguishers and how to use them.
- If a fire occurs, turn off the oxygen. Then get the client to safety.
- Remind the client and family members about oxygen safety. Report safety hazards immediately.

14. Tell your supervisor immediately.
15. Nostrils, ears, and cheekbones.
16. To add water vapour to the water so that the oxygen will not dry the client's airway's mucous membranes.
17. a. An artificial airway inserted through the mouth and into the pharynx.
    b. An airway inserted through a nostril and into the pharynx.
    c. An airway inserted through the mouth or nose and into the trachea.
    d. An airway inserted through a surgical incision into the trachea.
18. a. Checking vital signs.
    b. Observing the client for signs of hypoxia and other respiratory problems.
    c. Reporting if an airway comes out or is dislodged.
    d. Providing oral hygiene frequently.
19. The person may write or use hand signals, magic slates, or communication boards.
20. a. Outer cannula
    b. Inner cannula
    c. Obturator
21. a. The client shows signs and symptoms of hypoxia or respiratory distress.
    b. If the outer cannula comes out.
22. *(Any seven of the following.)*
    - Dressings do not have loose gauze or lint
    - The stoma or tube is covered when outdoors
    - The stoma is not covered with plastic, leather, or similar materials
    - Tub baths are taken, not showers
    - The client is helped with shampooing so that water does not enter the stoma
    - Swimming is not allowed
    - The client wears medical alert jewellery and carries a medical alert ID card
23. before/during/after
24. a. A drop in pulse rate or a pulse rate less than 60 beats per minute
    b. Irregular cardiac rhythms
    c. A drop or rise in blood pressure
    d. Respiratory distress
    e. A drop in the SpO2

25. hyperventilate the lungs before suctioning
26. Because the person depends on others for basic needs.
27. a. Changes in vital signs
    b. Signs and symptoms of hypoxia and respiratory distress, and complaints of pain or difficulty breathing.
    c. Changes in chest drainage, such as increase in drainage or the appearance of bright red drainage
    d. If bubbling in the drainage system increases, decreases, or stops.
    e. If any part of the system is loose or disconnected.
    f. If a chest tube comes out.
28. a. Cover the insertion site with sterile petrolatum gauze.
    b. Stay with the person, then follow the nurse's directions.
29. e
30. c
31. d
32. a
33. b
34. f
35. a
36. c
37. b
38. c
39. b
40. d
41. c
42. d
43. F; The sensor can be attached to a finger, toe, nose, earlobe, or the forehead.
44. T
45. F; Support workers do not administer medications, and oxygen is considered a medication.
46. F; The physician decides on the type of oxygen administration device.
47. F; Never remove the device used to administer oxygen.
48. F; Never shut off oxygen flow.
49. T
50. T
51. T
52. T
53. F; It is done through an endotracheal tube or through a tracheostomy tube.
54. F; Sterile technique is used.
55. F; Do not change settings on the machine.
56. F; The drainage system is kept below the level of the person's chest.
57. T

Crossword

Across

2. Tachypnea
7. Hyperventilation
9. Suction
11. Bradypnea
12. Hypoxemia
14. Pollutant
15. Orthopnea
17. Dyspnea

Down

1. Pneumothorax
3. Pleural effusion
4. Hemothorax
5. Hypoventilation
6. Hemoptysis
8. Intubation
16. Allergy

Chapter 44

1. b
2. d
3. a
4. c
5. a. Why the position is needed.
   b. How to assume the position
   c. How the body is draped for warmth and privacy
   d. How long the person will stay in the position
6. a. An empty bladder lets the examiner feel the abdominal organs.
   b. A full bladder can change the normal position and shape of organs.
7. To protect the person's privacy. Only the body part being examined is exposed.
8. a. For the legal protection of the patient and the physician.
   b. For the psychological comfort of the patient.
9. a. To hold the child still during some parts of the examination.
   b. To comfort the child.
10. a. disposable items
    b. supplies for the next exam
    c. reusable items according to employer policy
    d. specimens to the designated area
11. a. Laryngeal mirror. Used to examine the mouth, teeth, and throat.
    b. Nasal speculum. Used to examine the inside of the nose.
    c. Ophthalmoscope. Used to examine the internal structures of the eye.
    d. Tuning fork. Used to test hearing.
    e. Vaginal speculum. Used to open the vagina so

it and the cervix can be examined.
    f. Otoscope. Used to examine the external ear and the eardrum.
    g. Percussion hammer. Used to tap body parts to test reflexes.

Chapter 45

1. b
2. c
3. a
4. b
5. c
6. a
7. a
8. b
9. b
10. a
11. b
12. a
13. The physician
14. Crying, being quiet and withdrawn, or constantly talking about other things.
15. a. Listen to the patient who voices fears or concerns about surgery.
    b. Refer any questions about the surgery or its results to the nurse.
    c. Explain to the patient procedures you will perform and why they are being done.
    d. Communicate effectively.
    e. Report to your supervisor verbal and nonverbal signs of patient fear or anxiety.
    f. Report to your supervisor a patient's request to see a spiritual adviser.
16. a. Disfigurement and scarring
    b. Disability
    c. Pain during surgery
    d. Dying during surgery
    e. Anesthesia and its effects
    f. Exposure
    g. Severe pain or discomfort after surgery
    h. Tubes, needles, and other equipment used for care
    i. Complications
    j. Prolonged recovery
    k. More surgery or treatments
    l. Separation from family and friends
17. a. Caring for children and other family members
    b. Pets or the house, lawn, and garden
    c. Monthly bills, loan payments, mortgages, or rent
    d. Insurance coverage for interruption of work
    e. Loss of control
18. Explain that you cannot give this information and

that you will get the supervisor to help him or her.

19. To reduce the risk of vomiting and aspiration during anesthesia and after surgery.

20. A loose tooth could fall out during anesthesia, and the child could aspirate the tooth.

21. anatomical dolls

22. stay with the child while anesthesia is given.

23. a. To reduce the number of microbes on the body at the time of surgery.
    b. So that the skin, lips, and nail beds can be observed for colour and circulation during and after surgery.
    c. To keep hair out of the face and the operative area.
    d. To promote comfort because the person is NPO and probably has a dry mouth.

24. Long hair is braided. Wigs, hairpieces, hairpins, clips, combs, and similar items are removed.

25. swallow water

26. Dentures, glasses, contact lenses, hearing aids, jewellery, and artificial eyes and prostheses.

27. A note on the patient's chart states what valuables were removed and where they are kept.

28. Secure the item in place with gauze or tape according to hospital policy.

29. microbes

30. incision site/large area around the site

31. In the direction of hair growth.

32. Any skin break is a possible infection site.

33. drowsiness and lightheadedness

34. a. Have the person void before receiving medications
    b. Raise bed rails
    c. Have the person remain in bed
    d. Offer the bedpan or urinal for voiding
    e. Keep the bed in the lowest position or raised to the highest position, according to hospital policy.

35. Regional anesthesia

36. *(Any six of he following.)*
    - Thermometer
    - Stethoscope
    - Sphygmomanometer
    - Kidney basin
    - Tissues
    - Waterproof bed protector
    - Vital signs flow sheet
    - I&O record
    - IV pole
    - Other items as directed by the nurse

37. a . Make a surgical bed
    b. Raise the bed to its highest position
    c. Lower bed rails
    d. Move furniture out of the way for the stretcher

38. To prevent respiratory and circulatory complications.

39. Leg exercises help prevent thrombi.

40. *(Any eight of the following.)*
    - Choking
    - A drop or rise in blood pressure
    - Bright red blood from the incision, drainage tubes, or suction tubes
    - A pulse rate of more than 100 or less than 60 beats per minute
    - A weak or irregular pulse
    - A rise or drop in body temperature
    - Hypoxia
    - The need for upper airway suctioning—signalled by tachypnea, dyspnea, moist-sounding respirations, gurgling or gasping, restlessness, or cyanosis
    - Shallow, slow breathing
    - Weak cough
    - Complaints of thirst
    - Cold, moist, clammy, or pale skin
    - Increased drainage on or under dressings or on bed linens
    - Complaints of pain or nausea
    - Vomiting
    - Confusion or disorientation
    - Other measurements and observations as directed by the nurse

41. Because older adults are at higher risk for postoperative respiratory complications.

42. Thrombi, pneumonia, atelectasis, constipation, and urinary tract infections

43. a. Have the person sit with the legs over the edge of the bed (dangle).
    b. Measure blood pressure and pulse. If they are stable, assist the person out of bed.

44. If the patient has a nasogastric tube

45. IV therapy/provide frequent oral hygiene

46. If the patient does not void within 8 hours, a catheterization is usually ordered.

47. a. The extent of surgery
    b. The incision site
    c. The presence of drainage tubes, casts, or other devices
    d. Positioning during surgery can cause muscle strains and discomfort

48. a. wound drainage and skin prep solutions can irritate the skin and cause discomfort
    b. NOP causes a dry mouth and breath odours
    c. Moist, clammy skin from blood pressure changes or elevated body temperatures cause discomfort.

49. a

50. b

51. c
52. c

Chapter 46

1. comfort to the person and the family
2. Because they may have never seen a dying person or a dead body; death seems mysterious and unknown.
3. a. No concept of death.
   b. They notice when people or pets die, but they may think that death is temporary.
   c. They know that death is final, although they may not think it will happen to them.
4. a. Listening
   b. Using touch to show caring and support.
5. Because the person's vision may be failing.
6. So you do not tire the person with questions needing long answers.
7. a. The person's mouth may feel dry, uncomfortable, or sore
   b. Swallowing may be difficult and uncomfortable.
8. a. Circulation fails when death is near. The pulse is fast, weak, and irregular. Blood pressure begins to fall.
   b. Body temperature rises. The person feels cool or cold, looks pale, and perspires heavily.
9. a. Skin care and bathing
   b. frequent changes of linens and garments
10. a. fecal incontinence or constipation
    b. urinary incontinence or urinary retention
11. a Provide skin care and personal hygiene
    b. Keep the person in good body alignment
    c. Offer back massages
    d. Assist with relaxation techniques
12. To relieve pain and suffering, improve comfort, and promote dignity.
13. A legal document in which a person states his or her wishes about future health care, treatment, and personal care.
14. a. To be treated as a living human being until death.
    b. To maintain a sense of hopefulness.
    c. To be cared for by those who can maintain a sense of hopefulness
    d. To express feelings and emotions about one's approaching death.
    e. To participate in decisions concerning one's own care.
    f. To expect continuing medical and nursing attention even after "cure" goals have been changed to "comfort" goals
    g. To not die alone.

h. To be free of pain.
i. To have questions answered honestly.
j. To not be deceived.
k. To have help from and for one's family in accepting death.
l. To die in peace and dignity.
m. To retain individuality and not be judged for personal decisions, which may be contrary to the beliefs of others.
n. To discuss and enlarge one's religious and/or spiritual experiences.
o. To expect that the sanctity of the human body will be respected after death.
p. To be cared for by caring, sensitive, knowledgeable people who attempt to understand the person's needs and will be able to gain some satisfaction in helping the person face death.

15. a. Movement, muscle tone, and sensation are lost, beginning in the feet and legs and then spreading to other parts.
    b. Peristalsis and other digestive functions slow. The person usually refuses to eat or drink.
    c. Body temperature rises. The person feels cool to touch, looks pale, and perspires heavily.
    d. Circulation fails. The pulse is fast, weak, and irregular.
    e. The respiratory system fails. Cheyne-Stokes respirations are common.
    f. Pain decreases as the person loses consciousness. Some people are conscious until the moment of death.
16. Mucus collects in the airway, causing a wet, gurgling sound as the person breathes (the death rattle).
17. The right to privacy still applies after death.
18. Apply moist cotton balls gently over the eyelids.
19. a
20. d
21. b
22. c
23. d
24. a
25. e
26. c
27. b
28. a
29. c
30. d
31. a
32. g
33. g
34. b
35. a
36. h

37. f
38. b
39. a
43. g
41. a
42. h
43. c
44. d
45. b
46. c
47. d

Chapter 47

1. a. To prevent death.
   b. To prevent injuries from becoming worse.
2. a. Your location—street address and city
   b. Telephone number from where you are calling
   c. What happened
   d. How many people need help
   e. Condition of the person, obvious injuries, and life-threatening situations
3. Proceed with rescue breathing.
4. Tap the person's shoulder and ask loudly in each ear, "Are you okay?" Tap infants on the feet to check for responsiveness.
5. a. Look to see if the person's chest rises and falls
   b. Listen for the escape of air.
   c. Feel for the flow of air on your cheek.
6. 2
7. At the carotid pulse site (neck)
8. No longer than 10 seconds.
9. At the brachial pulse site (inner arm)
10. jaw-thrust manoeuvre
11. mouth and nose
12. To keep the airway open and allow fluids to drain from the mouth. It also prevents the tongue from falling toward the back of the throat.
13. Clutching the throat
14. Place the fist in the middle of the abdomen, slightly above the navel but well below the end of the breastbone.
15. Perform chest thrusts.
16. Place a sterile dressing or clean material over the wound and apply pressure with your hand.
17. Apply pressure over the artery above the bleeding site, using your first three fingers.
18. a. Pain
    b. Shock
    c. Vomiting blood
    d. Coughing up blood
    e. Loss of responsiveness
19. a. Have the person sit or lie down before fainting occurs.

b. If sitting, have the person bend forward and place the head between the knees.
   c. If the person is lying down, elevate his or her legs and loosen tight clothing.
   d. If fainting has occurred, keep the person lying down and elevate the legs.
   e. Do note let the person get up until symptoms have subsided for about 5 minutes.
20. dermis and part of the epidermis/the dermis and the entire epidermis
21. a. Activating the EMS system
    b. Stopping the burning process—removing the source of the burn while securing your own safety.
    c. Removing hot clothing that is not sticking to the skin.
    d. Providing rescue breathing and CPR as needed.
    e. Cooling the burned skin with cool water, not ice.
    f. Loosely covering the burn wounds with a clean, dry covering.
    g. Covering the person with a blanket or coat to prevent heat loss.
    h. Watching for signs of shock.
22. The affected side is limp, and the cheek appears puffy. Position the person on the unaffected side.
23. Try to keep onlookers away from the person. Do not tell onlookers about the situation or the person's care, treatment, or condition.
24. a
25. a
26. d
27. a
28. a
29. c
30. d
31. a
32. b
33. c
34. c
35. a
36. The person is choking.
37. a. Activate the EMS system
    b. Begin the Heimlich Manoeuvre
38. Shock
39. a. Activate the EMS system
    b. Keep the person lying down
    c. Maintain an open airway.
    d. Control hemorrhage
    e. Keep the person warm. Place blankets over and under the person if possible.
40. anaphylactic shock
41. a. Activate the EMS system
    b. keep the person lying down

c. Keep the airway open
d. Begin CPR if cardiac arrest occurs.

Chapter 48

1. i
2. m
3. k
4. a
5. n
6. o
7. d
8. h
9. c
10. e
11. l
12. f
13. b
14. g
15. J
16. self
17. slow
18. around
19. bad, difficult, abnormal
20. outer, outside
21. white
22. large
23. new
24. above, over
25. one
26. gland
27. vessel
28. bronchus, bronchi
29. skull
30. duodenum
31. intestines
32. woman
33. mammary gland, breast
34. spinal cord, bone marrow
35. pus
36. condition, usually abnormal
37. producing, causing
38. inflammation
39. tumour
40. speaking
41. falling, sagging, dropping, down
42. paralysis
43. enlargement
44. examination using a scope
45. maintenance, maintaining a constant level
46. abd
47. ac
48. pc
49. c̄

50. CA
51. dc
52. LLQ
53. qd
54. ROM
55. without
56. morning
57. cancer
58. water
59. every
60. weight
61. height
62. wheel chair
63. with
64. at once, immediately
65. oxygen
66. abdomen
67. cerebral vascular accident
68. bid
69. CBR
70. NPO
71. prn
72. qhs
73. ROM
74. RLQ
75. SSE
76. tid
77. qid
78. qod
79. LLQ
80. VS
81. b
82. a
83. d
84. b
85. c
86. d
87. a
88. b
89. c
90. a
91. hepato (root) megaly (suffix) Enlarged liver
92. hemi (prefix) plegia (suffix) Paralysis of one side of the body
93. Chol (root) cyst (root) ectomy (suffix) Excision of gallbladder
94. Laparo (root) tomy (suffix) Incision into the abdomen
95. Brady (prefix) cardia (root) Slow heart rate
96. Neuro (root) pathy (suffix) Disease of the nervous system
97. Tachy (prefix) pnea (root) Rapid breathing
98. Poly (prefix) uria (suffix) Excessive urination
99. Pyo (root) rrhea (suffix) Discharge of pus

100. Dys (prefix) phagia (root) Difficulty swallowing
101. Erythro (prefix) cyto (root) penia (suffix) Deficiency of red blood cells
102. Leuko (prefix) cyte (root) White blood cell
103. Broncho (root) scopy (suffix) Examination of the bronchi using a scope
104. en (prefix) cephalo (root) pathy (suffix) A disease of the brain
105. Stomat (root) itis (suffix) Inflammation of the mouth

Chapter 49

1. F; A résumé should be concise.
2. T
3. F; A cover letter should be one page.
4. T
5. T
6. F; Complete the entire application
7. F; Contacting people you know is an effective way to find a job.
8. F; Employers are very concerned with dependability.
9. F; Be truthful, but you may want attach a note of explanation.
10. F; You can ask these questions if you are offered the position.
11. c
12. d
13. a. Chronological résumé. Highlights employment history, starting with the most current employment and working backward.
    b. Functional résumé. Highlights skills or functions and briefly lists positions held.
14. a. Is the information relevant?
    b. Have I been completely honest?
    c. Have I expressed myself clearly?
    d. Is my résumé consistent?
    e. Is my résumé correct?
15. a. Employment advertisements
    b. The Internet
    c. College career services
    d. Personal contacts.
16. a. Relevant skills and qualities
    b. Accomplishments
    c. A respectful, capable, and professional tone
    d. Your mailing address
    e. Your signature
17. a. Someone with the educational qualifications for the job.
    b. Someone who has the skills necessary to do the job, or who is able to learn these skills
    c. Someone to whom clients and co-workers will respond well.
    d. Someone who is reliable, responsible, and motivated.
18. a. Preparing possible questions and answers
    b. Practicing—focusing on listening skills, relaxation techniques, and responses to questions
    c. Planning—deciding what you are going to wear, the route you will take to get there, and preparing a fresh copy of your résumé.
    d. Making a good impression—preparing your grooming and clothing
19. *(Any six of the following.)*
    - Use a firm handshake.
    - Do not use the interviewer's first name.
    - Project a confident image.
    - Listen carefully.
    - Take your time.
    - Answer questions honestly.
    - Speak positively about your previous job.
    - Use experiences to support opinions.
    - Ask the right questions.
    - Thank the interviewer for his or her time.
20. a. Find out if the offer is conditional.
    b. Find out if the job begins with a trial period.
21. a. express your thanks for the interview
    b. Show your interest in the position
    c. Sign your name

(Questions 22 to end 27 are not specifically covered in the textbook, but are useful topics to cover in class.)